Pediatric Oncology

Series Editors

Dominik Schneider, Department of Pediatrics, Klinikum Dortmund, Dortmund, Nordrhein-Westfalen, Germany

Dirk Reinhardt, Department of Pediatrics III, University of Duisburg-Essen, Essen, Germany

This series provides up-to-date information on important topics in pediatric oncology, from the diagnosis and treatment of particular forms of disease through to, for example, radiation oncology, supportive care, and survivorship. The entire spectrum of clinical management is covered with the aim of equipping readers with the latest knowledge relevant to daily practice. In addition, clinical, methodological, and research issues are addressed. The series benefits from homogeneous design and consistently high quality of illustrations. The volume editors are internationally renowned authorities and contributing authors have been selected for their expertise in the subjects discussed. *Pediatric Oncology* will serve pediatric oncologists, fellows, and residents both as a comprehensive source of information and as a quick reference. The series will also be of interest to pediatricians and general practitioners.

Gabriele Escherich • Valentino Conter
Editors

Acute Lymphoblastic Leukemia in Children and Adolescents

Springer

Editors
Gabriele Escherich
Dept of Ped. Hematology and Oncology
University Medical Center
Hamburg-Eppendorf
Hamburg, Germany

Valentino Conter
Ospedale S. Gerardo
University of Milano-Bicocca
Monza, Italy

ISSN 1613-5318 ISSN 2191-0812 (electronic)
Pediatric Oncology
ISBN 978-3-031-71179-4 ISBN 978-3-031-71180-0 (eBook)
https://doi.org/10.1007/978-3-031-71180-0

This Springer imprint is published by the registered company Springer Nature Switzerland AG
The registered company address is: Gewerbestrasse 11, 6330 Cham, Switzerland

Preface

Acute lymphoblastic leukemia (ALL) is the most frequent cancer—in childhood and adolescence—and a paradigm for the continuous progress of the whole pediatric oncology, demanding a thorough understanding and dynamic approach from clinicians. As the medical landscape evolves, with progress in diagnostic technologies and new treatment modalities, new research findings require a constant updating of the management of this challenging disease.

This book provides a comprehensive overview and practical insights into the complexities of ALL diagnosis and treatment. Physicians will find it as a compendium of the latest research findings, treatment guidelines, and emerging trends in ALL in children, exploring the current research on predisposing factors and molecular genetics aimed to tailor treatment approaches to optimize outcomes for our young patients. In particular, the latest research results in the rapidly developing field of immunotherapeutic approaches are comprehensively presented here.

In a rapidly evolving field such as oncology, staying abreast of the latest developments is imperative, and this textbook acts as a reliable resource for those seeking to enhance their knowledge and refine their clinical practice.

We are deeply indebted to numerous wonderful colleagues in basic, clinical, statistical, and epidemiological research, many of whom have contributed to this project and to the international collaboration, crucial for the progress made over the past decades. We would like to take this opportunity to thank all the authors without whom this book would not have been realized. Our special thanks go to all those families and patients who have participated in clinical trials and thus paved the way for success in research into this disease.

It is to all these children and families that we humbly and gratefully dedicate this book.

Hamburg, Germany — Gabriele Escherich
Monza, Italy — Valentino Conter

The original version of the book has been revised. A correction to this book can be found at https://doi.org/10.1007/978-3-031-71180-0_24

Contents

Part I

Epidemiology and Predisposition of ALL

Genetic Predisposition for Acute Lymphoblastic Leukemia

1

Ulrik Kristoffer Stoltze, Triantafyllia Brozou, Kjeld Schmiegelow, and Arndt Borkhardt

1.1 Introduction

Acute lymphoblastic leukemia (ALL) is the most common malignant disease in children and adolescents, and yet, the underlying etiology remains mostly obscure [1–4]. As for virtually all cancers, childhood ALL is evidently a result of an accumulation of genetic aberrations that drive a single somatic cell toward uncontrolled proliferation [5, 6]. This unchecked proliferation chokes normal hematopoiesis and displaces the healthy bone marrow and may cause significant extramedullary dissemination, which, in turn, leads to the classical clinical manifestations of ALL. Although the best contemporary antileukemic therapy has led to overall survival rates above 90%, a deeper understanding of ALL etiology may ultimately pave the way for prophylactic measures [7].

Curiously, evidence suggests that the most common ALL subtypes (*ETV6::RUNX1* translocation or high hyperdiploidy) is frequently initiated in utero, where early chromosomal aberrations in lymphoblastic precursor cells establish a preleukemic state with clonal expansion which occasionally progresses to overt leukemia [8, 9]. Why some children harbor preleukemic clones and why only some progress is largely unknown, and even more broadly underlying causes are for the most part elusive. However, genetic predisposition has been increasingly recognized as a pivotal etiological factor in childhood ALL, albeit the association with preleukemic states remains to be mapped.

In recent decades the ability to identify both common and rare genetic variants has increased exponentially with the advent of next-generation sequencing (NGS) and other DNA sequencing technologies—shedding new light on the germline genetic basis for leukemogenesis. In this chapter, we review both common and rare germline DNA variants that can predispose some children to development of ALL.

1.2 Empirical Evidence of ALL Heritability

Typically, heritability of disease is studied by investigating diagnoses in monozygotic versus fraternal twins. In such twin research, concordance rates are compared, indicating whether a condition has a genetic basis. However, due to the occurrence of placental cross-circulation of (pre) malignant leukemic cells, particularly in mono-

U. K. Stoltze (✉) · K. Schmiegelow
Righospitalet, Copenhagen, Denmark
e-mail: ulrik.kristoffer.stoltze@regionh.dk; Kjeld.Schmiegelow@regionh.dk

T. Brozou · A. Borkhardt
University Hospital Düsseldorf, Düsseldorf, Germany
e-mail:
Triantafyllia.Brozou@med.uni-duesseldorf.de;
Arndt.Borkhardt@med.uni-duesseldorf.de

G. Escherich, V. Conter (eds.), *Acute Lymphoblastic Leukemia in Children and Adolescents*, Pediatric Oncology, https://doi.org/10.1007/978-3-031-71180-0_1

zygotic twins, any deduction of genetic predisposition will be falsely inflated by this inherently nongenetic event [9, 10]. Accordingly, the standardized incidence ratio (SIR) for twins, where one has ALL, is 162.3 (95% confidence interval: 70.2–320.4) [11], and further studies are needed to tease apart which cases are a product of a single leukemogenic event and which are two truly independent occurrences of ALL. Hence explorations of childhood ALL heritability tend to rely on less ideal methods of investigation.

Relatively small sample sizes have made it difficult to conduct studies on the likelihood of leukemia in offspring of childhood leukemia survivors [12–16]. Consequently, studies on the risk in siblings of afflicted children provide the current best estimates of ALL heritability. However, such studies have significant limitations, e.g., that twins with leukemia must be excluded before estimating disease heritability due to the described in utero spread, and also that it is challenging to differentiate between purely genetic effects and other causative effects driven by a shared environment. Nevertheless, the largest study of ALL risk among siblings of 3994 afflicted individuals found ten singletons, i.e., nontwin, incidents of ALL in siblings, yielding a significantly increased SIR of 3.2 (95% confidence interval: 1.5–5.9) [11].

Further cooperating this evidence of heritability, a study, also using registry data from the Nordic countries, found increased SIRs for all family relations investigated (first-degree relative, offspring, sibling, niece/nephew), although each finding was nonsignificant [16]. Of note, another study looked at 54 sibships with two or more cases of ALL, and, importantly, counted any disease in twins as a single event. The authors described an unexpectedly high ALL subtype concordance, yet the leukemias in this cohort looked like ALL in general with respect to age, tumor burden at diagnosis, and cure rates, suggesting that whatever shared etiology is present in each family seemingly drives a molecularly specific type of leukemogenesis, and furthermore that yet unknown factors may be protecting against recurrence of ALL within families, since families with two or more cases of ALL are very rare [17].

Taken together, available evidence indicates that ALL is heritable. Deeper molecular studies of children and adolescents with the disease have uncovered at least some of the causes of this heritability, namely, rare and common genetic variants that lead to an increased risk of ALL. These are reviewed in the sections below.

1.3 Rare Variants and High-Penetrance ALL Predisposition

Rare genetic variants are most often defined as any genetic alteration that is present in less than one percent of the human gene pool. Such variants are also termed mutations, although this term generally implies some level of pathogenicity. In the following, variants that cause ALL with a high level of confidence, are referred to as pathogenic variants.

With the advent and continued improvement of modern DNA sequencing technologies, both research-based and clinical whole exome or whole genome sequencing of children with cancer has become increasingly widespread, although mostly in high-income nations [18]. The sequencing data has allowed exploration of rare genetic causes of ALL at a previously unattainable scale. One of the more striking realizations was that far more children with cancer have an underlying genetic cause than was originally understood. Historically, just a small number of cases, many of them overtly syndromic, were recognized as having a cancer predisposition syndrome (CPS). Now, children may be diagnosed with a CPS shortly after or even prior to a cancer diagnosis—and many have no other symptoms or family history (see Table 1.1 and Fig. 1.3). This underscores that both researchers and clinical pediatric oncologists, either studying or caring for children with ALL, must have an understanding of the CPSs underlying ALL (see Fig. 1.1).

Table 1.1 Overt and covert genetic syndromes associated with moderate to very high risk of ALL

Syndrome	Gene(s)	Heritability	ALL risk	Common clinical features	Associated ALL subtype	Commonly associated cancers	Approximate incidence
Ataxia–telangiectasia	*ATM*	Recessive	High (>1%)	OVERT: Cerebellar ataxia, apraxia, telangiectasia	T-ALL	NHL, BC, OV, GC, STS	1 in 80,000
Bloom syndrome	*BLM*	Recessive	High (>1%)	OVERT: Short stature, skin lesions, infections, male infertility		Epithelial, AML, NHL	Extremely rare
Constitutional mismatch repair deficiency	4 genes	Recessive	Very high (>5%)	COVERT: CALM, hyperpigmentation		Gliomas, NHL, GI, PNET, MB	1 in 775,000
ETV6 ALL susceptibility	*ETV6*	Dominant	Very high (>5%)	COVERT: Thrombocytopenia	B-ALL	Likely ST	Unknown
Fanconi anemia	19 genes	Recessive	Moderate (<1%)	OVERT: Short stature, CALM. None in 25–40%		AML, MDS, GU, head/neck ST	1 in 100,000
IKZF1 ALL susceptibility	*IKZF1*	Dominant	Likely very high (>5%)	COVERT: Immunodeficiency	B-ALL		Unknown
Li–Fraumeni syndrome	*TP53*	Dominant	High (>1%)	COVERT: None	Hypodiploid ALL	OS, ACC, CNS, STS	1 in 5000
Neurofibromatosis 1	*NF1*	Dominant	Moderate (<1%)	OVERT: CALM, freckling, neurofibromas, learning disabilities		MPNST, JMML, MDS, GIST	1 in 3000
Nijmegen breakage syndrome	*NBN*	Recessive	Very high (>5%)	OVERT: Microcephaly, short stature, pulmonary infections	T-ALL	NHL	Extremely rare
Noonan syndrome	13 genes	Dominant (gain-of-function)	Moderate (<1%)	OVERT: Short stature, congenital heart defect, developmental delay		AML	1 in 1000
PAX5 ALL susceptibility	*PAX5*	Dominant	Very high (>5%)	COVERT: None	B-ALL	None	Unknown
RUNX1 ALL susceptibility	*RUNX1*	Dominant	Likely high (>1%)	COVERT: None	T-ALL	AML, MDS	Unknown

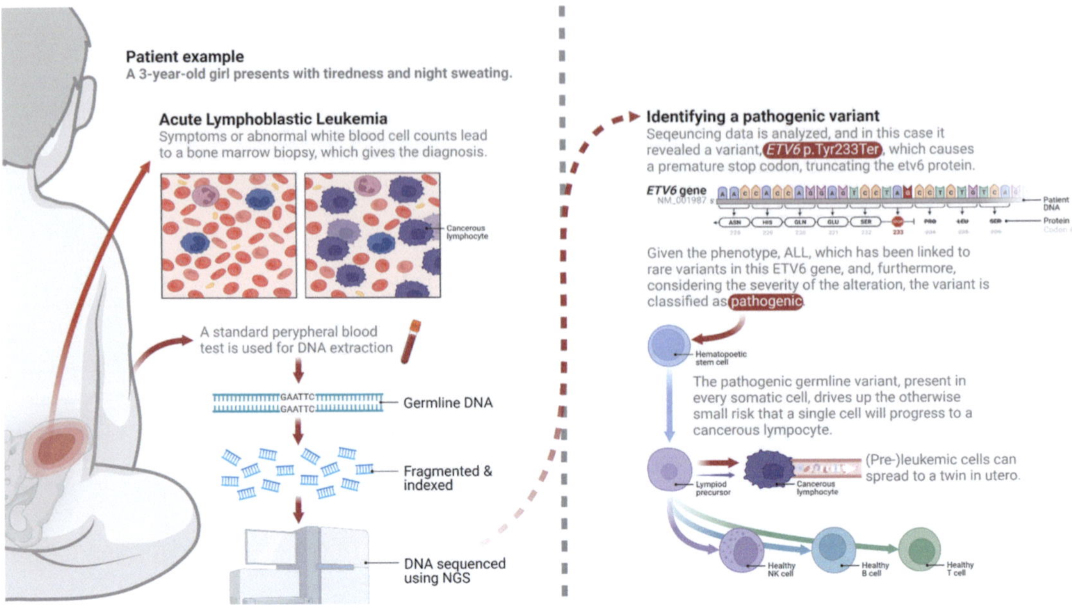

Fig. 1.1 Example of workflow identifying a high-penetrance ALL predisposition variant in a patient

1.3.1 ALL Predisposition Syndromes

1.3.1.1 Overt ALL Predisposition Syndromes

Prior to the discovery and clinical implementation of chromosomal and molecular testing, ALL predisposition was generally only noted for children that had an overt syndrome, i.e., a condition either characteristic or severe enough to be easily recognizable in the clinic (see Table 1.1 and Fig. 1.3). These overt syndromes, outlined below, have highly disparate noncancer phenotypes, and yet, more recent studies have highlighted that the commonality of ALL predisposition is likely due to each associated gene playing a key role in either the homologous recombination (HR) DNA repair pathway or the RAS/MAPK pathway.

1.3.1.1.1 Ataxia-Telangiectasia (A-T)

Lymphoid cancers have been closely linked to germline variants in the *ATM* gene, either in the heterozygous form or in the context of genuine A-T with biallelic *ATM* variants [19]. In two cohort studies of a total of 542 patients with either genetically confirmed biallelic *ATM* variants or clinical A-T, 21 patients (4%) had ALL, predominantly of the T-cell subtype [20, 21]. This gives an approximate odds ratio (OR) of 70 for ALL risk, yet considering the severe noncancer phenotype, with ataxia and development deficits typically presenting before the fourth year of life, cancer, such as ALL, is only rarely the presenting symptom of the syndrome. Importantly, likely due to the *ATM* gene's role in the homologous recombination (HR) DNA repair pathway, A-T patients are susceptible to secondary malignant neoplasms as a consequence of DNA damage caused by ionizing radiation and radiomimetic chemotherapeutic agents [22]. To accommodate the impaired DNA repair in A-T, doses of select chemotherapeutic drugs may be decreased by 25–50%, the most DNA-damaging drugs should be avoided if feasible, and extended recovery intervals between treatments should be considered [23].

1.3.1.1.2 Bloom Syndrome (BSyn)

In addition to pre- and post-natal growth deficiencies and other noncancer phenotypic traits, BSyn is characterized by a high risk of early-onset, typically lymphoid, cancer, often metasynchronously [24]. In the latest report from the Bloom Syndrome Registry, 13 out of 290 (4%)

had ALL, with one being secondary to a previous cancer, and at least two cases of ALL being diagnosed prior to the underlying BSyn [25–27]. This equates to an approximate ALL risk OR of 90. Of note, *BLM,* like *ATM*, is involved in DNA repair of double-strand breaks by the HR pathway. Accordingly, individuals with Bloom syndrome also have increased toxicity of chemotherapy and radiation, and anticancer therapies are often reduced, with both lower doses and/or fewer cycles of chemotherapy, but validated guidelines are lacking [25].

1.3.1.1.3 Fanconi Anemia (FA)

FA is caused by biallelic pathogenic germline variants in one of 19 FANC genes, all related to the FA core protein complex, either as direct structural components or as functional mediators. While risk of leukemia or other hematological (pre)malignancy is extremely high, with approx. 10% absolute risk per year of life, only a few are lymphoid in origin [28, 29]. In a literature-based registry of 1300 patients with FA, only seven patients (<1%) were diagnosed with ALL [30]. Similarly, in a recent registry-based study of German children with FA, just one patient out of 421 had ALL [31]. The noncancer phenotype associated with FA includes skeletal deformations, short stature, and café-au-lait macules (CALM), yet up to 40% of patients present without overt sign of the syndrome [32]. Interestingly, the FA DNA repair pathway has been increasingly linked to the HR pathway and the leukemogenesis associated with the germline variant of FANC genes may be molecularly related to that of *BLM* and *ATM* [33]. This too confers an inordinate sensitivity to radiation and chemotherapy that has led to use of adapted transplantation protocols, using radiation-free conditioning regimens, even in cases of unrelated donors [32].

1.3.1.1.4 Nijmegen Breakage Syndrome (NBS)

NBS is an extremely rare condition caused by biallelic pathogenic variants in the *NBN* gene. Around 90% of patients with the condition have at least one copy of the Slavic founder variant, a five base pair deletion, and hence the condition is most common in the Slavic countries, yet has been described elsewhere [34–36]. In a Polish study six patients with NBS were observed among 403 children with ALL (none had NBS among 7706 ethnically similar controls), while a German, Austrian, and Swiss study found four patients with NBS among 4939 children with ALL [23, 34]. Of note, the former study also found that patients with ALL had a higher rate of heterozygous carriers than controls, with an OR of 3.01 (95% confidence interval: 2.42–3.85). Similarly to *ATM*, *NBN* plays a vital role in the HR pathway and is strongly associated with ALL of the T-cell lineage [23, 37]. Once again, it follows that patients with NBS should avoid radiation when possible.

1.3.1.1.5 Neurofibromatosis Type 1 (NF1)

NF1 is a relatively common genetic condition caused by monoallelic pathogenic variants in the *NF1* gene, with a prevalence of at least one in 3000 births [38, 39]. Given this frequency, some co-occurrences with ALL are to be expected, yet two studies have provided population-based estimates indicating that significantly more children with ALL than expected have NF1 [23, 40]. Collectively, the two studies report on 10,664 children with ALL, of which 20 had NF1, versus the three to four that would be expected, resulting in a moderately increased OR of 5.4 (95% confidence interval: 2.8–9.4). Unlike the conditions discussed above, *NF1* is not known to be involved in DNA repair [41]. Rather, the gene functions as an inhibitor of the RAS/MAPK pathway, yet it is still advised that radiation is avoided when possible, as multiple treatment-related incidents of malignant transformation of benign tumors have been reported (see Fig. 1.2) [42–44].

1.3.1.1.6 Noonan Syndrome (NS) and Others

ALL has been observed in children with multiple other underlying syndromes, more notably RASopathies, such as NS. Two cases of childhood ALL were first observed among 632 German patients with NS, and subsequently another six children with ALL were observed in a French study of another 1176 patients [45, 46].

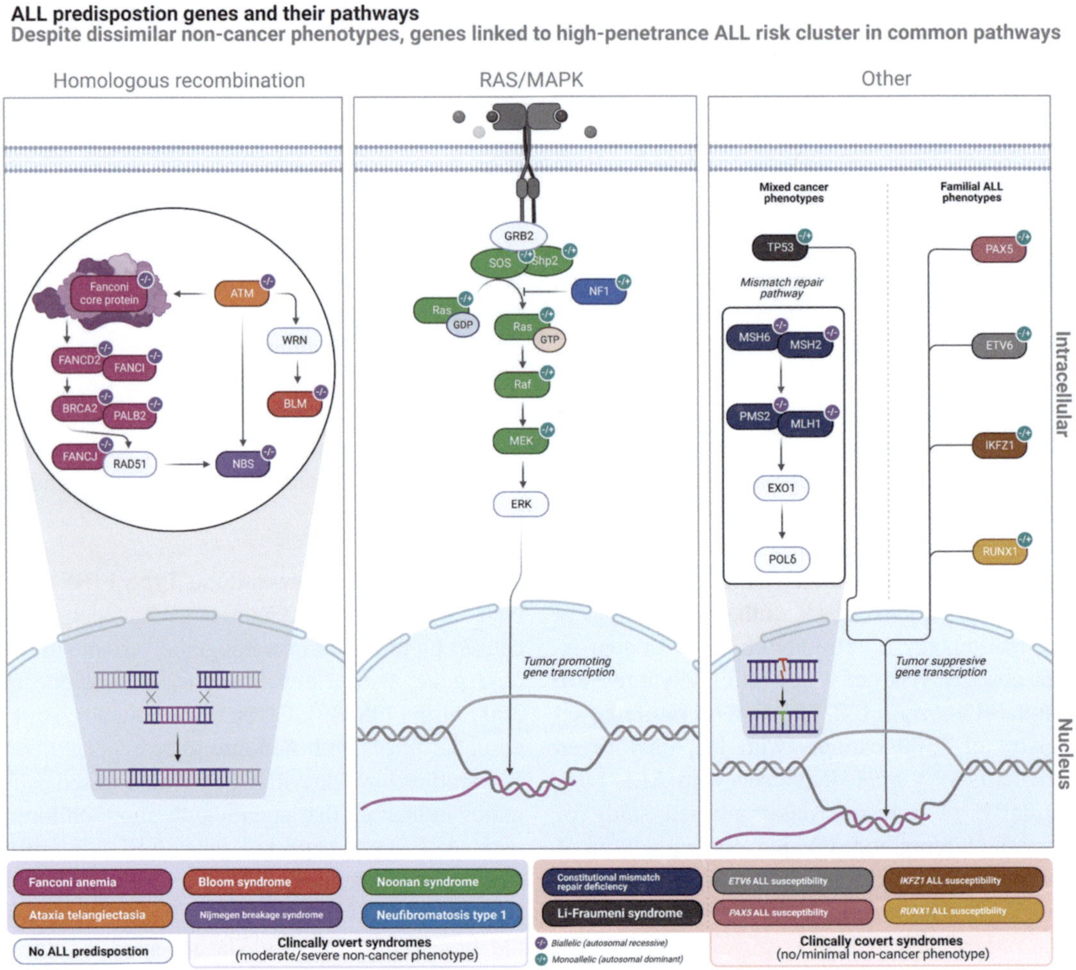

Fig. 1.2 Genes/proteins linked to ALL predisposition and their pathways

NS is classically caused by pathogenic gain-of-function variants in the central signal-transducing genes of the RAS/MAPK pathway, in which *NF1* acts as a negative regulator (see Fig. 1.2) [47, 48]. While a slight increase of ALL is apparent for NS, many other syndromes have been anecdotally linked to ALL, including familial myeloproliferative/lymphoproliferative neoplasms (*DDX41*) [49], thrombocythemia 3 (*JAK2*) [50], SHORT syndrome (*PIK3R1*) [51], Netherton syndrome (*SPINK5*) [52], Cornelia de Lange syndrome (*NIPBL*) [53], ataxia–pancytopenia syndrome (*SAMD9L*) [54], Emberger syndrome (*GATA2*) [55], and at least seven other genetic conditions [8]. ALL has also been linked to rare germline variants in the *TRAF3IP3* [56].

1.3.1.2 Covert ALL Predisposition Syndromes

1.3.1.2.1 Familial ALL Syndromes

PAX5 ALL Susceptibility

Studies of families with familial ALL have led to the discovery that pathogenic germline variants in the *PAX5* gene cause a seemingly very high, yet still incomplete, penetrance of ALL specifically. Possibly with the expectation of *ETV6* ALL susceptibility, discussed below, *PAX5* ALL susceptibility appears to be distinct in that it only predisposes to ALL, with no other cancer or non-cancer phenotype. Collectively, 34 carriers of pathogenic variants in the *PAX5* have been reported in the literature, of which 18 had ALL (53%, all B-cell precursors) and 16 were unaffected [57–60]. These cases represent five families, with just two recurrent hotspot missense variants, the c.547G > A:p.Gly183Ser and the c.113G > A:p.Arg38His variant. Somatically, *PAX5* alterations have been shown to be an early and central event in B lymphoid leukemogenesis, and patients with such *PAX5*-driven ALL have been suggested to constitute a separate subtype, with implications for both prognosis and treatment [61].

ETV6 ALL Susceptibility

The somatic fusion event known as t(12;21)(p13;q22), a *ETV6*::*RUNX1* fusion, was among the first molecular subtypes described in ALL, and thus alterations in the *ETV6* gene, historically known as *TEL*, has long been recognized as a somatic driver of lymphoid leukemogenesis [62, 63]. Only within the last few years have pathogenic germline variants in *ETV6* been identified as predisposing to childhood ALL. Initially, such variants were discovered in kindreds with familial ALL, and now more than 20 kindreds have been described as having germline *ETV6* variants [64–67]. Following this, a systematic genetic study of 4405 patients with pediatric ALL revealed 31 germline, mainly missense, variants in 35 (1%) of the ALL cases, and a more recent study of these variants has confirmed that at least 22 had tumor suppressor activity in vitro [68, 69]. Pathogenic variants in the gene tend to cluster in the ETS domain, and carriers have mild to severe thrombocytopenia, and about 30% of carriers are thought to develop leukemia, typically later in childhood and with a tendency for hyperdiploid subtypes [67].

IKZF1 ALL Susceptibility

Like *ETV6*, the *IKZF1* gene also plays a vital role in lymphoid development and somatic loss of activity of the protein product, IKAROS, is associated with high-risk B-cell precursor ALL, often positive for the *BCR*::*ABL1* fusion (Philadelphia chromosome) [70, 71]. Pathogenic germline variants in the gene have recently been linked to hereditary hypogammaglobulinemia and immunodeficiency in six families with 29 carriers; two (7%) of which included a carrier with ALL [72]. A subsequent systematic genetic study of 4963 patients with ALL found 27 rare germline variants in *IKZF1* in 43 patients (1%), almost exclusively in patients with B-cell ALL [73].

RUNX1 ALL Susceptibility

Pathogenic germline variants in the *RUNX1* gene were associated with familial platelet disorder more than a decade ago and often patients with this disorder develop myeloid cancers, however, typically later in life [74]. As described above, somatically, *RUNX1* forms a fusion transcript with *ETV6* driving a large proportion of B-cell leukemias, yet other somatic alterations of the gene are also common across ALL of both B- and T-cell lineages [75, 76]. With an outset in this somatic observation, a systematic genetic study of 6190 patients with childhood ALL performed targeted sequencing of the *RUNX1* gene [77]. The study revealed 31 carriers of 18 rare germline variants, and functional analyses of the variants further revealed that only six of the rare variants, all in patients with ALL of the T-cell lineage, resulted in loss of RUNX1 activity. Lastly, patients with T-cell ALL and germline *RUNX1* variants tended to have somatic loss of *JAK2*.

1.3.1.2.2 Covert Syndromes with Mixed Cancer Phenotypes

Li–Fraumeni Syndrome (LFS)

Pathogenic germline variants in the *TP53* gene, one of the most somatically mutated genes in cancers generally, cause LFS. The condition is among the most common childhood CPSs, causing perhaps as many as 2% of all early life cancers [78, 79]. LFS is associated with up to 40% risk of cancer before adulthood, and cancers may arise in virtually any tissue, including the bone marrow. In a French study of 415 patients with LFS, 12 developed leukemia (3%, all children) [80]. LFS-associated ALL tends to be hypodiploid, and in fact nearly half of children with this ALL subtype have a pathogenic germline *TP53* variant, and most of the remaining hypodiploid cases had somatic mutations in *TP53* [81, 82]. Tumor surveillance has been demonstrated to confer a survival benefit for patients with LFS, yet the study did not see this benefit extend to hematological malignancies [83, 84].

Constitutional Mismatch Repair Deficiency (CMMRD)

Pathogenic monoallelic variants in the mismatch repair (MMR) genes, *MSH6*, *MSH2*, *PMS2* and *MLH1*, have long been known to cause Lynch syndrome, a CPS affecting around 1 in 300 adults [85]. Biallelic variants, however, cause one of the most devastating childhood CPSs, CMMRD, that lead to a high risk of early cancers in most tissues, including ALL [86]. In a recent, international, prospective study of tumor surveillance interventions in this patient group, seven out of 110 patients developed ALL (6%, aged 3–18 years at diagnosis) [87]. The study found that surveillance gives an overall survival benefit; however, again this finding did not extend to hematological malignancies, for which both early diagnosis and the modalities to screen for leukemia are unlikely to have a clinical impact on prognosis [88]. Importantly, CMMRD is not entirely covert. A noncancer phenotype, consisting primarily of CALMs (similar yet more angular than those found in patients with NF1) or other changes in skin pigmentation, is present in at least 60% of patients with CMMRD, but it is often overlooked prior to the emergence of one or multiple cancers [86].

1.3.2 ALL Predisposition in Pediatric Pancancer Studies

The largest pediatric pancancer study to date included 588 patients with leukemia (both lymphoid and myeloid), of whom 26 (4.4%) had an identifiable pathogenic germline variant in a cancer predisposition gene [78]. Across 11 larger pediatric pancancer studies, a total of 4833 children with cancer underwent either extensive or targeted sequencing [78, 89–98]. Although not representative of the populations, these studies provide the perhaps best indication of which rare germline variants are most prevalent in clinical pediatric oncology/hematology. In total, the studies reported 74 pathogenic variants in patients with ALL (see Table 1.2).

Pathogenic variants were most commonly found in the *TP53* gene, with a total of 18 patients reported. However, this number is derived from cohorts with a clear overrepresentation of hypodiploid ALL in two studies, and these two studies also had an overlap of four patients with ALL [78, 92]. The other nine studies reported only three patients with ALL and a pathogenic germline variant in *TP53* [94, 97, 98]. Among the other genes linked to ALL predisposition, just ten patients with ALL had a variant that may be directly linked to leukemogenesis. Taken together, this evidence is somewhat sobering, and underscores that high-penetrance variants in children and adolescents with ALL, although present, is a rare phenomenon, at least based on the current level of evidence and understanding of genetic risk. As it appears, rare germline variants tend to play a far smaller role in the etiology of childhood ALL than in childhood CNS tumors and solid cancers [99–102].

1.3.3 Not Inherited, Yet Heritable

Recent abilities to perform extensive DNA sequencing on very large numbers of healthy individuals has led to an unprecedented characterization of genetic variation in the human gene pool as a whole. A recent study of 141,456 human exomes or genomes uncovered a tendency for some genes to show an unexpectedly low number of loss-of-function (LoF) variants [103]. These genes were termed *constrained* and LoF variants within them are understood to have been under considerable evolutionary pressure. Considering that the natural history of ALL is fatal, and that the disease is predominantly found in children, any genetic event conferring a high risk to this condition should in theory have a disadvantage in terms of reproductive propagation. Empirical evidence of this phenomenon was recently described, and indeed, the seven genes (*IKZF1*, *PAX5*, *ETV6*, *TP53*, *NF1*, *RUNX1*, and *FANCB*)

Table 1.2 Pathogenic germline variants in patients with ALL in pediatric pancancer studies

Gene(s)	Pathogenic variants in patients with any cancer	Pathogenic variants in patients with ALL	Studies where gene was included (patients)
Ataxia telangiectasia	*ATM*: 13 (2 biallelic)	***ATM*: 3 (0 biallelic)**	11 (*n* = 4833)
Bloom syndrome	*BLM*: 3 (0 biallelic)	***BLM*: 1 (0 biallelic)**	10 (*n* = 4043)
Fanconi anemia	*BRCA2*: 25 (1 biallelic) *PALB2*: 8 (0 biallelic) *FANCA*: 5 (0 biallelic) *FANCM*: 4 (0 biallelic) *FANCC*: 3 (0 biallelic) *FANCI*: 3 (0 biallelic) *BRIP1*: 2 (0 biallelic) *FANCD2*: 2 (0 biallelic) *FANCL*: 2 (0 biallelic) *ERCC4*: 1 (0 biallelic) *FANCG*: 1 (0 biallelic) *RAD51C*: 1 (0 biallelic) *SLX4*: 1 (0 biallelic)	***BRCA2*: 5 (0 biallelic)** ***FANCI*: 3 (0 biallelic)** ***ERCC4*: 1 (0 biallelic)** ***FANCD2*: 1 (0 biallelic)** ***FANCM*: 1 (0 biallelic)** ***PALB2*: 1 (0 biallelic)**	10 (*n* = 4043)
Nijmegen breakage syndrome	*NBN:* 2 (0 biallelic)	***NBN:* 0 (0 biallelic)**	10 (*n* = 4043)
Neurofibromatosis type 1	*NF1*: 40	***NF1*: 2**	11 (*n* = 4833)
Noonan syndrome	*KRAS*: 3 *PTPN11*: 2 *NRAS*: 1 *SOS1*: 1	***KRAS*: 2** ***PTPN11*: 2** ***NRAS*: 1**	8 (*n* = 3142)
PAX5 ALL susceptibility	*PAX5*: 0	***PAX5*: 0**	9 (*n* = 3893)
ETV6 ALL susceptibility	*ETV6*: 0	***ETV6*: 0**	7 (*n* = 2732)
IKZF1 ALL susceptibility	*IKZF1: 1*	***IKZF1*: 1**	5 (*n* = 1681)
RUNX1 ALL susceptibility	*RUNX1: 4*	***RUNX1:* 2**	11 (*n* = 4833)
Li–Fraumeni syndrome	*TP53*: 98	***TP53*: 18**	11 (*n* = 4833)
Constitutional mismatch repair deficiency	*PMS2*: 22 (2 biallelic) *MSH6*: 10 (2 biallelic) *MSH2*: 8 (0 biallelic) *MLH1*: 2 (0 biallelic)	***PMS2*: 2 (0 biallelic)**	11 (*n* = 4833) [*MLH1*: 10 (*n* = 4043)]
20 other genes with pathogenic variants in patients with ALL	N/A	**28 variants[a]**	N/A

[a]*MUTYH* (4), *WRN* (4), *APC* (2), *CHEK2* (2), *RECQL4* (2), *BRCA1*, *CDH1*, *DDB2*, *ERCC2*, *ERCC3*, *ERCC5*, *LZTR1*, *NF2*, *NOP10*, *PTCH1*, *RET*, *SH2B3*, *VHL*, and WT1

specifically associated with monoallelic, loss-of-function ALL predisposition show marked constraint (see Fig. 1.3b) [99, 104, 105].

Long-term curative treatment of ALL is a relatively modern phenomenon, and it is interesting to note that such cures will likely affect the propagation of causative germline variants, a situation that has presumably not happened previously in human evolution [7]. Counter to this development, diagnoses of underlying ALL predisposition syndromes may motivate some parents or ALL survivors to undergo preimplantation genetic testing, ensuring that pathogenic variants in genes related to high ALL risk are not passed on [106]. This is relevant, even in children with de novo variants, which, while not inherited, still are heritable once the child reaches reproductive age.

Along with continued studies of familial ALL, employment of rare, and partly deleterious, variant burden analysis, and deepened understanding of the somatic genomic landscape of ALL, analysis of genes with high level of constraint might lead to discovery of hitherto unknown high-penetrance ALL predisposition genes.

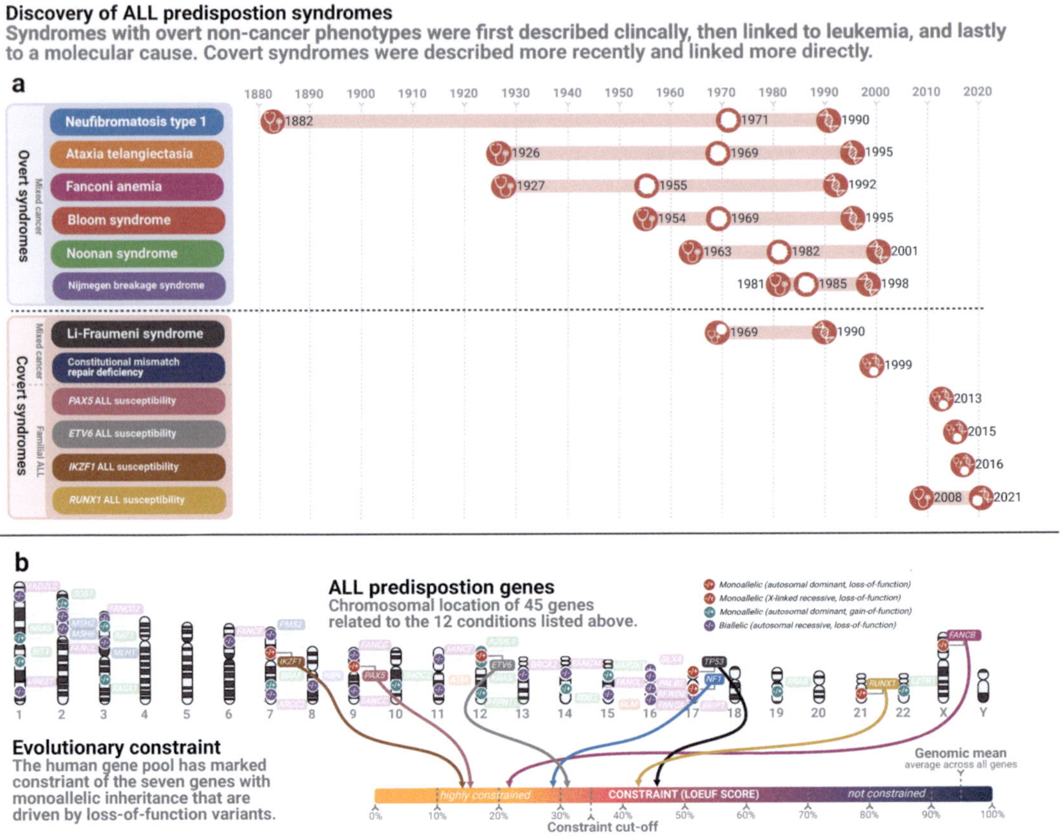

Fig. 1.3 (**a**): Discovery of ALL predisposition genes, chromosomal location, and evolutionary constraint. (**b**): Gene associated with ALL predispositions, highlighting genes with associated monoallelic ALL predisposition and the highly constrained nature of these genes, when compared with the genomic average

1.4 Common Variants and Low-Penetrance ALL Predisposition

Before the extensive DNA sequencing studies that led to many of the discoveries outlined above were technologically and economically feasible, more narrow genome-wide association (GWA) studies were used to investigate common variants' association with ALL. GWA studies rely on array data characterizing single nucleotide polymorphisms (SNPs), which are defined as a variant with an allele frequency (AF) in the human gene pool of more than 5%. Correlating the AFs of SNPs in cohorts with childhood ALL vs. those in a control cohort, several studies have demonstrated that a total of 14 independent SNPs across eight genes are associated with childhood ALL development (see Table 1.3) [107–117].

For all the identified SNPs associated with ALL risk, the high frequency of the risk allele in both affected and unaffected individuals means that the influence on absolute ALL risk is very modest, with ORs that are typically lower than 2. Nevertheless, due to the abundance of the SNPs their effects may still explain a sizable portion of ALL cases, with one study estimating that SNPs may account for around a quarter of total variation in ALL risk [118]. Still, for the individual, any clinical relevance or actionability of ALL risk SNP profiling has not materialized.

Table 1.3 GWAS results

Gene	Rsid (reference)	OR (95% CI)	Associated subtype, OR (95% CI)	RAF
ARID5B	rs7089424 rs10821936 rs10994982	1.65 (1.54–1.76) 1.91 (1.6–2.2) 1.86 (1.71–2.03)	HeH, 2.17 (1.5–3.1)	0.37 0.36 0.57
BCL11A-PAPOLG	rs2665658	N/A	*TCF3-PBX1* ALL, 4.00 (2.5–6.5)	0.37
CDKN2A	rs17756311 rs3731217 rs3731249	1.36 (1.18–1.56) 0.71 (0.64–0.78) 2.99 (2.21–4.26)		0.06 0.13 0.01
CEBPE	rs2239633 rs4982731	1.31 (1.22–1.42) 1.36 (1.24–1.48)		0.64 0.33
GATA3	rs3824662	1.31 (1.21–1.41)	Ph-like, 3.85 (2.7–5.4)	0.20
IKZF1	rs4132601 rs11978267	1.71 (1.58–1.85) 1.59 (1.45–1.74)		0.22 0.23
PIP4K2A	rs7088318 rs10828317	1.40 (1.28–1.53) 1.23 (1.15–1.32)	HeH	0.59 0.02

14 SNPs associated with ALL risk. Risk allele frequencies are global frequencies from the 1000 Genomes Project. SNP, single nucleotide polymorphism; *HeH* high-hyperdiploid, *OR* odds ratio; 95% CI, 95% confidence interval, *RAF* risk allele frequency, *Ph-like* Philadelphia-like ALL

The consistency with which certain genetic loci associated with ALL risk in GWA studies performed across disparate geographies and ethnicities, coupled with the fact that genes (e.g., *IKZF1* and *CDKN2A*) in close proximity to the identified SNPs are known to play key roles in somatic leukemogenesis, leaves little question that these associations have a bona fide biological basis. Yet attempts to describe the molecular mechanism driving these observed associations have been largely fruitless. Even early on, this component of GWA research has drawn criticism that, despite the fact that it was impossible to know in advance, GWA studies, at least in other disease entities, were ultimately not clinically meaningful [119]. Less derisively, genetic predisposition in general may be viewed more as a continuum, meaning that any sharp dichotomy into rare and common variants may not be conducive to etiological research [120]. Rather, extensive nucleotide-by-nucleotide sequencing of patients with ALL, now being undertaken across most developed nations, may elucidate currently unknown risk variants residing in the gulf between ultra-rare variants, like those described in the previous section, and the highly common ones listed above.

1.5 Future Directions

Since host genome variants clearly plays a role for leukemogenesis, research is needed to determine (i) if all children with ALL should be screened for these variants, (ii) to which extent host genome variants influences the response to treatment (change of cure and toxicity risks [121]), and (iii) interactions between the variants and our exposome (e.g., in utero exposures, childhood infections, and gut microbiome profiles) influences the risk of childhood ALL.

References

1. SEER Cancer Statistics review 1975–2012. National Cancer Institute.
2. Hjalgrim LL, Rostgaard K, Schmiegelow K, Söderhäll S, Kolmannskog S, Vettenranta K, et al. Age- and sex-specific incidence of childhood leukemia by immunophenotype in the Nordic countries. J Natl Cancer Inst. 2003;95(20):1539–44.
3. Steliarova-Foucher E, Parkin DM, Kramárová E, Draper GJ, Masuyer E. International incidence of childhood cancer. Lyon: IARC Scientific Publications; 1998.
4. Klco JM, Mullighan CG. Advances in germline predisposition to acute leukemias and myeloid neoplasms. Nat Rev Cancer. 2021;21(2):122–37.

5. Tomasetti C, Li L, Vogelstein B. Stem cell divisions, somatic mutations, cancer etiology, and cancer prevention. Science. 2017;355(6331):1330–4.
6. Mullighan CG. The genomic landscape of acute lymphoblastic leukemia in children and young adults. Hematol Am Soc Hematol Educ Program. 2014;2014(1):174–80.
7. Pui CH, Evans WE. A 50-year journey to cure childhood acute lymphoblastic leukemia. Semin Hematol. 2013;50(3):185–96.
8. Tulstrup M, Stoltze UK, Schmiegelow K, Yang JJ. Epidemiology and etiology of childhood ALL. In: Vora A, editor. Childhood acute lymphoblastic leukemia. Cham: Springer International Publishing; 2017. p. 1–27. https://doi.org/10.1007/978-3-319-39708-5_1.
9. MacMahon B, Levy MA. Prenatal origin of childhood leukemia*. N Engl J Med. 1964;270(21):1082–5.
10. Maia AT, van der Velden VHJ, Harrison CJ, Szczepanski T, Williams MD, Griffiths MJ, et al. Prenatal origin of hyperdiploid acute lymphoblastic leukemia in identical twins. Leukemia. 2003;17(11):2202–6.
11. Kharazmi E, da Silva Filho MI, Pukkala E, Sundquist K, Thomsen H, Hemminki K. Familial risks for childhood acute lymphocytic leukaemia in Sweden and Finland: far exceeding the effects of known germline variants. Br J Haematol. 2012;159(5):585–8.
12. Sankila R, Olsen JH, Anderson H, Garwicz S, Glattre E, Hertz H, Langmark F, Lanning M, Møller T, Tulinius H. Risk of cancer among offspring of childhood-cancer survivors. N Engl J Med. 1998;338:1339–44.
13. Hawkins MM, Draper GJ, Winter DL. Cancer in the offspring of survivors of childhood leukaemia and non-Hodgkin lymphomas. Br J Cancer. 1995;71(6):1335–9.
14. Hawkins M, Draper G, Smith R. Cancer among 1,348 offspring of survivors of childhood cancer. Int J Cancer. 1989;43:975–8.
15. Mulvihill JJ, Connelly RR, Austin DF, Cook JW, Holmes FF, Krauss MR, et al. Cancer in offspring of long-term survivors of childhood and adolescent cancer. Lancet. 1987;330(2283):813.
16. Madanat-Harjuoja LM, Pitkäniemi J, Hirvonen E, Malila N, Diller LR. Linking population-based registries to identify familial cancer risk in childhood cancer. Cancer. 2020;126(13):3076–83.
17. Schmiegelow K, Lausten Thomsen U, Baruchel A, Pacheco CE, Pieters R, Pombo-de-Oliveira MS, et al. High concordance of subtypes of childhood acute lymphoblastic leukemia within families: lessons from sibships with multiple cases of leukemia. Leukemia. 2012;26(4):675–81.
18. ICGC/TCGA Pan-Cancer Analysis of Whole Genomes Consortium. Pan-cancer analysis of whole genomes. Nature. 2020;578(7793):82–93.
19. Reiman A, Srinivasan V, Barone G, Last JI, Wootton LL, Davies EG, et al. Lymphoid tumours and breast cancer in ataxia telangiectasia; substantial protective effect of residual ATM kinase activity against childhood tumours. Br J Cancer. 2011;105(4):586–91.
20. Suarez F, Mahlaoui N, Canioni D, Andriamanga C, Dubois d'Enghien C, Brousse N, et al. Incidence, presentation, and prognosis of malignancies in ataxia-telangiectasia: a report from the French national registry of primary immune deficiencies. J Clin Oncol Off J Am Soc Clin Oncol. 2015;33(2):202–8.
21. Morrell D, Cromartie E, Swift M. Mortality and cancer incidence in 263 patients with ataxia-telangiectasia. J Natl Cancer Inst. 1986;77(1):89–92.
22. Gatti R. Ataxia-Telangiectasia. In: Pagon RA, Adam MP, Ardinger HH, et al., editors. GeneReviews®. Seattle: University of Washington; 1999. p. 1993–2016.
23. Schütte P, Möricke A, Zimmermann M, Bleckmann K, Reismüller B, Attarbaschi A, et al. Preexisting conditions in pediatric ALL patients: Spectrum, frequency and clinical impact. Eur J Med Genet. 2016;59(3):143–51.
24. Flanagan M, Cunniff CM. Bloom syndrome. In: Adam MP, Mirzaa GM, Pagon RA, Wallace SE, Bean LJ, Gripp KW, et al., editors. GeneReviews®. Seattle: University of Washington; 2022.
25. Sugrañes TA, Flanagan M, Thomas C, Chang VY, Walsh M, Cunniff C. Age of first cancer diagnosis and survival in bloom syndrome. Genet Med Off J Am Coll Med Genet. 2022;24(7):1476–84.
26. Adams M, Jenney M, Lazarou L, White R, Birdsall S. Acute myeloid leukaemia after treatment for acute lymphoblastic leukaemia in girl with bloom syndrome. J Genet Syndr Gene Ther. 2014;4(8)
27. Werner-Favre C, Wyss M, Cabrol C, Felix F, Guenin R, Laufer D, et al. Cytogenetic study in a mentally retarded child with bloom syndrome and acute lymphoblastic leukemia. Am J Med Genet. 1984;18(2):215–21.
28. Shimamura A, Alter BP. Pathophysiology and management of inherited bone marrow failure syndromes. Blood Rev. 2010;24(3):101–22.
29. Rosenberg PS, Greene MH, Alter BP. Cancer incidence in persons with Fanconi anemia. Blood. 2003;101(3):822–6.
30. Alter BP. Cancer in Fanconi anemia, 1927-2001. Cancer. 2003;97(2):425–40.
31. Dutzmann CM, Spix C, Popp I, Kaiser M, Erdmann F, Erlacher M, et al. Cancer in children with Fanconi anemia and ataxia-telangiectasia – a Nationwide register-based cohort study in Germany. J Clin Oncol. 2022;40(1):32–9.
32. Mehta PA, Ebens C. Fanconi Anemia. In: Adam MP, Mirzaa GM, Pagon RA, Wallace SE, Bean LJ, Gripp KW, et al., editors. GeneReviews®. Seattle: University of Washington; 1993.
33. Michl J, Zimmer J, Tarsounas M. Interplay between Fanconi anemia and homologous recombination pathways in genome integrity. EMBO J. 2016;35(9)
34. Pastorczak A, Stolarska M, Trelińska J, Zawitkowska J, Kowalczyk J, Mlynarski W. Nijmegen break-

age syndrome (NBS) as a risk factor for CNS involvement in childhood acute lymphoblastic leukemia. Pediatr Blood Cancer. 2011;57(1):160–2.
35. Pasic S, Vujic D, Fiorini M, Notarangelo LD. T-cell lymphoblastic leukemia/lymphoma in Nijmegen breakage syndrome. Haematologica. 2004;89(8):91–2.
36. Varon R, Vissinga C, Platzer M, Cerosaletti KM, Chrzanowska KH, Saar K, et al. Nibrin, a novel DNA double-strand break repair protein, is mutated in Nijmegen breakage syndrome. Cell. 1998;93(3):467–76.
37. Yamamoto H, Hirasawa A. Homologous recombination deficiencies and hereditary tumors. Int J Mol Sci. 2021;23(1):348.
38. Evans DG, Howard E, Giblin C, Clancy T, Spencer H, Huson SM, et al. Birth incidence and prevalence of tumor-prone syndromes: estimates from a UK family genetic register service. Am J Med Genet A. 2010;152(2):327–32.
39. Lammert M, Friedman JM, Kluwe L, Mautner VF. Prevalence of neurofibromatosis 1 in German children at elementary school enrollment. Arch Dermatol. 2005;141(1):71–4.
40. Stiller CA, Chessells JM, Fitchett M. Neurofibromatosis and childhood leukaemia/lymphoma: a population-based UKCCSG study. Br J Cancer. 1994;70(5):969–72.
41. Kiuru M, Busam KJ. The NF1 gene in tumor syndromes and melanoma. Lab Investig. 2017;97(2):146–57.
42. Krishnatry R, Zhukova N, Guerreiro Stucklin AS, Pole JD, Mistry M, Fried I, et al. Clinical and treatment factors determining long-term outcomes for adult survivors of childhood low-grade glioma: a population-based study. Cancer. 2016;122(8):1261–9.
43. Kleinerman RA. Radiation-sensitive genetically susceptible pediatric sub-populations. Pediatr Radiol. 2009;39(Suppl 1):S27–31.
44. Madden JR, Rush SZ, Stence N, Foreman NK, Liu AK. Radiation-induced gliomas in 2 pediatric patients with neurofibromatosis type 1: case study and summary of the literature. J Pediatr Hematol Oncol. 2014;36(2):e105–8.
45. Kratz CP, Franke L, Peters H, Kohlschmidt N, Kazmierczak B, Finckh U, Bier A, Eichhorn B, Blank C, Kraus C, Kohlhase J. Cancer spectrum and frequency among children with Noonan, Costello, and cardio-facio-cutaneous syndromes. Br J Cancer. 2015;14(112):1392–7.
46. Cavé H, Caye A, Strullu M, Aladjidi N, Vignal C, Ferster A, et al. Acute lymphoblastic leukemia in the context of RASopathies. Eur J Med Genet. 2016;59(3):173–8.
47. Roberts AE. Noonan Syndrome. In: Adam MP, Mirzaa GM, Pagon RA, Wallace SE, Bean LJ, Gripp KW, et al., editors. GeneReviews®. Seattle: University of Washington; 1993.
48. Anastasaki C, Orozco P, Gutmann DH. RAS and beyond: the many faces of the neurofibromatosis type 1 protein. Dis Model Mech. 2022;15(2):dmm049362.
49. Shin WY, Yoon SY, Park R, Kim JA, Song HH, Bang HI, et al. A novel bi-alleleic DDX41 mutations in B-cell lymphoblastic leukemia: case report. BMC Med Genet. 2022;15(1):46.
50. Carreño-Tarragona G, Varghese LN, Sebastián E, Gálvez E, Marín-Sánchez A, López-Muñoz N, et al. A typical acute lymphoblastic leukemia JAK2 variant, R683G, causes an aggressive form of familial thrombocytosis when germline. Leukemia. 2021;35(11):3295–8.
51. Marzollo A, Maestrini G, La Starza R, Elia L, Malfona F, Pierini T, et al. A novel germline variant in PIK3R1 results in SHORT syndrome associated with TAL/LMO T-cell acute lymphoblastic leukemia. Am J Hematol. 2020;95(12):E335–8.
52. Skoczen S, Stepien K, Mlynarski W, Centkowski P, Kwiecinska K, Korostynski M, et al. Genetic signature of acute lymphoblastic leukemia and Netherton syndrome co-incidence-first report in the literature. Front Oncol. 2019;9:1477.
53. Fazio G, Massa V, Grioni A, Bystry V, Rigamonti S, Saitta C, et al. First evidence of a paediatric patient with Cornelia de Lange syndrome with acute lymphoblastic leukaemia. J Clin Pathol. 2019;72(8):558–61.
54. Cheah JJC, Brown AL, Schreiber AW, Feng J, Babic M, Moore S, et al. A novel germline SAMD9L mutation in a family with ataxia-pancytopenia syndrome and pediatric acute lymphoblastic leukemia. Haematologica. 2019;104(7):e318–21.
55. Esparza O, Xavier AC, Atkinson TP, Hill BC, Whelan K. A unique phenotype of T-cell acute lymphoblastic leukemia in a patient with GATA2 haploinsufficiency. Pediatr Blood Cancer. 2019;66(6):e27649.
56. Pommert L, Burns R, Furumo Q, Pulakanti K, Brandt J, Burke MJ, et al. Novel germline TRAF3IP3 mutation in a dyad with familial acute B lymphoblastic leukemia. Cancer Rep Hoboken NJ. 2021;4(3):e1335.
57. Duployez N, Jamrog LA, Fregona V, Hamelle C, Fenwarth L, Lejeune S, et al. Germline PAX5 mutation predisposes to familial B-cell precursor acute lymphoblastic leukemia. Blood. 2021;137(10):1424–8.
58. Shah S, Schrader KA, Waanders E, Timms AE, Vijai J, Miething C, et al. A recurrent germline PAX5 mutation confers susceptibility to pre-B cell acute lymphoblastic leukemia. Nat Genet. 2013;45(10):1226–31.
59. Auer F, Rüschendorf F, Gombert M, Husemann P, Ginzel S, Izraeli S, et al. Inherited susceptibility to pre B-ALL caused by germline transmission of PAX5 c.547G\textgreaterA. Leukemia. 2014;28(5):1136–8.
60. Yazdanparast S, Khatami SR, Galehdari H, Jaseb K. One missense mutation in exon 2 of the PAX5 gene in Iran. Genet Mol Res. 2015;14(4):17768–75.

61. Gu Z, Churchman ML, Roberts KG, Moore I, Zhou X, Nakitandwe J, et al. PAX5-driven subtypes of B-progenitor acute lymphoblastic leukemia. Nat Genet. 2019;51(2):296–307.
62. Raimondi SC, Privitera E, Williams DL, Look AT, Behm F, Rivera GK, et al. New recurring chromosomal translocations in childhood acute lymphoblastic leukemia. Blood. 1991;77(9):2016–22.
63. Shurtleff SA, Buijs A, Behm FG, Rubnitz JE, Raimondi SC, Hancock ML, et al. TEL/AML1 fusion resulting from a cryptic t(12;21) is the most common genetic lesion in pediatric ALL and defines a subgroup of patients with an excellent prognosis. Leukemia. 1995;9(12):1985–9.
64. Noetzli L, Lo RW, Lee-Sherick AB, Callaghan M, Noris P, Savoia A, et al. Germline mutations in ETV6 are associated with thrombocytopenia, red cell macrocytosis and predisposition to lymphoblastic leukemia. Nat Genet. 2015;47(5):535–8.
65. Zhang MY, Churpek JE, Keel SB, Walsh T, Lee MK, Loeb KR, et al. Germline ETV6 mutations in familial thrombocytopenia and hematologic malignancy. Nat Genet. 2015;47(2):180–5.
66. Topka S, Vijai J, Walsh MF, Jacobs L, Maria A, Villano D, et al. Germline ETV6 mutations confer susceptibility to acute lymphoblastic leukemia and thrombocytopenia. PLoS Genet. 2015;11(6):e1005262.
67. Di Paola J, Porter CC. ETV6-related thrombocytopenia and leukemia predisposition. Blood. 2019;134(8):663–7.
68. Moriyama T, Metzger ML, Wu G, Nishii R, Qian M, Devidas M, et al. Germline genetic variation in ETV6 and risk of childhood acute lymphoblastic leukaemia: a systematic genetic study. Lancet Oncol. 2015;16(16):1659–66.
69. Nishii R, Baskin-Doerfler R, Yang W, Oak N, Zhao X, Yang W, et al. Molecular basis of ETV6-mediated predisposition to childhood acute lymphoblastic leukemia. Blood. 2021;137(3):364–73.
70. Martinelli G, Iacobucci I, Storlazzi CT, Vignetti M, Paoloni F, Cilloni D, et al. IKZF1 (Ikaros) deletions in BCR-ABL1-positive acute lymphoblastic leukemia are associated with short disease-free survival and high rate of cumulative incidence of relapse: a GIMEMA AL WP report. J Clin Oncol Off J Am Soc Clin Oncol. 2009;27(31):5202–7.
71. Mullighan CG, Su X, Zhang J, Radtke I, Phillips L, Miller CB, et al. Deletion of IKZF1 and prognosis in acute lymphoblastic leukemia. N Engl J Med. 2009;360(5):470–80.
72. Kuehn HS, Boisson B, Cunningham-Rundles C, Reichenbach J, Stray-Pedersen A, Gelfand EW, et al. Loss of B cells in patients with heterozygous mutations in IKAROS. N Engl J Med. 2016;374(11):1032–43.
73. Churchman ML, Qian M, te Kronnie G, Zhang R, Yang W, Zhang H, et al. Germline genetic IKZF1 variation and predisposition to childhood acute lymphoblastic leukemia. Cancer Cell. 2018;33(5):937–948.e8.
74. Owen CJ, Toze CL, Koochin A, Forrest DL, Smith C, Stevens JM, et al. Five new pedigrees with inherited RUNX1 mutations causing familial platelet disorder with propensity to myeloid malignancy. Blood. 2008;112(12):4639–45.
75. Grossmann V, Kern W, Harbich S, Alpermann T, Jeromin S, Schnittger S, et al. Prognostic relevance of RUNX1 mutations in T-cell acute lymphoblastic leukemia. Haematologica. 2011;96(12):1874–7.
76. Della Gatta G, Palomero T, Perez-Garcia A, Ambesi-Impiombato A, Bansal M, Carpenter ZW, et al. Reverse engineering of TLX oncogenic transcriptional networks identifies RUNX1 as tumor suppressor in T-ALL. Nat Med. 2012;18(3):436–40.
77. Li Y, Yang W, Devidas M, Winter SS, Kesserwan C, Yang W, et al. Germline RUNX1 variation and predisposition to childhood acute lymphoblastic leukemia. J Clin Invest. 2021;131(17):e147898.
78. Zhang J, Walsh MF, Wu G, Edmonson MN, Gruber TA, Easton J, et al. Germline mutations in predisposition genes in pediatric cancer. N Engl J Med. 2015;373(24):2336–46.
79. Kratz CP, Achatz MI, Brugieres L, Frebourg T, Garber JE, Greer MLC, et al. Cancer screening recommendations for individuals with Li-Fraumeni syndrome. Clin Cancer Res. 2017;23(11):e38–45.
80. Bougeard G, Renaux-Petel M, Flaman JM, Charbonnier C, Fermey P, Belotti M, et al. Revisiting Li-Fraumeni syndrome from TP53 mutation carriers. J Clin Oncol. 2015;33(21):2345–52.
81. Holmfeldt L, Wei L, Diaz-Flores E, Walsh M, Zhang J, Ding L, et al. The genomic landscape of hypodiploid acute lymphoblastic leukemia. Nat Genet. 2013;45(3):242–52.
82. Winter G, Kirschner-Schwabe R, Groeneveld-Krentz S, Escherich G, Möricke A, von Stackelberg A, et al. Clinical and genetic characteristics of children with acute lymphoblastic leukemia and Li-Fraumeni syndrome. Leukemia. 2021;35(5):1475–9.
83. Villani A, Shore A, Wasserman JD, Stephens D, Kim RH, Druker H, et al. Biochemical and imaging surveillance in germline TP53 mutation carriers with Li-Fraumeni syndrome: 11 year follow-up of a prospective observational study. Lancet Oncol. 2016;12(6):559–67.
84. Ballinger ML, Best A, Mai PL, Khincha PP, Loud JT, Peters JA, et al. Baseline surveillance in Li-Fraumeni syndrome using whole-body magnetic resonance imaging. JAMA Oncol. 2017;3:1634.
85. Lynch HT, Snyder CL, Shaw TG, Heinen CD, Hitchins MP. Milestones of Lynch syndrome: 1895-2015. Nat Rev Cancer. 2015;15(3):181–94.
86. Wimmer K, Kratz CP, Vasen HF, Caron O, Colas C, Entz-Werle N, et al. Diagnostic criteria for constitutional mismatch repair deficiency syndrome: suggestions of the European consortium "care for CMMRD" (C4CMMRD). J Med Genet. 2014;51(6):355–65.

87. Durno C, Ercan AB, Bianchi V, Edwards M, Aronson M, Galati M, et al. Survival benefit for individuals with constitutional mismatch repair deficiency undergoing surveillance. J Clin Oncol. 2021;39(25):2779–90.
88. Porter CC, Druley TE, Erez A, Kuiper RP, Onel K, Schiffman JD, et al. Recommendations for surveillance for children with leukemia-predisposing conditions. Clin Cancer Res Off J Am Assoc Cancer Res. 2017;23(11):e14–22.
89. Parsons DW, Roy A, Yang Y, Wang T, Scollon S, Bergstrom K, et al. Sequencing for children with solid tumors. JAMA Oncol. 2016;1200:1–9.
90. Mody RJ, Wu YM, Lonigro RJ, Cao X, Roychowdhury S, Vats P, et al. Integrative clinical sequencing in the management of refractory or relapsed cancer in youth. JAMA. 2015;314(9):913.
91. Oberg JA, Glade Bender JL, Sulis ML, Pendrick D, Sireci AN, Hsiao SJ, et al. Implementation of next generation sequencing into pediatric hematology-oncology practice: moving beyond actionable alterations. Genome Med. 2016;8:133.
92. Gröbner SN, Worst BC, Weischenfeldt J, Buchhalter I, Kleinheinz K, Rudneva VA, et al. The landscape of genomic alterations across childhood cancers. Nature. 2018;555(7696):321–7.
93. Wong M, Mayoh C, Lau LMS, Khuong-Quang DA, Pinese M, Kumar A, et al. Whole genome, transcriptome and methylome profiling enhances actionable target discovery in high-risk pediatric cancer. Nat Med. 2020;26(11):1742–53.
94. Byrjalsen A, Hansen TVO, Stoltze UK, Mehrjouy MM, Barnkob NM, Hjalgrim LL, et al. Nationwide germline whole genome sequencing of 198 consecutive pediatric cancer patients reveals a high incidence of cancer prone syndromes. PLoS Genet. 2020;16(12)
95. Fiala EM, Jayakumaran G, Mauguen A, Kennedy JA, Bouvier N, Kemel Y, et al. Prospective pan-cancer germline testing using MSK-IMPACT informs clinical translation in 751 patients with pediatric solid tumors. Nat Cancer. 2021;2:357–65.
96. Newman S, Nakitandwe J, Kesserwan CA, Azzato EM, Wheeler DA, Rusch M, et al. Genomes for kids: the scope of pathogenic mutations in pediatric cancer revealed by comprehensive DNA and RNA sequencing. Cancer Discov. 2021;11(12):3008–27.
97. von Stedingk K, Stjernfelt KJ, Kvist A, Wahlström C, Kristoffersson U, Stenmark-Askmalm M, et al. Prevalence of germline pathogenic variants in 22 cancer susceptibility genes in Swedish pediatric cancer patients. Sci Rep. 2021;11(1):5307.
98. Wagener R, Taeubner J, Walter C, Yasin L, Alzoubi D, Bartenhagen C, et al. Comprehensive germline-genomic and clinical profiling in 160 unselected children and adolescents with cancer. Eur J Hum Genet. 2021;29(8):1301–11.
99. Stoltze UK, Foss-Skiftesvik J, van Overeem Hansen T, Byrjalsen A, Sehested A, Scheie D, Mikkelsen TS, Rasmussen S, Bak M, Okkels H, Callesen MT. Population-based whole-genome sequencing with constrained gene analysis identifies predisposing germline variants in children with central nervous system tumors. medRxiv. 2022.
100. Klco JM, Mullighan CG. Advances in germline predisposition to acute leukaemias and myeloid neoplasms. Nat Rev Cancer. 2021;21(2): 122–37.
101. Foss-Skiftesvik J, Stoltze UK, van Overeem HT, Ahlborn LB, Sørensen E, Ostrowski SR, et al. Redefining germline predisposition in children with molecularly characterized ependymoma: a population-based 20-year cohort. Acta Neuropathol Commun. 2022;10(1):123.
102. Foss-Skiftesvik J, Stoltze UK. Genetic predisposition to central nervous system tumors in children – what the neurosurgeon should know. Acta Neurochir. 2022;164:3025.
103. Karczewski KJ, Francioli LC, Tiao G, Cummings BB, Alföldi J, Wang Q, et al. The mutational constraint spectrum quantified from variation in 141,456 humans. Nature. 2020;581(7809):434–43.
104. Stoltze UK, Foss-Skiftesvik J, van Overeem Hansen T, Rasmussen S, Karczewski KJ, Wadt KAW, et al. The evolutionary impact of childhood cancer on the human gene pool. Nat Commun. 2024;15(1):1881. https://doi.org/10.1038/s41467-024-45975-9. PMID: 38424437
105. Stoltze UK, Foss-Skiftesvik J, van Overeem Hansen T, Byrjalsen A, Sehested A, Scheie D, et al. Genetic predisposition and evolutionary traces of pediatric cancer risk: a prospective 5-year population-based genome sequencing study of children with CNS tumors. Neuro Oncol . 2023;25(4):761–773. https://doi.org/10.1093/neuonc/noac187. PMID: 35902210
106. Villy MC, Frydman N, Moutou C, Thierry G, Raad J, Colas C, et al. Preimplantation genetic testing in patients with genetic susceptibility to cancer. Fam Cancer. 2022;22:119.
107. Treviño LR, Yang W, French D, Hunger SP, Carroll WL, Devidas M, et al. Germline genomic variants associated with childhood acute lymphoblastic leukemia. Nat Genet. 2009;41(9):1001–5.
108. Xu H, Yang W, Perez-Andreu V, Devidas M, Fan Y, Cheng C, et al. Novel susceptibility variants at 10p12.31-12.2 for childhood acute lymphoblastic leukemia in ethnically diverse populations. J Natl Cancer Inst. 2013;105(10):733–42.
109. Migliorini G, Fiege B, Hosking FJ, Ma Y, Kumar R, Sherborne AL, et al. Variation at 10p12.2 and 10p14 influences risk of childhood B-cell acute lymphoblastic leukemia and phenotype. Blood. 2013;122(19):3298–307.
110. Perez-Andreu V, Roberts KG, Harvey RC, Yang W, Cheng C, Pei D, et al. Inherited GATA3 variants are associated with Ph-like childhood acute lymphoblastic leukemia and risk of relapse. Nat Genet. 2013;45(12):1494–8.
111. Xu H, Zhang H, Yang W, Yadav R, Morrison AC, Qian M, et al. Inherited coding variants at the

CDKN2A locus influence susceptibility to acute lymphoblastic leukaemia in children. Nat Commun. 2015;6:7553.
112. Ellinghaus E, Stanulla M, Richter G, Ellinghaus D, te Kronnie G, Cario G, et al. Identification of germline susceptibility loci in ETV6-RUNX1-rearranged childhood acute lymphoblastic leukemia. Leuk Off J Leuk Soc Am Leuk Res Fund UK. 2012;26(5):902–9.
113. Prasad RB, Hosking FJ, Vijayakrishnan J, Papaemmanuil E, Koehler R, Greaves M, et al. Verification of the susceptibility loci on 7p12.2, 10q21.2, and 14q11.2 in precursor B-cell acute lymphoblastic leukemia of childhood. Blood. 2010;115(9):1765–7.
114. Sherborne AL, Hosking FJ, Prasad RB, Kumar R, Koehler R, Vijayakrishnan J, et al. Variation in CDKN2A at 9p21.3 influences childhood acute lymphoblastic leukemia risk. Nat Genet. 2010;42(6):492–4.
115. Walsh KM, De Smith AJ, Hansen HM, Smirnov IV, Gonseth S, Endicott AA, Xiao J, Rice T, Fu CH, McCoy LS, Lachance DH. A heritable missense polymorphism in CDKN2A confers strong risk of childhood acute lymphoblastic leukemia and is preferentially selected during clonal evolution. Cancer Res. 2015;75(22):4884–94.
116. Moriyama T, Relling MV, Yang JJ. Inherited genetic variation in childhood acute lymphoblastic leukemia. Blood. 2015;125(26):3988–96.
117. Lee SHR, Qian M, Yang W, Diedrich JD, Raetz E, Yang W, et al. Genome-wide association study of susceptibility loci for TCF3-PBX1 acute lymphoblastic leukemia in children. JNCI J Natl Cancer Inst. 2020;113(7):933–7.
118. Enciso-Mora V, Hosking FJ, Sheridan E, Kinsey SE, Lightfoot T, Roman E, et al. Common genetic variation contributes significantly to the risk of childhood B-cell precursor acute lymphoblastic leukemia. Leukemia. 2012;26(10):2212–5.
119. Couzin-Frankel J. Major heart disease genes prove elusive. Science. 2010;328(5983):1220–1.
120. Visscher PM, Goddard ME, Derks EM, Wray NR. Evidence-based psychiatric genetics, AKA the false dichotomy between common and rare variant hypotheses. Mol Psychiatry. 2012;17(5):474–85.
121. Schmiegelow K, Müller K, Mogensen SS, Mogensen PR, Wolthers BO, Stoltze UK, et al. Non-infectious chemotherapy-associated acute toxicities during childhood acute lymphoblastic leukemia therapy. F1000Research. 2017;6

Part II

Biology and Diagnostics of ALL

2 Genomic Basis of B-Cell Precursor Acute Lymphoblastic Leukemia

Shunsuke Kimura, Monique L. Den Boer, and Charles G. Mullighan

2.1 Chromosomal Abnormalities

2.1.1 High Hyperdiploid ALL

High hyperdiploid ALL is one of the most common genetic subtypes of pediatric leukemia, accounting for approximately 25–30% of B-cell precursor (BCP-) ALL among children, with a median age of diagnosis ranging from 3 to 5 years (Fig. 2.1) [6, 9, 10]. High hyperdiploidy is defined as the gain of at least five chromosomes (typically a chromosomal modal number of 51–67). Criteria for diagnosing hyperdiploidy vary and include detection of double trisomy of chromosomes 4 and 10 (which detects the majority but not all cases) or DNA index ≥1.16 as measured by flow cytometry. These criteria exhibit an imperfect correlation [11, 12]. Furthermore, concurrent additional alterations with hyperdiploidy were reported, including *BCR::ABL1*, *TCF3::PBX1*, and *KMT2A::AFF1* [11]. The chromosomal gains are nonrandom, most commonly involving X, 4, 6, 10, 14, 17, 18, and 21 [9]. Mechanistically, this phenomenon results from an impaired condensin complex, leading to chromosome hypocondensation and mislocalization of components of the chromosome passenger complex (CPC), including survivin and aurora B kinase (AURKB), during early mitosis. The compromised AURKB activity gives rise to defects in the spindle assembly checkpoint and chromosome misalignments at the metaphase plate. Consequently, pronounced deficiencies in chromosome segregation occur, leading to nonmodal karyotypes [13].

Overall, high hyperdiploidy is associated with favorable outcomes, but outcome varies according to the pattern of aneuploidy and associated genomic features. Triple trisomy (+4, +10, +17), presence of +17 and + 18, and the absence of +5/+20 in conjunction with +17 or + 18 are associated with positive outcomes. Conversely, *SETD2* alterations are associated with a higher relapse rate (Table 2.1) [5, 12, 14, 15]. Due to the absence of an established consensus for the definition of high hyperdiploid ALL and prognostic markers, the criteria employed to classify the favorable prognostic subset within this subtype vary across clinical trials. For example, the Children's Oncology Group (COG) has adopted triple trisomy in AALL0331 [16]. However, this subgroup accounts for only two-thirds of high hyperdiploid cases. Genomically, most cases involve activating mutations in the receptor tyrosine kinase (RTK)/Ras pathway (*KRAS*, *NRAS*, *FLT3*, *PTPN11*), as well as histone modifier

S. Kimura · C. G. Mullighan (✉)
Department of Pathology, Hematological Malignancies Program, St. Jude Children's Research Hospital, Memphis, TN, USA
e-mail: charles.mullighan@stjude.org

M. L. Den Boer
Princess Máxima Center for Pediatric Oncology, Utrecht, The Netherlands

G. Escherich, V. Conter (eds.), *Acute Lymphoblastic Leukemia in Children and Adolescents*, Pediatric Oncology, https://doi.org/10.1007/978-3-031-71180-0_2

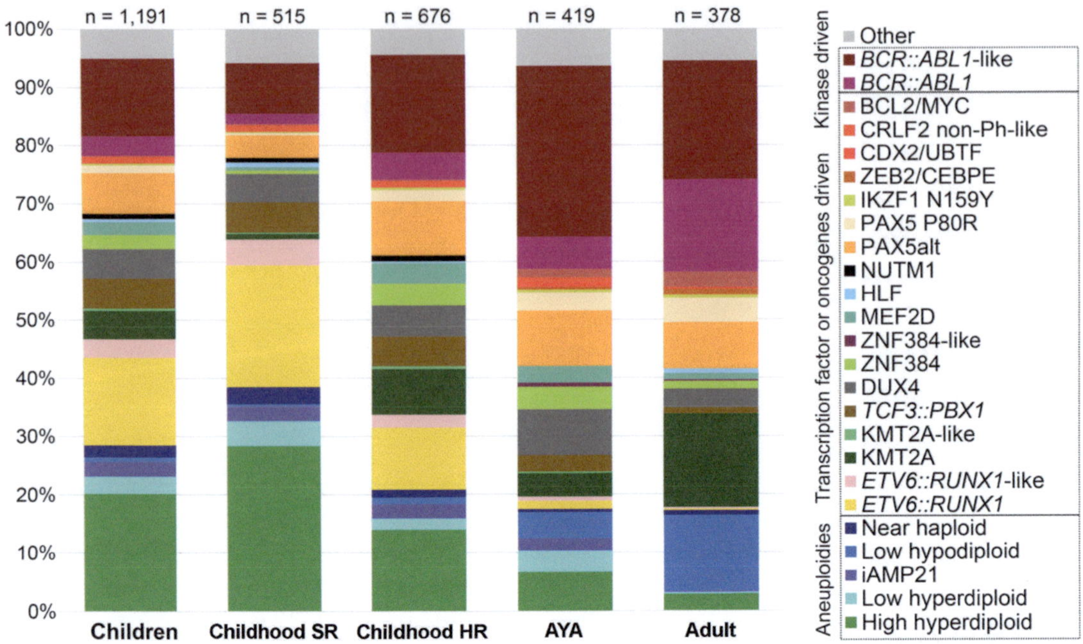

Fig. 2.1 Distribution of BCP-ALL subtypes within age group. The frequency of each B-ALL subtype [6] is shown in children (1191 cases, −15 years), standard-risk children (Children SR, 515 cases), high-risk children (Children HR, 676 cases), adolescents and young adult (AYA, 419 cases, 16–39 years), and adult (378 cases, 40– years). SR and HR are defined according to NCI criteria

genes (*CREBBP*, *WHSC1*, *SETD2*) [5, 9, 11, 17]. Alterations in *CREBBP* frequently cluster in the histone acetyltransferase (HAT) domain, result in resistance to glucocorticoids, and are selected for during disease progression [18]. Notably, the mutational signature associated with ultraviolet (UV) is enriched in high hyperdiploid ALL. These UV-induced mutations are often manifest on just one of three triploid chromosomes, suggesting that copy number gains precede UV exposure [5]. The predominant scenario of aneuploidy generation involves an early synchronous pattern, observed in roughly 80% of cases, where chromosomal gains precede the acquisition of point mutations [5].

The gene expression profiles (Fig. 2.2) of high hyperdiploid ALL and near haploid ALL are highly similar, in part due to the increased relative dosage of chromosomes 10, 14, 18, and 21, which are commonly acquired in high hyperdiploid ALL but usually remain intact in near haploid cases [5, 6]. As a result, gene expression profiles provide limited accuracy in distinguishing between these two aneuploidy categories that carry significantly different prognostic implications. Mutation-wise, both subtypes frequently exhibit alterations in *CREBBP* and Ras pathway genes, albeit affecting different members; *NRAS*, *KRAS*, and *PTPN11* in high hyperdiploid ALL, and *NF1* deletions in near haploid ALL [5, 9, 19].

2.1.2 Hypodiploid ALL

Hypodiploid ALL represents a subtype of BCP-ALL that is more common in adults than children, characterized by fewer than 44 chromosomes. This subtype is further divided into two main distinct subtypes based on the extent of aneuploidy: low-hypodiploid ALL (30–39 chromosomes or DNA index 0.65–0.82) and near-haploid ALL (24–29 chromosomes or DNA index below 0.65) [19]. High-hypodiploid ALL (40–44 chromosomes) is heterogeneous that differs from low-hypodiploid ALL and near-haploid ALL in terms of genomic alterations,

Table 2.1 Novel or potential therapeutic approaches for each BCP-ALL subtype

Subtype	Risk	Novel or potential therapeutic approaches
Chromosomal abnormalities, aneuploidy		
Hyperdiploid	Good	Identify high-risk cases by the combination of chromosome gains
Hypodiploid	Poor	PI3K and BCL2 inhibitors, Src kinase inhibitors (dasatinib, ponatinib) for *PAG1* deletion
iAMP21	Intermediate	High-risk treatment, JAK/STAT inhibitors, check germline alterations (Robertsonian, ring chr 21)
Transcription factor (TF) or oncogene-driven		
ETV6::RUNX1	Good	Identify high-risk cases (*TBL1XR1* mutations)
TCF3::PBX1	Intermediate	Src kinase inhibitors, ROR1 inhibitors
HLF-rearranged (*TCF3::HLF*)	Poor	Aurora A kinase inhibitors, BCL2 inhibitors, Src kinase inhibitors, EP300 inhibitors
KMT2A-rearranged	Poor	DOT1L inhibitors, Menin inhibitors, targeting CD72
DUX4-rearranged	Good	Reduce intensity?
MEF2D-rearranged	Intermediate	HDAC inhibitors, Src kinase inhibitors, bortezomib
ZNF384-rearranged	Intermediate	FLT3 inhibitors
PAX5-driven (PAX5 alt/P80R)	Intermediate	Unknown
CDX2/UBTF	Poor	Unknown
NUTM1-rearranged	Good	Bromodomain inhibitors
IKZF1 N159	Intermediate	Retinoids, FAK inhibitors, check germline IKZF1 N159 alterations
MYC-rearranged (BCL2/MYC)	Poor	Unknown
Kinase-driven		
BCR::ABL1 (Ph+)	Poor	Kinase inhibitors, retinoids, FAK inhibitors
BCR::ABL1-like (Ph-like)	Poor	Kinase inhibitors, TRK inhibitors, FLT3 inhibitors, JAK/STAG inhibitors, immune therapy
Others or provisional entities		
ETV6::RUNX1-like	Intermediate	Check germline *ETV6*/*PAX5* alterations
Hyper-mutation	Relapse	Checkpoint blockade

expression profiles, and clinical outcomes, and does not represent a distinct subtype of B-ALL [19]. Despite the improvement of outcome through therapy stratified by minimal residual disease (MRD), both low-hypodiploid and near-haploid ALL continue to carry an unfavorable prognosis, except for cases achieving MRD-negative status by the end of induction therapy (EOI) (Table 2.1) [20–23]. The presence of distinct CD10 positivity (positive for near-haploid and positive/negative for low-hypodiploid ALL) might correspond to the cell of origin, pro-B or earlier stage in low-hypodiploid ALL [19, 22]. Similar to high hyperdiploid ALL, the pattern of chromosome loss in hypodiploid ALL is nonrandom, frequently involving chromosomes 3, 7, 9, 15, 16, and 17 [19]. Notably, chromosome 21 is never lost. In near-haploid ALL, retained disomies typically encompass chromosomes 8, 10, 14, 18, 21, and X/Y, mirroring the gained chromosomes in high-hyperdiploid ALL [19].

Masked hypodiploidy is a common phenomenon in hypodiploid ALL that may be mistaken for high hyperdiploidy that reflects duplication of the aneuploid genome [22, 24]. Masked hypodiploidy may be mistaken for high hyperdiploidy; however, the patterns of chromosomal gain and loss of heterozygosity (LOH) differ: diploid and tetraploid chromosomes in masked hypodiploidy versus a combination of triploid and certain tetraploid chromosomes (21, X) in high hyperdiploidy [24]. In addition, the identification of masked hypodiploidy is simplified through techniques such as SNP array or genomic sequencing, which readily detect LOH across most chromosomes (Fig. 2.3) [24].

Almost all low-hypodiploid ALL cases encompass biallelic *TP53* alterations affecting

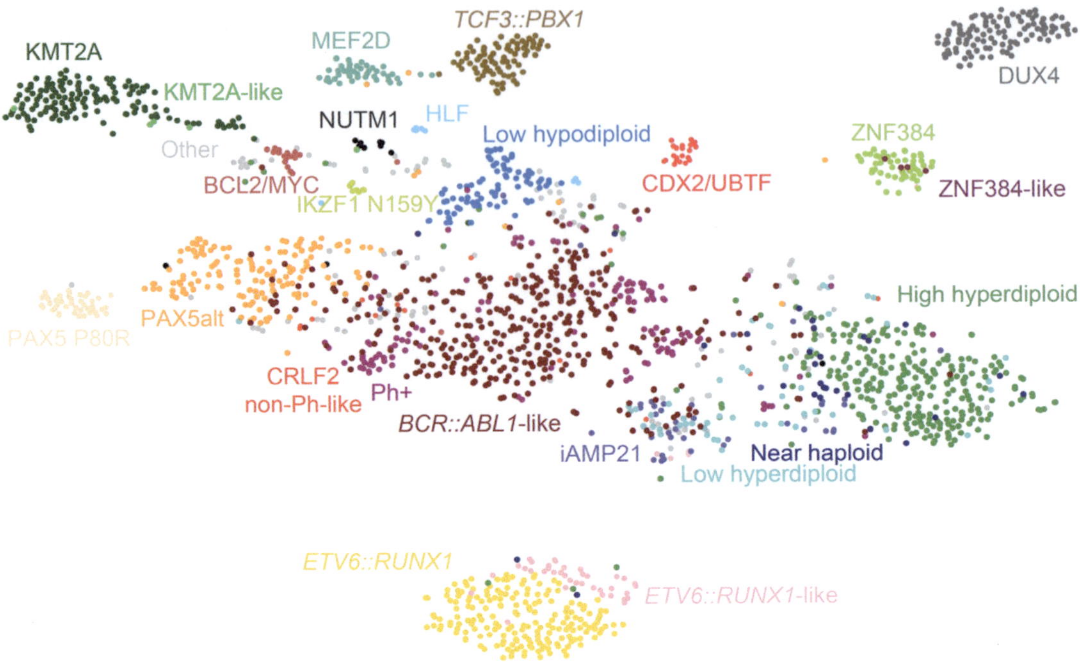

Fig. 2.2 The main subtypes of BCP-ALL. Gene expression profiles of BCP-ALL based on whole-transcriptome sequencing showing tSNE plot of 2004 cases [6, 117] by using the top 1000 most variable genes on the basis of median absolute deviation with a perplexity score of 30. Each dot represents a sample. The major ALL subtypes are highlighted in different colors

the DNA-binding domain, with nearly half being constitutional in children, potentially indicating the presence of Li-Fraumeni syndrome [19, 25]. Conversely, nearly all adult cases show somatic biallelic TP53 inactivation, although *TP53* mutations were identified in 34% of remission samples, suggesting the existence of preexisting *TP53* mutant clonal hematopoiesis [26]. The TP53 status affects treatment choice since *TP53* mutations were recently shown less responsive to CD19 chimeric antigen receptor (CAR) T-cell-mediated immunotherapy [27, 28].

Frequent additional alterations involve *RB1*, *IKZF2*, and *CDKN2A/B*. The occurrence of near-haploid ALL is largely confined to children and is genomically characterized by alterations in RTK/Ras pathway (particularly *NF1*), histone modifier genes (*CREBBP*), and *IKZF3*. Moreover, *PAG1* deletions are present in 10% of near-haploid cases, suggesting deregulation of Src-family kinases that might be targeted using Src inhibitors like dasatinib [5, 19]. The effectiveness of PI3K and BCL2 inhibitors, along with the synergistic effect of cyclin-dependent kinase (CDK) and BCL2 inhibitors, has been demonstrated in preclinical studies, presenting promising therapeutic avenues for hypodiploid ALL (Table 2.1) [19, 29, 30].

2.1.3 Intrachromosomal Amplification of Chromosome 21 (iAMP21)

BCP-ALL with iAMP21 accounts for roughly 1–2% of pediatric ALL cases. This subtype tends to manifest in older children, with a median age of 9 years, and typically displays a low white blood cell count (Fig. 2.1) [31–34]. The current definition of iAMP21 by fluorescence in situ hybridization (FISH) entails either (1) the presence of three or more extra copies of the *RUNX1* gene on a single abnormal chromosome 21 or (2) the occurrence of five or more copies of the *RUNX1* gene region per interphase cell [32, 33]. For the clinical identification of iAMP21, FISH probes targeting the *ETV6::RUNX1* fusion are

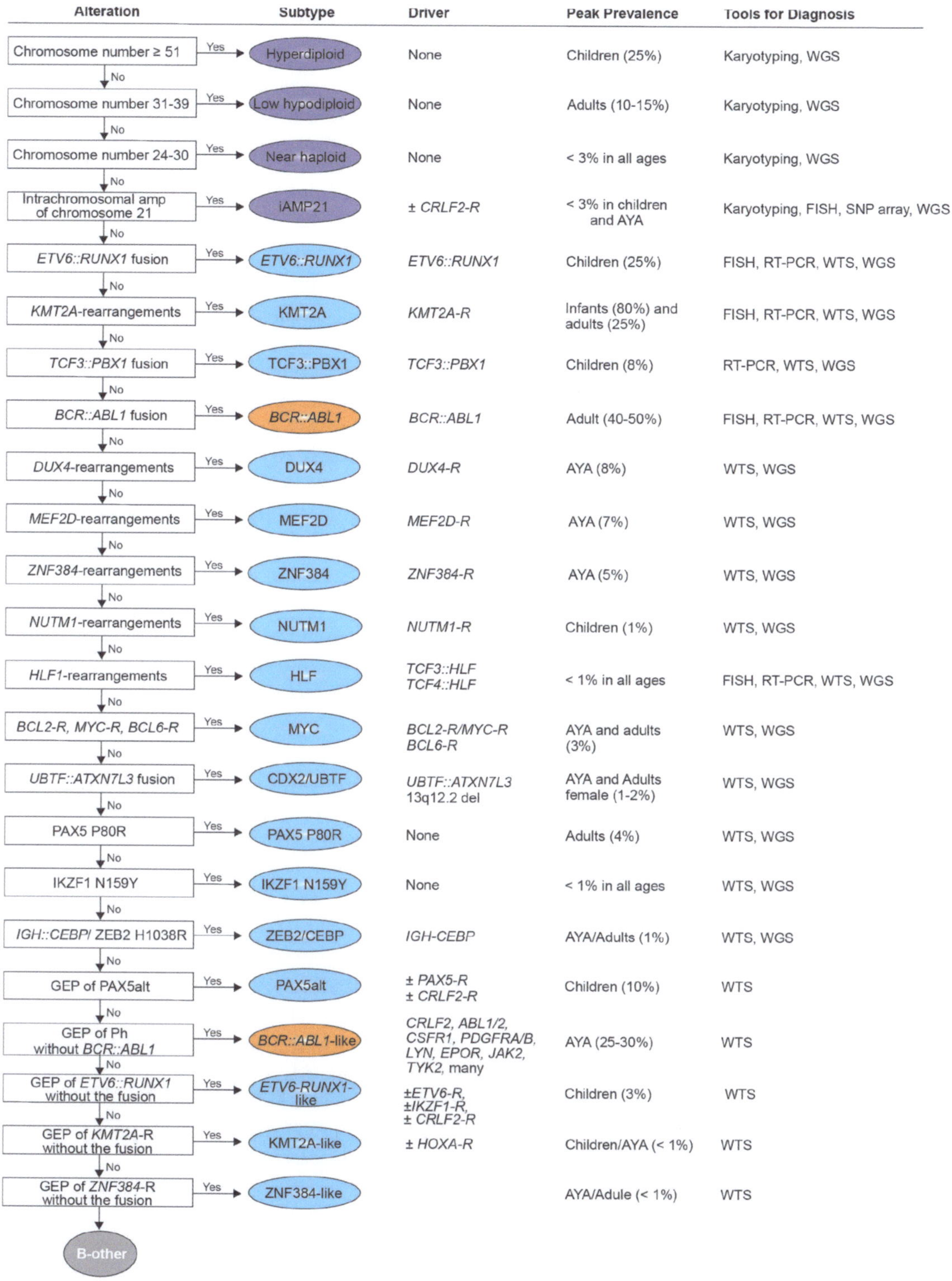

Fig. 2.3 A schematic algorithm for BCP-ALL subtyping, prevalence, and tools for the diagnosis [165]. This figure overviews how we can define each BCP-ALL subtype by using karyotyping, whole-genome sequencing (WGS), whole-transcriptome sequencing (WTS), fluorescence in situ hybridization (FISH), and reverse transcription-polymerase chain reaction (RT-PCR), and single-nucleotide polymorphism (SNP) array. Each subtype is colored based on defining genetic events: aneuploidies or gross chromosomal abnormalities (purple), transcription factor or oncogene-driven (blue), and kinase-driven (orange)

employed, as *RUNX1* usually resides within the shared region of chromosome 21 amplification. These probes, spanning approximately 40 Mb from *TIAM1* and *HMGN1*, encompass several genes implicated in the pathogenesis of BCP-ALL (*CHAF1B*, *DYRK1A*, *ERG*, *HMGN1*, *RUNX1*) [35]. Nonetheless, approximately 9% of iAMP21 cases do not align with the FISH definition and necessitate alternative methods such as chromosomal microarray and whole-genome sequencing. Accurate identification of iAMP21 holds significance, given that patients with iAMP21 exhibit unfavorable outcomes with standard-risk treatment but could overcome with intensive high-risk treatment [31, 36]. Mechanistically, the genesis of iAMP21 is attributed to the consequences of breakage–fusion–bridge cycles and chromothripsis [37]. The varied nature of the iAMP21-chromosome revealed through single-cell analysis suggests progressive amplification of iAMP21 over a period of time [35]. Though uncommon, constitutional structural chromosomal abnormalities such as Robertsonian translocation rob(15;21), isodicentric chromosome 21 idic(21), or a germline ring chromosome 21, are linked with an elevated risk of iAMP21 [38]. Concurrent genetic lesions encompass deletions within the histone gene region at 6p22.2, copy number neutral LOH of 12q, and alterations in genes of the JAK-STAT pathway (*SH2B3, IL7R, P2RY8::CRLF2*), implying the potential utility of ruxolitinib as a targeted therapeutic agent (Table 2.1) [5, 35]. Similar to high hyperdiploid ALL, iAMP21 is associated with an enrichment of UV-related mutational signatures. However, in contrast to high hyperdiploid ALL, UV-induced mutations occur prior to most chromosomal gains in cases of iAMP21 [5].

2.2 Transcription Factor or Oncogene-Driven BCP-ALL

2.2.1 *ETV6::RUNX1* and *ETV6::RUNX1*-Like ALL

The fusion gene *ETV6::RUNX1*, is the most common translocation in pediatric BCP-ALL, occurring in 20–25% of cases (Fig. 2.1) [6, 39–41]. *ETV6::RUNX1* leukemia exhibits exhibit CD27^{pos} and CD44$^{low-neg}$, and a favorable clinical course [16, 39, 42]. The genesis of this fusion gene arises from the t(12:21)(p13:q22) translocation, which is typically cryptic and necessitates the application of FISH or fusion gene detection through PCR- or sequencing-based techniques for accurate diagnosis. The detection of *ETV6::RUNX1* in unselected normal cord blood underscores its prenatal origin [43]. However, the presence of the *ETV6::RUNX1* fusion alone is not sufficient to precipitate overt leukemia, as a substantial variation of leukemia onset has been observed even in identical twins, along with a long latency for the acquisition of secondary mutations and heterogeneity in the subclonal composition at the time of leukemia [39, 44]. Experimental models utilizing mouse transplantation with retroviral *ETV6::RUNX1* expression have shown a low incidence of leukemia development with a long latency [45]. Transduction of *ETV6::RUNX1* into human cord blood hematopoietic progenitors leads to the emergence of the aberrant CD34^{+}CD38^{-}CD19^{+} population, indicative of an early stage of B-cell lineage before commitment, coupled with aberrant autophagosome formation [46–48]. The progression to full leukemia likely requires acquisition of secondary alterations, including deletions involving the normal alleles of *ETV6*, *PAX5*, *TBL1XR1*, *CDKN2A/B*, and *BTG1*, many of which are associated with aberrant RAG-mediated genomic recombination [5, 49, 50]. Among these alterations, *TBL1XR1* alteration is linked with inferior outcomes, being exclusively identified in *ETV6::RUNX1* ALL and not in *ETV6::RUNX1*-like ALL (Table 2.1) [5]. *IKZF1* is rarely deleted in *ETV6::RUNX1* ALL, and is not associated with unfavorable outcomes in contrast to *BCR::ABL1* and *BCR::ABL1*-like ALL in which it is more frequently altered [51, 52].

ETV6::RUNX1-like ALL constitutes a subtype that phenocopies *ETV6::RUNX1* ALL in terms of expression profiles, immunophenotype (CD27^{pos} and CD44$^{low-neg}$), and mutational signature (APOBEC), but distinctively lacks *ETV6::RUNX1* fusion [6, 53–55]. In place of the

ETV6::RUNX1 fusion, about 40% of *ETV6::RUNX1*-like ALL cases exhibit deletions or rearrangements of genes encoding transcription factors, including the ETS family (e.g., *ETV6*, *ERG*, and *FLI1*), *IKZF1*, and *TCF3* [6, 53–55]. *ETV6::RUNX1*-like ALL is associated with germline *ETV6* variants, accompanied by additional somatic alterations in *PAX5* and *ETV6* within the normal allele (Table 2.1) [56]. In contrast to *ETV6::RUNX1* ALL, *ETV6::RUNX1*-like ALL is associated with poor outcomes marked by high levels of MRD [5].

2.2.2 *TCF3*-Rearranged ALL (*TCF3::PBX1* and *TCF3::HLF*)

The fusion gene *TCF3::PBX1* is generated by the t(1;19)(q23;p13) translocation and is identified in approximately 5–6% of pediatric BCP-ALL patients (Fig. 2.1) [57, 58]. *TCF3::PBX1* ALL is characterized by a pre-B immunophenotype that exhibits cytoplasmic μ heavy chain expression, indicative of pre-B-cell receptor (BCR) signaling. This particular signaling pathway presents a potential target for Src kinase inhibitors including dasatinib and ponatinib, but not imatinib [59]. Combined therapy with ROR1 inhibition might offer a synergistic effect by countering the compensatory increase in *ROR1* expression induced by dasatinib treatment (Table 2.1) [59, 60]. Conditional activation of *TCF3::PBX1* leads to enhanced self-renewal and leukemia development accompanied by somatic alterations in *PAX5*, JAK-STAT, and Ras pathways, following a pre-leukemic phase [61]. Although human *TCF3::PBX1* ALL generally lacks JAK-STAT pathway gene mutations, subclonal alterations in Ras pathway gene and deletions involving *PAX5* and *CDKN2A* are found [17, 61] Notably, *CDKN2A* deletions in *TCF3::PBX1* ALL are associated with unfavorable outcomes [5]. The pathogenesis of *TCF3::PBX1* ALL involve interaction between PBX1 and HOXB7 [62], and a role of TCF3::PBX1 as a co-activator for RUNX1, that results in activation of RUNX1-related gene programs through a RUNX1 autoregulatory loop [63].

The translocation (17;19)(q22;p13) gives rise to a rare *TCF3::HLF* fusion, which is associated with an extremely dismal prognosis [64]. Despite common *TCF3* rearrangements, *TCF3::HLF* ALL has a distinct gene expression profile from *TCF3::PBX1* ALL (Fig. 2.2) with enrichment of stem cell and myeloid features. There are differences in the mutational landscape, marked by recurrent *PAX5* and *CDKN2A/B* deletions, as well as Ras signaling mutations [6, 64]. The *TCF3::HLF* fusion contains the transactivation domains within TCF3 and the DNA binding and dimerization domains in HLF, driving lymphoid differentiation [65–67]. Functioning as a pioneer TF, the TCF3::HLF fusion protein cooperates with ERG and recruits EP300, thereby activating MYC and promoting a hematopoietic stem cell-like state. Encouraging results have emerged from a preclinical study involving the EP300 inhibitor A-485, which inactivates TCF3::HLF binding enhancers [66]. Apart from inhibiting BCL2 (venetoclax), pre-B-cell receptor signaling (Src family inhibitors), and BIRC5, high expression of aurora A kinase (AURKA) might hold therapeutic promise for *TCF3::HLF* ALL (Table 2.1) [64, 67, 68].

2.2.3 *KMT2A*-Rearranged ALL

KMT2A-rearranged ALL represents a distinctive subtype within high-risk BCP-ALL, characterized by both lymphoid and myeloid features. This subgroup is defined by the rearrangement of the *KMT2A* (*MLL1*) gene located on chromosome 11q23 with more than 100 different partner genes. *KMT2A* rearrangements are known to occur in utero and they exhibit a high prevalence among infants diagnosed with ALL [69]. The clinical spectrum also encompasses a secondary peak of incidence in adult cases, comprising more than 10% of adult ALL instances (Fig. 2.1) [69, 70]. Exposure to topoisomerase II inhibitors is known to induce *KMT2A* rearrangement, developing therapy-related leukemia [71]. Absence of CD10 expression, accompanied by the presence of myeloid markers, is a typical feature of *KMT2A*-rearranged ALL. This feature aligns with lineage plasticity and reflects an early B-cell differentiation stage, encompassing early lymphocyte precursor (ELP) and pro-B state [72]. Prevalent translocations within this subtype include t(4;11)(q21;q23), *KMT2A::AFF1*, along with t(11;19) and t(9;11) [69, 73]. Some translocations exhibit lineage preference, exemplified by *KMT2A::AFF1* in BCP-ALL and *KMT2A::MLLT4* in T-ALL [69, 73]. The difference in partner genes is linked with different prognostic outcomes, with *KMT2A::AFF1*-rearranged leukemia showing inferior outcomes [73]. A multi-omic analysis of infant ALL proposed two subtypes, the IRX and HOXA subtypes, each characterized by the specific partner genes involved [74–77]. Although infant ALL harbors few genomic alterations, perturbations in PI3K and Ras pathways are found prominently and are often subclonal, underscoring their collaborative role in leukemogenesis and their potential as targets [77–80]. At the molecular level, the interaction between KMT2A and its fusion partners orchestrates the formation of a large multi-protein complex including DOT1L, a histone 3 lysine 79 methyltransferase, leading to epigenetic dysregulation and aberrant transcriptional activity. The targeted inhibition against this complex by using inhibitors of DOT1L, bromodomain, Menin, and polycomb repressive complex, is promising, although no durable remission has yet been achieved with these agents (Table 2.1) [81–83]. Although some CD19-targeted immunotherapies have yielded disappointing results in *KMT2A*-rearranged ALL due to lineage plasticity and immune escape [84], the low incidence of relapse-with no CD19-negative escape-after treatment with the Interfant-06 backbone and blinatumomab is promising [85]. Exploring new markers, including CD72, might have therapeutic potential for this high-risk subtype [86].

2.2.4 *DUX4*-Rearranged ALL

DUX4-rearranged ALL represents a distinct subtype arising from the cryptic translocation of the *DUX4* gene on chromosomes 4q/10q to enhancers, most commonly at the immunoglobulin heavy chain locus (IGH) locus. This translocation results in the overexpression of a 3′ truncated DUX4 protein [55, 87, 88]. Accounting for around 5% of BCP-ALL, *DUX4*-rearranged ALL exhibits a slight peak in AYAs. This subtype exhibits a unique immunophenotype characterized by positivity for CD2 and CD371, which may be used as a promising surrogate marker for identifying this subtype (Fig. 2.1) [6, 89]. The high CD371 expression may offer an alternative target for drug-conjugated antibodies in these cases [89]. Frequently observed genomic aberrations include deletions affecting *ERG* and *IKZF1*, as well as alterations involving epigenetic modifiers [5, 87, 88, 90]. *ERG* deletions are commonly employed as a surrogate marker for this subtype. However, these deletions are secondary events and not universally present across all cases [87, 91]. The *DUX4* rearrangements trigger the elevated expression of a 5′ fragment of DUX4, which in turn binds to an intronic region of *ERG* gene. This interplay leads to transcriptional deregulation of *ERG*, and culminates in intragenic *ERG* deletions and the expression of a noncanonical ERG 3′ fragment (ERGalt). ERGalt retains the DNA-binding and transactivating domain of ERG and exerts a dominant negative effect, contributing to lymphoid lineage shift and ultimately, transformation [87]. Despite the high MRD level at EOI, *DUX4*-rearranged ALL is associated with a favorable prognosis, irrespective of *IKZF1* alterations [87, 88, 92, 93]. Gene expression profiles further subclassified this *DUX4*-rearranged ALL into two developmentally different subtypes; one with the enrichment of alterations in *ERG* and *TBL1XR1*, high *NFATC4* expression, and excellent prognosis; and the other subtype with alterations in *NRAS*, *IKZF1*, and *KMT2D*, high expression of *FLT3* and *CEBPA* as well as higher incidence of relapse yet can be salvaged [5].

2.2.5 *MEF2D*-Rearranged ALL

MEF2D-rearranged ALL is found in up to 5% of BCP-ALL and is characterized by fusion genes of N-terminal *MEF2D* to various partner genes, such as *BCL9* and *HNRNPUL1* (Fig. 2.1) [94–96]. Deletions affecting *CDKN2A/B* genes are recurrently observed in this subtype [5]. *MEF2D*-rearranged ALL exhibits a unique immunophenotype, featuring positivity for CD38, CD5, and cytoplasmic μ chain with low/absent CD10 expression [94–96]. Although most cases exhibit negative MRD status at EOI, outcomes for *MEF2D*-rearranged ALL tend to be inferior. However, the exception is *MEF2D::HRNPUL1*, which exhibits relatively high CD10 expression and late pre-B stage [97].

MEF2D fusion protein enhances the transcriptional activity of MEF2D. This is achieved through an autoregulatory loop of core regulatory circuitry and evasion mechanism from miRNA-mediated degradation. Consequently, B-cell differentiation is impaired, and MEF2D targets including HDAC9 were dysregulated, and histone deacetylase inhibitors showed anti-leukemic efficacy [95, 98, 99]. Integration of pre-BCR signaling by MEF2D fusion-core regulatory circuitry might raise Src inhibitors as potential targets (Table 2.1) [98]. Additionally, SREBF1, a critical component of core regulatory circuitry, could be a promising target for this subtype [98].

2.2.6 *ZNF384*-Rearranged Leukemia

ZNF384 rearrangements delineate a subtype of leukemia with lineage ambiguity, exhibiting a distinct gene expression profile and characteristic immunophenotype characterized by weak CD10 and aberrant myeloid markers such as CD13 or CD33. (Fig. 2.2) [100, 101]. Notably, the manifestation of *ZNF384*-rearranged leukemia can span the spectrum from BCP-ALL to B/myeloid mixed phenotype acute leukemia (MPAL), depending on the myeloperoxidase expression at diagnosis [101]. Moreover, the immunophenotype of *ZNF384*-rearranged leukemia frequently exhibits multiclonality, often displaying lineage plasticity as the disease progresses and transitions between predominant expression of myeloid or lymphoid markers [100]. A mouse xenotransplantation model also demonstrated this lineage plasticity by reconstituting immunophenotypic diversity from flow-sorted subpopulations [100].

Secondary genetic alterations within *ZNF384*-rearranged leukemia encompass Ras pathway mutations, *ETV6* deletions, and *CDKN2A/B* deletions. However, these alterations remain consistent across various immunophenotypic subclones [5]. The detection of *ZNF384* rearrangements within a subset of hematopoietic progenitor cells (HPC) from diagnostic samples, coupled with the identification of twin *ZNF384*-rearranged leukemia cases, supports the notion that *ZNF384* rearrangements are founder events in HPC, serving as a possible cell of origin [100, 102]. Thus, *ZNF384*-rearranged leukemia is a single entity, irrespective of the immunophenotype (BCP-ALL or MPAL) at diagnosis.

The rearrangements involving *ZNF384* instigate the formation of fusion oncoproteins that usually retain the entire coding regions of ZNF384 [88, 103, 104]. N-terminus fusion partners include a variety of TFs such as *TAF15* and *TCF3*, and chromatin modifiers like *CREBBP* and *EP300* [101, 104]. An *Ep300::Znf384* knock-in mouse model revealed that ZNF384 fusion oncoproteins induce hematopoietic expansion, myeloid lineage skewing, and self-renewal. These results underscore that *ZNF384* rearrangements serve as founder alterations [104]. Furthermore, ZNF384 fusion oncoproteins interact with intergenic enhancer elements at the *FLT3* locus, leading to an overexpression of *FLT3*, which in turn manifests sensitivity to FLT3 inhibitors (Table 2.1) [105]. In this regard, FLT3 inhibitors might be a potential target therapy for this subtype, although lineage-directed conventional chemotherapy and recent immunotherapies (CAR T-cell therapy and blinatumomab) may cause lineage switch due to lineage plasticity.

2.2.7 *PAX5*-Driven ALL (PAX5alt and PAX5 P80R)

PAX5-driven ALL is classified into two subtypes, PAX5alt and PAX5 P80R, characterized by loss-of-function and/or dominant negative alterations in *PAX5*, an essential transcription factor in B-cell differentiation [6–8, 106–108]. These subtypes have distinct gene expression profiles (Fig. 2.2) and *PAX5* alterations that have essential roles in leukemogenesis as initiating or cooperating lesions.

PAX5alt encompasses a range of alterations, including rearrangements, focal intragenic amplifications (PAX5amp), and sequence mutations [6, 109]. These sequence mutations typically exclude P80R except for cases with rare heterozygous P80R mutation [5, 6]. Despite the diversity of alterations, PAX5alt cases share common gene expression profiles in BCP-ALL, although granularity exists within the PAX5alt subtype, as *PAX5::ETV6* and PAX5 R38H/R140L cases emerge as distinct groups [5, 6, 53]. *PAX5* rearrangements typically maintain the C-terminus DNA-binding domain and fuse with over 20 different partner genes, including *PAX5::ETV6* [6, 110]. Exceptions are *PAX5::JAK2* cases exclusively found in *BCR::ABL1*-like ALL and *PAX5::ZCCHC7* observed in several other subtypes [5, 6]. The lesions of PAX5amp are variable but consistently involve exon 5, leading to an in-frame duplication of the DNA-binding domain, frequently accompanied by *CDKN2A/B* alterations and trisomy 5 [6, 109]. Non-silent *PAX5* sequence mutations are generally compound heterozygous, found with multiple alterations including PAX5amp, PAX5 fusions, or structural variants [6]. The most prevalent compound heterozygosity in PAX5alt involves R38H and R140L in the DNA-binding paired domain [6]. The same concomitant alteration pattern was also observed in BCP-ALL with the germline R38H variant [111]. Alongside *PAX5* alterations, PAX5alt cases have concomitant alterations of cell cycle regulation genes (*CDKN2A*, *RB1*, *BTG1*), B-cell development genes (*IKZF1*), and transcriptional/epigenetic regulators (*KDM6A*, *KMT2A*, *ATRX*) [6].

The other subtype of PAX5-driven ALL, PAX5 P80R, is characterized by a nonsilent hot spot mutation in the paired domain of *PAX5*. PAX5 P80R yields distinct gene expression profiles, which can be defined by the sequence mutation (Fig. 2.2) [6, 112, 113]. Notably, PAX5 P80R is typically hemizygous, often found with concomitant inactivation of wild-type *PAX5* allele by deletion, loss-of-function mutation, or copy-neutral LOH [6, 113]. The heterozygous $Pax5^{P80R/+}$ knockin mouse model, which develops transplantable BCP-ALL, also exhibits the inactivation of the wild-type *Pax5* allele. This highlights the importance of biallelic *PAX5* alterations in PAX5 P80R and suggests the PAX5 P80R mutation as leukemia initiating events [6]. Additional co-lesions in PAX5 P80R encompass Ras and JAK-STAT pathway genes, *CDKN2A/B* and *SETD2* [5, 6]. Besides a subset of PAX5alt fusion genes (*PAX5::NOL4L*, *PAX5::ASXL1*), the structural rearrangements of chromosomal arms 9p and 20q found in PAX5 P80R may be associated with dic(9:20) [112, 114, 115]. A specific feature of PAX5 P80R might be the disruption of CD58 enhancer activity. The loss of CD58 expression leads to impaired T-cell activation induced by blinatumomab, potentially conferring CD19 positive resistance in blinatumomab treatment in vitro experimental models, although this should be tested in clinical settings [116].

2.2.8 CDX2/UBTF ALL

BCP-ALL with *UBTF::ATXN7L3/PAN3,CDX2* is a rare subtype of BCP-ALL characterized by distinct gene expression profiles (Fig. 2.2). This subtype commonly harbors two alterations, *UBTF::ATXN7L3* fusion and a deletion around *FLT3* region that deregulates *CDX2* expression [117–119]. Therefore, this entity is succinctly called "CDX2/UBTF ALL" to reflect these dual distinct alterations [7, 8]. Predominantly affecting AYAs and females (Fig. 2.1), CDX2/UBTF ALL has a characteristic immunophenotype with partial or negative CD10 expression, CD20 negativity, and positivity for CD34, CD38, and cytoplasmic IgM [117–119]. Patients with CDX2/UBTF ALL tend to exhibit positive MRD at EOI and represent a higher relapse rate [117–119]. The two driver lesions arise from dual microdeletions at 13q12.2 (*PAN3*, *FLT3*, and *CDX2* region) and 17q21.31 (*UBTF* and *ATXN7L3* region), both caused by aberrant RAG activity [117–119]. The deletions at 13q12.2 are distinct from other subtypes of B-ALL. Type I deletions, observed in non-CDX2/UBTF cases, spare the

FLT3 promoter, and lead to elevated *FLT3* expression [120]; and type II deletions, encompassing the *FLT3* promoter, result in *CDX2* overexpression at the expense of *FLT3* expression [117–119]. In both deletions, retargeting of the *PAN3* enhancer leads to aberrant *FLT3* or *CDX2* expression. The other micro-deletions on chromosome 17 yield the in-frame *UBTF::ATXN7L3* fusion, detectable by RT-PCR (Fig. 2.3). Additional genomic alterations comprise gains of 1q, *PAX5* alterations, and *CXCR4* truncating mutations [117–119, 121]. A unique feature of CDX2/UBTF ALL is the presence of two distinct clonal, genomic subtype-defining driver events. Examination of variant frequency suggested *CDX2* dysregulation appears to arise first [117]. The underlying mechanism of leukemogenesis from these dual alterations remains an area of future investigation.

2.2.9 NUTM1-Rearranged ALL

NUTM1-rearranged ALL is a subtype of rare pediatric BCP-ALL, with a prominent presence in infant ALL carrying germline *KMT2A* [6, 53, 122–124]. Unlike *KMT2A*-rearranged infant ALL, *NUTM1*-rearranged infant ALL displays an excellent prognosis [92, 122]. This subtype is characterized by an aberrant expression of *NUTM1*, induced by fusion with various different partner genes such as *ACIN1*, *AFF1*, *ATAD5*, *BRD9*, *CHD4*, *CUX1*, *IKZF1*, *RUNX1*, *SLC12A6*, and *ZNF618* [124]. The majority of *NUTM1* coding region is retained in these fusion genes, typically including the NUT domain that plays an important role in the regulation of histone acetylation [125]. In the cases with *BRD9::NUTM1*, histone deacetylase inhibitors or bromodomain inhibitors hold clinical promise (Table 2.1) [125, 126].

2.2.10 IKZF1 N159Y

A unique subtype of mutation-driven ALL is defined by heterozygous IKZF1 N159Y mutations, which are accompanied by distinct gene expression profiles (Fig. 2.2). The upregulation of *YAP1* and *SALL1* characterizes this subtype, and this feature is not observed in other subtypes of ALL with *IKZF1* deletions as secondary events [5, 6]. The N159 mutation is located at the critical DNA-binding domain of the second zinc fingers. The strong conservation of this residue across species implies a pivotal role [127]. While germline mutations of *IKZF1* give rise to combined immunodeficiency due to haploinsufficiency or familial pediatric ALL, patients harboring germline mutations at N159 residue (N159S, N159T) exhibit a dominant-negative effect and display more severe early-onset clinical manifestations [128, 129]. Moreover, all IKZF1 N159 germline mutations are de novo, with no asymptomatic individuals identified [129]. Therefore, IKZF1 N159Y might entail unique mechanisms for driving leukemia, in addition to nuclear mislocalization causing aberrant leukemic cell adhesion and drug resistance [127, 128].

2.3 Kinase-Driven BCP-ALL

2.3.1 *BCR::ABL1* (Ph+) and *BCR::ABL1*-Like (Ph-Like) ALL

The Philadelphia (Ph) chromosome is a derivative chromosome 22 that arises from the reciprocal t(9;22)(q34;q11) translocation [130, 131]. Although the frequency of *BCR::ABL1* ALL is low in children (2–5%), it becomes more frequent with age, constituting the most prevalent genetic subgroup in adults, with an incidence of 20–25% (Fig. 2.1) [132]. Historically, *BCR::ABL1* ALL has been associated with a dismal prognosis; however, the use of TKIs has greatly improved the outcome [133, 134]. Secondary cooperative lesions involve *IKZF1* and *CDKN2A/B*, with over 50% of cases showing these alterations, which cooperate in lymphoid leukemogenesis [49, 135, 136]. *IKZF1* alterations are included in the criteria of "IKZF1^{plus}," a recently established marker of high-risk ALL, and *BCR::ABL1* ALL cases with *IKZF1* alterations are associated with an unfavorable outcome irrespective of TKI treatment [137]. Alterations of *IKZF1* confer stem cell-like features, including self-renewal and increased stromal adhesion, which can potentially be reversed with retinoid receptor agonists to reintroduce the wild type IKZF1 expression or focal adhesion kinase inhibitors to hinder downstream integrin signaling pathways (Table 2.1) [138]. Importantly, *BCR::ABL1* fusion is also a hallmark of chronic myeloid leukemia (CML), with its lymphoid blast crisis often closely resembling *BCR::ABL1* ALL. There is a prevalence of the major-BCR::ABL1 fusion transcript (p210) for CML and the minor-BCR::ABL1 fusion transcripts (p190) for BCP-ALL [139]. However, leveraging DNA-based MRD monitoring by combining Ig/T-cell receptor (TCR) and genomic *BCR::ABL1* fusion can uncover a "CML-like" *BCR::ABL1* ALL resembling lymphoid blast crisis. This can be identified through the discordance of MRD level between these markers due to the presence of *BCR::ABL1* fusion in non-ALL hematopoietic cells [140, 141]. Although their outcomes are similar, the difference in their treatment response might imply biological difference between *BCR::ABL1* ALL and CML-like ALL [142].

BCR::ABL1-like ALL is a high-risk subgroup that phenocopies *BCR::ABL1* ALL in terms of gene expression profile and unfavorable prognosis. However, this subtype is characterized by alternative kinase-activating alterations rather than *BCR::ABL1* fusion (Fig. 2.2) [143, 144].

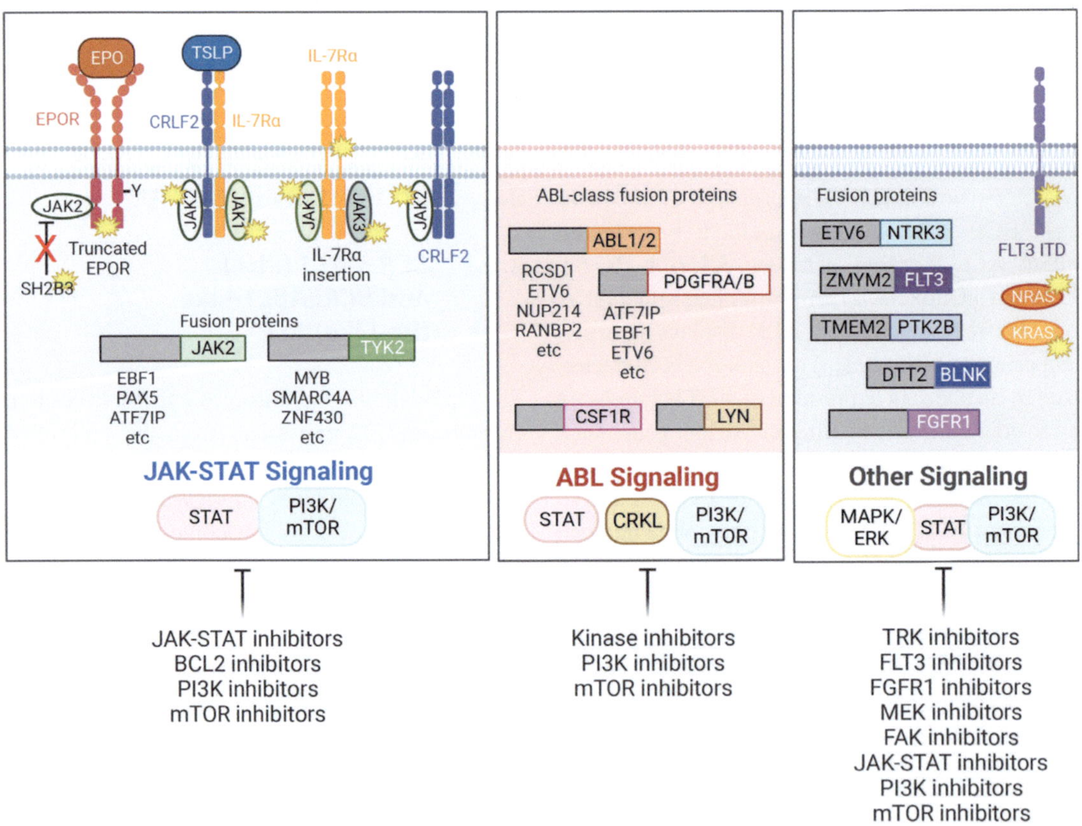

Fig. 2.4 A schematic showing the activation of kinase signaling and cytokine receptor in *BCR::ABL1*-like (Ph-like) ALL and potential targets. *BCR::ABL1*-like (Ph-like) ALL cases are characterized by activation of JAK-STAT signaling, ABL-class fusions, and other rare fusions. Activation of JAK-STAT signaling includes alterations of *CRLF2*, *JAK1/2*, *IL7RA*, *EPOR*, and accounts for approximately 70% of *BCR::ABL1*-like ALL cases. ABL-class fusions are observed in 10–15% which can be druggable by kinase inhibitors including dasatinib. The rest of cases include rare fusions involving *NTRK3*, *FLT3*, *BLNK*, *FGFR1*, and Ras signaling

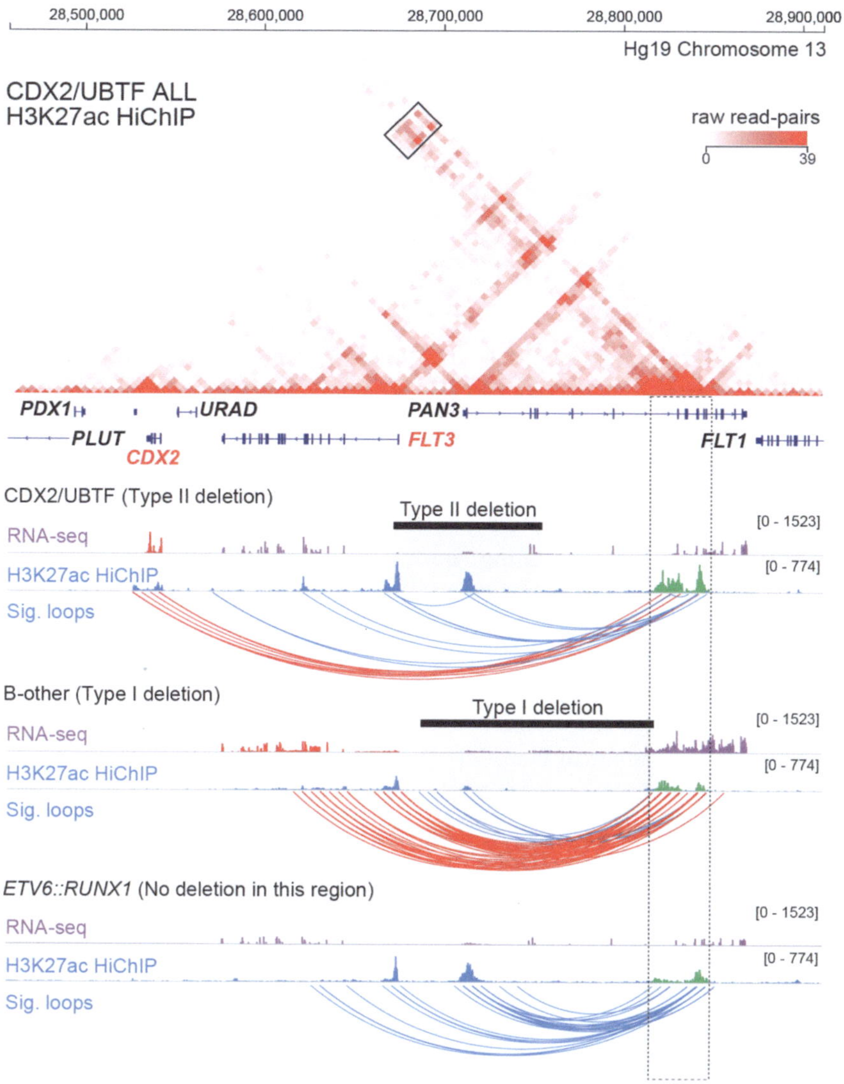

Fig. 2.5 H3K27ac HiChIP showing enhancer retargeting in CDX2/UBTF ALL [117]. Enhancer region is annotated in green (*PAN3*) and retargeted genes (*CDX2* and *FLT3*) are colored in red. The heatmap shows raw read counts for all pairwise 5 kb genomic bins. Significant (false discovery rate, 0.01) loops called with MAPS are shown as blue arcs. Representative cases of CDX2/UBTF ALL (type II deletion), type I deletion (B-other ALL), and no deletion in chromosome 13q12.2 (*ETV6::RUNX1* ALL) from the top to the bottom. Enhancer on *PAN3* gene is retargeting *CDX2* (in CDX2/UBTF ALL) and *FLT3* (in type I deletion), respectively

BCR::ABL1-like ALL tends to be more prevalent in adults, males, and individuals with Down syndrome, and is associated with unfavorable outcomes marked by persistent MRD positivity [131, 145–147]. Despite this, a standardized approach to defining this subtype in clinical practice has yet to be established, largely due to the considerable genomic heterogeneity within *BCR::ABL1*-like ALL. However, the diverse genomic alterations in *BCR::ABL1*-like ALL share the common attribute of activating cytokine receptor and kinase signaling pathways. These pathways are amenable to targeting through available TKIs, and they can be categorized into three types (Fig. 2.4): (1) activation of JAK-STAT signaling by alterations of *CRLF2*, *JAK1/2*,

IL7RA, or *EPOR* (70%); (2) ABL-class fusions involving *ABL1/2*, *CSF1R*, *LYN*, *PDGFRA/B* (10–15%); and (3) other rare fusions involving *NTRK3*, *FLT3*, *BLNK*, and *FGFR1* [131, 146–150]. Moreover, *BCR::ABL1*-like ALL exhibits recurrent alterations of Ras signaling (*NRAS*, *KRAS*, and *PTPN11*), and copy number alterations in genes related to B-cell differentiation (*IKZF1*, *PAX5*, *EBF1*, and *ETV6*) and cell cycle regulators (*CDKN2A/B*, *TP53*, and *RB1*) [6, 150]. Among these genomic events, *CRLF2* alterations are the most prevalent, encompassing roughly 50% of *BCR::ABL1*-like ALL cases. *CRLF2* alterations include cryptic rearrangements between *CRLF2* and the IGH locus, focal deletions in pseudoautosomal region 1 (PAR1) of chromosomes Xp22 and Yp11 resulting in *P2RY8::CRLF2*, and less commonly single-nucleotide variant (SNV) at CRLF2 F232C [146, 151–155]. PAR1 region alterations are used as a surrogate marker for *P2RY8::CRLF2*, and serve as one of the defining criteria for "IKZF1^{plus}," which is defined by co-occurrence of the *IKZF1* deletion with deletion of *CDKN2A*, *CDKN2B*, *PAX5*, and/or PAR1 region in the absence of *ERG* deletion [137]. However, a caveat in "IKZF1^{plus}" definition is that *IGH::CRLF2* and *CRLF2* SNVs are not detectable by using single-nucleotide polymorphism (SNP) or multiplex ligation-dependent probe amplification (MLPA) arrays [146]. Among *BCR::ABL1*-like ALL, cases with *JAK2* and *EPOR* rearrangements/alterations are generally associated with inferior prognosis compared to cases with other alterations [131].

Several clinical trials are currently underway to assess the effectiveness of FDA-approved TKIs in frontline studies. These studies include JAK inhibitors (ruxolitinib) for JAK-STAT activating alterations, imatinib/dasatinib/ponatinib for ABL-class fusions, TRK inhibitors (larotrectinib, PLX7486) for *NTRK3* fusions, and FLT3 inhibitors for *FLT3* alterations (Table 2.1) [149, 156–159]. Furthermore, several immunotherapeutic approaches are exhibiting encouraging outcomes, including blinatumomab (bispecific anti-CD3/CD19 monoclonal antibody), inotuzumab (CD22 antibody–drug conjugate) and CAR T-cell therapy targeting CD19 [146, 149].

2.4 Other Subtypes of BCP-ALL

BCP-ALL cases with ZEB2 hotspot H1038R mutation and *IGH::CEBPE* alterations define a rare BCP-ALL subtype, exhibiting comparable gene expression profiles based on unsupervised clustering [53]. However, ZEB2 H1038R and *IGH::CEBPE* commonly do not co-occur [53, 115]. In contrast to PAX5 P80R and IKZF1 N159Y, ZEB2 H1038R might not serve as a founder alteration, because some ZEB2 H1038R mutations are also identified in other BCP-ALL subtypes including *DUX4*- and *ZNF384*-rearranged ALL [53, 160]. Other features of this subtype include *NRAS* mutations and upregulation of *LMO1* [53].

Translocations involving IGH (less frequently light chain loci) and *MYC*, which lead to aberrant expression of *MYC* oncogene, serve as a hallmark of mature B-cell malignancies including Burkitt lymphoma (BL) and diffuse large B-cell lymphomas. Such translocations are also identified in immature B-ALL (BCP-ALL), though they are rare [6, 161–163]. In contrast to BL, *IGH::MYC* in BCP-ALL can manifest as either clonal or subclonal events [164]. BCP-ALL harboring *IGH::MYC* are categorized into three types: (1) cases with BCP-ALL specific drivers (e.g., *KMT2A*-R, *DUX4*-R) which exhibit expression profiles akin to the concurrent driver genes; (2) cases with concurrent *BCL2* and/or *BCL6* rearrangements, exhibiting "double/triple hit" lymphoma features (BCL2/MYC); and (3) cases lacking disease defining drivers [164]. The determination of appropriate treatment strategies (ALL-directed, BL-directed, or hybrid protocols) in BCP-ALL with *IGH::MYC* may be intricate due to the limited understanding.

Mutations involving IDH1 R132C and IDH2 R140Q define a rare subtype of BCP-ALL, characterized by distinct gene expression profiles [121]. While these mutations may be initiating events to drive leukemia, further functional studies are required. In line with the roles of IDH1/2 in cellular metabolism and epigenetic regulation, IDH1 R132C and IDH2 R140Q ALL display hypermethylated profiles that can distinguish from other subtypes of BCP-ALL [121].

2.5 Conclusion

In recent years, an impressive increase in the knowledge about the genetic landscape of BCP-ALL has been achieved. This steep learning curve started with deciphering new subtypes using Affymetrix gene expression profiling and accelerated with the development of next generation sequencing techniques. Nowadays, about 25 different genetic drivers of BCP-ALL have been identified, with often concomitant lesions in Ras and JAK-STAT activating pathways that drive proliferation. Some lesions provide clear targets for treatment, such as TKIs for ABL-class and JAK-class mutated leukemias or HDAC inhibitors for *MEF2D*-rearranged leukemias. For the majority of genetic aberrations, however, targeted drugs are lacking. The emerging field of cell-based immunotherapies like CD19-directed blinatumomab and CAR T cells, may provide a good alternative to targeted drugs. However, knowledge about the genetic aberrations characterizing BCP-ALL is still needed since this may affect the choice of immunotherapeutics (e.g., expected blinatumomab/CAR T resistance in case of PAX5 P80R and *TP53* mutated leukemias) and alternative therapeutics like targeted agents are still needed in case of reappearance of (immunotherapy resistant) leukemic cells.

References

1. Mullighan CG. How advanced are we in targeting novel subtypes of ALL? Best Pract Res Clin Haematol. 2019;32:101095. https://doi.org/10.1016/j.beha.2019.101095.
2. Kimura S, Mullighan CG. Molecular markers in ALL: clinical implications. Best Pract Res Clin Haematol. 2020;33:101193. https://doi.org/10.1016/j.beha.2020.101193.
3. Iacobucci I, Kimura S, Mullighan CG. Biologic and therapeutic implications of genomic alterations in acute lymphoblastic leukemia. J Clin Med. 2021;10 https://doi.org/10.3390/jcm10173792.
4. Boer JM, den Boer ML. BCR-ABL1-like acute lymphoblastic leukaemia: from bench to bedside. Eur J Cancer. 2017;82:203–18. https://doi.org/10.1016/j.ejca.2017.06.012.
5. Brady SW, Roberts KG, Gu Z, Shi L, Pounds S, Pei D, Cheng C, Dai Y, Devidas M, Qu C, et al. The genomic landscape of pediatric acute lymphoblastic leukemia. Nat Genet. 2022;54:1376–89. https://doi.org/10.1038/s41588-022-01159-z.
6. Gu Z, Churchman ML, Roberts KG, Moore I, Zhou X, Nakitandwe J, Hagiwara K, Pelletier S, Gingras S, Berns H, et al. PAX5-driven subtypes of B-progenitor acute lymphoblastic leukemia. Nat Genet. 2019;51:296–307. https://doi.org/10.1038/s41588-018-0315-5.
7. Arber DA, Orazi A, Hasserjian RP, Borowitz MJ, Calvo KR, Kvasnicka HM, Wang SA, Bagg A, Barbui T, Branford S, et al. International consensus classification of myeloid neoplasms and acute Leukemias: integrating morphologic, clinical, and genomic data. Blood. 2022;140:1200–28. https://doi.org/10.1182/blood.2022015850.
8. Duffield AS, Mullighan CG, Borowitz MJ. International consensus classification of acute lymphoblastic leukemia/lymphoma. Virchows Arch. 2023;482:11–26. https://doi.org/10.1007/s00428-022-03448-8.
9. Paulsson K, Lilljebjorn H, Biloglav A, Olsson L, Rissler M, Castor A, Barbany G, Fogelstrand L, Nordgren A, Sjogren H, et al. The genomic landscape of high hyperdiploid childhood acute lymphoblastic leukemia. Nat Genet. 2015;47:672–6. https://doi.org/10.1038/ng.3301.
10. Paulsson K, Johansson B. High hyperdiploid childhood acute lymphoblastic leukemia. Genes Chromosomes Cancer. 2009;48:637–60. https://doi.org/10.1002/gcc.20671.
11. Haas OA, Borkhardt A. Hyperdiploidy: the longest known, most prevalent, and most enigmatic form of acute lymphoblastic leukemia in children. Leukemia. 2022;36:2769–83. https://doi.org/10.1038/s41375-022-01720-z.
12. Enshaei A, Vora A, Harrison CJ, Moppett J, Moorman AV. Defining low-risk high hyperdiploidy in patients with paediatric acute lymphoblastic leukaemia: a retrospective analysis of data from the UKALL97/99 and UKALL2003 clinical trials. Lancet Haematol. 2021;8:e828–39. https://doi.org/10.1016/S2352-3026(21)00304-5.
13. Molina O, Vinyoles M, Granada I, Roca-Ho H, Gutierrez-Aguera F, Valledor L, Lopez-Lopez CM, Rodriguez-Gonzalez P, Trincado JL, Menendez ST, et al. Impaired condensin complex and Aurora B kinase underlie mitotic and chromosomal defects in hyperdiploid B-cell ALL. Blood. 2020;136:313–27. https://doi.org/10.1182/blood.2019002538.
14. Heerema NA, Sather HN, Sensel MG, Zhang T, Hutchinson RJ, Nachman JB, Lange BJ, Steinherz PG, Bostrom BC, Reaman GH, et al. Prognostic impact of trisomies of chromosomes 10, 17, and 5 among children with acute lymphoblastic leukemia and high hyperdiploidy (> 50 chromosomes). J Clin Oncol. 2000;18:1876–87. https://doi.org/10.1200/JCO.2000.18.9.1876.
15. Schultz KR, Pullen DJ, Sather HN, Shuster JJ, Devidas M, Borowitz MJ, Carroll AJ, Heerema NA, Rubnitz JE, Loh ML, et al. Risk- and response-

based classification of childhood B-precursor acute lymphoblastic leukemia: a combined analysis of prognostic markers from the pediatric oncology group (POG) and children's cancer group (CCG). Blood. 2007;109:926–35. https://doi.org/10.1182/blood-2006-01-024729.

16. Mattano LA Jr, Devidas M, Maloney KW, Wang C, Friedmann AM, Buckley P, Borowitz MJ, Carroll AJ, Gastier-Foster JM, Heerema NA, et al. Favorable Trisomies and ETV6-RUNX1 predict cure in Low-risk B-cell acute lymphoblastic leukemia: results from children's oncology group trial AALL0331. J Clin Oncol. 2021;39:1540–52. https://doi.org/10.1200/JCO.20.02370.
17. Jerchel IS, Hoogkamer AQ, Aries IM, Steeghs EMP, Boer JM, Besselink NJM, Boeree A, van de Ven C, de Groot-Kruseman HA, de Haas V, et al. RAS pathway mutations as a predictive biomarker for treatment adaptation in pediatric B-cell precursor acute lymphoblastic leukemia. Leukemia. 2018;32:931–40. https://doi.org/10.1038/leu.2017.303.
18. Mullighan CG, Zhang J, Kasper LH, Lerach S, Payne-Turner D, Phillips LA, Heatley SL, Holmfeldt L, Collins-Underwood JR, Ma J, et al. CREBBP mutations in relapsed acute lymphoblastic leukaemia. Nature. 2011;471:235–9. https://doi.org/10.1038/nature09727.
19. Holmfeldt L, Wei L, Diaz-Flores E, Walsh M, Zhang J, Ding L, Payne-Turner D, Churchman M, Andersson A, Chen SC, et al. The genomic landscape of hypodiploid acute lymphoblastic leukemia. Nat Genet. 2013;45:242–52. https://doi.org/10.1038/ng.2532.
20. Mullighan CG, Jeha S, Pei D, Payne-Turner D, Coustan-Smith E, Roberts KG, Waanders E, Choi JK, Ma X, Raimondi SC, et al. Outcome of children with hypodiploid ALL treated with risk-directed therapy based on MRD levels. Blood. 2015;126:2896–9. https://doi.org/10.1182/blood-2015-09-671131.
21. Safavi S, Paulsson K. Near-haploid and low-hypodiploid acute lymphoblastic leukemia: two distinct subtypes with consistently poor prognosis. Blood. 2017;129:420–3. https://doi.org/10.1182/blood-2016-10-743765.
22. Molina O, Bataller A, Thampi N, Ribera J, Granada I, Velasco P, Fuster JL, Menendez P. Near-haploidy and low-hypodiploidy in B-cell acute lymphoblastic leukemia: when less is too much. Cancers (Basel). 2021;14:32. https://doi.org/10.3390/cancers14010032.
23. Pui CH, Rebora P, Schrappe M, Attarbaschi A, Baruchel A, Basso G, Cave H, Elitzur S, Koh K, Liu HC, et al. Outcome of children with Hypodiploid acute lymphoblastic leukemia: a retrospective multinational study. J Clin Oncol. 2019;37:770–9. https://doi.org/10.1200/JCO.18.00822.
24. Carroll AJ, Shago M, Mikhail FM, Raimondi SC, Hirsch BA, Loh ML, Raetz EA, Borowitz MJ, Wood BL, Maloney KW, et al. Masked hypodiploidy: hypodiploid acute lymphoblastic leukemia (ALL) mimicking hyperdiploid ALL in children: a report from the children's oncology group. Cancer Genet. 2019;238:62–8. https://doi.org/10.1016/j.cancergen.2019.07.009.
25. Qian M, Cao X, Devidas M, Yang W, Cheng C, Dai Y, Carroll A, Heerema NA, Zhang H, Moriyama T, et al. TP53 germline variations influence the predisposition and prognosis of B-cell acute lymphoblastic leukemia in children. J Clin Oncol. 2018;36:591–9. https://doi.org/10.1200/JCO.2017.75.5215.
26. Kim R, Bergugnat H, Larcher L, Duchmann M, Passet M, Gachet S, Cuccuini W, Lafage-Pochitaloff M, Pastoret C, Grardel N, et al. Adult Low-Hypodiploid acute lymphoblastic leukemia emerges from Preleukemic TP53-mutant clonal hematopoiesis. Blood Cancer Discov. 2023;4:134–49. https://doi.org/10.1158/2643-3230.BCD-22-0154.
27. Pan J, Tan Y, Deng B, Tong C, Hua L, Ling Z, Song W, Xu J, Duan J, Wang Z, et al. Frequent occurrence of CD19-negative relapse after CD19 CAR T and consolidation therapy in 14 TP53-mutated r/r B-ALL children. Leukemia. 2020;34:3382–7. https://doi.org/10.1038/s41375-020-0831-z.
28. Zhang X, Lu XA, Yang J, Zhang G, Li J, Song L, Su Y, Shi Y, Zhang M, He J, et al. Efficacy and safety of anti-CD19 CAR T-cell therapy in 110 patients with B-cell acute lymphoblastic leukemia with high-risk features. Blood Adv. 2020;4:2325–38. https://doi.org/10.1182/bloodadvances.2020001466.
29. Pariury H, Fandel J, Bachl S, Ang KK, Markossian S, Wilson CG, Braun BS, Popescu B, Wohlfeil M, Beckman K, et al. Venetoclax and dinaciclib elicit synergistic preclinical efficacy against hypodiploid acute lymphoblastic leukemia. Haematologica. 2023;108:1272–83. https://doi.org/10.3324/haematol.2022.281443.
30. Diaz-Flores E, Comeaux EQ, Kim KL, Melnik E, Beckman K, Davis KL, Wu K, Akutagawa J, Bridges O, Marino R, et al. Bcl-2 is a therapeutic target for hypodiploid B-lineage acute lymphoblastic leukemia. Cancer Res. 2019;79:2339–51. https://doi.org/10.1158/0008-5472.CAN-18-0236.
31. Heerema NA, Carroll AJ, Devidas M, Loh ML, Borowitz MJ, Gastier-Foster JM, Larsen EC, Mattano LA Jr, Maloney KW, Willman CL, et al. Intrachromosomal amplification of chromosome 21 is associated with inferior outcomes in children with acute lymphoblastic leukemia treated in contemporary standard-risk children's oncology group studies: a report from the children's oncology group. J Clin Oncol. 2013;31:3397–402. https://doi.org/10.1200/JCO.2013.49.1308.
32. Koleilat A, Smadbeck JB, Zepeda-Mendoza CJ, Williamson CM, Pitel BA, Golden CL, Xu X, Greipp PT, Ketterling RP, Hoppman NL, et al. Characterization of unusual iAMP21 B-lymphoblastic leukemia (iAMP21-ALL) from the Mayo clinic and children's oncology group. Genes Chromosomes Cancer. 2022;61:710–9. https://doi.org/10.1002/gcc.23084.

33. Harrison CJ, Moorman AV, Schwab C, Carroll AJ, Raetz EA, Devidas M, Strehl S, Nebral K, Harbott J, Teigler-Schlegel A, et al. An international study of intrachromosomal amplification of chromosome 21 (iAMP21): cytogenetic characterization and outcome. Leukemia. 2014;28:1015–21. https://doi.org/10.1038/leu.2013.317.
34. Harrison CJ. Blood spotlight on iAMP21 acute lymphoblastic leukemia (ALL), a high-risk pediatric disease. Blood. 2015;125:1383–6. https://doi.org/10.1182/blood-2014-08-569228.
35. Gao Q, Ryan SL, Iacobucci I, Ghate PS, Cranston RE, Schwab CJ, Elsayed AH, Shi L, Pounds SB, Lei S, et al. The genomic landscape of acute lymphoblastic leukemia with intrachromosomal amplification of chromosome 21. Blood. 2023;142:711–23. https://doi.org/10.1182/blood.2022019094.
36. Moorman AV, Robinson H, Schwab C, Richards SM, Hancock J, Mitchell CD, Goulden N, Vora A, Harrison CJ. Risk-directed treatment intensification significantly reduces the risk of relapse among children and adolescents with acute lymphoblastic leukemia and intrachromosomal amplification of chromosome 21: a comparison of the MRC ALL97/99 and UKALL2003 trials. J Clin Oncol. 2013;31:3389–96. https://doi.org/10.1200/JCO.2013.48.9377.
37. Li Y, Schwab C, Ryan S, Papaemmanuil E, Robinson HM, Jacobs P, Moorman AV, Dyer S, Borrow J, Griffiths M, et al. Constitutional and somatic rearrangement of chromosome 21 in acute lymphoblastic leukaemia. Nature. 2014;508:98–102. https://doi.org/10.1038/nature13115.
38. Harrison CJ, Schwab C. Constitutional abnormalities of chromosome 21 predispose to iAMP21-acute lymphoblastic leukaemia. Eur J Med Genet. 2016;59:162–5. https://doi.org/10.1016/j.ejmg.2016.01.006.
39. Sundaresh A, Williams O. Mechanism of ETV6-RUNX1 leukemia. Adv Exp Med Biol. 2017;962:201–16. https://doi.org/10.1007/978-981-10-3233-2_13.
40. Shurtleff SA, Buijs A, Behm FG, Rubnitz JE, Raimondi SC, Hancock ML, Chan GC, Pui CH, Grosveld G, Downing JR. TEL/AML1 fusion resulting from a cryptic t(12;21) is the most common genetic lesion in pediatric ALL and defines a subgroup of patients with an excellent prognosis. Leukemia. 1995;9:1985–9.
41. Borkhardt A, Cazzaniga G, Viehmann S, Valsecchi MG, Ludwig WD, Burci L, Mangioni S, Schrappe M, Riehm H, Lampert F, et al. Incidence and clinical relevance of TEL/AML1 fusion genes in children with acute lymphoblastic leukemia enrolled in the German and Italian multicenter therapy trials. Associazione Italiana Ematologia Oncologia Pediatrica and the Berlin-Frankfurt-Munster study group. Blood. 1997;90:571–7.
42. Vaskova M, Mejstrikova E, Kalina T, Martinkova P, Omelka M, Trka J, Stary J, Hrusak O. Transfer of genomics information to flow cytometry: expression of CD27 and CD44 discriminates subtypes of acute lymphoblastic leukemia. Leukemia. 2005;19:876–8. https://doi.org/10.1038/sj.leu.2403706.
43. Mori H, Colman SM, Xiao Z, Ford AM, Healy LE, Donaldson C, Hows JM, Navarrete C, Greaves M. Chromosome translocations and covert leukemic clones are generated during normal fetal development. Proc Natl Acad Sci USA. 2002;99:8242–7. https://doi.org/10.1073/pnas.112218799.
44. Wiemels JL, Ford AM, Van Wering ER, Postma A, Greaves M. Protracted and variable latency of acute lymphoblastic leukemia after TEL-AML1 gene fusion in utero. Blood. 1999;94:1057–62.
45. Bernardin F, Yang Y, Cleaves R, Zahurak M, Cheng L, Civin CI, Friedman AD. TEL-AML1, expressed from t(12;21) in human acute lymphocytic leukemia, induces acute leukemia in mice. Cancer Res. 2002;62:3904–8.
46. Castor A, Nilsson L, Astrand-Grundstrom I, Buitenhuis M, Ramirez C, Anderson K, Strombeck B, Garwicz S, Bekassy AN, Schmiegelow K, et al. Distinct patterns of hematopoietic stem cell involvement in acute lymphoblastic leukemia. Nat Med. 2005;11:630–7. https://doi.org/10.1038/nm1253.
47. Hong D, Gupta R, Ancliff P, Atzberger A, Brown J, Soneji S, Green J, Colman S, Piacibello W, Buckle V, et al. Initiating and cancer-propagating cells in TEL-AML1-associated childhood leukemia. Science. 2008;319:336–9. https://doi.org/10.1126/science.1150648.
48. Polak R, Bierings MB, van der Leije CS, Sanders MA, Roovers O, Marchante JRM, Boer JM, Cornelissen JJ, Pieters R, den Boer ML, et al. Autophagy inhibition as a potential future targeted therapy for ETV6-RUNX1-driven B-cell precursor acute lymphoblastic leukemia. Haematologica. 2019;104:738–48. https://doi.org/10.3324/haematol.2018.193631.
49. Mullighan CG, Goorha S, Radtke I, Miller CB, Coustan-Smith E, Dalton JD, Girtman K, Mathew S, Ma J, Pounds SB, et al. Genome-wide analysis of genetic alterations in acute lymphoblastic leukaemia. Nature. 2007;446:758–64. https://doi.org/10.1038/nature05690.
50. Papaemmanuil E, Rapado I, Li Y, Potter NE, Wedge DC, Tubio J, Alexandrov LB, Van Loo P, Cooke SL, Marshall J, et al. RAG-mediated recombination is the predominant driver of oncogenic rearrangement in ETV6-RUNX1 acute lymphoblastic leukemia. Nat Genet. 2014;46:116–25. https://doi.org/10.1038/ng.2874.
51. Ostergaard A, Enshaei A, Pieters R, Vora A, Horstmann MA, Escherich G, Johansson B, Heyman M, Schmiegelow K, Hoogerbrugge PM, et al. The prognostic effect of IKZF1 deletions in ETV6::RUNX1 and high hyperdiploid childhood acute lymphoblastic leukemia. Hema. 2023;7:e875. https://doi.org/10.1097/HS9.0000000000000875.
52. van der Veer A, Waanders E, Pieters R, Willemse ME, Van Reijmersdal SV, Russell LJ, Harrison CJ,

Evans WE, van der Velden VH, Hoogerbrugge PM, et al. Independent prognostic value of BCR-ABL1-like signature and IKZF1 deletion, but not high CRLF2 expression, in children with B-cell precursor ALL. Blood. 2013;122:2622–9. https://doi.org/10.1182/blood-2012-10-462358.
53. Li JF, Dai YT, Lilljebjorn H, Shen SH, Cui BW, Bai L, Liu YF, Qian MX, Kubota Y, Kiyoi H, et al. Transcriptional landscape of B cell precursor acute lymphoblastic leukemia based on an international study of 1,223 cases. Proc Natl Acad Sci USA. 2018;115:E11711–20. https://doi.org/10.1073/pnas.1814397115.
54. Zaliova M, Kotrova M, Bresolin S, Stuchly J, Stary J, Hrusak O, Te Kronnie G, Trka J, Zuna J, Vaskova M. ETV6/RUNX1-like acute lymphoblastic leukemia: a novel B-cell precursor leukemia subtype associated with the CD27/CD44 immunophenotype. Genes Chromosomes Cancer. 2017;56:608–16. https://doi.org/10.1002/gcc.22464.
55. Lilljebjorn H, Henningsson R, Hyrenius-Wittsten A, Olsson L, Orsmark-Pietras C, von Palffy S, Askmyr M, Rissler M, Schrappe M, Cario G, et al. Identification of ETV6-RUNX1-like and DUX4-rearranged subtypes in paediatric B-cell precursor acute lymphoblastic leukaemia. Nat Commun. 2016;7:11790. https://doi.org/10.1038/ncomms11790.
56. Nishii R, Baskin-Doerfler R, Yang W, Oak N, Zhao X, Yang W, Hoshitsuki K, Bloom M, Verbist K, Burns M, et al. Molecular basis of ETV6-mediated predisposition to childhood acute lymphoblastic leukemia. Blood. 2021;137:364–73. https://doi.org/10.1182/blood.2020006164.
57. Jeha S, Pei D, Raimondi SC, Onciu M, Campana D, Cheng C, Sandlund JT, Ribeiro RC, Rubnitz JE, Howard SC, et al. Increased risk for CNS relapse in pre-B cell leukemia with the t(1;19)/TCF3-PBX1. Leukemia. 2009;23:1406–9. https://doi.org/10.1038/leu.2009.42.
58. Inaba H, Pui CH. Advances in the diagnosis and treatment of pediatric acute lymphoblastic leukemia. J Clin Med. 2021;10 https://doi.org/10.3390/jcm10091926.
59. Bicocca VT, Chang BH, Masouleh BK, Muschen M, Loriaux MM, Druker BJ, Tyner JW. Crosstalk between ROR1 and the pre-B cell receptor promotes survival of t(1;19) acute lymphoblastic leukemia. Cancer Cell. 2012;22:656–67. https://doi.org/10.1016/j.ccr.2012.08.027.
60. Karvonen H, Perttila R, Niininen W, Hautanen V, Barker H, Murumagi A, Heckman CA, Ungureanu D. Wnt5a and ROR1 activate non-canonical Wnt signaling via RhoA in TCF3-PBX1 acute lymphoblastic leukemia and highlight new treatment strategies via Bcl-2 co-targeting. Oncogene. 2019;38:3288–300. https://doi.org/10.1038/s41388-018-0670-9.
61. Duque-Afonso J, Feng J, Scherer F, Lin CH, Wong SH, Wang Z, Iwasaki M, Cleary ML. Comparative genomics reveals multistep pathogenesis of E2A-PBX1 acute lymphoblastic leukemia. J Clin Invest. 2015;125:3667–80. https://doi.org/10.1172/JCI81158.
62. Chang CP, de Vivo I, Cleary ML. The Hox cooperativity motif of the chimeric oncoprotein E2a-Pbx1 is necessary and sufficient for oncogenesis. Mol Cell Biol. 1997;17:81–8. https://doi.org/10.1128/MCB.17.1.81.
63. Pi WC, Wang J, Shimada M, Lin JW, Geng H, Lee YL, Lu R, Li D, Wang GG, Roeder RG, et al. E2A-PBX1 functions as a coactivator for RUNX1 in acute lymphoblastic leukemia. Blood. 2020;136:11–23. https://doi.org/10.1182/blood.2019003312.
64. Fischer U, Forster M, Rinaldi A, Risch T, Sungalee S, Warnatz HJ, Bornhauser B, Gombert M, Kratsch C, Stutz AM, et al. Genomics and drug profiling of fatal TCF3-HLF-positive acute lymphoblastic leukemia identifies recurrent mutation patterns and therapeutic options. Nat Genet. 2015;47:1020–9. https://doi.org/10.1038/ng.3362.
65. Inaba T, Roberts WM, Shapiro LH, Jolly KW, Raimondi SC, Smith SD, Look AT. Fusion of the leucine zipper gene HLF to the E2A gene in human acute B-lineage leukemia. Science. 1992;257:531–4. https://doi.org/10.1126/science.1386162.
66. Huang Y, Mouttet B, Warnatz HJ, Risch T, Rietmann F, Frommelt F, Ngo QA, Dobay MP, Marovca B, Jenni S, et al. The leukemogenic TCF3-HLF complex rewires enhancers driving cellular identity and self-renewal conferring EP300 vulnerability. Cancer Cell. 2019;36:630-644 e639. https://doi.org/10.1016/j.ccell.2019.10.004.
67. Huang Y, Bourquin JP. Targeting the oncogenic activity of TCF3-HLF in leukemia. Mol Cell Oncol. 2020;7:1709391. https://doi.org/10.1080/23723556.2019.1709391.
68. Leonard J, Wolf JS, Degnin M, Eide CA, LaTocha D, Lenz K, Wilmot B, Mullighan CG, Loh M, Hunger SP, et al. Aurora a kinase as a target for therapy in TCF3-HLF rearranged acute lymphoblastic leukemia. Haematologica. 2021;106:2990–4. https://doi.org/10.3324/haematol.2021.278692.
69. Meyer C, Larghero P, Almeida Lopes B, Burmeister T, Groger D, Sutton R, Venn NC, Cazzaniga G, Corral Abascal L, Tsaur G, et al. The KMT2A recombinome of acute leukemias in 2023. Leukemia. 2023;37:988–1005. https://doi.org/10.1038/s41375-023-01877-1.
70. Winters AC, Bernt KM. MLL-rearranged Leukemias-an update on science and clinical approaches. Front Pediatr. 2017;5:4. https://doi.org/10.3389/fped.2017.00004.
71. Andersen MK, Christiansen DH, Jensen BA, Ernst P, Hauge G, Pedersen-Bjergaard J. Therapy-related acute lymphoblastic leukaemia with MLL rearrangements following DNA topoisomerase II inhibitors, an increasing problem: report on two new cases and review of the literature since 1992. Br J Haematol. 2001;114:539–43. https://doi.org/10.1046/j.1365-2141.2001.03000.x.

72. Brown P, Pieters R, Biondi A. How I treat infant leukemia. Blood. 2019;133:205–14. https://doi.org/10.1182/blood-2018-04-785980.
73. Attarbaschi A, Moricke A, Harrison CJ, Mann G, Baruchel A, De Moerloose B, Conter V, Devidas M, Elitzur S, Escherich G, et al. Outcomes of childhood noninfant acute lymphoblastic leukemia with 11q23/KMT2A rearrangements in a modern therapy era: a retrospective international study. J Clin Oncol. 2023;41:1404–22. https://doi.org/10.1200/JCO.22.01297.
74. Armstrong SA, Staunton JE, Silverman LB, Pieters R, den Boer ML, Minden MD, Sallan SE, Lander ES, Golub TR, Korsmeyer SJ. MLL translocations specify a distinct gene expression profile that distinguishes a unique leukemia. Nat Genet. 2002;30:41–7. https://doi.org/10.1038/ng765.
75. Yeoh EJ, Ross ME, Shurtleff SA, Williams WK, Patel D, Mahfouz R, Behm FG, Raimondi SC, Relling MV, Patel A, et al. Classification, subtype discovery, and prediction of outcome in pediatric acute lymphoblastic leukemia by gene expression profiling. Cancer Cell. 2002;1:133–43. https://doi.org/10.1016/s1535-6108(02)00032-6.
76. Stam RW, Schneider P, Hagelstein JA, van der Linden MH, Stumpel DJ, de Menezes RX, de Lorenzo P, Valsecchi MG, Pieters R. Gene expression profiling-based dissection of MLL translocated and MLL germline acute lymphoblastic leukemia in infants. Blood. 2010;115:2835–44. https://doi.org/10.1182/blood-2009-07-233049.
77. Isobe T, Takagi M, Sato-Otsubo A, Nishimura A, Nagae G, Yamagishi C, Tamura M, Tanaka Y, Asada S, Takeda R, et al. Multi-omics analysis defines highly refractory RAS burdened immature subgroup of infant acute lymphoblastic leukemia. Nat Commun. 2022;13:4501. https://doi.org/10.1038/s41467-022-32266-4.
78. Andersson AK, Ma J, Wang J, Chen X, Gedman AL, Dang J, Nakitandwe J, Holmfeldt L, Parker M, Easton J, et al. The landscape of somatic mutations in infant MLL-rearranged acute lymphoblastic leukemias. Nat Genet. 2015;47:330–7. https://doi.org/10.1038/ng.3230.
79. Valentine MC, Linabery AM, Chasnoff S, Hughes AE, Mallaney C, Sanchez N, Giacalone J, Heerema NA, Hilden JM, Spector LG, et al. Excess congenital non-synonymous variation in leukemia-associated genes in MLL- infant leukemia: a children's oncology group report. Leukemia. 2014;28:1235–41. https://doi.org/10.1038/leu.2013.367.
80. Driessen EM, van Roon EH, Spijkers-Hagelstein JA, Schneider P, de Lorenzo P, Valsecchi MG, Pieters R, Stam RW. Frequencies and prognostic impact of RAS mutations in MLL-rearranged acute lymphoblastic leukemia in infants. Haematologica. 2013;98:937–44. https://doi.org/10.3324/haematol.2012.067983.
81. Chen CW, Koche RP, Sinha AU, Deshpande AJ, Zhu N, Eng R, Doench JG, Xu H, Chu SH, Qi J, et al. DOT1L inhibits SIRT1-mediated epigenetic silencing to maintain leukemic gene expression in MLL-rearranged leukemia. Nat Med. 2015;21:335–43. https://doi.org/10.1038/nm.3832.
82. Krivtsov AV, Evans K, Gadrey JY, Eschle BK, Hatton C, Uckelmann HJ, Ross KN, Perner F, Olsen SN, Pritchard T, et al. A Menin-MLL inhibitor induces specific chromatin changes and eradicates disease in models of MLL-rearranged leukemia. Cancer Cell. 2019;36:660-673 e611. https://doi.org/10.1016/j.ccell.2019.11.001.
83. Issa GC, Aldoss I, DiPersio J, Cuglievan B, Stone R, Arellano M, Thirman MJ, Patel MR, Dickens DS, Shenoy S, et al. The menin inhibitor revumenib in KMT2A-rearranged or NPM1-mutant leukaemia. Nature. 2023;615:920–4. https://doi.org/10.1038/s41586-023-05812-3.
84. Gardner R, Wu D, Cherian S, Fang M, Hanafi LA, Finney O, Smithers H, Jensen MC, Riddell SR, Maloney DG, et al. Acquisition of a CD19-negative myeloid phenotype allows immune escape of MLL-rearranged B-ALL from CD19 CAR-T-cell therapy. Blood. 2016;127:2406–10. https://doi.org/10.1182/blood-2015-08-665547.
85. van der Sluis IM, de Lorenzo P, Kotecha RS, Attarbaschi A, Escherich G, Nysom K, Stary J, Ferster A, Brethon B, Locatelli F, et al. Blinatumomab added to chemotherapy in infant lymphoblastic leukemia. N Engl J Med. 2023;388:1572–81. https://doi.org/10.1056/NEJMoa2214171.
86. Khabirova E, Jardine L, Coorens THH, Webb S, Treger TD, Engelbert J, Porter T, Prigmore E, Collord G, Piapi A, et al. Single-cell transcriptomics reveals a distinct developmental state of KMT2A-rearranged infant B-cell acute lymphoblastic leukemia. Nat Med. 2022;28:743–51. https://doi.org/10.1038/s41591-022-01720-7.
87. Zhang J, McCastlain K, Yoshihara H, Xu B, Chang Y, Churchman ML, Wu G, Li Y, Wei L, Iacobucci I, et al. Deregulation of DUX4 and ERG in acute lymphoblastic leukemia. Nat Genet. 2016;48:1481–9. https://doi.org/10.1038/ng.3691.
88. Yasuda T, Tsuzuki S, Kawazu M, Hayakawa F, Kojima S, Ueno T, Imoto N, Kohsaka S, Kunita A, Doi K, et al. Recurrent DUX4 fusions in B cell acute lymphoblastic leukemia of adolescents and young adults. Nat Genet. 2016;48:569–74. https://doi.org/10.1038/ng.3535.
89. Schinnerl D, Mejstrikova E, Schumich A, Zaliova M, Fortschegger K, Nebral K, Attarbaschi A, Fiser K, Kauer MO, Popitsch N, et al. CD371 cell surface expression: a unique feature of DUX4-rearranged acute lymphoblastic leukemia. Haematologica. 2019;104:e352–5. https://doi.org/10.3324/haematol.2018.214353.
90. Zaliova M, Stuchly J, Winkowska L, Musilova A, Fiser K, Slamova M, Starkova J, Vaskova M, Hrusak O, Sramkova L, et al. Genomic landscape of pediatric B-other acute lymphoblastic leukemia in a consecutive European cohort. Haematologica.

2019;104:1396–406. https://doi.org/10.3324/haematol.2018.204974.

91. Zaliova M, Potuckova E, Hovorkova L, Musilova A, Winkowska L, Fiser K, Stuchly J, Mejstrikova E, Starkova J, Zuna J, et al. ERG deletions in childhood acute lymphoblastic leukemia with DUX4 rearrangements are mostly polyclonal, prognostically relevant and their detection rate strongly depends on screening method sensitivity. Haematologica. 2019;104:1407–16. https://doi.org/10.3324/haematol.2018.204487.
92. Jeha S, Choi J, Roberts KG, Pei D, Coustan-Smith E, Inaba H, Rubnitz JE, Ribeiro RC, Gruber TA, Raimondi SC, et al. Clinical significance of novel subtypes of acute lymphoblastic leukemia in the context of minimal residual disease-directed therapy. Blood Cancer Discov. 2021;2:326–37. https://doi.org/10.1158/2643-3230.bcd-20-0229.
93. Li Z, Lee SHR, Chin WHN, Lu Y, Jiang N, Lim EH, Coustan-Smith E, Chiew KH, Oh BLZ, Koh GS, et al. Distinct clinical characteristics of DUX4- and PAX5-altered childhood B-lymphoblastic leukemia. Blood Adv. 2021;5:5226–38. https://doi.org/10.1182/bloodadvances.2021004895.
94. Suzuki K, Okuno Y, Kawashima N, Muramatsu H, Okuno T, Wang X, Kataoka S, Sekiya Y, Hamada M, Murakami N, et al. MEF2D-BCL9 fusion gene is associated with high-risk acute B-cell precursor lymphoblastic leukemia in adolescents. J Clin Oncol. 2016;34:3451–9. https://doi.org/10.1200/JCO.2016.66.5547.
95. Gu Z, Churchman M, Roberts K, Li Y, Liu Y, Harvey RC, McCastlain K, Reshmi SC, Payne-Turner D, Iacobucci I, et al. Genomic analyses identify recurrent MEF2D fusions in acute lymphoblastic leukaemia. Nat Commun. 2016;7:13331. https://doi.org/10.1038/ncomms13331.
96. Ohki K, Kiyokawa N, Saito Y, Hirabayashi S, Nakabayashi K, Ichikawa H, Momozawa Y, Okamura K, Yoshimi A, Ogata-Kawata H, et al. Clinical and molecular characteristics of MEF2D fusion-positive B-cell precursor acute lymphoblastic leukemia in childhood, including a novel translocation resulting in MEF2D-HNRNPH1 gene fusion. Haematologica. 2019;104:128–37. https://doi.org/10.3324/haematol.2017.186320.
97. Ohki K, Butler ER, Kiyokawa N, Hirabayashi S, Bergmann AK, Moricke A, Boer JM, Cave H, Cazzaniga G, Yeoh AEJ, et al. Clinical characteristics and outcomes of B-cell precursor ALL with MEF2D rearrangements: a retrospective study by the Ponte di Legno childhood ALL working group. Leukemia. 2023;37:212–6. https://doi.org/10.1038/s41375-022-01737-4.
98. Tsuzuki S, Yasuda T, Kojima S, Kawazu M, Akahane K, Inukai T, Imaizumi M, Morishita T, Miyamura K, Ueno T, et al. Targeting MEF2D-fusion oncogenic transcriptional circuitries in B-cell precursor acute lymphoblastic leukemia. Blood Cancer Discov. 2020;1:82–95. https://doi.org/10.1158/2643-3230.BCD-19-0080.
99. Hirano D, Hayakawa F, Yasuda T, Tange N, Yamamoto H, Kojima Y, Morishita T, Imoto N, Tsuzuki S, Mano H, et al. Chromosomal translocation-mediated evasion from miRNA induces strong MEF2D fusion protein expression, causing inhibition of PAX5 transcriptional activity. Oncogene. 2019;38:2263–74. https://doi.org/10.1038/s41388-018-0573-9.
100. Alexander TB, Gu Z, Iacobucci I, Dickerson K, Choi JK, Xu B, Payne-Turner D, Yoshihara H, Loh ML, Horan J, et al. The genetic basis and cell of origin of mixed phenotype acute leukaemia. Nature. 2018;562:373–9. https://doi.org/10.1038/s41586-018-0436-0.
101. Hirabayashi S, Butler ER, Ohki K, Kiyokawa N, Bergmann AK, Moricke A, Boer JM, Cave H, Cazzaniga G, Yeoh AEJ, et al. Clinical characteristics and outcomes of B-ALL with ZNF384 rearrangements: a retrospective analysis by the Ponte di Legno childhood ALL working group. Leukemia. 2021;35:3272–7. https://doi.org/10.1038/s41375-021-01199-0.
102. Bueno C, Tejedor JR, Bashford-Rogers R, Gonzalez-Silva L, Valdes-Mas R, Agraz-Doblas A, Diaz de la Guardia R, Ribera J, Zamora L, Bilhou-Nabera C, et al. Natural history and cell of origin of TCF3-ZN F384 and PTPN11 mutations in monozygotic twins with concordant BCP-ALL. Blood. 2019;134:900–5. https://doi.org/10.1182/blood.2019000893.
103. Hirabayashi S, Ohki K, Nakabayashi K, Ichikawa H, Momozawa Y, Okamura K, Yaguchi A, Terada K, Saito Y, Yoshimi A, et al. ZNF384-related fusion genes define a subgroup of childhood B-cell precursor acute lymphoblastic leukemia with a characteristic immunotype. Haematologica. 2017;102:118–29. https://doi.org/10.3324/haematol.2016.151035.
104. Dickerson KM, Qu C, Gao Q, Iacobucci I, Gu Z, Yoshihara H, Backhaus EA, Chang Y, Janke LJ, Xu B, et al. ZNF384 fusion oncoproteins drive lineage aberrancy in acute leukemia. Blood Cancer Discov. 2022;3:240–63. https://doi.org/10.1158/2643-3230.BCD-21-0163.
105. Zhao X, Wang P, Diedrich JD, Smart B, Reyes N, Yoshimura S, Zhang J, Yang W, Barnett K, Xu B, et al. Epigenetic activation of the FLT3 gene by ZNF384 fusion confers a therapeutic susceptibility in acute lymphoblastic leukemia. Nat Commun. 2022;13:5401. https://doi.org/10.1038/s41467-022-33143-w.
106. Somasundaram R, Prasad MA, Ungerback J, Sigvardsson M. Transcription factor networks in B-cell differentiation link development to acute lymphoid leukemia. Blood. 2015;126:144–52. https://doi.org/10.1182/blood-2014-12-575688.
107. Dang J, Wei L, de Ridder J, Su X, Rust AG, Roberts KG, Payne-Turner D, Cheng J, Ma J, Qu C, et al. PAX5 is a tumor suppressor in mouse mutagenesis models of acute lymphoblastic leukemia.

Blood. 2015;125:3609–17. https://doi.org/10.1182/blood-2015-02-626127.
108. Jia Z, Gu Z. PAX5 alterations in B-cell acute lymphoblastic leukemia. Front Oncol. 2022;12:1023606. https://doi.org/10.3389/fonc.2022.1023606.
109. Schwab C, Nebral K, Chilton L, Leschi C, Waanders E, Boer JM, Zaliova M, Sutton R, Ofverholm II, Ohki K, et al. Intragenic amplification of PAX5: a novel subgroup in B-cell precursor acute lymphoblastic leukemia? Blood Adv. 2017;1:1473–7. https://doi.org/10.1182/bloodadvances.2017006734.
110. Nebral K, Denk D, Attarbaschi A, Konig M, Mann G, Haas OA, Strehl S. Incidence and diversity of PAX5 fusion genes in childhood acute lymphoblastic leukemia. Leukemia. 2009;23:134–43. https://doi.org/10.1038/leu.2008.306.
111. Duployez N, Jamrog LA, Fregona V, Hamelle C, Fenwarth L, Lejeune S, Helevaut N, Geffroy S, Caillault A, Marceau-Renaut A, et al. Germline PAX5 mutation predisposes to familial B-cell precursor acute lymphoblastic leukemia. Blood. 2021;137:1424–8. https://doi.org/10.1182/blood.2020005756.
112. Passet M, Boissel N, Sigaux F, Saillard C, Bargetzi M, Ba I, Thomas X, Graux C, Chalandon Y, Leguay T, et al. PAX5 P80R mutation identifies a novel subtype of B-cell precursor acute lymphoblastic leukemia with favorable outcome. Blood. 2019;133:280–4. https://doi.org/10.1182/blood-2018-10-882142.
113. Bastian L, Schroeder MP, Eckert C, Schlee C, Tanchez JO, Kampf S, Wagner DL, Schulze V, Isaakidis K, Lazaro-Navarro J, et al. PAX5 biallelic genomic alterations define a novel subgroup of B-cell precursor acute lymphoblastic leukemia. Leukemia. 2019;33:1895–909. https://doi.org/10.1038/s41375-019-0430-z.
114. Coyaud E, Struski S, Prade N, Familiades J, Eichner R, Quelen C, Bousquet M, Mugneret F, Talmant P, Pages MP, et al. Wide diversity of PAX5 alterations in B-ALL: a Groupe francophone de Cytogenetique Hematologique study. Blood. 2010;115:3089–97. https://doi.org/10.1182/blood-2009-07-234229.
115. Schwab C, Cranston RE, Ryan SL, Butler E, Winterman E, Hawking Z, Bashton M, Enshaei A, Russell LJ, Kingsbury Z, et al. Integrative genomic analysis of childhood acute lymphoblastic leukaemia lacking a genetic biomarker in the UKALL2003 clinical trial. Leukemia. 2023;37:529–38. https://doi.org/10.1038/s41375-022-01799-4.
116. Li Y, Moriyama T, Yoshimura S, Zhao X, Li Z, Yang X, Paietta E, Litzow MR, Konopleva M, Yu J, et al. PAX5 epigenetically orchestrates CD58 transcription and modulates blinatumomab response in acute lymphoblastic leukemia. Sci Adv. 2022;8:eadd6403. https://doi.org/10.1126/sciadv.add6403.
117. Kimura S, Montefiori L, Iacobucci I, Zhao Y, Gao Q, Paietta EM, Haferlach C, Laird AD, Mead PE, Gu Z, et al. Enhancer retargeting of CDX2 and UBTF::ATXN7L3 define a subtype of high-risk B-progenitor acute lymphoblastic leukemia. Blood. 2022;139:3519–31. https://doi.org/10.1182/blood.2022015444.
118. Bastian L, Hartmann AM, Beder T, Hanzelmann S, Kassens J, Bultmann M, Hoeppner MP, Franzenburg S, Wittig M, Franke A, et al. UBTF::ATXN7L3 gene fusion defines novel B cell precursor ALL subtype with CDX2 expression and need for intensified treatment. Leukemia. 2022;36:1676–80. https://doi.org/10.1038/s41375-022-01557-6.
119. Passet M, Kim R, Gachet S, Sigaux F, Chaumeil J, Galland A, Sexton T, Quentin S, Hernandez L, Larcher L, et al. Concurrent CDX2 cis-deregulation and UBTF::ATXN7L3 fusion define a novel high-risk subtype of B-cell ALL. Blood. 2022;139:3505–18. https://doi.org/10.1182/blood.2021014723.
120. Yang M, Safavi S, Woodward EL, Duployez N, Olsson-Arvidsson L, Ungerback J, Sigvardsson M, Zaliova M, Zuna J, Fioretos T, et al. 13q12.2 deletions in acute lymphoblastic leukemia lead to upregulation of FLT3 through enhancer hijacking. Blood. 2020;136:946–56. https://doi.org/10.1182/blood.2019004684.
121. Yasuda T, Sanada M, Kawazu M, Kojima S, Tsuzuki S, Ueno H, Iwamoto E, Iijima-Yamashita Y, Yamada T, Kanamori T, et al. Two novel high-risk adult B-cell acute lymphoblastic leukemia subtypes with high expression of CDX2 and IDH1/2 mutations. Blood. 2021; https://doi.org/10.1182/blood.2021011921.
122. Boer JM, Valsecchi MG, Hormann FM, Antic Z, Zaliova M, Schwab C, Cazzaniga G, Arfeuille C, Cave H, Attarbaschi A, et al. Favorable outcome of NUTM1-rearranged infant and pediatric B cell precursor acute lymphoblastic leukemia in a collaborative international study. Leukemia. 2021;35:2978–82. https://doi.org/10.1038/s41375-021-01333-y.
123. Hormann FM, Hoogkamer AQ, Beverloo HB, Boeree A, Dingjan I, Wattel MM, Stam RW, Escherich G, Pieters R, den Boer ML, et al. NUTM1 is a recurrent fusion gene partner in B-cell precursor acute lymphoblastic leukemia associated with increased expression of genes on chromosome band 10p12.31-12.2. Haematologica. 2019;104:e455–9. https://doi.org/10.3324/haematol.2018.206961.
124. McEvoy CR, Fox SB, Prall OWJ. Emerging entities in NUTM1-rearranged neoplasms. Genes Chromosomes Cancer. 2020;59:375–85. https://doi.org/10.1002/gcc.22838.
125. French CA. NUT carcinoma: clinicopathologic features, pathogenesis, and treatment. Pathol Int. 2018;68:583–95. https://doi.org/10.1111/pin.12727.
126. French C. NUT midline carcinoma. Nat Rev Cancer. 2014;14:149–50. https://doi.org/10.1038/nrc3659.
127. Churchman ML, Low J, Qu C, Paietta EM, Kasper LH, Chang Y, Payne-Turner D, Althoff MJ, Song G, Chen SC, et al. Efficacy of Retinoids in IKZF1-mutated BCR-ABL1 acute lymphoblastic leukemia. Cancer Cell. 2015;28:343–56. https://doi.org/10.1016/j.ccell.2015.07.016.
128. Churchman ML, Qian M, Te Kronnie G, Zhang R, Yang W, Zhang H, Lana T, Tedrick P, Baskin R,

Verbist K, et al. Germline genetic IKZF1 variation and predisposition to childhood acute lymphoblastic leukemia. Cancer Cell. 2018;33:937–48. https://doi.org/10.1016/j.ccell.2018.03.021.

129. Boutboul D, Kuehn HS, Van de Wyngaert Z, Niemela JE, Callebaut I, Stoddard J, Lenoir C, Barlogis V, Farnarier C, Vely F, et al. Dominant-negative IKZF1 mutations cause a T, B, and myeloid cell combined immunodeficiency. J Clin Invest. 2018;128:3071–87. https://doi.org/10.1172/JCI98164.
130. Bernt KM, Hunger SP. Current concepts in pediatric Philadelphia chromosome-positive acute lymphoblastic leukemia. Front Oncol. 2014;4:54. https://doi.org/10.3389/fonc.2014.00054.
131. Roberts KG, Gu Z, Payne-Turner D, McCastlain K, Harvey RC, Chen IM, Pei D, Iacobucci I, Valentine M, Pounds SB, et al. High frequency and poor outcome of Philadelphia chromosome-like acute lymphoblastic leukemia in adults. J Clin Oncol. 2017;35:394–401. https://doi.org/10.1200/JCO.2016.69.0073.
132. Slayton WB, Schultz KR, Silverman LB, Hunger SP. How we approach Philadelphia chromosome-positive acute lymphoblastic leukemia in children and young adults. Pediatr Blood Cancer. 2020;67:e28543. https://doi.org/10.1002/pbc.28543.
133. Slayton WB, Schultz KR, Kairalla JA, Devidas M, Mi X, Pulsipher MA, Chang BH, Mullighan C, Iacobucci I, Silverman LB, et al. Dasatinib plus intensive chemotherapy in children, adolescents, and young adults with Philadelphia chromosome-positive acute lymphoblastic leukemia: results of children's oncology group trial AALL0622. J Clin Oncol. 2018;36:2306–14. https://doi.org/10.1200/JCO.2017.76.7228.
134. Shen S, Chen X, Cai J, Yu J, Gao J, Hu S, Zhai X, Liang C, Ju X, Jiang H, et al. Effect of Dasatinib vs Imatinib in the treatment of pediatric Philadelphia chromosome-positive acute lymphoblastic leukemia: a randomized clinical trial. JAMA Oncol. 2020;6:358–66. https://doi.org/10.1001/jamaoncol.2019.5868.
135. Mullighan CG, Miller CB, Radtke I, Phillips LA, Dalton J, Ma J, White D, Hughes TP, Le Beau MM, Pui CH, et al. BCR-ABL1 lymphoblastic leukaemia is characterized by the deletion of Ikaros. Nature. 2008;453:110–4. https://doi.org/10.1038/nature06866.
136. Iacobucci I, Storlazzi CT, Cilloni D, Lonetti A, Ottaviani E, Soverini S, Astolfi A, Chiaretti S, Vitale A, Messa F, et al. Identification and molecular characterization of recurrent genomic deletions on 7p12 in the IKZF1 gene in a large cohort of BCR-ABL1-positive acute lymphoblastic leukemia patients: on behalf of Gruppo Italiano Malattie Ematologiche dell'Adulto acute leukemia working party (GIMEMA AL WP). Blood. 2009;114:2159–67. https://doi.org/10.1182/blood-2008-08-173963.
137. Stanulla M, Dagdan E, Zaliova M, Moricke A, Palmi C, Cazzaniga G, Eckert C, Te Kronnie G, Bourquin JP, Bornhauser B, et al. IKZF1(plus) defines a new minimal residual disease-dependent very-poor prognostic profile in pediatric B-cell precursor acute lymphoblastic leukemia. J Clin Oncol. 2018;36:1240–9. https://doi.org/10.1200/JCO.2017.74.3617.
138. Churchman ML, Evans K, Richmond J, Robbins A, Jones L, Shapiro IM, Pachter JA, Weaver DT, Houghton PJ, Smith MA, et al. Synergism of FAK and tyrosine kinase inhibition in Ph(+) B-ALL. JCI Insight. 2016;1 https://doi.org/10.1172/jci.insight.86082.
139. Adnan-Awad S, Kim D, Hohtari H, Javarappa KK, Brandstoetter T, Mayer I, Potdar S, Heckman CA, Kytola S, Porkka K, et al. Characterization of p190-Bcr-Abl chronic myeloid leukemia reveals specific signaling pathways and therapeutic targets. Leukemia. 2021;35:1964–75. https://doi.org/10.1038/s41375-020-01082-4.
140. Hovorkova L, Zaliova M, Venn NC, Bleckmann K, Trkova M, Potuckova E, Vaskova M, Linhartova J, Machova Polakova K, Fronkova E, et al. Monitoring of childhood ALL using BCR-ABL1 genomic breakpoints identifies a subgroup with CML-like biology. Blood. 2017;129:2771–81. https://doi.org/10.1182/blood-2016-11-749978.
141. Pfeifer H, Cazzaniga G, van der Velden VHJ, Cayuela JM, Schafer B, Spinelli O, Akiki S, Avigad S, Bendit I, Borg K, et al. Standardisation and consensus guidelines for minimal residual disease assessment in Philadelphia-positive acute lymphoblastic leukemia (Ph + ALL) by real-time quantitative reverse transcriptase PCR of e1a2 BCR-ABL1. Leukemia. 2019;33:1910–22. https://doi.org/10.1038/s41375-019-0413-0.
142. Zuna J, Hovorkova L, Krotka J, Koehrmann A, Bardini M, Winkowska L, Fronkova E, Alten J, Koehler R, Eckert C, et al. Minimal residual disease in BCR::ABL1-positive acute lymphoblastic leukemia: different significance in typical ALL and in CML-like disease. Leukemia. 2022;36:2793–801. https://doi.org/10.1038/s41375-022-01668-0.
143. Den Boer ML, van Slegtenhorst M, De Menezes RX, Cheok MH, Buijs-Gladdines JG, Peters ST, Van Zutven LJ, Beverloo HB, Van der Spek PJ, Escherich G, et al. A subtype of childhood acute lymphoblastic leukaemia with poor treatment outcome: a genome-wide classification study. Lancet Oncol. 2009;10:125–34. https://doi.org/10.1016/S1470-2045(08)70339-5.
144. Mullighan CG, Su X, Zhang J, Radtke I, Phillips LA, Miller CB, Ma J, Liu W, Cheng C, Schulman BA, et al. Deletion of IKZF1 and prognosis in acute lymphoblastic leukemia. N Engl J Med. 2009;360:470–80. https://doi.org/10.1056/NEJMoa0808253.
145. Li Z, Chang TC, Junco JJ, Devidas M, Li Y, Yang W, Huang X, Hedges DJ, Cheng Z, Shago M, et al. Genomic landscape of down syndrome-associated acute lymphoblastic leukemia. Blood. 2023; https://doi.org/10.1182/blood.2023019765.

146. Iacobucci I, Roberts KG. Genetic alterations and therapeutic targeting of Philadelphia-like acute lymphoblastic leukemia. Genes (Basel). 2021;12 https://doi.org/10.3390/genes12050687.
147. Roberts KG, Pei D, Campana D, Payne-Turner D, Li Y, Cheng C, Sandlund JT, Jeha S, Easton J, Becksfort J, et al. Outcomes of children with BCR-ABL1-like acute lymphoblastic leukemia treated with risk-directed therapy based on the levels of minimal residual disease. J Clin Oncol. 2014;32:3012–20. https://doi.org/10.1200/JCO.2014.55.4105.
148. Iacobucci I, Li Y, Roberts KG, Dobson SM, Kim JC, Payne-Turner D, Harvey RC, Valentine M, McCastlain K, Easton J, et al. Truncating erythropoietin receptor rearrangements in acute lymphoblastic leukemia. Cancer Cell. 2016;29:186–200. https://doi.org/10.1016/j.ccell.2015.12.013.
149. Maese L, Raetz EA. Can Ph-like ALL be effectively targeted? Best Pract Res Clin Haematol. 2019;32:101096. https://doi.org/10.1016/j.beha.2019.101096.
150. Roberts KG, Li Y, Payne-Turner D, Harvey RC, Yang YL, Pei D, McCastlain K, Ding L, Lu C, Song G, et al. Targetable kinase-activating lesions in Ph-like acute lymphoblastic leukemia. N Engl J Med. 2014;371:1005–15. https://doi.org/10.1056/NEJMoa1403088.
151. Loh ML, Zhang J, Harvey RC, Roberts K, Payne-Turner D, Kang H, Wu G, Chen X, Becksfort J, Edmonson M, et al. Tyrosine kinome sequencing of pediatric acute lymphoblastic leukemia: a report from the children's oncology group TARGET project. Blood. 2013;121:485–8. https://doi.org/10.1182/blood-2012-04-422691.
152. Russell LJ, Jones L, Enshaei A, Tonin S, Ryan SL, Eswaran J, Nakjang S, Papaemmanuil E, Tubio JM, Fielding AK, et al. Characterisation of the genomic landscape of CRLF2-rearranged acute lymphoblastic leukemia. Genes Chromosomes Cancer. 2017;56:363–72. https://doi.org/10.1002/gcc.22439.
153. Mullighan CG, Collins-Underwood JR, Phillips LA, Loudin MG, Liu W, Zhang J, Ma J, Coustan-Smith E, Harvey RC, Willman CL, et al. Rearrangement of CRLF2 in B-progenitor- and down syndrome-associated acute lymphoblastic leukemia. Nat Genet. 2009;41:1243–6. https://doi.org/10.1038/ng.469.
154. Hertzberg L, Vendramini E, Ganmore I, Cazzaniga G, Schmitz M, Chalker J, Shiloh R, Iacobucci I, Shochat C, Zeligson S, et al. Down syndrome acute lymphoblastic leukemia, a highly heterogeneous disease in which aberrant expression of CRLF2 is associated with mutated JAK2: a report from the international BFM study group. Blood. 2010;115:1006–17. https://doi.org/10.1182/blood-2009-08-235408.
155. Yoda A, Yoda Y, Chiaretti S, Bar-Natan M, Mani K, Rodig SJ, West N, Xiao Y, Brown JR, Mitsiades C, et al. Functional screening identifies CRLF2 in precursor B-cell acute lymphoblastic leukemia. Proc Natl Acad Sci USA. 2010;107:252–7. https://doi.org/10.1073/pnas.0911726107.
156. Tanasi I, Ba I, Sirvent N, Braun T, Cuccuini W, Ballerini P, Duployez N, Tanguy-Schmidt A, Tamburini J, Maury S, et al. Efficacy of tyrosine kinase inhibitors in Ph-like acute lymphoblastic leukemia harboring ABL-class rearrangements. Blood. 2019;134:1351–5. https://doi.org/10.1182/blood.2019001244.
157. Schewe DM, Lenk L, Vogiatzi F, Winterberg D, Rademacher AV, Buchmann S, Henry D, Bergmann AK, Cario G, Cox MC. Larotrectinib in TRK fusion-positive pediatric B-cell acute lymphoblastic leukemia. Blood Adv. 2019;3:3499–502. https://doi.org/10.1182/bloodadvances.2019000700.
158. Tasian SK, Loh ML, Hunger SP. Philadelphia chromosome-like acute lymphoblastic leukemia. Blood. 2017;130:2064–72. https://doi.org/10.1182/blood-2017-06-743252.
159. Inaba H, Azzato EM, Mullighan CG. Integration of next-generation sequencing to treat acute lymphoblastic leukemia with targetable lesions: the St. Jude Children's Research Hospital approach. Front Pediatr. 2017;5:258. https://doi.org/10.3389/fped.2017.00258.
160. Zaliova M, Potuckova E, Lukes J, Winkowska L, Starkova J, Janotova I, Sramkova L, Stary J, Zuna J, Stanulla M, et al. Frequency and prognostic impact of ZEB2 H1038 and Q1072 mutations in childhood B-other acute lymphoblastic leukemia. Haematologica. 2021;106:886–90. https://doi.org/10.3324/haematol.2020.249094.
161. Dunleavy K. Double-hit lymphoma: optimizing therapy. Hematology Am Soc Hematol Educ Program. 2021;2021:157–63. https://doi.org/10.1182/hematology.2021000247.
162. Lopez C, Burkhardt B, Chan JKC, Leoncini L, Mbulaiteye SM, Ogwang MD, Orem J, Rochford R, Roschewski M, Siebert R. Burkitt lymphoma. Nat Rev Dis Primers. 2022;8:78. https://doi.org/10.1038/s41572-022-00404-3.
163. Wagener R, Lopez C, Kleinheinz K, Bausinger J, Aukema SM, Nagel I, Toprak UH, Seufert J, Altmuller J, Thiele H, et al. IG-MYC (+) neoplasms with precursor B-cell phenotype are molecularly distinct from Burkitt lymphomas. Blood. 2018;132:2280–5. https://doi.org/10.1182/blood-2018-03-842088.
164. Bomken S, Enshaei A, Schwalbe EC, Mikulasova A, Dai Y, Zaka M, Fung KTM, Bashton M, Lim H, Jones L, et al. Molecular characterization and clinical outcome of B-cell precursor acute lymphoblastic leukemia with IG-MYC rearrangement. Haematologica. 2023;108:717–31. https://doi.org/10.3324/haematol.2021.280557.
165. Paietta E, Roberts KG, Wang V, Gu Z, Buck GAN, Pei D, Cheng C, Levine RL, Abdel-Wahab O, Cheng Z, et al. Molecular classification improves risk assessment in adult BCR-ABL1-negative B-ALL. Blood. 2021;138:948–58. https://doi.org/10.1182/blood.2020010144.

Genetic and Epigenetic Profiles in T-ALL

3

Büşra Erarslan Uysal and Andreas E. Kulozik

3.1 Introduction

Acute lymphoblastic leukemia (ALL) is the most common childhood malignancy and arises from B- or T-lineage lymphoid progenitors. T-cell acute lymphoblastic leukemias originate from malignant hematopoietic cells carrying immature T-cell markers. T-ALL accounts for 10–15% of newly diagnosed pediatric and 20–25% of adult ALL patients [1, 2]. The hematology of T-ALL is typically characterized by elevated white blood cell (WBC) counts with peripheral blasts, neutropenia, anemia, and thrombocytopenia. The prevalence in males is approximately twice that in females [3–8]. Moreover, T-ALL patients frequently present with central nervous system (CNS) infiltration and mediastinal thymic masses [3–8].

T-ALL was classified as an aggressive and high-risk form of leukemia during the early 1980s, when combination therapy was newly developed. At the time, cure rates were only around 10% [1, 2]. However, the development of risk-adapted therapies in subsequent years has led to a significant improvement in cure rates, which now approach 85% in children [3–7], but remain much lower (around 60%) in adults [8–10]. Unfortunately, about 20% of patients suffer from relapse, which is the main cause of death from T-ALL [11–15].

The prognosis and risk stratification of ALL are influenced by several factors, including the patient's clinical characteristics such as CNS involvement at the time of diagnosis, WBC counts of $\geq 50 \times 10^9$/L, male sex, age (infant age or $\geq$ 10 years), race (African American or Hispanic), and cytogenetic and genetic abnormalities [16]. However, serial measurements of minimal residual disease (MRD) have emerged as the most useful prognostic marker in T-ALL. This measurement is based on clone specific immunoglobulin and T-cell receptor (TCR) gene rearrangements, which are detected by polymerase chain reaction (PCR) or on flow cytometric analysis of leukemia-specific surface antigens [16].

Treatment intensity is stratified based on MRD in all modern treatment protocols. However, some patients classified as MRD standard risk receive treatment with insufficient intensity and subsequently relapse. Conversely, some classified as MRD high risk are likely overtreated [17]. Although MRD stratified treatment intensity has markedly improved prognosis,

B. Erarslan Uysal · A. E. Kulozik (✉)
Molecular Medicine Partnership Unit (MMPU), European Molecular Biology Laboratory (EMBL) and University of Heidelberg, Heidelberg, Germany

Department of Pediatric Oncology, Hematology, and Immunology, University of Heidelberg, and Hopp Children's Cancer Center (KiTZ) Heidelberg, Heidelberg, Germany
e-mail: busra.erarslan@embl.de; andreas.kulozik@med.uni-heidelberg.de

G. Escherich, V. Conter (eds.), *Acute Lymphoblastic Leukemia in Children and Adolescents*, Pediatric Oncology, https://doi.org/10.1007/978-3-031-71180-0_3

accurately predicting patient outcomes remains a challenge. Additionally, the relapse risk within certain MRD groups varies between genetic subgroups of T-ALL [18, 19].

In terms of genetic and epigenetic background, T-cell leukemia is a highly heterogeneous disease resulting from accumulation of aberrations which disrupt key tumor suppressor, oncogenic, and developmental pathways responsible for normal growth, proliferation, differentiation, and survival of thymocytes [20–22]. As a result, developing thymocytes are arrested at different stages of T-cell maturation. T-ALLs can be classified into subgroups characterized by either driver oncogenic events and distinct gene expression profiles or by immunophenotypes which reflect stage of developmental arrest, yet there are genetic and epigenetic abnormalities common to each subgroup [20–22].

In this chapter, driver oncogenic events will be distinguished according to their distribution and the result of their deregulation as type A and type B abnormalities as first proposed by van Vlierberghe et al. [23]. Type A abnormalities are the consequence of fusion and rearrangement events which place transcription factors (TF) under the control of a T-cell receptor enhancer [24, 25]. In addition to chromosomal rearrangements, structural variations (SV) and mutations in noncoding/enhancer regions can also lead to deregulation of these transcription factors. Deregulated TFs are mutually exclusive and include homeobox genes (TLX1/3, HOXA, NKX2–1/5), basic helix–loop–helix (bHLH) family of TFs (TAL1/2, LYL1) and LIM-only domain proteins (LMO1/2/3). Type B abnormalities, on the other hand, are not mutually exclusive and are shared by multiple genetic subgroups [24, 25]. These abnormalities affect a variety of genes such as TF tumor suppressor genes such as RUNX1, BCL11B, and WT1; epigenetic regulators such as PHF6, EZH2, and KDM6A; ribosomal proteins; and translation regulators such as RPL5, RPL10, and CNDT3. Mutations and copy number alterations (CNA) which lead to deregulation of oncogenic pathways like NOTCH, PI3K/AKT, IL-7R/JAK/STAT and cellular processes (cell cycle or apoptosis) are also classified into type B abnormalities because of their distribution across all genetic subgroups [24, 25].

Another classification of T-ALLs is based on the stage of developmental arrest of thymocytes. The following three subgroups are defined based on clinical immunophenotypes: mature/late cortical T-ALL, cortical and early cortical T-ALL, and immature/early T-cell precursor ALL [26–28]. Driver oncogenic events introduced in the previous paragraph are non-randomly distributed across all immunophenotypic subgroups. For instance, overexpression of the TAL1 oncogene is enriched in T-ALLs whose immunophenotype resembles late stages of T-cell maturation (sCD3, CD4, and CD8 positive). As a separate entity, early T-cell precursor ALLs (ETP-ALL; CD4 and CD8 negative) are characterized by more diverse alterations in HOXA, BCL11B, and LMO1/2 genes.

The identification of genetic and epigenetic aberrations driving T-ALL carries the potential of establishing more accurate risk stratification, developing therapeutic approaches targeted to genetic subtypes and thereby reducing risk of relapse in T-ALL. In this chapter, we will review molecular aberrations driving the leukemogenesis of T-ALL and affect treatment response and prognosis. Some of these aberrations have been included into an update of the International Consensus Classification (ICC) of ALL [29].

3.2 Type A: Mutually Exclusive Abnormalities in Transcription Factor Oncogenes

More than 90% of acute precursor T-cell leukemias can be categorized into subgroups according to the overexpression of T-cell related transcription factors which are critical for hematopoiesis and T-cell development, maturation, and differentiation. Commonly deregulated TFs include homeobox genes (TLX1, TLX2, TLX3, HOXA, NKX2–1, NKX2–5), basic helix–loop–helix family of TFs (TAL1, TAL2, LYL1), and LIM-only domain proteins (LMO1, LMO2,

LMO3) [20, 30–32]. Chromosomal translocations reposition these TF oncogenes close to a T-cell receptor locus enhancer and thereby induce their overexpression. Alternatively, structural variations as well as small insertions and deletions (InDel) in enhancer regions of these genes can drive their aberrant expression [20, 30–32]. These T-ALL specific TF oncogenes also result in unique profiles of gene expression, chromatin accessibility, and methylation. Recent integrative analyses of omic datasets revealed that translocated and/or mutated TF oncogenes are the main source not only of genomic but also of epigenomic heterogeneity among T-ALLs [33–35].

3.2.1 bHLH Factors and LMO Genes

The transcription factors TAL1 and TAL2 belong to the class II bHLH family and form heterodimers with the class I bHLH proteins (E47, E2A, and HEB) [36]. Heterodimers then bind to other TFs such as LMO1, LMO2, GATA3, and RUNX1 to form transcriptional complexes [36]. During normal hematopoiesis, TAL1 and LMO2 expression need to be silenced at early stages of lineage commitment to allow initiation of T-cell receptor rearrangements and normal differentiation program [36–38].

T-ALL patients with upregulated TAL and LMO genes are grouped together, because these two genes, functioning in the same regulatory complex, are dysregulated together in approximately 80% of TAL1-driven T-ALLs [30, 39, 40] as well as leave highly similar genomic and epigenomic signatures [33, 34]. The TAL/LMO subgroup of T-ALL is the largest one characterizing 30–45% of pediatric and 10–15% of adult cases [24, 31, 41, 42].

3.2.1.1 TAL Genes

Acting as a master regulatory protein involved in T-cell differentiation and leukemogenesis, TAL1's oncogenic transforming potential was illustrated several times in transgenic mice which developed T-cell malignancies upon TAL1 overexpression [43–45]. In terms of gene expression profiles and immunophenotype, T-ALLs with TAL1-rearrangement are associated with the late cortical/mature stages of thymic differentiation [30, 46].

Table 3.1 Major alterations leading to TAL1 activation

Alteration	References
Translocation to TCRA/D loci	[47–49]
Small InDel at neighboring SIL gene	[50]
Heterogenous somatic InDel in its regulatory region creating an MYB binding site	[32, 51]
Upregulation of related genes as a result of chromosomal rearrangements (TAL2, LYL1, BHLHB1)	[52–55]

The most common mechanism driving upregulation of the T-cell acute leukemia 1 (TAL1) gene is an interchromosomal translocation event that repositions this gene close to the enhancer of the TCRA/D loci (Table 3.1) [47–49]. Another common mechanism is a small deletion at the neighboring gene SIL, which positions TAL1 under the control of a regulatory element of SIL (Table 3.1) [50]. More recently, heterogeneous somatic InDels were identified in an intergenic regulatory region upstream of TAL1, which creates a de novo binding site for MYB, which in turn drives monoallelic overexpression of TAL1 (Table 3.1) [32, 51]. Additionally, but rarely, TAL1-related genes such as TAL2, LYL1, and BHLHB1 are also upregulated as a result of chromosomal rearrangements placing them under control of T-cell receptor regulatory regions (Table 3.1) [52–55].

Overexpressed TAL1 inhibits homodimer formation of the class I bHLH TF E47 by forming TAL1-E47 heterodimers, and thereby preventing E47's normal function of negative regulation of proliferation [56]. TAL1 has several regulatory partner transcription factors, which are important for regulation of normal hematopoiesis and carry oncogenic potential, such as GATA3, RUNX1, MYB, and ETS family proteins (Table 3.2) [38, 57]. They positively regulate each other and form an autoregulatory feedback loop which, as a result, induces cell proliferation and helps maintain leukemogenic transcriptional programs (Table 3.2) [32, 38]. Other TAL1 targets with oncogenic potential include GI-MAP proteins,

Table 3.2 Consequences of TAL1 activation

Consequences of TAL1 activation	References
Prevention of negative regulation of proliferation by E47	[56]
Induction of cell proliferation by its TF partners (GATA3, RUNX1, MYB and ETS family proteins)	[32, 38, 57]
Activation of targets with oncogenic potential (GI-MAP proteins, TRIB2, MIR223, NKX3.1, and ARID5B)	[58–62]

Table 3.3 Common genetic and epigenetic aberrations inducing LMO1 and LMO2 activation

Major aberrations inducing LMO activation	References
Chromosomal translocations	[63–65]
Mutations in noncoding regions leading de novo TF activator binding sites	[66, 67]
Small InDels in genes' proximity	[68, 69]
Deacetylation of Lys 74 and 78	[70]

TRIB2, MIR223, NKX3.1, and ARID5B (Table 3.2) [58–62]. The latter co-occupies its targets with the TAL1 regulatory complex and promotes expression of oncogenes, as well as induces T-cell tumor formation in zebrafish when overexpressed [62].

3.2.1.2 LMO Genes

LMO2 belongs to the TAL1 transcriptional complex and its overexpression has comparable downstream effects of autoregulation of oncogenic transcriptional programs. Overexpression of LIM-only domain genes LMO1 and LMO2 is also driven by similar mechanisms which are (1) chromosomal translocations (t(11;14)(p15;q11) and t(11;14)(p13;q11)) in about 10% of T-ALLs [63–65], (2) mutations within noncoding genomic regions creating de novo binding sites for MYB, ETS1 or RUNX1 in ~5% of T-ALLs [66, 67], and (3) small chromosomal deletions in the vicinity of the LMO2 locus in ~5% of T-ALLs (Table 3.3) [68, 69]. In addition to genomic alterations, deacetylation on lysine 74 and 78 was recently found to give rise to over-activation of LMO2 and thereby the TAL1 transcriptional complex (Table 3.3) [70].

DNA binding properties of TAL1 are not required to collaborate with LMO2 to cause T-cell leukemia. However, LMO2 expression accelerates the onset of leukemia in TAL1 transgenic mice [71]. In addition to its shared downstream effects with TAL1, LMO2 upregulation confers self-renewal capacity to preleukemic thymocytes, which mediates accumulation of additional mutations required for leukemic transformation in vivo [72]. Although TAL1 is dispensable for LMO2-driven leukemia, experiments in transgenic mice showed that LYL1 is critical for all of the oncogenic effects of LMO2, including upregulation of stem cell-like gene signatures and aberrant self-renewal capability of normal T cells [73, 74]. The oncogenic potential of LMO2 is further highlighted by four patients with X-linked severe combined immunodeficiency (X-SCID) who received gene therapy developed T-ALL as a result of LMO2 upregulation which was induced by retrovirus vector integration into the LMO2 promoter [75–77].

3.2.2 Homeobox Genes

Class I homeobox genes (HOX) encode transcription factors with highly conserved DNA binding domains. HOX-TFs serve as master regulators of early embryogenesis, body patterning, and cell lineage specification as they provide cells with regional information along the main body axis [78]. HOX genes have also been found to be critical for normal hematopoiesis and leukemogenesis. They are expressed in hematopoietic stem cells (HSCs) and possess lineage- and developmental stage-restricted patterns [79]. For instance, HOXA and HOXB genes are predominantly expressed in early T-cell and in erythroid precursors, respectively [79]. Similar to HOX genes, NKL-class homeobox genes, including TLX1 to TLX3 and NKX2–1 to NKX2–5, encode TFs that regulate basic processes in tissue and organ development [80]. Additionally, they have been implicated in cellular processes important for oncogenesis, namely, proliferation, differentiation, and apoptosis [80]. Depending on the cellular context, NKL homeobox genes can act as oncogenes or tumor suppressors [80].

T-ALLs that do not show aberrant expression of oncogenic TAL or LMO TFs are driven by deregulated homeobox genes. In approximately 30% of children, T-ALL is driven by dysregulation of one of the NKL genes [80]. Unlike the TAL/LMO subgroup, the homeobox subgroup of T-ALLs are not grouped together, because HOXA, TLX1/2/3, and NKX2–1/5 dysregulation gives rise to distinct gene expression and epigenomic signatures [33, 34, 42, 81, 82].

3.2.2.1 HOXA Cluster Genes

Upregulation of HOXA cluster genes can be driven by both *cis*- and *trans*-acting mechanisms. The oncogenic roles of these genes were first implicated in 2003 in T-ALL patients with MLL rearrangements and increased expression of HOXA9, HOXA10, HOXC6 and HOX cofactor MEIS1 [83]. In 2005, two independent studies discovered the first *cis*-acting mechanism; an inversion or a translocation on chromosome 7 targeting HOXA cluster genes and the TCRB locus led to ectopic activation of HOXA5–11 genes [84, 85]. Another mechanism acting in *cis* was reported a little later; HOXA activation in a T-ALL patient was driven by a translocation juxtaposing the HOXA cluster to the TCRD locus [86].

Trans-acting mechanisms associated with increased expression of HOXA cluster genes include SET-NUP214 [87], MLLT10-PICALM (also known as AF10-CALM) [88], MLLT10-NAP1L1 [89], MLLT10-XPO1 [90] and MLLT10-HNRNPH1, and -DDX3X fusion events (Table 3.4) [91]. The SET-NUP214 fusion product was shown to transcriptionally activate specific HOXA genes through binding to their promoter regions [87]. Within the HOXA subgroup of T-ALL, MLLT10-translocated cases exhibited a specific gene expression profile that differed from those with MLL-rearranged, SET-NUP214 and inversions of chromosome 7. These T-ALLs were further characterized by elevated expressions of HHEX and MEF2C that are highly expressed in normal HSCs and ETP [41, 91].

Table 3.4 Common abnormalities resulting in activation of HOXA cluster genes

Major abnormalities driving HOXA activation	References
Inversion targeting HOXA cluster and the TCRB genes	[84, 85]
Translocation to TCRD locus	[86]
SET-NUP214, MLLT10-PICALM, MLLT10-NAP1L1, MLLT10-XPO1, MLLT10-HNRNPH1, and MLLT10-DDX3X fusions	[87–91]

In a cohort of 209 adult T-ALL patients, 55 HOXA-positive cases had a significantly higher frequency of the ETP-ALL immunophenotype, chemoresistance, and positivity for MRD when compared to HOXA-negative cases [92]. Within the HOXA-positive group, the 5-year overall survival rate was significantly less in ETP-ALLs than in other immunophenotypes, whereas within the HOXA-negative group, no difference in prognosis was identified [92]. In a cohort of 100 pediatric T-ALL patients, 26 patients were identified with HOXA activation [93]. Patients with MLL-rearrangements, but not MLLT10, were strongly associated with inferior event free survival (EFS) and induction failure [93]. Similarly, those T-ALLs exhibiting an ETP-ALL expression profile were associated with inferior EFS and enriched for MLL-rearranged cases [93]. Finally, the worst outcome (induction failure, refractory disease, and relapse) was strongly associated with a combination of MLL rearrangements and an ETP-ALL immunophenotype [93]. Although ETPs have been initially classified as high-risk group with poor prognosis and high prevalence of chemoresistance [94, 95], comparative and retrospective analyses of ETP- and non-ETP-ALL patients have shown that prognosis and outcome of patients in these two groups are similar to each other [96–100].

HOXA cluster genes activate their own expression as well as transcription of critical genes enhancing cell proliferation and survival such as c-MYB, MEIS1, KIT, FLT3, CDK6, and SOX4 [79]. Rapid development of both AML and T-ALL was observed in mouse models with transduced HOXA9 and JAK3 carrying activating mutations, and the same phenotype was identified in mouse models harboring constitutive active STAT5B and HOXA9 expression [101].

3.2.2.2 NK-Like (NKL) Homeobox Genes

NKL homeobox genes are considered not to be expressed during normal T-cell development. However, one study examining expression of NKL genes in previously published datasets of diverse hematopoietic lineages (differentiating and mature T cells, B cells, NK cells, myeloid cells and so on) has defined an NKL code in hematopoiesis [102]. Although no NKL activity was detectable in double positive (DP) or single positive (SP) T cells, expression of TLX2, NKX3–1, HLX, HHEX, and VENTX was identified in double negative T-cell precursors (DN) [102]. Deregulation of NKL homeobox genes is common, affecting approx. 30% of all T-ALL. Aberrant expression of NKL genes is mainly driven by chromosomal rearrangements that involve TCR genes in addition to rare inversions, deletions or promoter hypermethylation. T-ALL patients with TLX or NKX rearrangements share a similar gene expression profile, mostly with the cortical immunophenotype [24, 30, 41].

TLX1, being the first NKL homeobox gene reported to be deregulated in T-ALL in 1991, is upregulated in 5–10% of pediatric and up to 30% of adult T-ALL patients as a result of translocation placing the gene under the control of TCR enhancers (Table 3.5) [30, 103–105]. This gene is normally not expressed in mature T cells, thymocytes, or HSCs. However, it plays a key role in early spleen and neural development [110, 111]. TLX1 can either block differentiation or promote proliferation of hematopoietic precursors. Experiments with differentiating embryonic stem cell (ESC) lines showed that TLX1 overexpression leads to immortalization of hematopoietic precursors [112–114]. Its overexpression in mouse thymus induced T-ALL with BCL11B and NOTCH1 mutations and promoted aneuploidy during T-cell transformation [115, 116]. It directly downregulated expression of mitotic genes including CHEK1 and induced loss of mitotic checkpoint control in thymocytes, thereby contributing to leukemogenesis [115, 116].

Table 3.5 Common aberrations leading to activation of NKL homeobox genes

Major aberrations leading to NKL activation	References
Chromosomal translocations involving TCR gene enhancers (TLX1)	[30, 103–105]
Translocation to the enhancer region of BCL11B (TLX3, NKX2–5)	[106–108]
Translocation to CDK6 or TCRA/D locus and deletions affecting WT1 and FBXW7 (TLX3)	[30, 107, 109]
Translocation to TCR loci or inversion to the IGH enhancer locus (NKXs)	[41]

Aberrant expression of TLX3 characterizes 25% of pediatric and 5% of adult T-ALLs and occurs as a result of its translocation to the enhancer region of BCL11B (Table 3.5) [106–108], a gene encoding a Zn-finger TF expressed in the course of T-cell commitment and upregulating several T-cell specific genes [117]. Other rare aberrations include translocation to CDK6 or the TCRA/D locus (Table 3.5). Other recurrent deletion events affect WT1 and FBXW7 [30, 107, 109]. TLX3 is not expressed in normal hematopoietic cells. TLX1 and TLX3 are closely related genes as demonstrated in unsupervised clustering analyses of transcriptome and epigenome datasets which positioned these genes close to each other [30, 33, 34, 41, 84]. Despite their substantial similarity, TLX1 or TLX3 have been reported to be associated with a differential clinical effect with T-ALLs carrying TLX1 rearrangements conferring a better prognosis than those with TLX3 rearrangements [103, 105, 118]. Another member of the TLX family, TLX2, is not expressed in normal thymocytes and is only rarely deregulated in T-ALLs [87, 119].

Aberrant expression of NKX2–1 and NKX2–2 characterize approx. 5% of pediatric T-ALLs whereas, NKX2–5 aberrations are only sporadically observed [41, 106]. None of these NKX family genes are expressed in normal T-cell development. However, they are involved in the development of the lung and the thyroid gland (NKX2–1), brain and pancreas (NKX2–2), and spleen and muscle (NKX2–5)

[120–122]. Upregulation of NKXs is driven by their translocation to T-cell receptor gene loci or by an inversion to the IGH enhancer locus (Table 3.5) [41]. NKX2–5 was also shown to be deregulated by juxtaposition to BCL11B in T-ALL cell lines [106]. NKX2–5 upregulation activates expression of MEF2C, myocyte enhancer factor, which is normally downregulated during T-cell maturation [41, 123]. Ectopic expression of MEF2C can block T-cell differentiation as well as inhibit BCL2-regulated apoptosis via repression of NR4A1 [123]. Similarly, aberrations of NKX2–1 and NKX2–2 genes also activate MEF2C expression [41]. Furthermore, MEF2C itself has appeared as an essential transcriptional oncogene, activated by alternative mechanisms such as deletions and translocations (discussed in more detail in the context of Type B abnormalities in the following section). Finally, NKX2–5 deregulation can cause cell survival through activation of NOTCH3 and cell proliferation through upregulation of miR-17-92 [124, 125].

3.3 Type B: Abnormalities Common in All Genetic Subgroups

In accordance with Alfred Knudson's two-hit hypothesis [126, 127], the development of leukemia requires additional genetic aberrations beyond the mutually exclusive chromosomal rearrangements discussed earlier. These aberrations can affect a wide range of protein families, such as transcription factors, cell cycle regulators, tumor suppressors, oncogenes, and proteins belonging to signaling pathways. They are present in all previously defined genetic subgroups, although not randomly, as some of these secondary aberrations are more prevalent in certain type-A subgroups. In addition to Knudson's concept of molecular evolution, recent studies have shown that single catastrophic events, such as chromothripsis, can also lead to the development of T-ALLs with a molecularly complex profile, likely without a long phase of prior molecular evolution [128, 129].

3.3.1 Oncogenic NOTCH1 Signaling

The NOTCH signaling pathway regulates interactions between physically adjacent cells, is evolutionarily conserved, and contributes to various aspects of development, including T-cell development [130–132]. It is essential to initiate the T-cell transcriptional machinery and lineage commitment, while proliferation and survival signals need to remain active during T-cell development [133, 134]. NOTCH1 is a transmembrane protein that is activated after binding of the ligands Jagged and Delta, expressed on the neighboring cells' surfaces. Proteolytic cleavage of NOTCH1, first by ADAM10 at its extracellular domain and then by γ-secretase at the intracellular domain, releases its activated intracellular NOTCH (ICN) domain, which then migrates to the nucleus and activates target genes expression [126, 127].

More than 70% of T-ALL patients harbor activating mutations of the NOTCH signaling pathway [31, 135, 136]. Despite being rare, two translocation events that juxtapose NOTCH1 to T-cell receptor loci TRAD or TRB were the first evidence of NOTCH1 contributing to T-cell leukemogenesis (Table 3.6) [137, 138]. NOTCH1 becomes constitutively active when it is translocated under the control of TCR enhancers. Three most abundant variants activate NOTCH signal-

Table 3.6 Main drivers of the activation of NOTCH signaling pathway

Major mechanisms leading to NKL activation	References
Translocation to TRAD or TRB loci resulting in constitutive expression of NOTCH1	[137, 138]
Somatic mutations or InDels at negative regulatory regions (esp. heterodimerization domain) resulting in constitutively active cleavage at the cell membrane	[139, 140]
Truncating PEST domain mutations resulting in increased stability of intracellular NOTCH (ICN)	[139, 140]
Inactivating mutations of the E3 ubiquitin ligase FBXW7 resulting in increased nuclear stability of intracellular NOTCH (ICN)	[141, 142]

ing. First, somatic mutations, insertions, or deletions at the negative regulatory region (NRR), particularly the heterodimerization domain of NOTCH1, induce its ligand-independent activation (Table 3.6) [139, 140]. As a result of NRR mutations, the NOTCH1 extracellular domain cannot be protected from cleavage by ADAM10 in the absence of ligand and becomes constitutively active. Second, truncating PEST domain mutations of NOTCH1 impair proteasomal degradation of intracellular NOTCH1, increase its half-life, and lead to constitutive activation of NOTCH signaling (Table 3.6) [139, 140]. Third, the NOTCH pathway can be activated by inactivating mutations of the E3 ubiquitin ligase FBXW7, which is responsible for mediating degradation of intracellular NOTCH1 (Table 3.6). As a result of deletions or loss-of-function (LoF) single-nucleotide variants (SNV) of FBXW7, intracellular NOTCH1 is stabilized in the nucleus [141, 142]. In addition, ectopic expression of delta-like ligand (DLL4) of NOTCH1 induced T-cell transformation in mice [143] and blockade of DLL4 in the microenvironment inhibited T-ALL growth and stimulated apoptosis in PDX mice [144].

Constitutively active NOTCH1 directly upregulates its target genes including MYC, CDKs, cyclin D3, p21, HES1, and PTCRA, which are involved in cell growth, proliferation, and anabolic pathways. More than 70% of NOTCH activating mutations are found in T-ALL patients harboring TLX1, TLX3, or NKX2–1 fusion genes [145]. Co-occurrence of mutations of the NOTCH negative regulatory region with NOTCH PEST domain or FBXW7 mutations are identified in >20% T-ALLs [136, 139]. Studies of transduced murine bone marrow cells with constitutively active forms of NOTCH1, showed different results; in some but not in others acute clonal leukemias were induced [146]. Additional aberrations need to be present for development of NOTCH1-induced T-ALL, such as loss of PHF6 or activation of KRAS [147, 148]. Unlike early evidence that NOTCH1 mutations can be early or leukemia initiating events [149], they are now considered to be acquired as late secondary events in leukemogenesis [150–153].

Because of the frequency of activating mutations and the prominent role of NOTCH signaling in T-cell differentiation, development, and proliferation, the predictive prognostic value of NOTCH1 has been extensively studied. When analyzing the results of different study groups, the prognostic effect of NOTCH1 activation has been variable. While in most studies a favorable effect on early treatment response has been found, improved long term outcome has been observed in some but not in other studies suggesting that the impact on NOTCH-pathway activation on long term outcome depends on (even subtle) differences of modern treatment protocols [136, 154–157]. Further, the favorable prognostic effect of NOTCH-activation can be counteracted by inactivation of the tumor suppressor PTEN [158], thus highlighting the complexity of molecular interactions even of a small number of oncogenes and tumor suppressor genes in T-ALL.

The frequency and the functional role of NOTCH1 pathway activation has spurred the development of NOTCH inhibitors for the treatment of T-ALL. The main categories of the small molecules tested in the NOTCH1-targeted therapy studies were (1) γ-Secretase inhibitors (GSI), (2) ADAM inhibitors, (3) monoclonal antibodies, (4) SERCA inhibitors and (5) other agents targeting NOTCH1. However, none of these candidates have so far been licensed to be used in clinical practice [159].

3.3.2 Cell Cycle Dysregulation Through Loss of CDKN2A and Other Regulators

Cyclin-dependent kinase inhibitor 2A (CDKN2A) encodes for two alternatively spliced transcripts; the p14 and p16 tumor suppressor genes. p14 (P14/ARF) induces apoptosis and cell cycle arrest during the transition from the G2 to the M phase by inhibiting MDM2, whose normal function is to induce ubiquitin-mediated degradation of p53 [160]. p16 (P16/INK4), on the other hand, leads to cell cycle arrest during the G1 phase by inhibiting CDK4/6, whose normal function is to phosphorylate RB, which then releases the E2F transcription factor, thus promoting entry into the S phase of cell cycle [160].

More than 70% of T-ALL patients harbor deletions of the CDKN2A/CDKN2B locus (9p21). Although less commonly, aberrations in other cell cycle regulators were also identified in T-ALL. Deletions of CDKN1B ($p27^{Kip1}$), which controls cell cycle progression at the G1 phase by preventing activation of cyclin E-CDK2 or cyclin D–CDK4 complexes, are present in 12% of a pediatric T-ALL cohort comprising 73 patients [161]. The frequency of 13q deletions targeting RB has been reported as 17% in an adult T-ALL cohort [95]. D-type cyclins CCND1, CCND2, and CCND3 are considered key regulators of G1-to-S transition by regulating cyclin-dependent kinases CDK4/6. Chromosomal translocation of CCND2 to T-cell receptor loci has been reported to result in its upregulation in 3/89 T-ALLs [162]. Moreover, mutations of CCND3 were found in 15 patients in a cohort of 264 pediatric and young adult T-ALLs [31].

3.3.3 Transcription Factor Oncogenes

Genes encoding transcription factors other than TALs, LMOs, or NKXs are also frequently mutated in T-ALL. However, these mutations do not define T-ALL genetic subtypes and therefore are categorized under type B abnormalities. First, transcription factors which function as oncogenes and then those functioning as tumor suppressors will be discussed.

3.3.3.1 MYC

MYC encodes a bHLH leucine zipper transcription factor that controls the expression of a broad range of genes involved in cell metabolism, ribosome biogenesis, DNA replication, cell cycle regulation, cell growth and proliferation [163]. MYC expression is dynamically regulated during T-cell differentiation, with increased expression at the DN3 to DN4 transition and reduced expression at the DP stage [163]. MYC is a direct NOTCH1 target and thus shares overlapping transcriptional targets of cell growth, proliferation, and self-renewal genes.

There are four main mechanisms which lead to MYC overexpression: (1) Activating mutations of NOTCH1 signaling also upregulate MYC expression [164]. (2) Loss-of-function mutations of FBXW7 stabilize and increase MYC protein levels because, similar to NOTCH1, proteasomal degradation of MYC is mediated by FBXW7 [165]. (3) In about 5% of T-ALLs, MYC upregulation results from a duplication of the T-cell-specific NOTCH1 MYC enhancer (N-Me) [166]. (4) In less than 1% of T-ALLs, chromosomal translocation which juxtaposes MYC and TCRA/D enhancer leads to its upregulation [167].

In a cohort of 196 pediatric and adult T-ALL patients, MYC translocations characterized a genetic subgroup of 6%, which were NOTCH1-independent and TAL/LMO driven [168]. In another smaller cohort of 25 pediatric T-ALLs, patients with MYC rearrangements represented a NOTCH1-independent subtype and were enriched for TAL/LMO activation. These T-ALLs frequently depended on PTEN deletions which will be discussed in Sect. 3.5.1 in more detail [169]. Strong oncogenic activity of MYC is confirmed in mouse and zebrafish leukemia models. Transgenic mice with constitutive MYC expression rapidly developed T-cell lymphoma of mature CD4+ CD8- T cells, a rarely seen malignancy in mouse models [170, 171]. Clonally derived T-ALL was induced in a transgenic zebrafish expressing mouse c-MYC under the control of the zebrafish RAG2 promoter [172].

3.3.3.2 MYB

MYB encodes a leucine zipper, a nuclear transcription factor that functions as a transcriptional activator and, rarely, as a repressor. MYB is a key factor in maintaining cell proliferation and survival during early hematopoiesis and is downregulated after lineage commitment [173].

First reported in 2007, MYB upregulation was found to be driven by the duplication of the whole MYB gene in 9/104 pediatric and adult T-ALL patients and in five T-ALL cell lines. MYB knockdown induced irreversible T-cell differentiation in the cell lines with MYB duplication but not in those without the duplication [174]. In the same year, a somatic duplication event and a translocation that juxtaposed the MYB and TCRB loci was reported. The translocation was frequently identified in young children (median age: 2.2 years) who showed a marked increase of cell proliferation and mitosis-related genes, whereas the duplication was found in association with other T-ALL subtypes [175]. MYB duplications occur at low frequency during normal thymopoiesis and are clonally selected during T-cell leukemogenesis [176]. A study in 2021 recapitulated that translocations occur rarely and only in children (3/331 patients) and duplications in both children and adults (14/331) [25]. Moreover, somatic mutations of MYB were found in 13/264 pediatric and young adults with T-ALL [31].

The TAL1 transcriptional complex directly activates the MYB oncogene and as a result, patients without MYB aberrations can also show MYB upregulation and are significantly enriched in the TAL/LMO subgroup [38, 60]. Other mechanisms which lead to overexpression of wild type MYB include downregulation of MYB-targeting microRNAs [177, 178] and posttranslational activation by the TAL1/miR-223/FBXW7 regulatory axis [60]. Moreover, an analysis of structural variants in single cells using Strand-seq revealed activation of the C-terminal domain of MYB (c-MYB) as a result of a subclonal chromothripsis event in one T-ALL patient [129].

3.3.3.3 SPI1 (PU.1)

SPI1 (PU.1) is a transcription factor that plays several roles during hematopoiesis mostly as an activator, occasionally as a repressor. SPI1 can regulate its target genes by directly binding to the promoter sequences or by changing the chromatin accessibility and recruiting the cofactors to the open chromatin regions [179]. It is expressed in the earliest stages of T-cell development and is sharply downregulated before any TCR-dependent steps, i.e., at the transition between DN2 and DN3 stages [179].

In a cohort of 181 children with T-ALL, 7 patients harbored new genomic rearrangements which juxtaposed SPI1 to the TCF7 or STMN1 loci driving its upregulation [135]. These patients showed a DN or CD8-single-positive immunophenotype, had unique gene expression profiles and a uniformly poor prognosis [135]. Constitutive SPI1 expression in mouse stem/progenitor cells induced proliferation and a differentiation block during DN3 transition [135]. SPI fusions alone are generally insufficient to drive leukemogenesis. However, a SPI1-TCF7 fusion together with activating NRAS mutations can drive an immature T-ALL in vivo using a mouse bone marrow transplant model [180].

Recently, 3/19 pediatric T-ALL patients were reported to be characterized by SPI1 overexpression and highly accessible SPI1 binding sites despite harboring a wild type copy of the gene [34]. These patients were deconvoluted to the DN2 stage of T-cell development in terms of their overall chromatin accessibility and showed distinct RNA expression profiles [34]. These results indicate that an increased accessibility of SPI1-binding motifs resulting in its overexpression may be an alternative mechanism leading to early developmental arrest.

3.3.3.4 MEF2C

Myocyte-specific enhancer factor 2C, Mef2c, is a MADS box transcription enhancer factor first identified to regulate muscle differentiation and to be essential for the development of other cell types such as cardiac lineage and neuronal cells [181]. Although HSCs and common myeloid and lymphoid progenitors (CMPs) show abundant expression, T cells virtually lack MEF2C expression [181].

As discussed in Sect. 2.2.2, MEF2C can be activated in T-cell leukemias as a result of aberrantly expressed NKL homeobox genes. MEF2C overexpression can also be driven by rearrangements and deletions in its promoter region [41] as well as by aberrations of its transcriptional activators and repressors [182]. A comprehensive study published in 2022 has shown that MEF2C upregulation blocks thymocyte differentiation by repressing the NOTCH-induced T-cell differentiation program while promoting the B-cell lineage program [183]. MEF2C has also been shown to induce IL-7R and BCL2 expression and to provide a survival advantage to an ETP-ALL cell line under limiting serum conditions [183]. MEF2C overexpression in murine progenitor cells blocked early T-cell differentiation and induced lymphoid tumors in mouse models [183]. Finally, salt-inducible kinase (SIK) inhibitors synergistically blocked MEF2C function and sensitized the cell line toward steroid treatment [183].

3.3.4 Transcription Factor Tumor Suppressors

3.3.4.1 BCL11B

Bcl11b is a zinc-finger transcription factor essential for T-cell lineage commitment, which does not occur until SPI1/PU.1 is downregulated and BCL11B is upregulated at the end of the DN2a stage. BCL11B is not expressed detectably in hematopoietic progenitors, whereas its expression is restricted to the post-commitment T-lineage and innate lymphoid cells [184]. BCL11B activation in T-cell precursors requires NOTCH signaling, TCF1, GATA3, and RUNX1 [185].

As discussed in Sect. 2.2.2, chromosomal translocations that juxtapose TLX3 or NKX2–5 genes to the BCL11B enhancer locus, at the cost of losing BCL11B expression, are characteristic of the NKL homeobox subgroup of T-ALL. In addition, somatic loss-of-function mutations or deletions of BCL11B are identified in 9–16% of T-ALL patients and in 30% of ETP patients [115, 186]. Loss-of-function studies in mouse models revealed that BCL11B regulates T-lineage commitment through upregulating T-lineage genes and downregulating stem, natural killer (NK), and myeloid genes [187]. Its inactivation in murine T-cell progenitors led to developmental arrest at the DN2 stage as well to promote aberrant self-renewal activity [188, 189].

Recently, allele-specific upregulation of BCL11B characterized a distinct subtype of ETPs and of acute leukemias of ambiguous lineage (ALAL) expressing myeloid, T lymphoid, and stem cell markers. This upregulation was driven by either (1) translocations that repositioned BCL11B to super-enhancers active in hematopoietic progenitors or (2) amplifications that generated a super-enhancer from a noncoding distal element [81]. Also, activating mutations of FLT3 were found in 80% BCL11B-activated ALAL and co-expression with BCL11B in HSPCs conferred self-renewal properties and blocked myeloid differentiation [81]. In a cohort of 915 AML and ALL patients, four types of translocations were identified, which led to the activation of BCL11B. BCL11B overexpression behaved as a disease marker that was identified at initial diagnosis and relapse but not at remission [42]. Patients with BCL11B upregulation showed a distinct RNA expression signature and were sensitive to tyrosine kinases and JAK/STAT inhibitors [42]. BCL11B-activated ETPs ALLs are a defined entity of the ICC of ALL [29].

3.3.4.2 RUNX1

Runx family transcription factors are highly conserved and involved in the development of diverse cell types including hematopoietic lineage cells. During hematopoietic differentiation RUNX1 functions as a transcriptional activator of a large number of genes including TCRs, cytokines, and cytokine receptors which regulate HSC fate, differentiation, and function. Depending on its cofactor interactions, RUNX1 can also function as a transcriptional repressor [190–192]. It can also act as an epigenetic regulator through mediating the increase in chromatin accessibility [193].

As discussed in Sect. 3.1, RUNX1 is one of the cofactors of transcriptional complexes formed by TAL and LMO type transcription factors. Therefore, it can be deregulated as a result of chromosomal rearrangements involving TAL and LMO genes. In addition, RUNX1 can also be deregulated by somatic mutations. In a cohort of 128 ALLs, 15 patients (13 T-ALL and 2 B-ALL) harbored 17 different RUNX1 mutations, which were associated with higher age and poor prognosis [194]. A reverse engineering approach analyzing global transcriptional networks of T-ALLs induced by TLX1 and TLX3 identified RUNX1 as a key mediator of leukemogenesis [195].

Moreover, heterozygous germline mutations in RUNX1 cause familial platelet disorder, which is inherited in an autosomal dominant fashion and is characterized by thrombocytopenia and predisposition to AML and T-ALL [196–198].

3.3.4.3 WT1

WT1 is a tumor suppressor TF playing an essential role in normal development of the urogenital system. Experiments with WT1-deficient mouse embryonic stem cells showed reduced hematopoietic potential caused by VEGF-dependent apoptosis of hematopoietic progenitor cells [199, 200].

Deletions and loss-of-function mutations in WT1 are found in ~10% of T-ALLs [201–204]. These mutations are mostly heterozygous frameshifts and are preferentially found in patients with TLX1, TLX3 or HOXA rearrangements [201, 202, 204]. Loss of WT1 conferred resistance to DNA damaging agents through attenuating the TP53-induced DNA damage response and through upregulating the apoptosis inhibitor XIAP [205]. Although WT1 mutations were reported not to signify poor prognosis in T-ALL [201, 202], they were associated with an inferior relapse-free survival in others [203, 205].

3.3.4.4 LEF1

LEF1 is a central transcriptional mediator of Wnt signaling, whose precisely controlled level of activation is essential for self-renewal, survival, development, and proliferation of hematopoietic stem cells [206]. Eight out of 91 pediatric T-ALL patients were identified with mutations and monoallelic or biallelic deletions of LEF1 gene at the time of diagnosis [207]. Patients with LEF1 inactivation showed increased expression of MYC and MYC target genes, as well as differentiation arrest at the early cortical stage [207]. In another cohort of 264 pediatric and young adults with T-ALLs, LEF1 mutations were most common in NKX2–1 rearranged patients [31].

3.3.4.5 GATA3

GATA3 is a member of a family of highly conserved zinc-finger transcription factors. It is involved in the transcriptional regulatory complexes of TAL and LMO genes discussed in Sect. 3.1, which are required for the development of early T-cell progenitors. Loss-of-function mutations disrupting its DNA-binding domain were identified exclusively in six ETP-ALL patients [89].

3.3.4.6 ETV6

ETV6 is a member of ETS family transcription factors and plays complex roles in hematopoietic stem cell differentiation and maturation [208, 209]. With a diverse range of aberrations including deletions, translocations, and somatic mutations, ETV6 is one of the most recurrently deregulated genes in hematological malignancies [210]. However, ETV6 mutations were only reported in 10 T-ALL patients, all of whom had an immature immunophenotype, in a cohort of 82 adult patients [208].

3.3.5 Oncogenic Activation of Signaling Pathways and Cellular Processes

Genetic aberrations leading to deregulation of transcription factors playing key roles in normal hematopoiesis frequently affect the activity of signaling pathways and cellular processes which are discussed below.

3.3.5.1 PI3K/AKT/mTOR Pathway

The phosphoinositide 3-kinase (PI3K), one of the most recurrent constitutively activated pathways in T-ALL, plays a key role in cell survival, proliferation, differentiation, apoptosis, and migration [211]. This pathway is normally activated by binding of growth factors to G protein-coupled receptors (GPCRs) and receptor tyrosine kinase (RTKs) [212]. PI3K phosphorylates and mediates activation of downstream effectors, one of which is AKT, which then either directly (GSK-3β, FOXO1, Bad, TSC2) or indirectly (mTOR) induces anti-apoptotic and proliferative signals [213]. The phosphatase PTEN inhibits the first step of the PI3K/AKT/mTOR pathway by dephosphorylating PIP3 to PIP2 [214]. During normal T-cell development, PI3K/AKT signaling is necessary to translate signals from the pre-TCR, NOTCH, and IL-7R into functional outcomes [215]. Inactivation of this pathway in mouse models results in a block of T-cell differentiation at the β-selection stage [216, 217].

With 30–40% frequency, constitutive activation of PI3K/AKT pathway is highly prevalent among T-ALLs [31] and mainly driven by deletions or loss-of-function mutations of PTEN, the main negative regulator of this pathway [186, 218]. Deletions and LoFs frequently occur in exon 7, which results in truncation and subsequent degradation of the protein [186, 218]. Further, deletion of a distal enhancer that interacts with the PTEN promoter was reported in 5/398 T-ALLs [219]. PTEN inactivation can also be induced by nongenetic mechanisms, such as CK2-mediated phosphorylation and reactive oxygen species-induced oxidation [220]. In a cohort of 212 adult T-ALL patients, PTEN mutations were almost exclusively associated with the TAL/LMO subgroup, and to co-occur with NOTCH1/FBXW7 mutations [221]. Alternative but less frequent mechanisms (overall ~2%) of activation of PI3K/AKT/mTOR signaling include activating mutations in AKT1, in the genes encoding the PIKC3A and PIK3CD catalytic and regulatory subunits of the PI3K complex [31, 222, 223] and a translocation inducing overexpression of IRS4, an AKT activator [224, 225].

Interestingly, in patients with NOTCH-activated T-ALL and PTEN inactivation the favorable treatment response that is typically seen in this type of T-ALL is antagonized [158]. Consistent with this observation, PTEN abnormalities have been associated with an increased risk of relapse [226] and a poor outcome [227] [161, 222, 228]. Recently, a child with Short syndrome harboring germline PIK3R1 mutations developed T-ALL at the age of 13 years. Leukemic blasts additionally acquired a PTEN deletion and a SIL-TAL1 fusion, conceptionally supporting the close cooperation between the TAL/LMO regulatory complex and the PI3K/AKT pathway [229].

Activation of AKT and inactivation of PTEN in hematopoietic progenitors or in early/late thymocytes induced T-ALL in mouse models [230–233]. Constitutive activation of PI3K/AKT/mTOR signaling is widespread and its inhibition in T-ALL cell lines, mouse models, and PDXs induced apoptosis and suppressed tumor growth [233–237]. Further, PTEN mutations were associated with glucocorticoid (GC) resistance in T-ALL patients [158], and PTEN loss and AKT activation induced GC resistance in mouse models [236]. Inhibition of the PI3K/AKT/mTOR axis has been shown to reverse GC resistance in T-ALL cell lines and mouse models [236, 238].

3.3.5.2 IL-7R and JAK/STAT Signaling

Interleukin 7 (IL-7) is produced by stromal cells in the bone marrow. The IL-7-Receptor is a heterodimeric receptor composed of IL-7Rα and IL-7Rγc chains which are essential for normal hematopoiesis and T-cell development [239]. Binding of IL-7 to its receptor induces phosphorylation of JAK1 and JAK3, which then phosphorylate STAT5 [239]. Activated STAT5 translocates to the nucleus where it transcriptionally regulates expression of its target genes, including Bcl-2, Bcl-XL, CyclinA, CyclinD2, and $p27^{kip}$, which are all involved in the regulation of cell proliferation, growth, and survival [239]. In addition to JAK/STAT, IL-7 binding to the receptor induces activation of PI3K/AKT and RAS/MAPK signaling pathways, whose anti-apoptotic and proliferative roles in T-ALL are discussed in the previous and following section, respectively [240].

Activation of IL-7R-mediated signaling was identified in 25% of patients in a cohort of 264 pediatric and young adult T-ALLs [31]. Its activation may occur in all subtypes, however, is enriched in HOXA and TLX subgroups [31, 241–243] and in ETP-ALLs (47% of cases) [89, 244]. Moreover, a negative association was observed between the TAL/LMO subgroup and activation of IL-7R signaling [243], which is in line with the results indicating that TAL1 may directly repress IL-7R [245].

With about 10%, somatic gain-of-function of IL-7Rα represents the most frequent mechanism activating IL-7R signaling. These mutations result in homodimerization of IL-7Rα subunits

[243]. Homodimerization then leads to ligand-independent, constitutive activation of the IL-7R-mediated signaling pathway, which induces cell transformation in vitro and tumor formation in vivo [89, 243, 246–248]. IL-7R-mediated signaling can also be activated by the gain of function mutations in its downstream effectors, namely, JAK1, JAK3, and STAT5B in 5–10% of T-ALLs [249–252]. In addition to gain-of-function mutations inactivation of negative regulators of this network have also been identified: (1) Inactivating mutations of PTPN2, a tyrosine phosphatase and negative regulator of STATs, were found in 6% T-ALLs [253]. (2) Inactivation of DNM2 was shown to impair endocytosis of the IL-7R, thus causing increased receptor density on the surface of leukemic cells [254]. (3) SH2B3, also known as lymphocyte adapter protein LNK, was found to be inactivated and to accelerate the development of NOTCH-induced T-ALL in mice [89, 255]. Moreover, NOTCH1, one of the most recurrently activated genes in T-ALL (discussed in detail in Sect. 4.1), is known to bind to the IL-7R promoter and to regulate its transcription and IL-7Rα expression [139, 256]. Finally, mutations in RPL10, a ribosomal protein gene (see Sect. 3.7. for details), promotes IL-7Rα expression and the components of downstream JAK/STAT signaling [257].

In addition to activation of the IL-7R, mutations of downstream effectors can also confer leukemogenic potential. A JAK3 kinase domain mutant induced a long-latency T-ALL in mice [258]. Treatment with tofacitinib, a JAK3-selective inhibitor, reduced white blood cell counts and resulted in apoptosis of leukemic cells [258]. Inhibition of JAK1/2 by ruxolitinib showed antileukemic activity in patient-derived xenograft models of ETP-ALL [259]. Expression of mutant JAK3 and HOXA9, whose overexpression co-occurs with JAK3 mutations, led to rapid development of leukemia with decrease in latency in mice [101]. Phosphoproteomic profiling identified key regulatory proteins of PI3K/Akt, RAS/MAPK and apoptotic signaling pathways to be significantly phosphorylated upon activating JAK3 in lymphocytes. JAK3-mutant T-ALLs showed increased sensitivity to combined treatment by tofacitinib and venetoclax, a Bcl2 inhibitor, in vitro and in vivo [260]. Moreover, a recurrent translocation targeting ZEB2, a zinc-finger E-box-binding TF, was identified in ETP-ALL and ZEB2 overexpression in mouse model induced ETP-like ALL together with transcriptional activation of IL-7-R and increased JAK/STAT signaling [244].

Notably, in a cohort of 12 patients, overexpression of IL-7R has been identified exclusively in patients ($n = 5$) who developed a type-1 relapse, which is characterized by the clonal evolution of major clone present at the time of initial diagnosis [33]. Although one out of five patients carried an activating IL-7R mutation, upregulation of components of the JAK/STAT pathway (IL-7R itself, its ligand HGF and SOCS1/2/3) has been identified, which possibly had a compensatory effect in the remaining four patients [33].

3.3.5.3 Ras/MAPK Pathway

The Ras/MAPK signaling pathway transmits extracellular signals to the cell nucleus where the expression of cell growth, proliferation, and survival genes are stimulated. Activation of the Ras signaling pathway is induced upon T-cell receptor stimulation and is of critical importance during T-cell differentiation [261].

In pediatric T-ALL, genetic aberrations that activate Ras/MAPK signaling are more prevalent at the time of relapse (~40%) than of first diagnosis (~15%) [204, 262]. Mechanisms of activation can be grouped into (1) inactivating mutations of negative regulators of the Ras pathway including NF1 and PTPN11 [263, 264], (2) hotspot mutations in NRAS, KRAS, and BRAF [95, 262] or (3) gain of function mutations of an upstream gene including FLT3 [95, 262, 263].

Ras pathway mutations are associated with resistance to chemotherapy and a poor overall survival [204, 262, 264]. Such mutations predict resistance to methotrexate in mouse and human mutant Ras-expressing leukemia cells but also improved the response to vincristine, demonstrating a previously unrecognized dual role of Ras mutations as drivers of both sensitivity and resistance to chemotherapy [264]. Moreover, Ras pathway mutated leukemias showed significant differential sensitivity to a mitogen-activated protein kinase inhibitor selumetinib, when compared with nonactivated ALL both in vivo and in vitro [262].

3.3.5.4 ABL Kinase

ABL1 encodes a ubiquitously expressed protein tyrosine kinase that is involved in cell division, adhesion, differentiation, and survival. Abl kinases are required for linking pre-T-cell receptor signaling to the activation of downstream genes, as well as for modulating T-cell development in mice [265, 266].

ABL1 is found to be activated in ~6% of T-ALL patients as a result of amplified episomes formed by extrachromosomal circularization of the DNA fragment between NUP214 and ABL1 genes [267]. BCR-ABL1, ETV6-ABL, and EML1-ABL1 fusion genes were also sporadically reported in T-ALL [267–271]. The NUP214-ABL1 fusion gene was identified almost exclusively in TLX1 or TLX3 subgroups of pediatric and adult T-ALLs harboring CDKN2A deletions and/or NOTCH mutations [267, 272]. PTPN2 was identified as a negative regulator of NUP214-ABL1 and was specifically deleted in TLX1-driven T-ALLs [253].

Although these data suggest that ABL fusion events are weak leukemia driving factors which need to be accompanied by additional mutations, they induce sensitivity to selected tyrosine kinase inhibitors (TKi), such as imatinib and dasatinib [273, 274]. ABL-class fusion events sporadically observed in T-ALL were also shown to be associated with clinical TKi sensitivity in ALL [275]. Activity of LCK, a member of the SRC family kinase, has been reported to be required for the proliferation and survival of T-ALL cells with a NUP214-ABL1 fusion [276]. LCK/calcineurin signaling axis is also particularly active in pediatric ETP-ALLs [277] and in T-ALLs with a prednisone poor response [278]. Notably, glucocorticoid resistance in the xenograft samples derived from these poor responders could be reversed by LCK inhibitors [278].

3.3.6 Aberrations in Epigenetic Regulators

3.3.6.1 PHF6

PHF6, located on the X chromosome, encodes a nucleolar protein implicated in chromatin remodeling through its interaction with the nucleosome remodeling and deacetylation (NuRD) complex [279]. It was shown to interact with upstream binding factor (UBF) and to suppress ribosomal RNA synthesis [280]. PHF6 also interacts with the PAF1 transcription complex in the control of neuronal migration in the brain [281]. Germline mutations of PHF6 cause the rare X-linked mental disability disorder Börjeson–Forssman–Lehmann syndrome (BFLS) [279–281].

Inactivating mutations and deletions of PHF6 were identified in ~16% (14/89) of pediatric and ~ 38% (16/42) of adult T-ALLs, almost exclusively in males, and were enriched within the TLX1 and TLX3 subgroups [31, 282]. A significant positive correlation between mutations in IL-7R/JAK signaling genes and in PHF6, as well as members of the PRC2 complex was identified [242]. A male BFLS patient developed T-ALL at the age of 7, indicating a cancer predisposing role for PHF6 [283]. An in vivo study revealed that PHF6 is an early mutational event in leukemia transformation. Its knockout in mice enhanced HSC long-term self-renewal and hematopoietic recovery after chemotherapy, and favored the development of NOTCH-induced T-ALL [148].

3.3.6.2 PRC2 Complex Genes EZH2, EED, and SUZ12

EZH2, EED, and SUZ12 encode the subunits of polycomb repressive complex 2 (PRC2), which is a major epigenetic regulator of transcriptional repression with methyltransferase activity toward lysine 27 on histone 3 (H3K27) [284]. (Loss-of-function mutations or deletions in one of these PRC2 complex genes were found in 25% of T-ALLs in a cohort of 68 adult patients [285] and have been reported to be particularly common in ETP-ALLs (42%) [89, 286]. Aberrations in PRC2 core components were found to be associated with mitochondrial-mediated apoptosis resistance in primary T-ALLs [287].

Functional consequences of loss of EZH2 have been more widely studied than other PRC2 components. Inactivation of EZH2 or EED was found to cooperate with oncogenic NRAS and with CDKN2A deletions to accelerate development of ETP-like ALL in a mouse model [288]. Another in vivo study showed that combined inactivation of EZH2 and RUNX1 in early lymphoid progenitors leads to expansion of preleukemic ETPs, which generated acute lymphomyeloid leukemia when combined with a FLT3 mutation, thus activating the RAS signaling pathway [289]. Loss of H3K27me3 caused by PRC2 inactivation has also been proposed to induce T-ALL through increased FLT3 transcription [286]. Loss of EZH2 in a *p53*-null mouse model induces ETP-ALL-like disease in mice, as well as DNA hypermethylation and CpG island promoter regions, leading to repression of critical T-cell differentiation genes like RUNX1 and BCL11B [290]. One study reported a reciprocal and complex association between PRC2 deficiency and CpG island hypermethylation profile in T-ALL [291]. Finally, similar to PHF6, inactivation of SUZ12 was found to cooperate with JAK3 mutant signaling to drive T-ALL development with increased PI3K/mTOR, VEGF, and WNT signaling in mice. JAK3/SUZ12 mutant leukemia cells showed increased sensitivity to histone deacetylase (HDAC) inhibitors [292].

3.3.6.3 KDM6A (UTX)

KDM6A (also known as UTX) is an X-linked epigenetic regulator with H3K27me3 demethylase activity and plays an important role in HOX gene regulation and animal body patterning [293]. KDM6A was shown to function as a tumor suppressor and to harbor loss-of-function mutations in 5–15% of T-ALLs [294, 295]. In a T-ALL cohort of 35 pediatric and adult patients (10 female and 25 male), inactivating KDM6A mutations were restricted to males (5/25) [295]. KDM6A escaped X-inactivation in female T-ALL blasts and in normal T cells, giving protection to females against loss of single copy of the gene [295]. Moreover, loss of KDM6A in a mouse model contributed to T-ALL that exhibited sensitivity to H3K37me3 inhibition [295]. Hypothetically, involvement of X-linked tumor suppressor genes such as PHF6 and KDM6A in T-ALL development may contribute to the skewed gender distribution of T-ALL toward males.

3.3.7 Ribosomal Proteins and Translation Regulators

Ribosomal proteins represent the structural components of the ribosome and are essential for ribosome assembly and function. They are among the most highly conserved proteins across all life forms [296]. In a cohort of 122 pediatric T-ALL patients, 12 (~10%) were identified with mutations affecting the ribosomal proteins RPL5 and RPL10 [297, 298]. In another cohort of 264 pediatric and young adults with T-ALL, 16 patients (6%) harbored RPL10 mutations that were enriched in NKX-subgroup [31].

Yeast and lymphoid cells carrying the RPL10 R98S mutation, the most prevalent in T-ALL, showed defects of ribosome biogenesis [297]. Experiments with transgenic mice and T-ALL xenograft models uncovered that JAK-STAT hyperactivation is induced upon cytokine stimulation in RPL10 R98S expressing cells [257]. T-ALL cells harboring RPL10 R98S mutations obtained a survival advantage under oxidative stress by mediating antiapoptotic BCL2 overexpression [299]. In addition, 7/89 adult T-ALL patients harbored mutations in CNOT3, a major cellular mRNA deadenylase whose knockdown caused tumors in a sensitized *Drosophila melanogaster* model [297]. Lastly, two contiguous genes involved in regulating RNA maturation and translation, SYNCRIP and SNHG5, were affected due to the deletion of 6q14 in 34/107 TAL1-driven T-ALL patients. Combined silencing of both genes in Tal1/Lmo1/Notch1-driven mouse model accelerated leukemogenesis [300]. Therefore, as is known for other ribosomopathies including those resulting in bone marrow failure and cancer predisposition [301], disturbance of the complex mechanism contributing to ribosomal function also contributes to T-ALL.

3.4 T-ALL Classification by the Stage of Developmentally Arrested T Cells

Although unique gene expression profiles are used to classify T-ALLs into genetic subgroups [36], immunophenotyping reflecting developmental arrest of differentiating thymocytes has been performed for decades and is still used for the classification of T-ALLs [33]. While some immunophenotypes, notably ETP-ALL and cortical T-ALL, have been linked to adverse and favorable prognosis, respectively [34, 302], it should be noted that immunophenotypic differences are insufficient to explain the prognostic significance of molecular-genetic and cytogenetic aberrations [303]. In fact, immunophenotypic classification of T-ALLs is losing its prognostic significance with modern MRD-based risk stratification and chemotherapy protocols, which could potentially be tailored to genetic aberrations in the future [304]. However, T-cell-specific surface markers, such as CD7 and CD1a, have recently emerged as potential targets for immunotherapy of resistant and relapsed T-ALL [305, 306], indicating the potential usefulness of immunophenotyping in designing innovative therapy.

3.4.1 Mature/Late Cortical T-ALL

T-ALLs with a characteristic CD3+, CD4+, and CD8+ immunophenotype, corresponding to late cortical stages of T-cell differentiation, are associated with activation of the TAL1 transcription factor (Fig. 3.1) [30]. Developmental arrest of TAL/LMO-driven T-ALLs at the late cortical stage is reflected by their gene expression profile, presenting upregulation of LCK, TCRA, TCRB, CD2, CD6, and CD3E [46, 307]. Although several early studies have reported that TAL-driven cortical T-ALLs show a good treatment response and a favorable prognosis [118, 308, 309], it has been shown that TAL rearrangements are related with poor outcome [22, 29, 310, 311]. As discussed in detail in previous paragraphs, genetic aberrations associated with the TAL/LMO subgroup include MYC translocations [168, 169], PTEN inactivating mutations [221, 229], 6q14-q16 deletions [300], and a low incidence of NOTCH1 mutations [168, 169].

3.4.2 Cortical and Early-Cortical T-ALL

T-ALLs with a characteristic of CD1a+, CD4+, and CD8+ immunophenotype, corresponding to

T-cell differentiation		Subtype	Frequency	Prognosis	Partner genes/other rearrangements	Common co-lesions
	Early T-cell progenitor (ETP)	BCL11B-activated	30% of ETP and T/M MPAL		BCL11B Enhancer Tandem Amplification at 14q32, ARID1B, CCDC26/ MYC, CDK6, STAB1, ETV6, ZEB2, RUNX1	FLT3-ITD, WT1
Double negative (DN)		LMO1/2-R	LMO1-R 5% LMO2-R 10%		TCR , cryptic deletion, enhancer/promoter mutations in LMO complex with bHLH factors	CDKN2A, NOTCH1, FBXW7, PTEN, LEF1
		HOXA	15–25%		HOXA::TCRB/TCRG , KMT2A-R, PICALM::MLLT10, SET::NUP214	
T-lineage commitment		SPI1-R	< 5%, pediatric	Very poor	STMN1, TCF7, BCL11B	NRAS, KRAS
β-selection	Early cortical	TLX3-R	20-25%, pediatric <5%, adult	Good	TCR , BCL11B, CDK6	CDKN2A, NOTCH1, FBXW7, PTEN
Double positive (DP)		TLX1-R	5-10%, pediatric <30%, adult	Good	TCR	PHF6, DNM2, BCL11B, RB1, CDKN1B
	Late cortical	NKX2-R	< 5%, pediatric		NKX2.1/NKX2.2/NKX2.5::TCR, BCL11B, CDK6	CDKN2A, NOTCH1, PHF6, LEF1, RPL10
		TAL1/2-R	30-40% of T-ALL TAL2 rare	Poor	TCRA/D, TCRB (TAL2), 1p32 deletion (STIL), intergenic SNV generating a TAL1-dergulating superenhancer	CDKN2A, NOTCH1, PTEN, USP7
		BHLH, other	<2%		TCRB::LYL1 TCR::BHLHB1, high LMO expression	

Fig. 3.1 The progression of events during T-cell maturation and most recent classification of T-ALLs according to genetic aberrations and stage of T-cell developmental arrest. Adapted from Duffield et al. [29] and Iacobucci et al. [22] (other than BCL11B-activated, all are provisional)

early cortical stages of T-cell differentiation, are associated with activation of TLX1, TLX3 or NKX2–1 homeobox genes (Fig. 3.1) [30]. Analyses of large pediatric and adult T-ALLs revealed that TLX1-driven T-ALLs result in better treatment outcome than other genetic subtypes [80, 105, 312, 313]. TLX/NKX subgroups have the highest frequency of NOTCH1 alterations and almost always harbor CDKN2A deletions [24, 31]. Other genetic aberrations associated with the TLX/NKX rearranged subgroup and early-cortical developmental arrest have been discussed in previous sections, include BCL11B rearrangements [115, 116], RPL10 mutations [31], NUP214-ABL1 fusion gene [267, 272, 314], and LEF1 mutations [31].

3.4.3 Immature/Early T-Cell Precursor ALL

Immature/Early T-cell precursor ALLs are recognized by a distinct and diverse gene expression profile and immunophenotype (Fig. 3.1). They are characterized by the lack of rearranged TCR and IG-genes, expression of cytoplasmic CD3 and CD7, at least one stem cell marker (CD34 or CD117) and/or myeloid markers (CD13, CD33, HLA-DE, CD11b, CD65) and no expression of CD1a, CD4, and CD8, as well as weak CD5 [27, 28]. In addition, near-ETP ALL has been defined by fulfilling ETP-ALL criteria but with normal CD5 expression [31]. ETP-ALL accounts for 40–50% of adult T-ALLs [95, 208, 315], whereas it is less prevalent in children with ~10% frequency [27, 28, 315]. ETPs have been initially classified as high-risk with chemotherapy resistance and poor prognosis [94, 95]. However, recent studies showed that the poor prognosis can be neutralized in modern treatment protocols [316, 317]. Similarly, comparative and/or retrospective analyses of ETP- and non-ETP-ALL patients have recently revealed that prognosis and outcome of patients in these two groups are similar [96–100].

Despite the commonalities in the expression of CD surface markers, ETP-ALLs exhibit a high degree of heterogeneity in their genomic and transcriptomic profiles, with aberrations and deregulations of various genes/pathways. Intriguingly, NOTCH1 activating mutations and CDKN2A loss-of-function mutations, which are the most common aberrations in T-ALL, are underrepresented in ETP-ALLs [24, 89, 145, 208]. Rearrangements and aberrant expression of HOXA cluster genes are found in almost half of the immature/early T-ALL subgroup [30, 83, 84, 87]. Activation of transcription enhancer factor MEF2C [41, 183, 318] and lack of BCL11B expression [319] are also characteristically observed in this subgroup. BCL11B-activated ETP-ALL has recently become one of the new ICC subgroups [29]. HOXA, MEF2C, and BCL11B aberrations altogether account for approximately half of ETP-ALLs [25].

Deletions or loss-of-function mutations in epigenetic regulators (EZH2, EED, SUZ12, SETD2, DNMT3A, IDH1/2) and in transcription factors regulating hematopoiesis and T-cell development (RUNX1, ETV6, and GATA3) are all associated with ETP-ALL [89, 208, 302]. As discussed in Sect. 3.5.4, LoF mutations in GATA3 were identified exclusively in ETP-ALL patients [89]. Activation of the JAK/STAT and of the RAS/MAPK pathways caused by aberrations of IL-7R, JAK1/3, and ZEB2 or by aberrations of NRAS, HRAS, KRAS, FLT3, and BRAF, respectively, are particularly prevalent in ETP-ALLs [31, 89, 259]. Other genetic aberrations associated with ETP-ALLs include SPI1 (PU.1) fusions, KMT2A rearrangements, PICALM-MLLT10 and SET-NUP214 fusion genes [31, 89, 135].

3.5 The Role of Cancer Predisposition in T-ALL

There is growing evidence that constitutional mutations in cancer predisposition genes (CPG) contribute to approximately 10% of all childhood malignancies [303, 304, 320, 321]. With the aim of identifying the role of predisposing constitutional variants in T-ALL, a recent study performed multi-omics analyses in 38 matched pairs of T-ALLs collected at the time of first diagnosis, remission, and relapse [33]. Profiles of SNVs and InDels derived from whole-exome sequencing (WES) data identified 18/38 patients with type-1 relapse [33] as characterized by all clonal mutations (AF > 30%) being preserved at relapse [322]. On the other hand, 20/38 patients were classified as type-2 [33], which is characterized by the major clone found at first diagnosis having been eradicated and the relapse having evolved from a minor ancestral clone [322].

At the time of relapse both types had acquired either mutations or an increased mRNA expression of known and novel drivers of multidrug resistance including NT5C2, MDR1 and MVP, and JAK/STAT activators [33]. Only T-ALLs later developing into type-1 relapse were characterized by overexpression of IL7-R [33]. When compared to type-2 relapses, type-1 relapses tend to remain more stable in their mutational spectrum, promoter methylation, and gene expression profile. Similarly, their chromatin accessibility profiles were more homogeneous predominantly resembling a single early normal T-cell population [33]. In marked contrast, T-ALLs later developing into type-2 relapse have typically undergone stronger chromatin remodeling as indicated by more complex chromatin accessibility profiles resembling a mixture of normal T-cell precursors already at the time of first diagnosis [33]. Type-2 relapses were also characterized by enrichment of somatic hypermutator phenotypes and constitutional mutations in cancer predisposition genes [33].

Although none of the type-1 patients were found to carry constitutional mutations in genes implicated in cancer predisposition, 7/20 type-2 patients were identified with nine constitutional heterozygous mutations in DNA repair and tumor suppressor genes. Comparison of the frequency of CPG mutations in remission samples of relapsing and nonrelapsing T-ALL patients did not indicate a significant difference between two groups in terms of gaining a higher risk of relapse [33]. Likewise, comparison of frequencies in noncancer and relapsing T-ALL patients showed an even distribution, indicating that the presence of constitutional CPG variants does not confer a higher risk of developing T-ALL [33]. This study has concluded that the constitutional mutations in CPGs are likely to shape the type of T-ALL relapse toward type 2 instead of type1 but do not increase the overall risk of developing T-ALL or a T-ALL relapse [33]. This was in line with the finding that type-2 relapses were more heterogeneous in terms of epi−/genetic profiles and have undergone extensive epi−/genetic remodeling during evolution to relapse, a process which could have been facilitated by constitutional variants in cancer predisposition genes [33].

3.6 Closing Remarks

The analysis of mutational, epigenomic, and transcriptomic profiles has revealed numerous leukemogenic mechanisms in pediatric and adult T-ALL. However, this gain of knowledge has only translated into the development of new treatment strategies for a minority of molecularly defined subgroups, and overall treatment outcome has not improved, particularly in resistant and relapsed T-ALL where the clinical need is dire. Several factors must be considered when accounting for this lack of correlation between biological insight and clinical progress. These include the specific effect of treatment on molecularly defined abnormalities, the weak correlation between mutational, epigenomic, and transcriptomic profiles and the cellular proteome, and protein activity [323, 324]. Further, many studies have not placed specific emphasis on the subclonal architecture of leukemias and the combinatorial effects of different leukemogenic mechanisms, which likely impact the effectiveness of targeted treatment strategies. Future studies will have to address these and very likely other parameters more directly, a challenge given the complex biology of the disease and the regulatory restrictions on clinical studies.

References

1. Greaves MF, Janossy G, Peto J, Kay H. Immunologically defined subclasses of acute lymphoblastic leukaemia in children: their relationship to presentation features and prognosis. Br J Haematol. 1981;48:179–97.
2. Thiel E. Cell surface markers in leukemia: biological and clinical correlations. Crit Rev Oncol Hematol. 1985;2:209–60.
3. Pui CH, Evans WE. Treatment of acute lymphoblastic leukemia. N Engl J Med. 2006;354:166–78.
4. Pui CH, Robison LL, Look AT. Acute lymphoblastic leukaemia. Lancet. 2008;371:1030–43.
5. Vrooman LM, Silverman LB. Childhood acute lymphoblastic leukemia: update on prognostic factors. Curr Opin Pediatr. 2009;21:1–8.
6. Hunger SP, Lu X, Devidas M, Camitta BM, Gaynon PS, Winick NJ, Reaman GH, Carroll WL. Improved survival for children and adolescents with acute lymphoblastic leukemia between 1990 and 2005: a report from the children's oncology group. J Clin Oncol. 2012;30:1663–9.
7. Conter V, Valsecchi MG, Parasole R, Putti MC, Locatelli F, Barisone E, Lo Nigro L, Santoro N, Arico M, Ziino O, Pession A, Testi AM, Micalizzi C, Casale F, Zecca M, Casazza G, Tamaro P, La Barba G, Notarangelo LD, Silvestri D, Colombini A, Rizzari C, Biondi A, Masera G, Basso G. Childhood high-risk acute lymphoblastic leukemia in first remission: results after chemotherapy or transplant from the AIEOP ALL 2000 study. Blood. 2014;123:1470–8.
8. Huguet F, Leguay T, Raffoux E, Thomas X, Beldjord K, Delabesse E, Chevallier P, Buzyn A, Delannoy A, Chalandon Y, Vernant JP, Lafage-Pochitaloff M, Chassevent A, Lheritier V, Macintyre E, Bene MC, Ifrah N, Dombret H. Pediatric-inspired therapy in adults with Philadelphia chromosome-negative acute lymphoblastic leukemia: the GRAALL-2003 study. J Clin Oncol. 2009;27:911–8.
9. Marks DI, Paietta EM, Moorman AV, Richards SM, Buck G, DeWald G, Ferrando A, Fielding AK, Goldstone AH, Ketterling RP, Litzow MR, Luger SM, McMillan AK, Mansour MR, Rowe JM, Tallman MS, Lazarus HM. T-cell acute lymphoblastic leukemia in adults: clinical features, immunophenotype, cytogenetics, and outcome from the large randomized prospective trial (UKALL XII/ECOG 2993). Blood. 2009;114:5136–45.
10. Stock W, Johnson JL, Stone RM, Kolitz JE, Powell BL, Wetzler M, Westervelt P, Marcucci G, DeAngelo DJ, Vardiman JW, McDonnell D, Mrozek K, Bloomfield CD, Larson RA. Dose intensification of daunorubicin and cytarabine during treatment of adult acute lymphoblastic leukemia: results of cancer and leukemia group B study 19802. Cancer. 2013;119:90–8.
11. Uderzo C, Dini G, Locatelli F, Miniero R, Tamaro P. Treatment of childhood acute lymphoblastic leukemia after the first relapse: curative strategies. Haematologica. 2000;85:47–53.
12. Einsiedel HG, von Stackelberg A, Hartmann R, Fengler R, Schrappe M, Janka-Schaub G, Mann G, Hahlen K, Gobel U, Klingebiel T, Ludwig WD, Henze G. Long-term outcome in children with relapsed ALL by risk-stratified salvage therapy: results of trial acute lymphoblastic leukemia-relapse study of the Berlin-Frankfurt-Munster group 87. J Clin Oncol. 2005;23:7942–50.
13. Tallen G, Ratei R, Mann G, Kaspers G, Niggli F, Karachunsky A, Ebell W, Escherich G, Schrappe M, Klingebiel T, Fengler R, Henze G, von Stackelberg A. Long-term outcome in children with relapsed acute lymphoblastic leukemia after time-point and site-of-relapse stratification and intensified short-course multidrug chemotherapy: results of trial ALL-REZ BFM 90. J Clin Oncol. 2010;28:2339–47.
14. Hof J, Krentz S, van Schewick C, Korner G, Shalapour S, Rhein P, Karawajew L, Ludwig WD, Seeger K, Henze G, von Stackelberg A, Hagemeier C, Eckert C, Kirschner-Schwabe R. Mutations and deletions of the TP53 gene predict nonresponse to treatment and poor outcome in first relapse of childhood acute lymphoblastic leukemia. J Clin Oncol. 2011;29:3185–93.
15. Sutton R, Shaw PJ, Venn NC, Law T, Dissanayake A, Kilo T, Haber M, Norris MD, Fraser C, Alvaro F, Revesz T, Trahair TN, Dalla-Pozza L, Marshall GM, O'Brien TA. Persistent MRD before and after allogeneic BMT predicts relapse in children with acute lymphoblastic leukaemia. Br J Haematol. 2015;168:395–404.
16. Schrappe M, Valsecchi MG, Bartram CR, Schrauder A, Panzer-Grumayer R, Moricke A, Parasole R, Zimmermann M, Dworzak M, Buldini B, Reiter A, Basso G, Klingebiel T, Messina C, Ratei R, Cazzaniga G, Koehler R, Locatelli F, Schafer BW, Arico M, Welte K, van Dongen JJ, Gadner H, Biondi A, Conter V. Late MRD response determines relapse risk overall and in subsets of childhood T-cell ALL: results of the AIEOP-BFM-ALL 2000 study. Blood. 2011;118:2077–84.
17. Teachey DT, Hunger SP. Predicting relapse risk in childhood acute lymphoblastic leukaemia. Br J Haematol. 2013;162:606–20.
18. Pui CH, Pei D, Raimondi SC, Coustan-Smith E, Jeha S, Cheng C, Bowman WP, Sandlund JT, Ribeiro RC, Rubnitz JE, Inaba H, Gruber TA, Leung WH, Yang JJ, Downing JR, Evans WE, Relling MV, Campana D. Clinical impact of minimal residual disease in children with different subtypes of acute lymphoblastic leukemia treated with response-adapted therapy. Leukemia. 2017;31:333–9.
19. O'Connor D, Enshaei A, Bartram J, Hancock J, Harrison CJ, Hough R, Samarasinghe S, Schwab C, Vora A, Wade R, Moppett J, Moorman AV, Goulden N. Genotype-specific minimal residual disease interpretation improves stratification in pediat-

ric acute lymphoblastic leukemia. J Clin Oncol. 2018;36:34–43.
20. Gianni F, Belver L, Ferrando A. The genetics and mechanisms of T-cell acute lymphoblastic leukemia. Cold Spring Harb Perspect Med. 2020;10:a035246.
21. Inaba H, Mullighan CG. Pediatric acute lymphoblastic leukemia. Haematologica. 2020;105:2524–39.
22. Iacobucci I, Kimura S, Mullighan CG. Biologic and therapeutic implications of genomic alterations in acute lymphoblastic leukemia. J Clin Med. 2021;10
23. Van Vlierberghe P, Pieters R, Beverloo HB, Meijerink JP. Molecular-genetic insights in paediatric T-cell acute lymphoblastic leukaemia. Br J Haematol. 2008;143:153–68.
24. La Starza R, Pierini V, Pierini T, Nofrini V, Matteucci C, Arniani S, Moretti M, Lema Fernandez AG, Pellanera F, Di Giacomo D, Storlazzi TC, Vitale A, Gorello P, Sammarelli G, Roti G, Basso G, Chiaretti S, Foa R, Schwab C, Harrison CJ, Van Vlierberghe P, Mecucci C. Design of a comprehensive fluorescence in situ hybridization assay for genetic classification of T-cell acute lymphoblastic leukemia. J Mol Diagn. 2020;22:629–39.
25. Bardelli V, Arniani S, Pierini V, Di Giacomo D, Pierini T, Gorello P, Mecucci C, La Starza R. T-cell acute lymphoblastic leukemia: biomarkers and their clinical usefulness. Genes (Basel). 2021;12
26. Bene MC, Castoldi G, Knapp W, Ludwig WD, Matutes E, Orfao A, van't Veer MB. Proposals for the immunological classification of acute leukemias. European Group for the Immunological Characterization of Leukemias (EGIL). Leukemia. 1995;9:1783–6.
27. Coustan-Smith E, Mullighan CG, Onciu M, Behm FG, Raimondi SC, Pei D, Cheng C, Su X, Rubnitz JE, Basso G, Biondi A, Pui CH, Downing JR, Campana D. Early T-cell precursor leukaemia: a subtype of very high-risk acute lymphoblastic leukaemia. Lancet Oncol. 2009;10:147–56.
28. Inukai T, Kiyokawa N, Campana D, Coustan-Smith E, Kikuchi A, Kobayashi M, Takahashi H, Koh K, Manabe A, Kumagai M, Ikuta K, Hayashi Y, Tsuchida M, Sugita K, Ohara A. Clinical significance of early T-cell precursor acute lymphoblastic leukaemia: results of the Tokyo children's cancer study group study L99-15. Br J Haematol. 2012;156:358–65.
29. Duffield AS, Mullighan CG, Borowitz MJ. International consensus classification of acute lymphoblastic leukemia/lymphoma. Virchows Arch. 2023;482:11–26.
30. Ferrando AA, Neuberg DS, Staunton J, Loh ML, Huard C, Raimondi SC, Behm FG, Pui CH, Downing JR, Gilliland DG, Lander ES, Golub TR, Look AT. Gene expression signatures define novel oncogenic pathways in T cell acute lymphoblastic leukemia. Cancer Cell. 2002;1:75–87.
31. Liu Y, Easton J, Shao Y, Maciaszek J, Wang Z, Wilkinson MR, McCastlain K, Edmonson M, Pounds SB, Shi L, Zhou X, Ma X, Sioson E, Li Y, Rusch M, Gupta P, Pei D, Cheng C, Smith MA, Auvil JG, Gerhard DS, Relling MV, Winick NJ, Carroll AJ, Heerema NA, Raetz E, Devidas M, Willman CL, Harvey RC, Carroll WL, Dunsmore KP, Winter SS, Wood BL, Sorrentino BP, Downing JR, Loh ML, Hunger SP, Zhang J, Mullighan CG. The genomic landscape of pediatric and young adult T-lineage acute lymphoblastic leukemia. Nat Genet. 2017;49:1211–8.
32. Mansour MR, Abraham BJ, Anders L, Berezovskaya A, Gutierrez A, Durbin AD, Etchin J, Lawton L, Sallan SE, Silverman LB, Loh ML, Hunger SP, Sanda T, Young RA, Look AT. Oncogene regulation. An oncogenic super-enhancer formed through somatic mutation of a noncoding intergenic element. Science. 2014;346:1373–7.
33. Richter-Pechanska P, Kunz JB, Rausch T, Erarslan-Uysal B, Bornhauser B, Frismantas V, Assenov Y, Zimmermann M, Happich M, von Knebel-Doeberitz C, von Neuhoff N, Kohler R, Stanulla M, Schrappe M, Cario G, Escherich G, Kirschner-Schwabe R, Eckert C, Avigad S, Pfister SM, Muckenthaler MU, Bourquin JP, Korbel JO, Kulozik AE. Pediatric T-ALL type-1 and type-2 relapses develop along distinct pathways of clonal evolution. Leukemia. 2022;36:1759–68.
34. Erarslan-Uysal B, Kunz JB, Rausch T, Richter-Pechanska P, van Belzen IA, Frismantas V, Bornhauser B, Ordonez-Rueada D, Paulsen M, Benes V, Stanulla M, Schrappe M, Cario G, Escherich G, Bakharevich K, Kirschner-Schwabe R, Eckert C, Loukanov T, Gorenflo M, Waszak SM, Bourquin JP, Muckenthaler MU, Korbel JO, Kulozik AE. Chromatin accessibility landscape of pediatric T-lymphoblastic leukemia and human T-cell precursors. EMBO Mol Med. 2020;12:e12104.
35. Richter-Pechanska P, Kunz JB, Bornhauser B, von Knebel Doeberitz C, Rausch T, Erarslan-Uysal B, Assenov Y, Frismantas V, Marovca B, Waszak SM, Zimmermann M, Seemann J, Happich M, Stanulla M, Schrappe M, Cario G, Escherich G, Bakharevich K, Kirschner-Schwabe R, Eckert C, Muckenthaler MU, Korbel JO, Bourquin JP, Kulozik AE. PDX models recapitulate the genetic and epigenetic landscape of pediatric T-cell leukemia. EMBO Mol Med. 2018;10
36. Murre C. Helix-loop-helix proteins and lymphocyte development. Nat Immunol. 2005;6:1079–86.
37. Porcher C, Chagraoui H, Kristiansen MS. SCL/TAL1: a multifaceted regulator from blood development to disease. Blood. 2017;129:2051–60.
38. Sanda T, Lawton LN, Barrasa MI, Fan ZP, Kohlhammer H, Gutierrez A, Ma W, Tatarek J, Ahn Y, Kelliher MA, Jamieson CH, Staudt LM, Young RA, Look AT. Core transcriptional regulatory circuit controlled by the TAL1 complex in human T cell acute lymphoblastic leukemia. Cancer Cell. 2012;22:209–21.
39. Rabbitts TH. Chromosomal translocations in human cancer. Nature. 1994;372:143–9.

40. Wadman I, Li J, Bash RO, Forster A, Osada H, Rabbitts TH, Baer R. Specific in vivo association between the bHLH and LIM proteins implicated in human T cell leukemia. EMBO J. 1994;13:4831–9.
41. Homminga I, Pieters R, Langerak AW, de Rooi JJ, Stubbs A, Verstegen M, Vuerhard M, Buijs-Gladdines J, Kooi C, Klous P, van Vlierberghe P, Ferrando AA, Cayuela JM, Verhaaf B, Beverloo HB, Horstmann M, de Haas V, Wiekmeijer AS, Pike-Overzet K, Staal FJ, de Laat W, Soulier J, Sigaux F, Meijerink JP. Integrated transcript and genome analyses reveal NKX2-1 and MEF2C as potential oncogenes in T cell acute lymphoblastic leukemia. Cancer Cell. 2011;19:484–97.
42. Di Giacomo D, La Starza R, Gorello P, Pellanera F, Kalender Atak Z, De Keersmaecker K, Pierini V, Harrison CJ, Arniani S, Moretti M, Testoni N, De Santis G, Roti G, Matteucci C, Bassan R, Vandenberghe P, Aerts S, Cools J, Bornhauser B, Bourquin JP, Piazza R, Mecucci C. 14q32 rearrangements deregulating BCL11B mark a distinct subgroup of T-lymphoid and myeloid immature acute leukemia. Blood. 2021;138:773–84.
43. Kelliher MA, Seldin DC, Leder P. Tal-1 induces T cell acute lymphoblastic leukemia accelerated by casein kinase IIalpha. EMBO J. 1996;15:5160–6.
44. Condorelli GL, Facchiano F, Valtieri M, Proietti E, Vitelli L, Lulli V, Huebner K, Peschle C, Croce CM. T-cell-directed TAL-1 expression induces T-cell malignancies in transgenic mice. Cancer Res. 1996;56:5113–9.
45. O'Neil J, Shank J, Cusson N, Murre C, Kelliher M. TAL1/SCL induces leukemia by inhibiting the transcriptional activity of E47/HEB. Cancer Cell. 2004;5:587–96.
46. Terstappen LW, Huang S, Picker LJ. Flow cytometric assessment of human T-cell differentiation in thymus and bone marrow. Blood. 1992;79:666–77.
47. Begley CG, Aplan PD, Davey MP, Nakahara K, Tchorz K, Kurtzberg J, Hershfield MS, Haynes BF, Cohen DI, Waldmann TA, et al. Chromosomal translocation in a human leukemic stem-cell line disrupts the T-cell antigen receptor delta-chain diversity region and results in a previously unreported fusion transcript. Proc Natl Acad Sci USA. 1989;86:2031–5.
48. Bernard O, Guglielmi P, Jonveaux P, Cherif D, Gisselbrecht S, Mauchauffe M, Berger R, Larsen CJ, Mathieu-Mahul D. Two distinct mechanisms for the SCL gene activation in the t(1;14) translocation of T-cell leukemias. Genes Chromosomes Cancer. 1990;1:194–208.
49. Chen Q, Yang CY, Tsan JT, Xia Y, Ragab AH, Peiper SC, Carroll A, Baer R. Coding sequences of the tal-1 gene are disrupted by chromosome translocation in human T cell leukemia. J Exp Med. 1990;172:1403–8.
50. Aplan PD, Lombardi DP, Ginsberg AM, Cossman J, Bertness VL, Kirsch IR. Disruption of the human SCL locus by "illegitimate" V-(D)-J recombinase activity. Science. 1990;250:1426–9.
51. Navarro JM, Touzart A, Pradel LC, Loosveld M, Koubi M, Fenouil R, Le Noir S, Maqbool MA, Morgado E, Gregoire C, Jaeger S, Mamessier E, Pignon C, Hacein-Bey-Abina S, Malissen B, Gut M, Gut IG, Dombret H, Macintyre EA, Howe SJ, Gaspar HB, Thrasher AJ, Ifrah N, Payet-Bornet D, Duprez E, Andrau JC, Asnafi V, Nadel B. Site- and allele-specific polycomb dysregulation in T-cell leukaemia. Nat Commun. 2015;6:6094.
52. Mellentin JD, Smith SD, Cleary ML. Lyl-1, a novel gene altered by chromosomal translocation in T cell leukemia, codes for a protein with a helix-loop-helix DNA binding motif. Cell. 1989;58:77–83.
53. Xia Y, Brown L, Yang CY, Tsan JT, Siciliano MJ, Espinosa R 3rd, Le Beau MM, Baer RJ. TAL2, a helix-loop-helix gene activated by the (7;9)(q34;q32) translocation in human T-cell leukemia. Proc Natl Acad Sci USA. 1991;88:11416–20.
54. Wang J, Jani-Sait SN, Escalon EA, Carroll AJ, de Jong PJ, Kirsch IR, Aplan PD. The t(14;21)(q11.2;q22) chromosomal translocation associated with T-cell acute lymphoblastic leukemia activates the BHLHB1 gene. Proc Natl Acad Sci USA. 2000;97:3497–502.
55. Homminga I, Vuerhard MJ, Langerak AW, Buijs-Gladdines J, Pieters R, Meijerink JP. Characterization of a pediatric T-cell acute lymphoblastic leukemia patient with simultaneous LYL1 and LMO2 rearrangements. Haematologica. 2012;97:258–61.
56. Park ST, Sun XH. The Tal1 oncoprotein inhibits E47-mediated transcription. Mechanism of inhibition. J Biol Chem. 1998;273:7030–7.
57. Nottingham WT, Jarratt A, Burgess M, Speck CL, Cheng JF, Prabhakar S, Rubin EM, Li PS, Sloane-Stanley J, Kong ASJ, de Bruijn MF. Runx1-mediated hematopoietic stem-cell emergence is controlled by a Gata/Ets/SCL-regulated enhancer. Blood. 2007;110:4188–97.
58. Liau WS, Tan SH, Ngoc PCT, Wang CQ, Tergaonkar V, Feng H, Gong Z, Osato M, Look AT, Sanda T. Aberrant activation of the GIMAP enhancer by oncogenic transcription factors in T-cell acute lymphoblastic leukemia. Leukemia. 2017;31:1798–807.
59. Tan SH, Yam AW, Lawton LN, Wong RW, Young RA, Look AT, Sanda T. TRIB2 reinforces the oncogenic transcriptional program controlled by the TAL1 complex in T-cell acute lymphoblastic leukemia. Leukemia. 2016;30:959–62.
60. Mansour MR, Sanda T, Lawton LN, Li X, Kreslavsky T, Novina CD, Brand M, Gutierrez A, Kelliher MA, Jamieson CH, von Boehmer H, Young RA, Look AT. The TAL1 complex targets the FBXW7 tumor suppressor by activating miR-223 in human T cell acute lymphoblastic leukemia. J Exp Med. 2013;210:1545–57.
61. Kusy S, Gerby B, Goardon N, Gault N, Ferri F, Gerard D, Armstrong F, Ballerini P, Cayuela JM, Baruchel A, Pflumio F, Romeo PH. NKX3.1 is a

direct TAL1 target gene that mediates proliferation of TAL1-expressing human T cell acute lymphoblastic leukemia. J Exp Med. 2010;207:2141–56.
62. Leong WZ, Tan SH, Ngoc PCT, Amanda S, Yam AWY, Liau WS, Gong Z, Lawton LN, Tenen DG, Sanda T. ARID5B as a critical downstream target of the TAL1 complex that activates the oncogenic transcriptional program and promotes T-cell leukemogenesis. Genes Dev. 2017;31:2343–60.
63. McGuire EA, Hockett RD, Pollock KM, Bartholdi MF, O'Brien SJ, Korsmeyer SJ. The t(11;14)(p15;q11) in a T-cell acute lymphoblastic leukemia cell line activates multiple transcripts, including Ttg-1, a gene encoding a potential zinc finger protein. Mol Cell Biol. 1989;9:2124–32.
64. Boehm T, Foroni L, Kaneko Y, Perutz MF, Rabbitts TH. The rhombotin family of cysteine-rich LIM-domain oncogenes: distinct members are involved in T-cell translocations to human chromosomes 11p15 and 11p13. Proc Natl Acad Sci USA. 1991;88:4367–71.
65. Royer-Pokora B, Loos U, Ludwig WD. TTG-2, a new gene encoding a cysteine-rich protein with the LIM motif, is overexpressed in acute T-cell leukaemia with the t(11;14)(p13;q11). Oncogene. 1991;6:1887–93.
66. Li Z, Abraham BJ, Berezovskaya A, Farah N, Liu Y, Leon T, Fielding A, Tan SH, Sanda T, Weintraub AS, Li B, Shen S, Zhang J, Mansour MR, Young RA, Look AT. APOBEC signature mutation generates an oncogenic enhancer that drives LMO1 expression in T-ALL. Leukemia. 2017;31:2057–64.
67. Rahman S, Magnussen M, Leon TE, Farah N, Li Z, Abraham BJ, Alapi KZ, Mitchell RJ, Naughton T, Fielding AK, Pizzey A, Bustraan S, Allen C, Popa T, Pike-Overzet K, Garcia-Perez L, Gale RE, Linch DC, Staal FJT, Young RA, Look AT, Mansour MR. Activation of the LMO2 oncogene through a somatically acquired neomorphic promoter in T-cell acute lymphoblastic leukemia. Blood. 2017;129:3221–6.
68. Van Vlierberghe P, van Grotel M, Beverloo HB, Lee C, Helgason T, Buijs-Gladdines J, Passier M, van Wering ER, Veerman AJ, Kamps WA, Meijerink JP, Pieters R. The cryptic chromosomal deletion del(11)(p12p13) as a new activation mechanism of LMO2 in pediatric T-cell acute lymphoblastic leukemia. Blood. 2006;108:3520–9.
69. Van Vlierberghe P, Beverloo HB, Buijs-Gladdines J, van Wering ER, Horstmann M, Pieters R, Meijerink JP. Monoallelic or biallelic LMO2 expression in relation to the LMO2 rearrangement status in pediatric T-cell acute lymphoblastic leukemia. Leukemia. 2008;22:1434–7.
70. Morishima T, Krahl AC, Nasri M, Xu Y, Aghaallaei N, Findik B, Klimiankou M, Ritter M, Hartmann MD, Gloeckner CJ, Stefanczyk S, Lindner C, Oswald B, Bernhard R, Hahnel K, Hermanutz-Klein U, Ebinger M, Handgretinger R, Casadei N, Welte K, Andre M, Muller P, Bajoghli B, Skokowa J. LMO2 activation by deacetylation is indispensable for hematopoiesis and T-ALL leukemogenesis. Blood. 2019;134:1159–75.
71. Draheim KM, Hermance N, Yang Y, Arous E, Calvo J, Kelliher MA. A DNA-binding mutant of TAL1 cooperates with LMO2 to cause T cell leukemia in mice. Oncogene. 2011;30:1252–60.
72. McCormack MP, Young LF, Vasudevan S, de Graaf CA, Codrington R, Rabbitts TH, Jane SM, Curtis DJ. The Lmo2 oncogene initiates leukemia in mice by inducing thymocyte self-renewal. Science. 2010;327:879–83.
73. McCormack MP, Shields BJ, Jackson JT, Nasa C, Shi W, Slater NJ, Tremblay CS, Rabbitts TH, Curtis DJ. Requirement for Lyl1 in a model of Lmo2-driven early T-cell precursor ALL. Blood. 2013;122:2093–103.
74. Gerby B, Tremblay CS, Tremblay M, Rojas-Sutterlin S, Herblot S, Hebert J, Sauvageau G, Lemieux S, Lecuyer E, Veiga DF, Hoang T. SCL, LMO1 and Notch1 reprogram thymocytes into self-renewing cells. PLoS Genet. 2014;10:e1004768.
75. Hacein-Bey-Abina S, de Saint Basile G, Cavazzana-Calvo M. Gene therapy of X-linked severe combined immunodeficiency. Methods Mol Biol. 2003;215:247–59.
76. Hacein-Bey-Abina S, Garrigue A, Wang GP, Soulier J, Lim A, Morillon E, Clappier E, Caccavelli L, Delabesse E, Beldjord K, Asnafi V, MacIntyre E, Dal Cortivo L, Radford I, Brousse N, Sigaux F, Moshous D, Hauer J, Borkhardt A, Belohradsky BH, Wintergerst U, Velez MC, Leiva L, Sorensen R, Wulffraat N, Blanche S, Bushman FD, Fischer A, Cavazzana-Calvo M. Insertional oncogenesis in 4 patients after retrovirus-mediated gene therapy of SCID-X1. J Clin Invest. 2008;118:3132–42.
77. Howe SJ, Mansour MR, Schwarzwaelder K, Bartholomae C, Hubank M, Kempski H, Brugman MH, Pike-Overzet K, Chatters SJ, de Ridder D, Gilmour KC, Adams S, Thornhill SI, Parsley KL, Staal FJ, Gale RE, Linch DC, Bayford J, Brown L, Quaye M, Kinnon C, Ancliff P, Webb DK, Schmidt M, von Kalle C, Gaspar HB, Thrasher AJ. Insertional mutagenesis combined with acquired somatic mutations causes leukemogenesis following gene therapy of SCID-X1 patients. J Clin Invest. 2008;118:3143–50.
78. Mark M, Rijli FM, Chambon P. Homeobox genes in embryogenesis and pathogenesis. Pediatr Res. 1997;42:421–9.
79. Alharbi RA, Pettengell R, Pandha HS, Morgan R. The role of HOX genes in normal hematopoiesis and acute leukemia. Leukemia. 2013;27:1000–8.
80. Homminga I, Pieters R, Meijerink JP. NKL homeobox genes in leukemia. Leukemia. 2012;26:572–81.
81. Montefiori LE, Bendig S, Gu Z, Chen X, Polonen P, Ma X, Murison A, Zeng A, Garcia-Prat L, Dickerson K, Iacobucci I, Abdelhamed S, Hiltenbrand R, Mead PE, Mehr CM, Xu B, Cheng Z, Chang TC, Westover T, Ma J, Stengel A, Kimura S, Qu C, Valentine MB,

Rashkovan M, Luger S, Litzow MR, Rowe JM, den Boer ML, Wang V, Yin J, Kornblau SM, Hunger SP, Loh ML, Pui CH, Yang W, Crews KR, Roberts KG, Yang JJ, Relling MV, Evans WE, Stock W, Paietta EM, Ferrando AA, Zhang J, Kern W, Haferlach T, Wu G, Dick JE, Klco JM, Haferlach C, Mullighan CG. Enhancer hijacking drives oncogenic BCL11B expression in lineage-ambiguous stem cell leukemia. Cancer Discov. 2021;11:2846–67.

82. Dadi S, Le Noir S, Payet-Bornet D, Lhermitte L, Zacarias-Cabeza J, Bergeron J, Villarese P, Vachez E, Dik WA, Millien C, Radford I, Verhoeyen E, Cosset FL, Petit A, Ifrah N, Dombret H, Hermine O, Spicuglia S, Langerak AW, Macintyre EA, Nadel B, Ferrier P, Asnafi V. TLX homeodomain oncogenes mediate T cell maturation arrest in T-ALL via interaction with ETS1 and suppression of TCRalpha gene expression. Cancer Cell. 2012;21:563–76.
83. Ferrando AA, Armstrong SA, Neuberg DS, Sallan SE, Silverman LB, Korsmeyer SJ, Look AT. Gene expression signatures in MLL-rearranged T-lineage and B-precursor acute leukemias: dominance of HOX dysregulation. Blood. 2003;102:262–8.
84. Soulier J, Clappier E, Cayuela JM, Regnault A, Garcia-Peydro M, Dombret H, Baruchel A, Toribio ML, Sigaux F. HOXA genes are included in genetic and biologic networks defining human acute T-cell leukemia (T-ALL). Blood. 2005;106:274–86.
85. Speleman F, Cauwelier B, Dastugue N, Cools J, Verhasselt B, Poppe B, Van Roy N, Vandesompele J, Graux C, Uyttebroeck A, Boogaerts M, De Moerloose B, Benoit Y, Selleslag D, Billiet J, Robert A, Huguet F, Vandenberghe P, De Paepe A, Marynen P, Hagemeijer A. A new recurrent inversion, inv(7)(p15q34), leads to transcriptional activation of HOXA10 and HOXA11 in a subset of T-cell acute lymphoblastic leukemias. Leukemia. 2005;19:358–66.
86. Bergeron J, Clappier E, Cauwelier B, Dastugue N, Millien C, Delabesse E, Beldjord K, Speleman F, Soulier J, Macintyre E, Asnafi V. HOXA cluster deregulation in T-ALL associated with both a TCRD-HOXA and a CALM-AF10 chromosomal translocation. Leukemia. 2006;20:1184–7.
87. Van Vlierberghe P, van Grotel M, Tchinda J, Lee C, Beverloo HB, van der Spek PJ, Stubbs A, Cools J, Nagata K, Fornerod M, Buijs-Gladdines J, Horstmann M, van Wering ER, Soulier J, Pieters R, Meijerink JP. The recurrent SET-NUP214 fusion as a new HOXA activation mechanism in pediatric T-cell acute lymphoblastic leukemia. Blood. 2008;111:4668–80.
88. Dik WA, Brahim W, Braun C, Asnafi V, Dastugue N, Bernard OA, van Dongen JJ, Langerak AW, Macintyre EA, Delabesse E. CALM-AF10+ T-ALL expression profiles are characterized by overexpression of HOXA and BMI1 oncogenes. Leukemia. 2005;19:1948–57.
89. Zhang J, Ding L, Holmfeldt L, Wu G, Heatley SL, Payne-Turner D, Easton J, Chen X, Wang J, Rusch M, Lu C, Chen SC, Wei L, Collins-Underwood JR, Ma J, Roberts KG, Pounds SB, Ulyanov A, Becksfort J, Gupta P, Huether R, Kriwacki RW, Parker M, McGoldrick DJ, Zhao D, Alford D, Espy S, Bobba KC, Song G, Pei D, Cheng C, Roberts S, Barbato MI, Campana D, Coustan-Smith E, Shurtleff SA, Raimondi SC, Kleppe M, Cools J, Shimano KA, Hermiston ML, Doulatov S, Eppert K, Laurenti E, Notta F, Dick JE, Basso G, Hunger SP, Loh ML, Devidas M, Wood B, Winter S, Dunsmore KP, Fulton RS, Fulton LL, Hong X, Harris CC, Dooling DJ, Ochoa K, Johnson KJ, Obenauer JC, Evans WE, Pui CH, Naeve CW, Ley TJ, Mardis ER, Wilson RK, Downing JR, Mullighan CG. The genetic basis of early T-cell precursor acute lymphoblastic leukaemia. Nature. 2012;481:157–63.
90. Bond J, Bergon A, Durand A, Tigaud I, Thomas X, Asnafi V, Spicuglia S, Macintyre E. Cryptic XPO1-MLLT10 translocation is associated with HOXA locus deregulation in T-ALL. Blood. 2014;124:3023–5.
91. Brandimarte L, Pierini V, Di Giacomo D, Borga C, Nozza F, Gorello P, Giordan M, Cazzaniga G, Te Kronnie G, La Starza R, Mecucci C. New MLLT10 gene recombinations in pediatric T-acute lymphoblastic leukemia. Blood. 2013;121:5064–7.
92. Bond J, Marchand T, Touzart A, Cieslak A, Trinquand A, Sutton L, Radford-Weiss I, Lhermitte L, Spicuglia S, Dombret H, Macintyre E, Ifrah N, Hamel JF, Asnafi V. An early thymic precursor phenotype predicts outcome exclusively in HOXA-overexpressing adult T-cell acute lymphoblastic leukemia: a Group for Research in adult acute lymphoblastic leukemia study. Haematologica. 2016;101:732–40.
93. Meijerink JP, Cante-Barrett K, Vroegindeweij E, Pieters R. HOXA-activated early T-cell progenitor acute lymphoblastic leukemia: predictor of poor outcome? Haematologica. 2016;101:654–6.
94. Gutierrez A, Dahlberg SE, Neuberg DS, Zhang J, Grebliunaite R, Sanda T, Protopopov A, Tosello V, Kutok J, Larson RS, Borowitz MJ, Loh ML, Ferrando AA, Winter SS, Mullighan CG, Silverman LB, Chin L, Hunger SP, Sallan SE, Look AT. Absence of Biallelic TCRγ deletion predicts early treatment failure in pediatric T-cell acute lymphoblastic leukemia. J Clin Oncol. 2010;28:3816–23.
95. Van Vlierberghe P, Ambesi-Impiombato A, De Keersmaecker K, Hadler M, Paietta E, Tallman MS, Rowe JM, Forne C, Rue M, Ferrando AA. Prognostic relevance of integrated genetic profiling in adult T-cell acute lymphoblastic leukemia. Blood. 2013;122:74–82.
96. Zhang Y, Qian J-J, Zhou Y-L, Huang X, Li J-H, Li X-Y, Li C-Y, Wang H-P, Lou Y-J, Meng H-T, Yu W-J, Tong H-Y, Jin J, Zhu H-H. Comparison of early T-cell precursor and non-ETP subtypes among 122 Chinese adults with acute lymphoblastic leukemia. Front Oncol. 2020;10
97. Morita K, Jain N, Kantarjian H, Takahashi K, Fang H, Konopleva M, El Hussein S, Wang F, Short NJ,

Maiti A, Sasaki K, Garcia-Manero G, Konoplev S, Ravandi F, Khoury JD, Jabbour E. Outcome of T-cell acute lymphoblastic leukemia/lymphoma: focus on near-ETP phenotype and differential impact of nelarabine. Am J Hematol. 2021;96:589–98.
98. Yoon J-H, Kim HS, Min GJ, Park S-S, Park S, Lee S-E, Cho B-S, Eom K-S, Kim Y-J, Kim H-J, Min C-K, Cho S-G, Lee JW, Kim M, Kim Y, Lee S. Cytogenetic and molecular characteristics and outcomes of adult patients with early T-cell precursor acute lymphoblastic leukemia. Eur J Haematol. 2023;110:137–48.
99. Chen J, Liu L, Ma R, Pang A, Yang D, Chen X, Wei J, He Y, Zhang R, Zhai W, Ma Q, Jiang E, Han M, Feng S. Comparison of characteristics and outcomes on ETP-ALL/LBL and non-ETP ALL patients receiving allogeneic hematopoietic stem cell transplantation. Front Oncol. 2022;12:1025885.
100. Onishi Y, Furukawa E, Kamata M, Fukatsu M, Kameoka Y, Hatta S, Hamada H, Oyake T, Kai T, Sukegawa M, Nakajima S, Yanagiya R, Yamaguchi K, Takahashi T, Harazaki Y, Izumi T, Murai K, Ito S, Ikezoe T, Ishizawa K, Takahashi N, Harigae H. Outcomes of adult patients with early T-cell precursor (ETP) acute lymphoblastic leukemia/lymphoma (ALL) and non-ETP T-ALL. Int J Hematol. 2023;
101. de Bock CE, Demeyer S, Degryse S, Verbeke D, Sweron B, Gielen O, Vandepoel R, Vicente C, Vanden Bempt M, Dagklis A, Geerdens E, Bornschein S, Gijsbers R, Soulier J, Meijerink JP, Heinaniemi M, Teppo S, Bouvy-Liivrand M, Lohi O, Radaelli E, Cools J. HOXA9 cooperates with activated JAK/STAT signaling to drive leukemia development. Cancer Discov. 2018;8:616–31.
102. Nagel S. The role of NKL Homeobox genes in T-cell malignancies. Biomedicines. 2021;9
103. Kees UR, Heerema NA, Kumar R, Watt PM, Baker DL, La MK, Uckun FM, Sather HN. Expression of HOX11 in childhood T-lineage acute lymphoblastic leukaemia can occur in the absence of cytogenetic aberration at 10q24: a study from the children's cancer group (CCG). Leukemia. 2003;17: 887–93.
104. Berger R, Dastugue N, Busson M, Van Den Akker J, Pérot C, Ballerini P, Hagemeijer A, Michaux L, Charrin C, Pages MP, Mugneret F, Andrieux J, Talmant P, Hélias C, Mauvieux L, Lafage-Pochitaloff M, Mozziconacci MJ, Cornillet-Lefebvre P, Radford I, Asnafi V, Bilhou-Nabera C, Nguyen Khac F, Léonard C, Speleman F, Poppe B, Bastard C, Taviaux S, Quilichini B, Herens C, Grégoire MJ, Cavé H, Bernard OA. t(5;14)/HOX11L2-positive T-cell acute lymphoblastic leukemia. A collaborative study of the Groupe Français de Cytogénétique Hématologique (GFCH). Leukemia. 2003;17:1851–7.
105. Ferrando AA, Neuberg DS, Dodge RK, Paietta E, Larson RA, Wiernik PH, Rowe JM, Caligiuri MA, Bloomfield CD, Look AT. Prognostic importance of TLX1 (HOX11) oncogene expression in adults with T-cell acute lymphoblastic leukaemia. Lancet. 2004;363:535–6.
106. Nagel S, Kaufmann M, Drexler HG, MacLeod RA. The cardiac homeobox gene NKX2-5 is deregulated by juxtaposition with BCL11B in pediatric T-ALL cell lines via a novel t(5;14)(q35.1;q32.2). Cancer Res. 2003;63:5329–34.
107. Bernard OA, Busson-LeConiat M, Ballerini P, Mauchauffe M, Della Valle V, Monni R, Nguyen Khac F, Mercher T, Penard-Lacronique V, Pasturaud P, Gressin L, Heilig R, Daniel MT, Lessard M, Berger R. A new recurrent and specific cryptic translocation, t(5;14)(q35;q32), is associated with expression of the Hox11L2 gene in T acute lymphoblastic leukemia. Leukemia. 2001;15:1495–504.
108. Van Vlierberghe P, Homminga I, Zuurbier L, Gladdines-Buijs J, van Wering ER, Horstmann M, Beverloo HB, Pieters R, Meijerink JP. Cooperative genetic defects in TLX3 rearranged pediatric T-ALL. Leukemia. 2008;22:762–70.
109. Asnafi V, Buzyn A, Thomas X, Huguet F, Vey N, Boiron JM, Reman O, Cayuela JM, Lheritier V, Vernant JP, Fiere D, Macintyre E, Dombret H. Impact of TCR status and genotype on outcome in adult T-cell acute lymphoblastic leukemia: a LALA-94 study. Blood. 2005;105:3072–8.
110. Kanzler B, Dear TN. Hox11 acts cell autonomously in spleen development and its absence results in altered cell fate of mesenchymal spleen precursors. Dev Biol. 2001;234:231–43.
111. Cheng L, Arata A, Mizuguchi R, Qian Y, Karunaratne A, Gray PA, Arata S, Shirasawa S, Bouchard M, Luo P, Chen CL, Busslinger M, Goulding M, Onimaru H, Ma Q. Tlx3 and Tlx1 are post-mitotic selector genes determining glutamatergic over GABAergic cell fates. Nat Neurosci. 2004;7:510–7.
112. Hawley RG, Fong AZ, Reis MD, Zhang N, Lu M, Hawley TS. Transforming function of the HOX11/TCL3 homeobox gene. Cancer Res. 1997;57:337–45.
113. Keller G, Wall C, Fong AZ, Hawley TS, Hawley RG. Overexpression of HOX11 leads to the immortalization of embryonic precursors with both primitive and definitive hematopoietic potential. Blood. 1998;92:877–87.
114. Hawley RG, Fong AZ, Lu M, Hawley TS. The HOX11 homeobox-containing gene of human leukemia immortalizes murine hematopoietic precursors. Oncogene. 1994;9:1–12.
115. De Keersmaecker K, Real PJ, Gatta GD, Palomero T, Sulis ML, Tosello V, Van Vlierberghe P, Barnes K, Castillo M, Sole X, Hadler M, Lenz J, Aplan PD, Kelliher M, Kee BL, Pandolfi PP, Kappes D, Gounari F, Petrie H, Van der Meulen J, Speleman F, Paietta E, Racevskis J, Wiernik PH, Rowe JM, Soulier J, Avran D, Cave H, Dastugue N, Raimondi S, Meijerink JP, Cordon-Cardo C, Califano A, Ferrando AA. The TLX1 oncogene drives aneuploidy in T cell transformation. Nat Med. 2010;16:1321–7.
116. Rakowski LA, Lehotzky EA, Chiang MY. Transient responses to NOTCH and TLX1/HOX11 inhibition

in T-cell acute lymphoblastic leukemia/lymphoma. PLoS One. 2011;6:e16761.
117. Montefiori LE, Mullighan CG. Redefining the biological basis of lineage-ambiguous leukemia through genomics: BCL11B deregulation in acute leukemias of ambiguous lineage. Best Pract Res Clin Haematol. 2021;34:101329.
118. Cavé H, Suciu S, Preudhomme C, Poppe B, Robert A, Uyttebroeck A, Malet M, Boutard P, Benoit Y, Mauvieux L, Lutz P, et al. Clinical significance of HOX11L2 expression linked to t(5;14)(q35;q32), of HOX11 expression, and of SIL-TAL fusion in childhood T-cell malignancies: results of EORTC studies 58881 and 58951. Blood. 2004;103:442–50.
119. Nagel S, Pommerenke C, Scherr M, Meyer C, Kaufmann M, Battmer K, MacLeod RA, Drexler HG. NKL homeobox gene activities in hematopoietic stem cells, T-cell development and T-cell leukemia. PLoS One. 2017;12:e0171164.
120. Kelly SE, Bachurski CJ, Burhans MS, Glasser SW. Transcription of the lung-specific surfactant protein C gene is mediated by thyroid transcription factor 1. J Biol Chem. 1996;271:6881–8.
121. Briscoe J, Sussel L, Serup P, Hartigan-O'Connor D, Jessell TM, Rubenstein JL, Ericson J. Homeobox gene Nkx2.2 and specification of neuronal identity by graded sonic hedgehog signalling. Nature. 1999;398:622–7.
122. Tanaka M, Chen Z, Bartunkova S, Yamasaki N, Izumo S. The cardiac homeobox gene Csx/Nkx2.5 lies genetically upstream of multiple genes essential for heart development. Development. 1999;126:1269–80.
123. Nagel S, Meyer C, Quentmeier H, Kaufmann M, Drexler HG, MacLeod RA. MEF2C is activated by multiple mechanisms in a subset of T-acute lymphoblastic leukemia cell lines. Leukemia. 2008;22:600–7.
124. Nagel S, Venturini L, Przybylski GK, Grabarczyk P, Meyer C, Kaufmann M, Battmer K, Schmidt CA, Drexler HG, Scherr M, Macleod RA. NK-like homeodomain proteins activate NOTCH3-signaling in leukemic T-cells. BMC Cancer. 2009;9:371.
125. Nagel S, Venturini L, Przybylski GK, Grabarczyk P, Schmidt CA, Meyer C, Drexler HG, Macleod RA, Scherr M. Activation of miR-17-92 by NK-like homeodomain proteins suppresses apoptosis via reduction of E2F1 in T-cell acute lymphoblastic leukemia. Leuk Lymphoma. 2009;50:101–8.
126. Bray SJ. Notch signalling in context. Nat Rev Mol Cell Biol. 2016;17:722–35.
127. Siebel C, Lendahl U. Notch signaling in development, tissue homeostasis, and disease. Physiol Rev. 2017;97:1235–94.
128. Sanders AD, Meiers S, Ghareghani M, Porubsky D, Jeong H, van Vliet M, Rausch T, Richter-Pechanska P, Kunz JB, Jenni S, Bolognini D, Longo GMC, Raeder B, Kinanen V, Zimmermann J, Benes V, Schrappe M, Mardin BR, Kulozik AE, Bornhauser B, Bourquin JP, Marschall T, Korbel JO. Single-cell analysis of structural variations and complex rearrangements with tri-channel processing. Nat Biotechnol. 2019;
129. Jeong H, Grimes K, Rauwolf KK, Bruch PM, Rausch T, Hasenfeld P, Benito E, Roider T, Sabarinathan R, Porubsky D, Herbst SA, Erarslan-Uysal B, Jann JC, Marschall T, Nowak D, Bourquin JP, Kulozik AE, Dietrich S, Bornhauser B, Sanders AD, Korbel JO. Functional analysis of structural variants in single cells using Strand-seq. Nat Biotechnol. 2022;
130. Yuan JS, Kousis PC, Suliman S, Visan I, Guidos CJ. Functions of notch signaling in the immune system: consensus and controversies. Annu Rev Immunol. 2010;28:343–65.
131. Abe N, Hozumi K, Hirano K, Yagita H, Habu S. Notch ligands transduce different magnitudes of signaling critical for determination of T-cell fate. Eur J Immunol. 2010;40:2608–17.
132. Seo W, Taniuchi I. Transcriptional regulation of early T-cell development in the thymus. Eur J Immunol. 2016;46:531–8.
133. Radtke F, Wilson A, Stark G, Bauer M, van Meerwijk J, MacDonald HR, Aguet M. Deficient T cell fate specification in mice with an induced inactivation of Notch1. Immunity. 1999;10:547–58.
134. Pui JC, Allman D, Xu L, DeRocco S, Karnell FG, Bakkour S, Lee JY, Kadesch T, Hardy RR, Aster JC, Pear WS. Notch1 expression in early lymphopoiesis influences B versus T lineage determination. Immunity. 1999;11:299–308.
135. Seki M, Kimura S, Isobe T, Yoshida K, Ueno H, Nakajima-Takagi Y, Wang C, Lin L, Kon A, Suzuki H, Shiozawa Y, Kataoka K, Fujii Y, Shiraishi Y, Chiba K, Tanaka H, Shimamura T, Masuda K, Kawamoto H, Ohki K, Kato M, Arakawa Y, Koh K, Hanada R, Moritake H, Akiyama M, Kobayashi R, Deguchi T, Hashii Y, Imamura T, Sato A, Kiyokawa N, Oka A, Hayashi Y, Takagi M, Manabe A, Ohara A, Horibe K, Sanada M, Iwama A, Mano H, Miyano S, Ogawa S, Takita J. Recurrent SPI1 (PU.1) fusions in high-risk pediatric T cell acute lymphoblastic leukemia. Nat Genet. 2017;49:1274–81.
136. Kox C, Zimmermann M, Stanulla M, Leible S, Schrappe M, Ludwig WD, Koehler R, Tolle G, Bandapalli OR, Breit S, Muckenthaler MU, Kulozik AE. The favorable effect of activating NOTCH1 receptor mutations on long-term outcome in T-ALL patients treated on the ALL-BFM 2000 protocol can be separated from FBXW7 loss of function. Leukemia. 2010;24:2005–13.
137. Grabher C, von Boehmer H, Look AT. Notch 1 activation in the molecular pathogenesis of T-cell acute lymphoblastic leukaemia. Nat Rev Cancer. 2006;6:347–59.
138. Suzuki S, Nagel S, Schneider B, Chen S, Kaufmann M, Uozumi K, Arima N, Drexler HG, MacLeod RA. A second NOTCH1 chromosome rearrangement: t(9;14)(q34.3;q11.2) in T-cell neoplasia. Leukemia. 2009;23:1003–6.

139. Weng AP, Ferrando AA, Lee W, Morris JP, Silverman LB, Sanchez-Irizarry C, Blacklow SC, Look AT, Aster JC. Activating mutations of NOTCH1 in human T cell acute lymphoblastic leukemia. Science. 2004;306:269–71.
140. Sulis ML, Williams O, Palomero T, Tosello V, Pallikuppam S, Real PJ, Barnes K, Zuurbier L, Meijerink JP, Ferrando AA. NOTCH1 extracellular juxtamembrane expansion mutations in T-ALL. Blood. 2008;112:733–40.
141. O'Neil J, Grim J, Strack P, Rao S, Tibbitts D, Winter C, Hardwick J, Welcker M, Meijerink JP, Pieters R, Draetta G, Sears R, Clurman BE, Look AT. FBW7 mutations in leukemic cells mediate NOTCH pathway activation and resistance to gamma-secretase inhibitors. J Exp Med. 2007;204:1813–24.
142. Thompson BJ, Buonamici S, Sulis ML, Palomero T, Vilimas T, Basso G, Ferrando A, Aifantis I. The SCFFBW7 ubiquitin ligase complex as a tumor suppressor in T cell leukemia. J Exp Med. 2007;204:1825–35.
143. Xiong H, Maraver A, Latkowski JA, Henderson T, Schlessinger K, Ding Y, Shen J, Tadokoro CE, Lafaille JJ. Characterization of two distinct lymphoproliferative diseases caused by ectopic expression of the notch ligand DLL4 on T cells. PLoS One. 2013;8:e84841.
144. Minuzzo S, Agnusdei V, Pusceddu I, Pinazza M, Moserle L, Masiero M, Rossi E, Crescenzi M, Hoey T, Ponzoni M, Amadori A, Indraccolo S. DLL4 regulates NOTCH signaling and growth of T acute lymphoblastic leukemia cells in NOD/SCID mice. Carcinogenesis. 2015;36:115–21.
145. Neumann M, Heesch S, Gokbuget N, Schwartz S, Schlee C, Benlasfer O, Farhadi-Sartangi N, Thibaut J, Burmeister T, Hoelzer D, Hofmann WK, Thiel E, Baldus CD. Clinical and molecular characterization of early T-cell precursor leukemia: a high-risk subgroup in adult T-ALL with a high frequency of FLT3 mutations. Blood Cancer J. 2012;2:e55.
146. Pear WS, Aster JC, Scott ML, Hasserjian RP, Soffer B, Sklar J, Baltimore D. Exclusive development of T cell neoplasms in mice transplanted with bone marrow expressing activated notch alleles. J Exp Med. 1996;183:2283–91.
147. Chiang MY, Xu L, Shestova O, Histen G, L'Heureux S, Romany C, Childs ME, Gimotty PA, Aster JC, Pear WS. Leukemia-associated NOTCH1 alleles are weak tumor initiators but accelerate K-ras-initiated leukemia. J Clin Invest. 2008;118:3181–94.
148. Wendorff AA, Quinn SA, Rashkovan M, Madubata CJ, Ambesi-Impiombato A, Litzow MR, Tallman MS, Paietta E, Paganin M, Basso G, Gastier-Foster JM, Loh ML, Rabadan R, Van Vlierberghe P, Ferrando AA. Phf6 loss enhances HSC self-renewal driving tumor initiation and leukemia stem cell activity in T-ALL. Cancer Discov. 2019;9:436–51.
149. Eguchi-Ishimae M, Eguchi M, Kempski H, Greaves M. NOTCH1 mutation can be an early, prenatal genetic event in T-ALL. Blood. 2008;111:376–8.
150. O'Neil J, Calvo J, McKenna K, Krishnamoorthy V, Aster JC, Bassing CH, Alt FW, Kelliher M, Look AT. Activating Notch1 mutations in mouse models of T-ALL. Blood. 2006;107:781–5.
151. Lin YW, Nichols RA, Letterio JJ, Aplan PD. Notch1 mutations are important for leukemic transformation in murine models of precursor-T leukemia/lymphoma. Blood. 2006;107:2540–3.
152. De Bie J, Demeyer S, Alberti-Servera L, Geerdens E, Segers H, Broux M, De Keersmaecker K, Michaux L, Vandenberghe P, Voet T, Boeckx N, Uyttebroeck A, Cools J. Single-cell sequencing reveals the origin and the order of mutation acquisition in T-cell acute lymphoblastic leukemia. Leukemia. 2018;32:1358–69.
153. Alberti-Servera L, Demeyer S, Govaerts I, Swings T, De Bie J, Gielen O, Brociner M, Michaux L, Maertens J, Uyttebroeck A, De Keersmaecker K, Boeckx N, Segers H, Cools J. Single-cell DNA amplicon sequencing reveals clonal heterogeneity and evolution in T-cell acute lymphoblastic leukemia. Blood. 2021;137:801–11.
154. Mansour MR, Sulis ML, Duke V, Foroni L, Jenkinson S, Koo K, Allen CG, Gale RE, Buck G, Richards S, Paietta E, Rowe JM, Tallman MS, Goldstone AH, Ferrando AA, Linch DC. Prognostic implications of NOTCH1 and FBXW7 mutations in adults with T-cell acute lymphoblastic leukemia treated on the MRC UKALLXII/ECOG E2993 protocol. J Clin Oncol. 2009;27:4352–6.
155. Clappier E, Collette S, Grardel N, Girard S, Suarez L, Brunie G, Kaltenbach S, Yakouben K, Mazingue F, Robert A, Boutard P, Plantaz D, Rohrlich P, van Vlierberghe P, Preudhomme C, Otten J, Speleman F, Dastugue N, Suciu S, Benoit Y, Bertrand Y, Cave H, Eortc CLG. NOTCH1 and FBXW7 mutations have a favorable impact on early response to treatment, but not on outcome, in children with T-cell acute lymphoblastic leukemia (T-ALL) treated on EORTC trials 58881 and 58951. Leukemia. 2010;24:2023–31.
156. Zuurbier L, Homminga I, Calvert V, te Winkel ML, Buijs-Gladdines JG, Kooi C, Smits WK, Sonneveld E, Veerman AJ, Kamps WA, Horstmann M, Petricoin EF 3rd, Pieters R, Meijerink JP. NOTCH1 and/or FBXW7 mutations predict for initial good prednisone response but not for improved outcome in pediatric T-cell acute lymphoblastic leukemia patients treated on DCOG or COALL protocols. Leukemia. 2010;24:2014–22.
157. Breit S, Stanulla M, Flohr T, Schrappe M, Ludwig WD, Tolle G, Happich M, Muckenthaler MU, Kulozik AE. Activating NOTCH1 mutations predict favorable early treatment response and long-term outcome in childhood precursor T-cell lymphoblastic leukemia. Blood. 2006;108:1151–7.
158. Bandapalli OR, Zimmermann M, Kox C, Stanulla M, Schrappe M, Ludwig WD, Koehler R, Muckenthaler MU, Kulozik AE. NOTCH1 activation clinically antagonizes the unfavorable effect of PTEN inactivation in BFM-treated children with precursor T-cell

acute lymphoblastic leukemia. Haematologica. 2013;98:928–36.
159. Zheng R, Li M, Wang S, Liu Y. Advances of target therapy on NOTCH1 signaling pathway in T-cell acute lymphoblastic leukemia. Exp Hematol Oncol. 2020;9:31.
160. Zhao R, Choi BY, Lee MH, Bode AM, Dong Z. Implications of genetic and epigenetic alterations of CDKN2A (p16(INK4a)) in cancer. EBioMedicine. 2016;8:30–9.
161. Remke M, Pfister S, Kox C, Toedt G, Becker N, Benner A, Werft W, Breit S, Liu S, Engel F, Wittmann A, Zimmermann M, Stanulla M, Schrappe M, Ludwig WD, Bartram CR, Radlwimmer B, Muckenthaler MU, Lichter P, Kulozik AE. High-resolution genomic profiling of childhood T-ALL reveals frequent copy-number alterations affecting the TGF-beta and PI3K-AKT pathways and deletions at 6q15-16.1 as a genomic marker for unfavorable early treatment response. Blood. 2009;114:1053–62.
162. Clappier E, Cuccuini W, Cayuela JM, Vecchione D, Baruchel A, Dombret H, Sigaux F, Soulier J. Cyclin D2 dysregulation by chromosomal translocations to TCR loci in T-cell acute lymphoblastic leukemias. Leukemia. 2006;20:82–6.
163. Sanchez-Martin M, Ferrando A. The NOTCH1-MYC highway toward T-cell acute lymphoblastic leukemia. Blood. 2017;129:1124–33.
164. Palomero T, Lim WK, Odom DT, Sulis ML, Real PJ, Margolin A, Barnes KC, O'Neil J, Neuberg D, Weng AP, Aster JC, Sigaux F, Soulier J, Look AT, Young RA, Califano A, Ferrando AA. NOTCH1 directly regulates c-MYC and activates a feed-forward-loop transcriptional network promoting leukemic cell growth. Proc Natl Acad Sci USA. 2006;103:18261–6.
165. Welcker M, Orian A, Jin J, Grim JE, Harper JW, Eisenman RN, Clurman BE. The Fbw7 tumor suppressor regulates glycogen synthase kinase 3 phosphorylation-dependent c-Myc protein degradation. Proc Natl Acad Sci USA. 2004;101:9085–90.
166. Herranz D, Ambesi-Impiombato A, Palomero T, Schnell SA, Belver L, Wendorff AA, Xu L, Castillo-Martin M, Llobet-Navas D, Cordon-Cardo C, Clappier E, Soulier J, Ferrando AA. A NOTCH1-driven MYC enhancer promotes T cell development, transformation and acute lymphoblastic leukemia. Nat Med. 2014;20:1130–7.
167. Erikson J, Finger L, Sun L, Ar-Rushdi A, Nishikura K, Minowada J, Finan J, Emanuel BS, Nowell PC, Croce CM. Deregulation of c-myc by translocation of the alpha-locus of the T-cell receptor in T-cell leukemias. Science. 1986;232:884–6.
168. La Starza R, Borga C, Barba G, Pierini V, Schwab C, Matteucci C, Lema Fernandez AG, Leszl A, Cazzaniga G, Chiaretti S, Basso G, Harrison CJ, te Kronnie G, Mecucci C. Genetic profile of T-cell acute lymphoblastic leukemias with MYC translocations. Blood. 2014;124:3577–82.
169. Milani G, Matthijssens F, Van Loocke W, Durinck K, Roels J, Peirs S, Thénoz M, Pieters T, Reunes L, Lintermans B, Vandamme N, Lammens T, Van Roy N, Van Nieuwerburgh F, Deforce D, Schwab C, Raimondi S, Dalla Pozza L, Carroll AJ III, De Moerloose B, Benoit Y, Goossens S, Berx G, Harrison CJ, Basso G, Cavé H, Sutton R, Asnafi V, Meijerink J, Mullighan C, Loh M, Van Vlierberghe P. Genetic characterization and therapeutic targeting of MYC-rearranged T cell acute lymphoblastic leukaemia. Br J Haematol. 2019;185:169–74.
170. Smith DP, Bath ML, Metcalf D, Harris AW, Cory S. MYC levels govern hematopoietic tumor type and latency in transgenic mice. Blood. 2006;108:653–61.
171. Smith DP, Bath ML, Harris AW, Cory S. T-cell lymphomas mask slower developing B-lymphoid and myeloid tumours in transgenic mice with broad haemopoietic expression of MYC. Oncogene. 2005;24:3544–53.
172. Langenau DM, Traver D, Ferrando AA, Kutok JL, Aster JC, Kanki JP, Lin S, Prochownik E, Trede NS, Zon LI, Look AT. Myc-induced T cell leukemia in transgenic zebrafish. Science. 2003;299:887–90.
173. Ramsay RG, Gonda TJ. MYB function in normal and cancer cells. Nat Rev Cancer. 2008;8:523–34.
174. Lahortiga I, De Keersmaecker K, Van Vlierberghe P, Graux C, Cauwelier B, Lambert F, Mentens N, Beverloo HB, Pieters R, Speleman F, Odero MD, Bauters M, Froyen G, Marynen P, Vandenberghe P, Wlodarska I, Meijerink JPP, Cools J. Duplication of the MYB oncogene in T cell acute lymphoblastic leukemia. Nat Genet. 2007;39:593–5.
175. Clappier E, Cuccuini W, Kalota A, Crinquette A, Cayuela JM, Dik WA, Langerak AW, Montpellier B, Nadel B, Walrafen P, Delattre O, Aurias A, Leblanc T, Dombret H, Gewirtz AM, Baruchel A, Sigaux F, Soulier J. The C-MYB locus is involved in chromosomal translocation and genomic duplications in human T-cell acute leukemia (T-ALL), the translocation defining a new T-ALL subtype in very young children. Blood. 2007;110:1251–61.
176. O'Neil J, Tchinda J, Gutierrez A, Moreau L, Maser RS, Wong K-K, Li W, McKenna K, Liu XS, Feng B, Neuberg D, Silverman L, DeAngelo DJ, Kutok JL, Rothstein R, DePinho RA, Chin L, Lee C, Look AT. Alu elements mediate MYB gene tandem duplication in human T-ALL. J Exp Med. 2007;204:3059–66.
177. Sanghvi VR, Mavrakis KJ, Van der Meulen J, Boice M, Wolfe AL, Carty M, Mohan P, Rondou P, Socci ND, Benoit Y, Taghon T, Van Vlierberghe P, Leslie CS, Speleman F, Wendel H-G. Characterization of a set of tumor suppressor microRNAs in T cell acute lymphoblastic leukemia. Sci Signal. 2014;7:ra111.
178. Mets E, Van der Meulen J, Van Peer G, Boice M, Mestdagh P, Van de Walle I, Lammens T, Goossens S, De Moerloose B, Benoit Y, Van Roy N, Clappier E, Poppe B, Vandesompele J, Wendel HG, Taghon T, Rondou P, Soulier J, Van Vlierberghe P, Speleman F. MicroRNA-193b-3p acts as a tumor suppressor by

targeting the MYB oncogene in T-cell acute lymphoblastic leukemia. Leukemia. 2015;29:798–806.
179. Rothenberg EV, Hosokawa H, Ungerback J. Mechanisms of action of hematopoietic transcription factor PU.1 in initiation of T-cell development. Front Immunol. 2019;10:228.
180. Van Thillo Q, De Bie J, Seneviratne JA, Demeyer S, Omari S, Balachandran A, Zhai V, Tam WL, Sweron B, Geerdens E, Gielen O, Provost S, Segers H, Boeckx N, Marshall GM, Cheung BB, Isobe K, Kato I, Takita J, Amos TG, Deveson IW, McCalmont H, Lock RB, Oxley EP, Garwood MM, Dickins RA, Uyttebroeck A, Carter DR, Cools J, de Bock CE. Oncogenic cooperation between TCF7-SPI1 and NRAS(G12D) requires β-catenin activity to drive T-cell acute lymphoblastic leukemia. Nat Commun. 2021;12:4164.
181. Canté-Barrett K, Pieters R, Meijerink JPP. Myocyte enhancer factor 2C in hematopoiesis and leukemia. Oncogene. 2014;33:403–10.
182. Nagel S, Venturini L, Meyer C, Kaufmann M, Scherr M, Drexler HG, Macleod RAF. Transcriptional deregulation of oncogenic myocyte enhancer factor 2C in T-cell acute lymphoblastic leukemia. Leuk Lymphoma. 2011;52:290–7.
183. Canté-Barrett K, Meijer MT, Cordo V, Hagelaar R, Yang W, Yu J, Smits WK, Nulle ME, Jansen JP, Pieters R, Yang JJ, Haigh JJ, Goossens S, Meijerink JPP. MEF2C opposes notch in lymphoid lineage decision and drives leukemia in the thymus. JCI Insight. 2022;7
184. Rothenberg EV. Programming for T-lymphocyte fates: modularity and mechanisms. Genes Dev. 2019;33:1117–35.
185. Kueh HY, Yui MA, Ng KKH, Pease SS, Zhang JA, Damle SS, Freedman G, Siu S, Bernstein ID, Elowitz MB, Rothenberg EV. Asynchronous combinatorial action of four regulatory factors activates Bcl11b for T cell commitment. Nat Immunol. 2016;17:956–65.
186. Gutierrez A, Kentsis A, Sanda T, Holmfeldt L, Chen S-C, Zhang J, Protopopov A, Chin L, Dahlberg SE, Neuberg DS, Silverman LB, Winter SS, Hunger SP, Sallan SE, Zha S, Alt FW, Downing JR, Mullighan CG, Look AT. The BCL11B tumor suppressor is mutated across the major molecular subtypes of T-cell acute lymphoblastic leukemia. Blood. 2011;118:4169–73.
187. Ha VL, Luong A, Li F, Casero D, Malvar J, Kim YM, Bhatia R, Crooks GM, Parekh C. The T-ALL related gene BCL11B regulates the initial stages of human T-cell differentiation. Leukemia. 2017;31:2503–14.
188. Ikawa T, Hirose S, Masuda K, Kakugawa K, Satoh R, Shibano-Satoh A, Kominami R, Katsura Y, Kawamoto H. An essential developmental checkpoint for production of the T cell lineage. Science. 2010;329:93–6.
189. Wakabayashi Y, Inoue J, Takahashi Y, Matsuki A, Kosugi-Okano H, Shinbo T, Mishima Y, Niwa O, Kominami R. Homozygous deletions and point mutations of the Rit1/Bcl11b gene in γ-ray induced mouse thymic lymphomas. Biochem Biophys Res Commun. 2003;301:598–603.
190. Swiers G, de Bruijn M, Speck NA. Hematopoietic stem cell emergence in the conceptus and the role of Runx1. Int J Dev Biol. 2010;54:1151–63.
191. Lizama CO, Hawkins JS, Schmitt CE, Bos FL, Zape JP, Cautivo KM, Borges Pinto H, Rhyner AM, Yu H, Donohoe ME, Wythe JD, Zovein AC. Repression of arterial genes in hemogenic endothelium is sufficient for haematopoietic fate acquisition. Nat Commun. 2015;6:7739.
192. Voon DC, Hor YT, Ito Y. The RUNX complex: reaching beyond haematopoiesis into immunity. Immunology. 2015;146:523–36.
193. Lichtinger M, Ingram R, Hannah R, Müller D, Clarke D, Assi SA, Lie-A-Ling M, Noailles L, Vijayabaskar MS, Wu M, Tenen DG, Westhead DR, Kouskoff V, Lacaud G, Göttgens B, Bonifer C. RUNX1 reshapes the epigenetic landscape at the onset of haematopoiesis. EMBO J. 2012;31:4318–33.
194. Vera G, Wolfgang K, Stefan H, Tamara A, Sabine J, Susanne S, Claudia H, Torsten H, Alexander K. Prognostic relevance of RUNX1 mutations in T-cell acute lymphoblastic leukemia. Haematologica. 2011;96:1874–7.
195. Della Gatta G, Palomero T, Perez-Garcia A, Ambesi-Impiombato A, Bansal M, Carpenter ZW, De Keersmaecker K, Sole X, Xu L, Paietta E, Racevskis J, Wiernik PH, Rowe JM, Meijerink JP, Califano A, Ferrando AA. Reverse engineering of TLX oncogenic transcriptional networks identifies RUNX1 as tumor suppressor in T-ALL. Nat Med. 2012;18:436–40.
196. Owen CJ, Toze CL, Koochin A, Forrest DL, Smith CA, Stevens JM, Jackson SC, Poon MC, Sinclair GD, Leber B, Johnson PR, Macheta A, Yin JA, Barnett MJ, Lister TA, Fitzgibbon J. Five new pedigrees with inherited RUNX1 mutations causing familial platelet disorder with propensity to myeloid malignancy. Blood. 2008;112:4639–45.
197. Preudhomme C, Renneville A, Bourdon V, Philippe N, Roche-Lestienne C, Boissel N, Dhedin N, André JM, Cornillet-Lefebvre P, Baruchel A, Mozziconacci MJ, Sobol H. High frequency of RUNX1 biallelic alteration in acute myeloid leukemia secondary to familial platelet disorder. Blood. 2009;113:5583–7.
198. Nishimoto N, Imai Y, Ueda K, Nakagawa M, Shinohara A, Ichikawa M, Nannya Y, Kurokawa M. T cell acute lymphoblastic leukemia arising from familial platelet disorder. Int J Hematol. 2010;92:194–7.
199. Alberta JA, Springett GM, Rayburn H, Natoli TA, Loring J, Kreidberg JA, Housman D. Role of the WT1 tumor suppressor in murine hematopoiesis. Blood. 2003;101:2570–4.
200. Cunningham TJ, Palumbo I, Grosso M, Slater N, Miles CG. WT1 regulates murine hematopoiesis via maintenance of VEGF isoform ratio. Blood. 2013;122:188–92.

201. Tosello V, Mansour MR, Barnes K, Paganin M, Sulis ML, Jenkinson S, Allen CG, Gale RE, Linch DC, Palomero T, Real P, Murty V, Yao X, Richards SM, Goldstone A, Rowe J, Basso G, Wiernik PH, Paietta E, Pieters R, Horstmann M, Meijerink JP, Ferrando AA. WT1 mutations in T-ALL. Blood. 2009;114:1038–45.
202. Renneville A, Kaltenbach S, Clappier E, Collette S, Micol JB, Nelken B, Lepelley P, Dastugue N, Benoît Y, Bertrand Y, Preudhomme C, Cavé H. Wilms tumor 1 (WT1) gene mutations in pediatric T-cell malignancies. Leukemia. 2010;24:476–80.
203. Sandra H, Nicola G, Andrea S, Jutta Ortiz T, Cornelia S, Thomas B, Stefan S, Olga B, Ulrich K, Antonia B, Dieter H, Eckhard T, Wolf-Karsten H, Claudia DB. Prognostic implications of mutations and expression of the Wilms tumor 1 (WT1) gene in adult acute T-lymphoblastic leukemia. Haematologica. 2010;95:942–9.
204. Richter-Pechanska P, Kunz JB, Hof J, Zimmermann M, Rausch T, Bandapalli OR, Orlova E, Scapinello G, Sagi JC, Stanulla M, Schrappe M, Cario G, Kirschner-Schwabe R, Eckert C, Benes V, Korbel JO, Muckenthaler MU, Kulozik AE. Identification of a genetically defined ultra-high-risk group in relapsed pediatric T-lymphoblastic leukemia. Blood Cancer J. 2017;7:e523.
205. Fulvio B, Erich P, Elena M, Alberto A-I, Sonia M, Roberta B, Valeria S, Giorgia P, Giuseppe B, Paola Z, Alberto A, Valeria T. WT1 loss attenuates the TP53-induced DNA damage response in T-cell acute lymphoblastic leukemia. Haematologica. 2018;103:266–77.
206. Ruan Y, Kim HN, Ogana H, Kim YM. Wnt signaling in leukemia and its bone marrow microenvironment. Int J Mol Sci. 2020;21
207. Gutierrez A, Sanda T, Ma W, Zhang J, Grebliunaite R, Dahlberg S, Neuberg D, Protopopov A, Winter SS, Larson RS, Borowitz MJ, Silverman LB, Chin L, Hunger SP, Jamieson C, Sallan SE, Look AT. Inactivation of LEF1 in T-cell acute lymphoblastic leukemia. Blood. 2010;115:2845–51.
208. Van Vlierberghe P, Ambesi-Impiombato A, Perez-Garcia A, Haydu JE, Rigo I, Hadler M, Tosello V, Della Gatta G, Paietta E, Racevskis J, Wiernik PH, Luger SM, Rowe JM, Rue M, Ferrando AA. ETV6 mutations in early immature human T cell leukemias. J Exp Med. 2011;208:2571–9.
209. Wang LC, Swat W, Fujiwara Y, Davidson L, Visvader J, Kuo F, Alt FW, Gilliland DG, Golub TR, Orkin SH. The TEL/ETV6 gene is required specifically for hematopoiesis in the bone marrow. Genes Dev. 1998;12:2392–402.
210. Feurstein S, Godley LA. Germline ETV6 mutations and predisposition to hematological malignancies. Int J Hematol. 2017;106:189–95.
211. Okkenhaug K, Vanhaesebroeck B. PI3K in lymphocyte development, differentiation and activation. Nat Rev Immunol. 2003;3:317–30.
212. Thorpe LM, Yuzugullu H, Zhao JJ. PI3K in cancer: divergent roles of isoforms, modes of activation and therapeutic targeting. Nat Rev Cancer. 2015;15:7–24.
213. Manning BD, Toker A. AKT/PKB signaling: navigating the network. Cell. 2017;169:381–405.
214. Georgescu MM. PTEN tumor suppressor network in PI3K-Akt pathway control. Genes Cancer. 2010;1:1170–7.
215. Juntilla MM, Koretzky GA. Critical roles of the PI3K/Akt signaling pathway in T cell development. Immunol Lett. 2008;116:104–10.
216. Swat W, Montgrain V, Doggett TA, Douangpanya J, Puri K, Vermi W, Diacovo TG. Essential role of PI3Kδ and PI3Kγ in thymocyte survival. Blood. 2006;107:2415–22.
217. Juntilla MM, Wofford JA, Birnbaum MJ, Rathmell JC, Koretzky GA. Akt1 and Akt2 are required for alphabeta thymocyte survival and differentiation. Proc Natl Acad Sci USA. 2007;104:12105–10.
218. Palomero T, Sulis ML, Cortina M, Real PJ, Barnes K, Ciofani M, Caparros E, Buteau J, Brown K, Perkins SL, Bhagat G, Agarwal AM, Basso G, Castillo M, Nagase S, Cordon-Cardo C, Parsons R, Zuniga-Pflucker JC, Dominguez M, Ferrando AA. Mutational loss of PTEN induces resistance to NOTCH1 inhibition in T-cell leukemia. Nat Med. 2007;13:1203–10.
219. Tottone L, Lancho O, Loh JW, Singh A, Kimura S, Roels J, Kuchmiy A, Strubbe S, Lawlor MA, da Silva-Diz V, Luo S, Gachet S, García-Prieto CA, Hagelaar R, Esteller M, Meijerink JPP, Soulier J, Taghon T, Van Vlierberghe P, Mullighan CG, Khiabanian H, Rocha PP, Herranz D. A tumor suppressor enhancer of PTEN in T-cell development and leukemia. Blood Cancer Discov. 2021;2:92–109.
220. Silva A, Yunes JA, Cardoso BA, Martins LR, Jotta PY, Abecasis M, Nowill AE, Leslie NR, Cardoso AA, Barata JT. PTEN posttranslational inactivation and hyperactivation of the PI3K/Akt pathway sustain primary T cell leukemia viability. J Clin Invest. 2008;118:3762–74.
221. Trinquand A, Tanguy-Schmidt A, Ben Abdelali R, Lambert J, Beldjord K, Lengliné E, De Gunzburg N, Payet-Bornet D, Lhermitte L, Mossafa H, Lhéritier V, Bond J, Huguet F, Buzyn A, Leguay T, Cahn J-Y, Thomas X, Chalandon Y, Delannoy A, Bonmati C, Maury S, Nadel B, Macintyre E, Ifrah N, Dombret H, Asnafi V. Toward a NOTCH1/FBXW7/RAS/PTEN–based oncogenetic risk classification of adult T-cell acute lymphoblastic leukemia: A Group for research in adult acute lymphoblastic leukemia study. J Clin Oncol. 2013;31:4333–42.
222. Gutierrez A, Sanda T, Grebliunaite R, Carracedo A, Salmena L, Ahn Y, Dahlberg S, Neuberg D, Moreau LA, Winter SS, Larson R, Zhang J, Protopopov A, Chin L, Pandolfi PP, Silverman LB, Hunger SP, Sallan SE, Look AT. High frequency of PTEN, PI3K, and AKT abnormalities in T-cell acute lymphoblastic leukemia. Blood. 2009;114:647–50.

223. Zuurbier L, Petricoin EF 3rd, Vuerhard MJ, Calvert V, Kooi C, Buijs-Gladdines JG, Smits WK, Sonneveld E, Veerman AJ, Kamps WA, Horstmann M, Pieters R, Meijerink JP. The significance of PTEN and AKT aberrations in pediatric T-cell acute lymphoblastic leukemia. Haematologica. 2012;97:1405–13.
224. Karrman K, Kjeldsen E, Lassen C, Isaksson M, Davidsson J, Andersson A, Hasle H, Fioretos T, Johansson B. The t(X;7)(q22;q34) in paediatric T-cell acute lymphoblastic leukaemia results in overexpression of the insulin receptor substrate 4 gene through illegitimate recombination with the T-cell receptor beta locus. Br J Haematol. 2009;144:546–51.
225. Kang DH, Kim SH, Jun JW, Lee YW, Shin HB, Ahn JY, Hong DS, Lee YK, Jeon BR. Simultaneous translocation of both TCR loci (14q11) with rare partner loci (Xq22 and 12p13) in a case of T-lymphoblastic leukemia. Ann Lab Med. 2012;32:220–4.
226. Paganin M, Grillo MF, Silvestri D, Scapinello G, Buldini B, Cazzaniga G, Biondi A, Valsecchi MG, Conter V, Te Kronnie G, Basso G. The presence of mutated and deleted PTEN is associated with an increased risk of relapse in childhood T cell acute lymphoblastic leukaemia treated with AIEOP-BFM ALL protocols. Br J Haematol. 2018;182:705–11.
227. Szarzyńska-Zawadzka B, Kunz JB, Sędek Ł, Kosmalska M, Zdon K, Biecek P, Bandapalli OR, Kraszewska-Hamilton M, Jaksik R, Drobna M, Kowalczyk JR, Szczepański T, Van Vlierberghe P, Kulozik AE, Witt M, Dawidowska M. PTEN abnormalities predict poor outcome in children with T-cell acute lymphoblastic leukemia treated according to ALL IC-BFM protocols. Am J Hematol. 2019;94:E93–e96.
228. Tesio M, Trinquand A, Ballerini P, Hypolite G, Lhermitte L, Petit A, Ifrah N, Baruchel A, Dombret H, Macintyre E, Asnafi V. Age-related clinical and biological features of PTEN abnormalities in T-cell acute lymphoblastic leukaemia. Leukemia. 2017;31:2594–600.
229. Marzollo A, Maestrini G, La Starza R, Elia L, Malfona F, Pierini T, Tretti Parenzan C, Coppe A, Bortoluzzi S, Biffi A, Mecucci C, Bresolin S, Testi AM. A novel germline variant in PIK3R1 results in SHORT syndrome associated with TAL/LMO T-cell acute lymphoblastic leukemia. Am J Hematol. 2020;95:E335–8.
230. Yilmaz ÖH, Valdez R, Theisen BK, Guo W, Ferguson DO, Wu H, Morrison SJ. Pten dependence distinguishes haematopoietic stem cells from leukaemia-initiating cells. Nature. 2006;441:475–82.
231. Zhang J, Grindley JC, Yin T, Jayasinghe S, He XC, Ross JT, Haug JS, Rupp D, Porter-Westpfahl KS, Wiedemann LM, Wu H, Li L. PTEN maintains haematopoietic stem cells and acts in lineage choice and leukaemia prevention. Nature. 2006;441:518–22.
232. Hagenbeek TJ, Spits H. T-cell lymphomas in T-cell-specific Pten-deficient mice originate in the thymus. Leukemia. 2008;22:608–19.
233. Hagenbeek TJ, Naspetti M, Malergue F, Garçon F, Nunès JA, Cleutjens KBJM, Trapman J, Krimpenfort P, Spits H. The loss of PTEN allows TCR αβ lineage Thymocytes to bypass IL-7 and pre-TCR–mediated signaling. J Exp Med. 2004;200:883–94.
234. Evangelisti C, Ricci F, Tazzari P, Tabellini G, Battistelli M, Falcieri E, Chiarini F, Bortul R, Melchionda F, Pagliaro P, Pession A, McCubrey JA, Martelli AM. Targeted inhibition of mTORC1 and mTORC2 by active-site mTOR inhibitors has cytotoxic effects in T-cell acute lymphoblastic leukemia. Leukemia. 2011;25:781–91.
235. Subramaniam PS, Whye DW, Efimenko E, Chen J, Tosello V, De Keersmaecker K, Kashishian A, Thompson MA, Castillo M, Cordon-Cardo C, Davé UP, Ferrando A, Lannutti BJ, Diacovo TG. Targeting nonclassical oncogenes for therapy in T-ALL. Cancer Cell. 2012;21:459–72.
236. Piovan E, Yu J, Tosello V, Herranz D, Ambesi-Impiombato A, Silva D, Ana C, Sanchez-Martin M, Perez-Garcia A, Rigo I, Castillo M, Indraccolo S, Cross JR, de Stanchina E, Paietta E, Racevskis J, Rowe JM, Tallman MS, Basso G, Meijerink JP, Cordon-Cardo C, Califano A, Ferrando AA. Direct reversal of glucocorticoid resistance by AKT inhibition in acute lymphoblastic leukemia. Cancer Cell. 2013;24:766–76.
237. Dail M, Wong J, Lawrence J, O'Connor D, Nakitandwe J, Chen S-C, Xu J, Lee LB, Akagi K, Li Q, Aster JC, Pear WS, Downing JR, Sampath D, Shannon K. Loss of oncogenic Notch1 with resistance to a PI3K inhibitor in T-cell leukaemia. Nature. 2014;513:512–6.
238. Wei G, Twomey D, Lamb J, Schlis K, Agarwal J, Stam RW, Opferman JT, Sallan SE, den Boer ML, Pieters R, Golub TR, Armstrong SA. Gene expression-based chemical genomics identifies rapamycin as a modulator of MCL1 and glucocorticoid resistance. Cancer Cell. 2006;10: 331–42.
239. Barata JT, Durum SK, Seddon B. Flip the coin: IL-7 and IL-7R in health and disease. Nat Immunol. 2019;20:1584–93.
240. Oliveira ML, Akkapeddi P, Ribeiro D, Melão A, Barata JT. IL-7R-mediated signaling in T-cell acute lymphoblastic leukemia: an update. Adv Biol Regul. 2019;71:88–96.
241. Canté-Barrett K, Spijkers-Hagelstein JA, Buijs-Gladdines JG, Uitdehaag JC, Smits WK, van der Zwet J, Buijsman RC, Zaman GJ, Pieters R, Meijerink JP. MEK and PI3K-AKT inhibitors synergistically block activated IL7 receptor signaling in T-cell acute lymphoblastic leukemia. Leukemia. 2016;30:1832–43.
242. Vicente C, Schwab C, Broux M, Geerdens E, Degryse S, Demeyer S, Lahortiga I, Elliott A, Chilton L, La Starza R, Mecucci C, Vandenberghe P, Goulden N, Vora A, Moorman AV, Soulier J, Harrison CJ, Clappier E, Cools J. Targeted sequencing identifies associations between IL7R-JAK mutations and

epigenetic modulators in T-cell acute lymphoblastic leukemia. Haematologica. 2015;100:1301–10.
243. Zenatti PP, Ribeiro D, Li W, Zuurbier L, Silva MC, Paganin M, Tritapoe J, Hixon JA, Silveira AB, Cardoso BA, Sarmento LM, Correia N, Toribio ML, Kobarg J, Horstmann M, Pieters R, Brandalise SR, Ferrando AA, Meijerink JP, Durum SK, Yunes JA, Barata JT. Oncogenic IL7R gain-of-function mutations in childhood T-cell acute lymphoblastic leukemia. Nat Genet. 2011;43:932–9.
244. Goossens S, Radaelli E, Blanchet O, Durinck K, Van der Meulen J, Peirs S, Taghon T, Tremblay CS, Costa M, Farhang Ghahremani M, De Medts J, Bartunkova S, Haigh K, Schwab C, Farla N, Pieters T, Matthijssens F, Van Roy N, Best JA, Deswarte K, Bogaert P, Carmichael C, Rickard A, Suryani S, Bracken LS, Alserihi R, Cante-Barrett K, Haenebalcke L, Clappier E, Rondou P, Slowicka K, Huylebroeck D, Goldrath AW, Janzen V, McCormack MP, Lock RB, Curtis DJ, Harrison C, Berx G, Speleman F, Meijerink JP, Soulier J, Van Vlierberghe P, Haigh JJ. ZEB2 drives immature T-cell lymphoblastic leukaemia development via enhanced tumour-initiating potential and IL-7 receptor signalling. Nat Commun. 2015;6: 5794.
245. Bornschein S, Demeyer S, Stirparo R, Gielen O, Vicente C, Geerdens E, Ghesquière B, Aerts S, Cools J, de Bock CE. Defining the molecular basis of oncogenic cooperation between TAL1 expression and Pten deletion in T-ALL using a novel pro-T-cell model system. Leukemia. 2018;32:941–51.
246. Bains T, Heinrich MC, Loriaux MM, Beadling C, Nelson D, Warrick A, Neff TL, Tyner JW, Dunlap J, Corless CL, Fan G. Newly described activating JAK3 mutations in T-cell acute lymphoblastic leukemia. Leukemia. 2012;26:2144–6.
247. Porcu M, Kleppe M, Gianfelici V, Geerdens E, De Keersmaecker K, Tartaglia M, Foa R, Soulier J, Cauwelier B, Uyttebroeck A, Macintyre E, Vandenberghe P, Asnafi V, Cools J. Mutation of the receptor tyrosine phosphatase PTPRC (CD45) in T-cell acute lymphoblastic leukemia. Blood. 2012;119:4476–9.
248. Shochat C, Tal N, Bandapalli OR, Palmi C, Ganmore I, te Kronnie G, Cario G, Cazzaniga G, Kulozik AE, Stanulla M, Schrappe M, Biondi A, Basso G, Bercovich D, Muckenthaler MU, Izraeli S. Gain-of-function mutations in interleukin-7 receptor-α (IL7R) in childhood acute lymphoblastic leukemias. J Exp Med. 2011;208:901–8.
249. Flex E, Petrangeli V, Stella L, Chiaretti S, Hornakova T, Knoops L, Ariola C, Fodale V, Clappier E, Paoloni F, Martinelli S, Fragale A, Sanchez M, Tavolaro S, Messina M, Cazzaniga G, Camera A, Pizzolo G, Tornesello A, Vignetti M, Battistini A, Cavé H, Gelb BD, Renauld JC, Biondi A, Constantinescu SN, Foà R, Tartaglia M. Somatically acquired JAK1 mutations in adult acute lymphoblastic leukemia. J Exp Med. 2008;205:751–8.
250. Zhang K, Wong P, Zhang L, Jacobs B, Borden EC, Aster JC, Bedogni B. A Notch1-neuregulin1 autocrine signaling loop contributes to melanoma growth. Oncogene. 2012;31:4609–18.
251. Bandapalli OR, Schuessele S, Kunz JB, Rausch T, Stutz AM, Tal N, Geron I, Gershman N, Izraeli S, Eilers J, Vaezipour N, Kirschner-Schwabe R, Hof J, von Stackelberg A, Schrappe M, Stanulla M, Zimmermann M, Koehler R, Avigad S, Handgretinger R, Frismantas V, Bourquin JP, Bornhauser B, Korbel JO, Muckenthaler MU, Kulozik AE. The activating STAT5B N642H mutation is a common abnormality in pediatric T-cell acute lymphoblastic leukemia and confers a higher risk of relapse. Haematologica. 2014;99:e188–92.
252. Kontro M, Kuusanmaki H, Eldfors S, Burmeister T, Andersson EI, Bruserud O, Brummendorf TH, Edgren H, Gjertsen BT, Itala-Remes M, Lagstrom S, Lohi O, Lundan T, Marti JM, Majumder MM, Parsons A, Pemovska T, Rajala H, Vettenranta K, Kallioniemi O, Mustjoki S, Porkka K, Heckman CA. Novel activating STAT5B mutations as putative drivers of T-cell acute lymphoblastic leukemia. Leukemia. 2014;28:1738–42.
253. Kleppe M, Lahortiga I, El Chaar T, De Keersmaecker K, Mentens N, Graux C, Van Roosbroeck K, Ferrando AA, Langerak AW, Meijerink JP, Sigaux F, Haferlach T, Wlodarska I, Vandenberghe P, Soulier J, Cools J. Deletion of the protein tyrosine phosphatase gene PTPN2 in T-cell acute lymphoblastic leukemia. Nat Genet. 2010;42:530–5.
254. Tremblay CS, Brown FC, Collett M, Saw J, Chiu SK, Sonderegger SE, Lucas SE, Alserihi R, Chau N, Toribio ML, McCormack MP, Chircop M, Robinson PJ, Jane SM, Curtis DJ. Loss-of-function mutations of dynamin 2 promote T-ALL by enhancing IL-7 signalling. Leukemia. 2016;30:1993–2001.
255. Perez-Garcia A, Ambesi-Impiombato A, Hadler M, Rigo I, LeDuc CA, Kelly K, Jalas C, Paietta E, Racevskis J, Rowe JM, Tallman MS, Paganin M, Basso G, Tong W, Chung WK, Ferrando AA. Genetic loss of SH2B3 in acute lymphoblastic leukemia. Blood. 2013;122:2425–32.
256. González-García S, García-Peydró M, Martín-Gayo E, Ballestar E, Esteller M, Bornstein R, de la Pompa JL, Ferrando AA, Toribio ML. CSL-MAML-dependent Notch1 signaling controls T lineage-specific IL-7R{alpha} gene expression in early human thymopoiesis and leukemia. J Exp Med. 2009;206:779–91.
257. Girardi T, Vereecke S, Sulima SO, Khan Y, Fancello L, Briggs JW, Schwab C, de Beeck JO, Verbeeck J, Royaert J, Geerdens E, Vicente C, Bornschein S, Harrison CJ, Meijerink JP, Cools J, Dinman JD, Kampen KR, De Keersmaecker K. The T-cell leukemia-associated ribosomal RPL10 R98S mutation enhances JAK-STAT signaling. Leukemia. 2018;32:809–19.
258. Degryse S, de Bock CE, Cox L, Demeyer S, Gielen O, Mentens N, Jacobs K, Geerdens E, Gianfelici

V, Hulselmans G, Fiers M, Aerts S, Meijerink JP, Tousseyn T, Cools J. JAK3 mutants transform hematopoietic cells through JAK1 activation, causing T-cell acute lymphoblastic leukemia in a mouse model. Blood. 2014;124:3092–100.
259. Maude SL, Dolai S, Delgado-Martin C, Vincent T, Robbins A, Selvanathan A, Ryan T, Hall J, Wood AC, Tasian SK, Hunger SP, Loh ML, Mullighan CG, Wood BL, Hermiston ML, Grupp SA, Lock RB, Teachey DT. Efficacy of JAK/STAT pathway inhibition in murine xenograft models of early T-cell precursor (ETP) acute lymphoblastic leukemia. Blood. 2015;125:1759–67.
260. Degryse S, de Bock CE, Demeyer S, Govaerts I, Bornschein S, Verbeke D, Jacobs K, Binos S, Skerrett-Byrne DA, Murray HC, Verrills NM, Van Vlierberghe P, Cools J, Dun MD. Mutant JAK3 phosphoproteomic profiling predicts synergism between JAK3 inhibitors and MEK/BCL2 inhibitors for the treatment of T-cell acute lymphoblastic leukemia. Leukemia. 2018;32:788–800.
261. Lapinski PE, King PD. Regulation of Ras signal transduction during T cell development and activation. Am J Clin Exp Immunol. 2012;1:147–53.
262. Irving J, Matheson E, Minto L, Blair H, Case M, Halsey C, Swidenbank I, Ponthan F, Kirschner-Schwabe R, Groeneveld-Krentz S, Hof J, Allan J, Harrison C, Vormoor J, von Stackelberg A, Eckert C. Ras pathway mutations are prevalent in relapsed childhood acute lymphoblastic leukemia and confer sensitivity to MEK inhibition. Blood. 2014;124:3420–30.
263. Balgobind BV, Van Vlierberghe P, van den Ouweland AM, Beverloo HB, Terlouw-Kromosoeto JN, van Wering ER, Reinhardt D, Horstmann M, Kaspers GJ, Pieters R, Zwaan CM, Van den Heuvel-Eibrink MM, Meijerink JP. Leukemia-associated NF1 inactivation in patients with pediatric T-ALL and AML lacking evidence for neurofibromatosis. Blood. 2008;111:4322–8.
264. Oshima K, Khiabanian H, da Silva-Almeida AC, Tzoneva G, Abate F, Ambesi-Impiombato A, Sanchez-Martin M, Carpenter Z, Penson A, Perez-Garcia A, Eckert C, Nicolas C, Balbin M, Sulis ML, Kato M, Koh K, Paganin M, Basso G, Gastier-Foster JM, Devidas M, Loh ML, Kirschner-Schwabe R, Palomero T, Rabadan R, Ferrando AA. Mutational landscape, clonal evolution patterns, and role of RAS mutations in relapsed acute lymphoblastic leukemia. Proc Natl Acad Sci USA. 2016;113:11306–11.
265. Gu JJ, Ryu JR, Pendergast AM. Abl tyrosine kinases in T-cell signaling. Immunol Rev. 2009;228:170–83.
266. Gu JJ, Zhang N, He YW, Koleske AJ, Pendergast AM. Defective T cell development and function in the absence of Abelson kinases. J Immunol. 2007;179:7334–43.
267. Graux C, Cools J, Melotte C, Quentmeier H, Ferrando A, Levine R, Vermeesch JR, Stul M, Dutta B, Boeckx N, Bosly A, Heimann P, Uyttebroeck A, Mentens N, Somers R, MacLeod RAF, Drexler HG, Look AT, Gilliland DG, Michaux L, Vandenberghe P, Wlodarska I, Marynen P, Hagemeijer A. Fusion of NUP214 to ABL1 on amplified episomes in T-cell acute lymphoblastic leukemia. Nat Genet. 2004;36:1084–9.
268. Van Limbergen H, Beverloo HB, van Drunen E, Janssens A, Hählen K, Poppe B, Van Roy N, Marynen P, De Paepe A, Slater R, Speleman F. Molecular cytogenetic and clinical findings in ETV6/ABL1-positive leukemia. Genes Chromosomes Cancer. 2001;30:274–82.
269. Quentmeier H, Cools J, MacLeod RAF, Marynen P, Uphoff CC, Drexler HG. e6-a2 BCR-ABL1 fusion in T-cell acute lymphoblastic leukemia. Leukemia. 2005;19:295–6.
270. De Keersmaecker K, Graux C, Odero MD, Mentens N, Somers R, Maertens J, Wlodarska I, Vandenberghe P, Hagemeijer A, Marynen P, Cools J. Fusion of EML1 to ABL1 in T-cell acute lymphoblastic leukemia with cryptic t(9;14)(q34;q32). Blood. 2005;105:4849–52.
271. De Keersmaecker K, Lahortiga I, Graux C, Marynen P, Maertens J, Cools J, Vandenberghe P. Transition from EML1-ABL1 to NUP214-ABL1 positivity in a patient with acute T-lymphoblastic leukemia. Leukemia. 2006;20:2202–4.
272. Graux C, Stevens-Kroef M, Lafage M, Dastugue N, Harrison CJ, Mugneret F, Bahloula K, Struski S, Grégoire MJ, Nadal N, Lippert E, Taviaux S, Simons A, Kuiper RP, Moorman AV, Barber K, Bosly A, Michaux L, Vandenberghe P, Lahortiga I, De Keersmaecker K, Wlodarska I, Cools J, Hagemeijer A, Poirel HA, on behalf of the, G. & the, B. Heterogeneous patterns of amplification of the NUP214-ABL1 fusion gene in T-cell acute lymphoblastic leukemia. Leukemia. 2009;23:125–33.
273. Quintás-Cardama A, Tong W, Manshouri T, Vega F, Lennon PA, Cools J, Gilliland DG, Lee F, Cortes J, Kantarjian H, Garcia-Manero G. Activity of tyrosine kinase inhibitors against human NUP214-ABL1-positive T cell malignancies. Leukemia. 2008;22:1117–24.
274. De Keersmaecker K, Versele M, Cools J, Superti-Furga G, Hantschel O. Intrinsic differences between the catalytic properties of the oncogenic NUP214-ABL1 and BCR-ABL1 fusion protein kinases. Leukemia. 2008;22:2208–16.
275. Moorman AV, Schwab C, Winterman E, Hancock J, Castleton A, Cummins M, Gibson B, Goulden N, Kearns P, James B, Kirkwood AA, Lancaster D, Madi M, McMillan A, Motwani J, Norton A, O'Marcaigh A, Patrick K, Bhatnagar N, Qureshi A, Richardson D, Stokley S, Taylor G, van Delft FW, Moppett J, Harrison CJ, Samarasinghe S, Vora A. Adjuvant tyrosine kinase inhibitor therapy improves outcome for children and adolescents with acute lymphoblastic leukaemia who have an ABL-class fusion. Br J Haematol. 2020;191:844–51.
276. De Keersmaecker K, Porcu M, Cox L, Girardi T, Vandepoel R, de Beeck JO, Gielen O, Mentens N,

Bennett KL, Hantschel O. NUP214-ABL1-mediated cell proliferation in T-cell acute lymphoblastic leukemia is dependent on the LCK kinase and various interacting proteins. Haematologica. 2014;99:85–93.
277. Serafin V, Lissandron V, Buldini B, Bresolin S, Paganin M, Grillo F, Andriano N, Palmi C, Cazzaniga G, Marmiroli S, Conter V, Basso G, Accordi B. Phosphoproteomic analysis reveals hyperactivation of mTOR/STAT3 and LCK/Calcineurin axes in pediatric early T-cell precursor ALL. Leukemia. 2017;31:1007–11.
278. Serafin V, Capuzzo G, Milani G, Minuzzo SA, Pinazza M, Bortolozzi R, Bresolin S, Porcù E, Frasson C, Indraccolo S, Basso G, Accordi B. Glucocorticoid resistance is reverted by LCK inhibition in pediatric T-cell acute lymphoblastic leukemia. Blood. 2017;130:2750–61.
279. Todd MA, Picketts DJ. PHF6 interacts with the nucleosome remodeling and deacetylation (NuRD) complex. J Proteome Res. 2012;11:4326–37.
280. Wang J, Leung JW, Gong Z, Feng L, Shi X, Chen J. PHF6 regulates cell cycle progression by suppressing ribosomal RNA synthesis. J Biol Chem. 2013;288:3174–83.
281. Zhang C, Mejia LA, Huang J, Valnegri P, Bennett EJ, Anckar J, Jahani-Asl A, Gallardo G, Ikeuchi Y, Yamada T, Rudnicki M, Harper JW, Bonni A. The X-linked intellectual disability protein PHF6 associates with the PAF1 complex and regulates neuronal migration in the mammalian brain. Neuron. 2013;78:986–93.
282. Van Vlierberghe P, Palomero T, Khiabanian H, Van der Meulen J, Castillo M, Van Roy N, De Moerloose B, Philippe J, Gonzalez-Garcia S, Toribio ML, Taghon T, Zuurbier L, Cauwelier B, Harrison CJ, Schwab C, Pisecker M, Strehl S, Langerak AW, Gecz J, Sonneveld E, Pieters R, Paietta E, Rowe JM, Wiernik PH, Benoit Y, Soulier J, Poppe B, Yao X, Cordon-Cardo C, Meijerink J, Rabadan R, Speleman F, Ferrando A. PHF6 mutations in T-cell acute lymphoblastic leukemia. Nat Genet. 2010;42:338–42.
283. Chao MM, Todd MA, Kontny U, Neas K, Sullivan MJ, Hunter AG, Picketts DJ, Kratz CP. T-cell acute lymphoblastic leukemia in association with Börjeson-Forssman-Lehmann syndrome due to a mutation in PHF6. Pediatr Blood Cancer. 2010;55:722–4.
284. Laugesen A, Højfeldt JW, Helin K. Role of the Polycomb repressive complex 2 (PRC2) in transcriptional regulation and cancer. Cold Spring Harb Perspect Med. 2016;6:a026575.
285. Ntziachristos P, Tsirigos A, Van Vlierberghe P, Nedjic J, Trimarchi T, Flaherty MS, Ferres-Marco D, da Ros V, Tang Z, Siegle J, Asp P, Hadler M, Rigo I, De Keersmaecker K, Patel J, Huynh T, Utro F, Poglio S, Samon JB, Paietta E, Racevskis J, Rowe JM, Rabadan R, Levine RL, Brown S, Pflumio F, Dominguez M, Ferrando A, Aifantis I. Genetic inactivation of the polycomb repressive complex 2 in T cell acute lymphoblastic leukemia. Nat Med. 2012;18:298–301.
286. Zhang J, Zhang Y, Zhang M, Liu C, Liu X, Yin J, Wu P, Chen X, Yang W, Zhang L, Guo Y, Zou Y, Chen Y, Cao Y, Cheng T, Zhu X. FLT3 pathway is a potential therapeutic target for PRC2-mutated T-cell acute lymphoblastic leukemia. Blood. 2018;132:2520–4.
287. Ariës IM, Bodaar K, Karim SA, Chonghaile TN, Hinze L, Burns MA, Pfirrmann M, Degar J, Landrigan JT, Balbach S, Peirs S, Menten B, Isenhart R, Stevenson KE, Neuberg DS, Devidas M, Loh ML, Hunger SP, Teachey DT, Rabin KR, Winter SS, Dunsmore KP, Wood BL, Silverman LB, Sallan SE, Van Vlierberghe P, Orkin SH, Knoechel B, Letai AG, Gutierrez A. PRC2 loss induces chemoresistance by repressing apoptosis in T cell acute lymphoblastic leukemia. J Exp Med. 2018;215:3094–114.
288. Danis E, Yamauchi T, Echanique K, Zhang X, Haladyna JN, Riedel SS, Zhu N, Xie H, Orkin SH, Armstrong SA, Bernt KM, Neff T. Ezh2 controls an early hematopoietic program and growth and survival signaling in early T cell precursor acute lymphoblastic leukemia. Cell Rep. 2016;14:1953–65.
289. Booth CAG, Barkas N, Neo WH, Boukarabila H, Soilleux EJ, Giotopoulos G, Farnoud N, Giustacchini A, Ashley N, Carrelha J, Jamieson L, Atkinson D, Bouriez-Jones T, Prinjha RK, Milne TA, Teachey DT, Papaemmanuil E, Huntly BJP, Jacobsen SEW, Mead AJ. Ezh2 and Runx1 mutations collaborate to initiate Lympho-myeloid leukemia in early Thymic progenitors. Cancer Cell. 2018;33:274–291.e8.
290. Wang C, Oshima M, Sato D, Matsui H, Kubota S, Aoyama K, Nakajima-Takagi Y, Koide S, Matsubayashi J, Mochizuki-Kashio M, Nakano-Yokomizo T, Bai J, Nagao T, Kanai A, Iwama A, Sashida G. Ezh2 loss propagates hypermethylation at T cell differentiation-regulating genes to promote leukemic transformation. J Clin Invest. 2018;128:3872–86.
291. Roels J, Thenoz M, Szarzynska B, Landfors M, De Coninck S, Demoen L, Provez L, Kuchmiy A, Strubbe S, Reunes L, Pieters T, Matthijssens F, Van Loocke W, Erarslan-Uysal B, Richter-Pechanska P, Declerck K, Lammens T, De Moerloose B, Deforce D, Van Nieuwerburgh F, Cheung LC, Kotecha RS, Mansour MR, Ghesquiere B, Van Camp G, Berghe WV, Kowalczyk JR, Szczepanski T, Dave UP, Kulozik AE, Goossens S, Curtis DJ, Taghon T, Dawidowska M, Degerman S, Van Vlierberghe P. Aging of preleukemic thymocytes drives CpG Island hypermethylation in T-cell acute lymphoblastic leukemia. Blood Cancer Discov. 2020;1:274–89.
292. Broux M, Prieto C, Demeyer S, Vanden Bempt M, Alberti-Servera L, Lodewijckx I, Vandepoel R, Mentens N, Gielen O, Jacobs K, Geerdens E, Vicente C, de Bock CE, Cools J. Suz12 inactivation cooperates with JAK3 mutant signaling in the development of T-cell acute lymphoblastic leukemia. Blood. 2019;134:1323–36.

293. Lan F, Bayliss PE, Rinn JL, Whetstine JR, Wang JK, Chen S, Iwase S, Alpatov R, Issaeva I, Canaani E, Roberts TM, Chang HY, Shi Y. A histone H3 lysine 27 demethylase regulates animal posterior development. Nature. 2007;449:689–94.
294. Ntziachristos P, Tsirigos A, Welstead GG, Trimarchi T, Bakogianni S, Xu L, Loizou E, Holmfeldt L, Strikoudis A, King B, Mullenders J, Becksfort J, Nedjic J, Paietta E, Tallman MS, Rowe JM, Tonon G, Satoh T, Kruidenier L, Prinjha R, Akira S, Van Vlierberghe P, Ferrando AA, Jaenisch R, Mullighan CG, Aifantis I. Contrasting roles of histone 3 lysine 27 demethylases in acute lymphoblastic leukaemia. Nature. 2014;514:513–7.
295. Van der Meulen J, Sanghvi V, Mavrakis K, Durinck K, Fang F, Matthijssens F, Rondou P, Rosen M, Pieters T, Vandenberghe P, Delabesse E, Lammens T, De Moerloose B, Menten B, Van Roy N, Verhasselt B, Poppe B, Benoit Y, Taghon T, Melnick AM, Speleman F, Wendel HG, Van Vlierberghe P. The H3K27me3 demethylase UTX is a gender-specific tumor suppressor in T-cell acute lymphoblastic leukemia. Blood. 2015;125:13–21.
296. Kang J, Brajanovski N, Chan KT, Xuan J, Pearson RB, Sanij E. Ribosomal proteins and human diseases: molecular mechanisms and targeted therapy. Signal Transduct Target Ther. 2021;6:323.
297. De Keersmaecker K, Atak ZK, Li N, Vicente C, Patchett S, Girardi T, Gianfelici V, Geerdens E, Clappier E, Porcu M, Lahortiga I, Luca R, Yan J, Hulselmans G, Vranckx H, Vandepoel R, Sweron B, Jacobs K, Mentens N, Wlodarska I, Cauwelier B, Cloos J, Soulier J, Uyttebroeck A, Bagni C, Hassan BA, Vandenberghe P, Johnson AW, Aerts S, Cools J. Exome sequencing identifies mutation in CNOT3 and ribosomal genes RPL5 and RPL10 in T-cell acute lymphoblastic leukemia. Nat Genet. 2013;45:186–90.
298. Tzoneva G, Perez-Garcia A, Carpenter Z, Khiabanian H, Tosello V, Allegretta M, Paietta E, Racevskis J, Rowe JM, Tallman MS, Paganin M, Basso G, Hof J, Kirschner-Schwabe R, Palomero T, Rabadan R, Ferrando A. Activating mutations in the NT5C2 nucleotidase gene drive chemotherapy resistance in relapsed ALL. Nat Med. 2013;19:368–71.
299. Kampen KR, Sulima SO, Verbelen B, Girardi T, Vereecke S, Rinaldi G, Verbeeck J, Op de Beeck J, Uyttebroeck A, Meijerink JP, Moorman AV, Harrison CJ, Spincemaille P, Cools J, Cassiman D, Fendt S-M, Vermeersch P, De Keersmaecker K. The ribosomal RPL10 R98S mutation drives IRES-dependent BCL-2 translation in T-ALL. Leukemia. 2019;33:319–32.
300. Gachet S, El-Chaar T, Avran D, Genesca E, Catez F, Quentin S, Delord M, Thérizols G, Briot D, Meunier G, Hernandez L, Pla M, Smits WK, Buijs-Gladdines JG, Van Loocke W, Menschaert G, André-Schmutz I, Taghon T, Van Vlierberghe P, Meijerink JP, Baruchel A, Dombret H, Clappier E, Diaz J-J, Gazin C, de Thé H, Sigaux F, Soulier J. Deletion 6q drives T-cell leukemia progression by ribosome modulation. Cancer Discov. 2018;8:1614–31.
301. Dörner K, Ruggeri C, Zemp I, Kutay U. Ribosome biogenesis factors-from names to functions. EMBO J. 2023;42:e112699.
302. Grossmann V, Haferlach C, Weissmann S, Roller A, Schindela S, Poetzinger F, Stadler K, Bellos F, Kern W, Haferlach T, Schnittger S, Kohlmann A. The molecular profile of adult T-cell acute lymphoblastic leukemia: mutations in RUNX1 and DNMT3A are associated with poor prognosis in T-ALL. Genes Chromosom Cancer. 2013;52:410–22.
303. Zhang J, Walsh MF, Wu G, Edmonson MN, Gruber TA, Easton J, Hedges D, Ma X, Zhou X, Yergeau DA, Wilkinson MR, Vadodaria B, Chen X, McGee RB, Hines-Dowell S, Nuccio R, Quinn E, Shurtleff SA, Rusch M, Patel A, Becksfort JB, Wang S, Weaver MS, Ding L, Mardis ER, Wilson RK, Gajjar A, Ellison DW, Pappo AS, Pui CH, Nichols KE, Downing JR. Germline mutations in predisposition genes in pediatric cancer. N Engl J Med. 2015;373:2336–46.
304. Stieglitz E, Loh ML. Genetic predispositions to childhood leukemia. Ther Adv Hematol. 2013;4:270–90.
305. Pan J, Tan Y, Wang G, Deng B, Ling Z, Song W, Seery S, Zhang Y, Peng S, Xu J, Duan J, Wang Z, Yu X, Zheng Q, Xu X, Yuan Y, Yan F, Tian Z, Tang K, Zhang J, Chang AH, Feng X. Donor-derived CD7 chimeric antigen receptor T cells for T-cell acute lymphoblastic leukemia: first-in-human, phase I trial. J Clin Oncol. 2021;39:3340–51.
306. Sánchez-Martínez D, Baroni ML, Gutierrez-Agüera F, Roca-Ho H, Blanch-Lombarte O, González-García S, Torrebadell M, Junca J, Ramírez-Orellana M, Velasco-Hernández T, Bueno C, Fuster JL, Prado JG, Calvo J, Uzan B, Cools J, Camos M, Pflumio F, Toribio ML, Menéndez P. Fratricide-resistant CD1a-specific CAR T cells for the treatment of cortical T-cell acute lymphoblastic leukemia. Blood. 2019;133:2291–304.
307. Rodewald H-R, Fehling HJ. Molecular and cellular events in early Thymocyte development 11Received for publication October 14, 1997. In: Dixon FJ, editor. Advances in immunology. Academic Press; 1998. p. 1–112.
308. Kikuchi A, Hayashi Y, Kobayashi S, Hanada R, Moriwaki K, Yamamoto K, Fujimoto J, Kaneko Y, Yamamori S. Clinical significance of TAL1 gene alteration in childhood T-cell acute lymphoblastic leukemia and lymphoma. Leukemia. 1993;7:933–8.
309. Bash RO, Crist WM, Shuster JJ, Link MP, Amylon M, Pullen J, Carroll AJ, Buchanan GR, Smith RG, Baer R. Clinical features and outcome of T-cell acute lymphoblastic leukemia in childhood with respect to alterations at the TAL1 locus: a pediatric oncology group study. Blood. 1993;81:2110–7.
310. Wang D, Zhu G, Wang N, Zhou X, Yang Y, Zhou S, Xiong J, He J, Jiang L, Li C, Xu D, Huang L, Zhou J. SIL-TAL1 rearrangement is related with poor out-

come: a study from a Chinese institution. PLoS One. 2013;8:e73865.
311. Haider Z, Larsson P, Landfors M, Köhn L, Schmiegelow K, Flaegstad T, Kanerva J, Heyman M, Hultdin M, Degerman S. An integrated transcriptome analysis in T-cell acute lymphoblastic leukemia links DNA methylation subgroups to dysregulated TAL1 and ANTP homeobox gene expression. Cancer Med. 2019;8:311–24.
312. Bergeron J, Clappier E, Radford I, Buzyn A, Millien C, Soler G, Ballerini P, Thomas X, Soulier J, Dombret H, Macintyre EA, Asnafi V. Prognostic and oncogenic relevance of TLX1/HOX11 expression level in T-ALLs. Blood. 2007;110:2324–30.
313. Paola B, Judith L-P, Jean Michel C, Vahid A, Myriam L, Virginie G, Yves P, Gérard M, Thierry L, Claudine S, Sylvie F, Anne H, François S, Marie Françoise A, Luc D, Guy L, André B. Impact of genotype on survival of children with T-cell acute lymphoblastic leukemia treated according to the French protocol FRALLE-93: the effect of TLX3/HOX11L2 gene expression on outcome. Haematologica. 2008;93:1658–65.
314. Hagemeijer A, Graux C. ABL1 rearrangements in T-cell acute lymphoblastic leukemia. Genes Chromosom Cancer. 2010;49:299–308.
315. Allen A, Sireci A, Colovai A, Pinkney K, Sulis M, Bhagat G, Alobeid B. Early T-cell precursor leukemia/lymphoma in adults and children. Leuk Res. 2013;37:1027–34.
316. Patrick K, Wade R, Goulden N, Mitchell C, Moorman AV, Rowntree C, Jenkinson S, Hough R, Vora A. Outcome for children and young people with early T-cell precursor acute lymphoblastic leukaemia treated on a contemporary protocol, UKALL 2003. Br J Haematol. 2014;166:421–4.
317. Bond J, Graux C, Lhermitte L, Lara D, Cluzeau T, Leguay T, Cieslak A, Trinquand A, Pastoret C, Belhocine M, Spicuglia S, Lheritier V, Leprêtre S, Thomas X, Huguet F, Ifrah N, Dombret H, Macintyre E, Boissel N, Asnafi V. Early response-based therapy stratification improves survival in adult early Thymic precursor acute lymphoblastic leukemia: A Group for Research on adult acute lymphoblastic leukemia study. J Clin Oncol. 2017;35:2683–91.
318. Zuurbier L, Gutierrez A, Mullighan CG, Cante-Barrett K, Gevaert AO, de Rooi J, Li Y, Smits WK, Buijs-Gladdines JG, Sonneveld E, Look AT, Horstmann M, Pieters R, Meijerink JP. Immature MEF2C-dysregulated T-cell leukemia patients have an early T-cell precursor acute lymphoblastic leukemia gene signature and typically have non-rearranged T-cell receptors. Haematologica. 2014;99:94–102.
319. Fang H, Wang W, El Hussein S, Morita K, Beird HC, Mitra A, Loghavi S, Lin P, Jabbour EJ, Khoury JD. B-cell lymphoma/leukaemia 11B (BCL11B) expression status helps distinguish early T-cell precursor acute lymphoblastic leukaemia/lymphoma (ETP-ALL/LBL) from other subtypes of T-cell ALL/LBL. Br J Haematol. 2021;194:1034–8.
320. Wong M, Mayoh C, Lau LMS, Khuong-Quang DA, Pinese M, Kumar A, Barahona P, Wilkie EE, Sullivan P, Bowen-James R, Syed M, Martincorena I, Abascal F, Sherstyuk A, Bolanos NA, Baber J, Priestley P, Dolman MEM, Fleuren EDG, Gauthier ME, Mould EVA, Gayevskiy V, Gifford AJ, Grebert-Wade D, Strong PA, Manouvrier E, Warby M, Thomas DM, Kirk J, Tucker K, O'Brien T, Alvaro F, McCowage GB, Dalla-Pozza L, Gottardo NG, Tapp H, Wood P, Khaw SL, Hansford JR, Moore AS, Norris MD, Trahair TN, Lock RB, Tyrrell V, Haber M, Marshall GM, Ziegler DS, Ekert PG, Cowley MJ. Whole genome, transcriptome and methylome profiling enhances actionable target discovery in high-risk pediatric cancer. Nat Med. 2020;26:1742–53.
321. Newman S, Nakitandwe J, Kesserwan CA, Azzato EM, Wheeler DA, Rusch M, Shurtleff S, Hedges DJ, Hamilton KV, Foy SG, Edmonson MN, Thrasher A, Bahrami A, Orr BA, Klco JM, Gu J, Harrison LW, Wang L, Clay MR, Ouma A, Silkov A, Liu Y, Zhang Z, Liu Y, Brady SW, Zhou X, Chang TC, Pande M, Davis E, Becksfort J, Patel A, Wilkinson MR, Rahbarinia D, Kubal M, Maciaszek JL, Pastor V, Knight J, Gout AM, Wang J, Gu Z, Mullighan CG, McGee RB, Quinn EA, Nuccio R, Mostafavi R, Gerhardt EL, Taylor LM, Valdez JM, Hines-Dowell SJ, Pappo AS, Robinson G, Johnson LM, Pui CH, Ellison DW, Downing JR, Zhang J, Nichols KE. Genomes for kids: the scope of pathogenic mutations in pediatric cancer revealed by comprehensive DNA and RNA sequencing. Cancer Discov. 2021;11:3008–27.
322. Kunz JB, Rausch T, Bandapalli OR, Eilers J, Pechanska P, Schuessele S, Assenov Y, Stutz AM, Kirschner-Schwabe R, Hof J, Eckert C, von Stackelberg A, Schrappe M, Stanulla M, Koehler R, Avigad S, Elitzur S, Handgretinger R, Benes V, Weischenfeldt J, Korbel JO, Muckenthaler MU, Kulozik AE. Pediatric T-lymphoblastic leukemia evolves into relapse by clonal selection, acquisition of mutations and promoter hypomethylation. Haematologica. 2015;
323. Ghazalpour A, Bennett B, Petyuk VA, Orozco L, Hagopian R, Mungrue IN, Farber CR, Sinsheimer J, Kang HM, Furlotte N, Park CC, Wen PZ, Brewer H, Weitz K, Camp DG 2nd, Pan C, Yordanova R, Neuhaus I, Tilford C, Siemers N, Gargalovic P, Eskin E, Kirchgessner T, Smith DJ, Smith RD, Lusis AJ. Comparative analysis of proteome and transcriptome variation in mouse. PLoS Genet. 2011;7:e1001393.
324. Liu Y, Beyer A, Aebersold R. On the dependency of cellular protein levels on mRNA abundance. Cell. 2016;165:535–50.

Clinical and Laboratory Features of Children and Young People with ALL

4

Rachael Hough and Ajay Vora

4.1 Clinical Features

Acute lymphoblastic leukaemia (ALL) is more common in boys than girls and is primarily a disease of young children (Table 4.1). Children and young people with ALL frequently present with symptoms and signs of pancytopenia due to marrow infiltration. Fever, often due to leukaemia rather than infection, is present in 60% of patients. A meta-analysis of more than 3000 children with childhood leukaemia [1] found that more than half presented with at least one of the following five features: palpable liver, palpable spleen, pallor, fever or bruising. Lymphadenopathy was noted in nearly a half of children and musculoskeletal pain was a presenting feature in 43% of cases. Young children with bone pain may present with a limp or refusal to bear weight. Bulky extramedullary disease, especially overt CNS disease, mediastinal mass and renal infiltrates are more common in T-lineage ALL. Mediastinal masses can cause superior vena cava (SVC) syndrome which can present with swelling of the face and upper limbs due to compression of the SVC. CNS involvement is usually leptomeningeal rather than parenchymal and may present with symptoms of meningism or cranial nerve palsies. Ocular involvement is more common at relapse than first presentation and can affect the retina, ocular nerve, orbit, cornea or anterior chamber with hypopyon. Painless enlargement of the scrotum may be due to a testicular infiltrate or hydrocele resulting from lymphatic obstruction. Rarely, the diagnosis is made in a child who has a blood count for minor, non-specific, symptoms.

4.2 Laboratory Features

A blood count at diagnosis shows varying degrees of pancytopenia which is generally more severe in B-lineage than T-lineage ALL. Initial leucocyte count (Table 4.1) ranges from 0.5 to $>1000 \times 10^9$/L (median 12×10^9/L); it is greater than 10×10^9/L in slightly over half of patients and greater than 100×10^9/L in 10–15% of patients. Most patients have circulating blasts, but they may be difficult to detect in those with leucopenia without careful scrutiny of a blood film ('aleukaemic leukaemia'). Reactive hypereosinophilia with pulmonary infiltration and cardiomyopathy is a feature of a rare sub-type of B-lineage ALL with t(5;14)(q31;q32)/*IGH-IL3*. Coagulopathy is less common than in acute myeloid leukaemia, usually mild, and not associated with severe haemorrhage except in patients with very high white

R. Hough (✉)
University College Hospital, London, UK
e-mail: rachaelhough@nhs.net

A. Vora
Great Ormond Street Hospital, London, UK
e-mail: Ajay.Vora@gosh.nhs.uk

G. Escherich, V. Conter (eds.), *Acute Lymphoblastic Leukemia in Children and Adolescents*, Pediatric Oncology, https://doi.org/10.1007/978-3-031-71180-0_4

Table 4.1 Characteristics of patients in UKALL 2003 (October 2003–June 2011)

Clinical feature		Number (%)
Total		3126
Sex		
	Male	1776 (57)
	Female	1350 (43)
Age (years)		
	Median	5 (1–24)
	<2	210 (7)
	2–9	2077 (66)
	10–15	610 (20)
	16–24	229 (7)
Immunophenotype		
	B-lineage	2733 (88)
	T-lineage	386 (12)
	Not known	7
NCI risk group		
	High	1310 (42)
	Standard	1816 (58)
WCC × 10^9/L:		
	Median (range)	12 (0.4–881)
	<10	1407 (45)
	10–19	502 (16)
	20–49	526 (17)
	50–99	315 (10)
	≥100	376 (12)

Modified from Toft et al. [5]
NCI National Cancer Institute, *WCC* white cell count

cell counts who are at risk of CNS haemorrhage due to leukostasis and tumour lysis. Elevated uric acid and phosphorus levels may be seen due to rapid tumour proliferation in patients with high tumour burden. An enlarged kidney can be detected in 30–50% of patients but has no prognostic or therapeutic implications. Raised liver enzymes due to leukaemic infiltration are present in 10–20% of patients, are usually mild and have no important clinical or prognostic consequences. A minority of patients may have cholestatic jaundice due to lymphadenopathy at the porta hepatis or portal tract infiltration. Abnormalities of the bone, such as metaphyseal banding, periosteal reactions, osteolysis, osteosclerosis or osteopenia with or without fractures, are present in half of the patients. As these changes do not affect treatment and outcome, routine diagnostic imaging studies (except for chest radiography to rule out mediastinal mass) is not necessary.

Leukaemic blast cells are identified morphologically at diagnosis in a cytospin of cerebrospinal fluid (CSF) in approximately one-third of cases, most of whom have no neurological symptoms. Only a minority of such cases (2–3%) fulfil the criteria for CNS leukaemia (CNS 3) which is defined by the presence of at least five leucocytes per microlitre of CSF and the detection of leukaemic blast cells, or by the presence of cranial nerve palsy. A recent Scandinavian group (NOPHO) study detected CSF blasts in newly diagnosed ALL patients by cytospin in 13.8% and by flow cytometry in 25.4% [2, 3]. Patients with T-ALL, high count ALL and traumatic lumbar punctures (defined as >10 RBC/μl) were more likely to have blasts detected by flow cytometry. CSF positivity, either detected by a cytospin or by flow cytometry, was associated with a higher risk of relapse. Further studies are planned to determine the prognostic value of CSF leukaemia detection by flow cytometry.

A dense infiltrate of lymphoblasts is usually detected in a marrow aspirate. Occasionally, the aspirate may be difficult to obtain and appear hypocellular with sparse blasts due to haemodilution. In such cases, a trephine invariably shows a dense infiltrate but in rare cases with 'aplastic' presentation (see Sect. 3) may also be severely hypocellular. Morphological analysis of leukaemic cells distinguishes three subtypes of ALL (L1, L2 and L3) according to the French–American–British (FAB) classification. Unlike in AML, the FAB classification has no prognostic or therapeutic relevance in ALL and, along with cytochemical staining, has been replaced by immunophenotypic and genotypic diagnostic investigation and classification. The immunophenotype of ALL can be characterized by flow cytometry of the peripheral blood, bone marrow and CSF or immunohistochemistry of bone marrow trephines. These techniques confirm the diagnosis of ALL and define whether the blasts are of B- or T-cell lineage. Analysis of genetic aberrations has traditionally used G-banding (karyotype) or fluorescence in situ hybridization (FISH) with molecular techniques being more widely used in recent years. Specific genetic abnormalities are clearly associated with differ-

Table 4.2 Frequency of presenting features according to age in NOPHO2008

Age group (years)	1–9 (%)	10–17 (%)	18–45 (%)	All (%)	P (%)
All	1022 (67.7)	266 (17.6)	221 (14.6)	1509 (100)	
Immunophenotype B	929 (90.9)	199 (74.8)	150 (67.9)	1278 (84.7)	**0.001**
T	93 (9.1)	67 (25.2)	71 (32.1)	231 (15.3)	
WBC < 100	897 (87.8)	221 (83.1)	182 (84.3)	1300 (86.4)	0.094
⩾ 100	125 (12.2)	45 (16.9)	34 (15.7)	204 (13.6)	
CNS status					
CNS 1	888 (87.1)	233 (87.9)	198 (92.1)	1319 (88)	0.12
CNS 2	91 (8.9)	17 (6.4)	11 (5.1)	119 (7.9)	
CNS 3	40 (3.9)	15 (5.7)	6 (2.8)	61 (4.1)	
t(12;21) Present	287 (28.5)	16 (6.1)	4 (1.9)	307 (20.8)	**0.001**
Absent	720 (71.5)	246 (93.9)	204 (98.1)	1170 (79.2)	
Hyperdiploid Present	336 (38.4)	42 (19.4)	23 (13)	401 (31.6)	**0.001**
Absent	540 (61.6)	174 (80.6)	154 (87)	868 (68.4)	
iAmp21 Present	15 (1.5)	15 (5.8)	4 (2)	34 (2.3)	**0.001**[c]
Absent	984 (98.5)	244 (94.2)	197 (98)	1425 (97.7)	

ent clinical outcomes with good risk cytogenetics including high hyperdiploidy, *ETV6-RUNX1* and *TCF3-PBX1* and high risk cytogenetics including hypodiploidy, *BCR-ABL1* and *KMT2A*.

Over the last two decades there has been an increasing use of paediatric or 'paediatric-inspired' protocols in adolescent and young adults (AYA) with ALL. These studies have shown that the presenting and diagnostic features described above for children are similar. However, the frequency of poor prognostic features, such as T-cell immunophenotype and deleterious genetic profiles [4–8], increases with increasing age (Table 4.2).

4.3 Differential Diagnosis

Immune thrombocytopenic purpura (ITP) is the most common benign condition to be associated with symptoms that raise concern about leukaemia. Severe skin haemorrhage in an otherwise well child with isolated severe thrombocytopenia and normal blood film without circulating blasts makes it possible to distinguish the condition from leukaemia in a vast majority of cases. The presence of mild anaemia due to nose or gum bleeding and activated lymphocytes on blood film due to a recent viral illness, may create diagnostic uncertainty in some cases but it should be possible for an experienced morphologist to exclude the presence of blasts on a blood film without resorting to a bone marrow aspirate. The mean corpuscular volume (MCV) of red blood cells is usually normal in patients with ALL but low in those with iron deficiency due to chronic bleeding and the latter can be identified by performing iron studies in the peripheral blood.

Pancytopenia due to aplastic anaemia is difficult to distinguish from 'aleukaemic leukaemia' without examination of a bone marrow aspirate and trephine. Rare cases of ALL present with an aplastic marrow without blasts, often accompanying severe sepsis, with spontaneous reconstitution of normal haemopoiesis on recovery from the infection. They re-present several weeks to months later with low counts and circulating lymphoblasts. Clonal rearrangements are invariably detected on retrospective examination of the initial marrow using sensitive genetic techniques and it i's likely that the 'aplastic' presentation of ALL in such cases is due to severe sepsis causing marrow aplasia followed by spontaneous remission due to a cytokine release phenomenon.

Bone pain, arthralgia and occasionally arthritis may mimic juvenile arthritis in a minority of patients.

Paediatric small round cell tumours that involve the bone marrow, including neuroblastoma, rhabdomyosarcoma and retinoblastoma, may be confused with ALL on marrow morphology but can be easily distinguished on flow cytometry or immune-histochemistry.

References

1. Clarke RT, Van den Bruel A, Bankhead C, Mitchell CD, Phillips B, Thompson MJ. Clinical presentation of childhood leukaemia: a systematic review and meta-analysis. Arch Dis Child. 2016;101(10):894–901. https://doi.org/10.1136/archdischild-2016-311251.
2. Thastrup M, Marquart HV, Levinsen M, et al. Flow cytometric analysis of cerebrospinal fluid improves detection of leukaemic blasts in infants with acute lymphoblastic leukaemia. Br J Haematol. 2021;195(1):119–22. https://doi.org/10.1111/bjh.17769.
3. Thastrup M, Marquart HV, Levinsen M, et al. Flow cytometric detection of leukemic blasts in cerebrospinal fluid predicts risk of relapse in childhood acute lymphoblastic leukemia: a Nordic Society of Pediatric Hematology and Oncology study. Leukemia. 2020;34(2):336–46. https://doi.org/10.1038/s41375-019-0570-1.
4. Hough R, Rowntree C, Goulden N, et al. Efficacy and toxicity of a paediatric protocol in teenagers and young adults with Philadelphia chromosome negative acute lymphoblastic leukaemia: results from UKALL 2003. Br J Haematol. 2016;172(3):439–51. https://doi.org/10.1111/bjh.13847.
5. Toft N, Birgens H, Abrahamsson J, et al. Results of NOPHO ALL2008 treatment for patients aged 1-45 years with acute lymphoblastic leukemia. Leukemia. 2018;32(3):606–15. https://doi.org/10.1038/leu.2017.265.
6. Nachman JB, La MK, Hunger SP, et al. Young adults with acute lymphoblastic leukemia have an excellent outcome with chemotherapy alone and benefit from intensive postinduction treatment: a report from the Children's oncology group. J Clin Oncol. 2009;27(31):5189–94. https://doi.org/10.1200/JCO.2008.20.8959.
7. Hocking J, Schwarer AP, Gasiorowski R, et al. Excellent outcomes for adolescents and adults with acute lymphoblastic leukemia and lymphoma without allogeneic stem cell transplant: the FRALLE-93 pediatric protocol. Leuk Lymphoma. 2014;55(12):2801–7. https://doi.org/10.3109/10428194.2014.894191.
8. Ribera JM, Oriol A, Sanz MA, et al. Comparison of the results of the treatment of adolescents and young adults with standard-risk acute lymphoblastic leukemia with the Programa Espanol de Tratamiento en Hematologia pediatric-based protocol ALL-96. J Clin Oncol. 2008;26(11):1843–9. https://doi.org/10.1200/JCO.2007.13.7265.

Immunological Diagnosis

5

Margarita Maurer-Granofszky
and Michael N. Dworzak

5.1 Overview of Immunophenotyping at Diagnosis

Immunophenotyping by FCM is applied in combination with cytogenetic and molecular testing to define the subtype of leukemia according to a growing list of clinically relevant categories, many but not all of which are established in the current WHO classification [1, 2]. Immunophenotyping is primarily used for acute leukemia (AL) lineage assignment. Acute lymphoblastic leukemia (ALL) needs to be distinguished from acute myeloid leukemia (AML) and the former can be further subdivided into leukemias of B or T lineage. This permits timely selection of the further diagnostic workup as well as prompt initiation of chemotherapy according to lineage-oriented paths. Importantly, leukemias which fulfill criteria of more than one lineage (variable terminology according to reference: AL of ambiguous lineage, ALAL; mixed phenotype AL, MPAL; biphenotypic AL, BAL) or without a clear lineage derivation (acute undifferentiated leukemia, AUL) do also exist.

In the process of immunophenotyping, panels of surface and intracellular antigens known to be expressed on hematopoietic cells in association with lineage, stage of differentiation, and/or malignant transformation are evaluated on the leukemic cells. Antigen expression rating considers both qualitative (positive or negative) as well as quantitative aspects (weak or strong expression; partial positivity on a blast subset) [3, 4]. In the late 1990s, a score system was established by the European Group for Immunological Classification of Leukemia (EGIL) that assigns different weight to different antigens for lineage assignment [5]. In this scoring system, AML and ALL subtypes exhibiting marker expression of only one lineage or with limited cross-lineage antigen expression, and those fulfilling criteria of BAL (if a score of >2 is achieved for at least two lineages) can be distinguished. The WHO classification later adopted this approach but modified the criteria to warrant diagnosis of MPAL by putting more weight on fewer but fundamental lineage antigens [2]. This approach has seen refinements over time to incorporate guidelines to quantify expression levels of these markers in order to avoid misinterpretation of marginal cross-lineage coexpression patterns as sign of MPAL [1, 2]. Currently, when making a diagnosis of

M. Maurer-Granofszky
St. Anna Children's Cancer Research Institute (CCRI), Vienna, Austria

M. N. Dworzak (✉)
St. Anna Children's Hospital, Department of Pediatrics, Medical University of Vienna, Vienna, Austria

St. Anna Children's Cancer Research Institute (CCRI), Vienna, Austria
e-mail: michael.dworzak@stanna.at

G. Escherich, V. Conter (eds.), *Acute Lymphoblastic Leukemia in Children and Adolescents*, Pediatric Oncology, https://doi.org/10.1007/978-3-031-71180-0_5

MPAL, lineage affiliation is assigned by strong CD19 expression and at least one additional B-lineage marker for B-, strong cyCD3/sCD3 expression for T- and strong myeloperoxidase or clear monocytic differentiation in case of myeloid lineage. Notably, a diagnosis of AL with differentiation into more than one lineage potentially implicates a conundrum with respect to treatment choice. Toward this end, the Associazione Italiana di Ematologia e Oncologia Pediatrica (AIEOP) and Berlin–Frankfurt–Münster (BFM) consortium established the concept and criteria for dominant lineage assignment, irrespective of whether a case fulfills also MPAL or BAL criteria [4]. This approach allows for assignment of the dominant lineage in cases of BAL/MPAL with a single blast clone, whereas only the very rare cases with blasts differentiating into separate lineage subsets (bilineal or complex MPAL) cannot be assigned to a dominant lineage. Along this reasoning, cases with a dominant lineage should primarily be treated along the treatment path available for this AL lineage [4, 6].

In addition to lineage assignment, immunophenotyping renders also information on the differentiation level of the blast population. Leukemic maturation levels in ALL are defined by different antigen patterns which show similarities but also differences compared to normal lymphopoiesis. The ALL maturational subclassification most broadly used in Europe is from EGIL [5]. In this system, B-ALLs can be subclassified into pro-B ALL (B-I), common-ALL (B-II), pre-B-ALL (B-III) and mature B-ALL (B-IV) and T-ALLs are further classified into pro-T (T-I), pre-T (T-II), cortical T (T-III), and mature T-ALL (T-IV). More recently, early T-cell precursor ALL (ETP) has been characterized as a fifth subgroup with only limited T-antigen expression (e.g., absent CD1a, CD3, CD4, CD8, weak/negative CD5) along with cross-lineage myeloid marker positivity but is a subset of T-I/T-II cases [7]. Although there is association between maturational stage and outcome (favorable in B-II, B-III, T-III), this does not render independent prognostic information because immunophenotypes are strongly related to genetic background in ALL which has more specific impact on outcome and treatment choice. Hence, maturational subclassification is generally not applied to risk stratification but can inform of underlying genetic lesions driving aberrant maturational patterns, as shown below.

Based on WHO [1, 2] and EGIL [5, 8] classification, the AIEOP-BFM group has established a consensus panel to meet the requirements for immunophenotypic diagnosis of pediatric ALL, MPAL, BAL as well as ETP discrimination (Table 5.1) [4].

Table 5.1 Mandatory diagnostic intracellular and surface antigens plus optional markers associated with genetic subtype or suitable for FCM-MRD assessment in pediatric ALL

Intracellular markers[a]	iCD3, iCD22, iCD79a, iIgM (μ-chain), iMPO, iLysozyme
Surface markers[a]	CD2, CD3, CD5, CD7; CD10, CD19, CD20; CD11b, CD11c, CD13, CD14, CD15, CD33, CD64, CD117; CD34, CD45, CD56, HLA-DR If T-ALL: CD1a, CD4, CD8, TCRαβ, TCRγδ If B-IV suspected: Kappa chain/lambda chain
Recommended additional/optional markers	All cases: NG2, CD38, CD99, CD371 If B-ALL: CD11a, CD22, CD24, CD27, CD44, CD58, CD66c, CD73, CD86, CD123, CRLF2 If T-ALL: CD48, iTdT If ALAL (AUL or MPAL): All involved lineage-associated markers should be evaluated If AUL, platelet/dendritic cell markers should be evaluated

Modified from [4]

ALAL ambiguous lineage acute leukemia, *ALL* acute lymphoblastic leukemia, *i* intracellular, *ETP* early T-cell precursor, *MPAL* mixed phenotype acute leukemia, *MPO* myeloperoxidase, *AUL* acute undifferentiated leukemia

[a]Mandatory markers for WHO, EGIL, ETP classifications

5.2 Markers with Implications for Measurable Residual Disease (MRD) Assessment

In pediatric ALL, MRD assessment by flow cytometry (FCM-MRD) is a well-established methodology to evaluate treatment response for risk stratification and to guide further treatment [9]. Significant efforts have been made by laboratory consortia such as the International-BFM FCM network [10, 11] or EuroFlow [12] to optimize and standardize FCM-MRD methodology in pediatric ALL and allow for multicentric application of the assay in internationally collaborative clinical trials. The basic objective of FCM-MRD is the sensitive and specific discrimination of residual leukemic blasts from normal hematopoietic cells. In ALL this is achieved via the leukemia-associated immunophenotype (LAIP) approach, which is based on the detection of leukemia specific phenotypic markers or marker profiles (antigen over- or under-expression or asynchronous marker constellations) that are tracked during follow-up [13]. It is important to note that such aberrant antigen expression in ALL follows generic, recurrent patterns which allows to screen for as well as discern malignant lymphoblasts even at low quantities in the case of suspicion, prior to formal diagnosis of ALL and without knowledge of its immunophenotype.

Nowadays, 8–13-color approaches are used for MRD assessment [14–17]. Usually, a set of commonly used backbone markers against lineage and maturational stage-associated antigens is complemented with LAIP markers for MRD detection. Careful marker selection as well as design of marker combinations for follow-up assessments demands their evaluation already at diagnosis.

In pediatric B-ALL, antigens including CD11a [13], CD38 [17], CD58 [18], CD123 [19, 20], CD371 [21, 22], CRLF2 [23], and NG2 [24] have proven to be particularly useful for the discrimination of leukemic blasts from normal BCPs (Table 5.1). Besides those also other markers like CD49f [25], CD73 [26, 27], CD81 [28], CD86 [26, 27], and CD304 [27] can be used. In contrast to B-ALL, there are fewer reports of FCM-panels for MRD assessment in T-ALL [29–31]. In the latter, typical panels consist of antibodies against broadly expressed leukocyte antigens (e.g., CD45, CD48) and common T-lineage antigens (e.g., CD3, CD4, CD5, CD7, CD8) combined with immaturity markers (CD34, CD99, iTdT) to identify T-cell lymphoblasts. Expression of antigens normally completely absent on T cells is less common in T-ALL and occurs mainly in ETP (e.g., expression of myeloid antigens like CD33 and/or CD117).

As the leukemia evolves and under therapeutic pressure, immunophenotypic features may change and antigens may appear down- or up-regulated due to either treatment-associated selection of blast subsets or drug-induced modulation of gene expression [29, 30, 32, 33]. Of further relevance in current clinical practice is antigenic escape along with immunotherapies. A potential loss of CD19, the primary blast cell gating marker in MRD-evaluation, demands assessment of alternative B-cell antigens like CD22 and CD24 already at diagnosis and in follow-up after CD19-directed immunotherapy [34]. Loss of CD19 expression on leukemic cells may also occur early during induction therapy in certain B-ALL subtypes (e.g., with *DUX4*-fusion, *ZNF384*-fusions or PAX5-P80R mutation) who show a propensity to undergo steroid-induced monocytoid transdifferentiation ("monocytic switch") [35]. In those cases, information on specific marker expression patterns (e.g., CD371) at diagnosis allows for selection of specific follow-up panels which are able to delineate switching monocytoid blasts not resembling lymphoblasts anymore [21, 22]. This type of transdifferentiation to eventually mature monocytes (with no need to change lymphoblast-oriented treatment) differs markedly from the type of lineage switch occurring in *KMT2A*-rearranged ALL. The latter type of switch may also appear early in induction (most probably on the basis of bilineal MPAL with a minor preexisting myeloid blast clone which escaped attention at diagnosis) or later on, either at relapse or after immunotherapies [36–38]. Such switch blasts usually fulfill criteria of immature myeloid blasts indistinguishable from AML and contain the same genetic lesion as the primary lymphoblastic disease. Hence, careful inspection of immunophenotyping analyses for the existence of minor additional myeloid blast subsets is especially warranted in cases of *KMT2A*-rearranged ALL.

5.3 Markers with Implications for Immunotherapy

Immunotherapeutic approaches targeting antigens on leukemic blasts nowadays play more and more role in the management of ALL. Hence, immunophenotyping is a prerequisite for choosing the immunotherapeutic strategy and must inform on both, level of antigen expression on blasts as well as whether the entire leukemic population or only a subset expresses the antigen of interest. Since antigen expression on blast cells is not a stable phenomenon [32, 33], immunophenotyping data from diagnosis are not sufficiently valid when planning interventions later during treatment and new options for treatment may appear especially during follow-up. This makes FCM-MRD a unique diagnostic assay not only regarding treatment response assessment but also with respect to selecting the targets for immunotherapy [33].

In the case of B-ALL, therapeutic antibodies against CD19 (e.g., blinatumomab), CD22 (e.g., inotuzumab), or against CD20 (e.g., rituximab) are used in clinical practice [39]. In T-ALL, Daratumumab, a human monoclonal antibody targeting CD38 is a therapeutic option since the antigen is expressed on T-ALL blasts and remains stable after chemotherapy [39–42] In the case of CD33 expressing ALL, also such a myeloid-directed immunotherapeutic approach (e.g., gemtuzumab) may be warranted.

In addition to specific monoclonal antibodies, autologous T lymphocytes equipped with chimeric antigen receptors (CAR) are an established treatment option in particular for relapsed or resistant disease. To date, CAR-T cell therapy has been most successful in B-ALL. CD19-targeted CAR-T cells were able to cure pediatric patients as the last resort after blinatumomab therapy [43]. There are also promising data from CD22 CAR-T-cell trials in children and AYA [44, 45]. In addition, CAR-T cells targeting CD20 [46] or CRLF2 [47, 48] have been developed. Although CD123- and CD371-directed CAR-T cells are currently considered mainly for targeting acute myeloid leukemia, it may also be an innovative treatment strategy for specific B-ALLs subtypes such as CD123-positive hyperdiploid and CD371-positive *DUX4*-rearranged B-ALL [19–22, 49]. In T-ALL, CAR-T cell therapy is less straightforward due to challenges based on both, protracted T-cell aplasia and fratricide (self-targeting), which need to be overcome via gene editing or transduction to decrease expression of the target antigen on the CAR-T cells themselves [50]. CAR-T cells targeting CD1a, CD2, CD5, CD7 as well as CD38 have already been studied in preclinical models and some of them, in particular against CD7, are currently under investigation in clinical trials.

Determination of the lack or preservation of antigen expression during or after immunotherapies is crucial for the further choice of treatment strategy. For example, CD19 negativity occurs after CD19 targeted therapy with Blinatumomab or CAR-T cells [51, 52]. Hence, information on the expression of other typical B-cell antigens like CD20, CD22, and CD24 is required either for choosing other possible immunotherapies or for blast cell gating [34].

5.4 Correlation Between Immunophenotype and Genotype

5.4.1 Genotype–Immunophenotype Correlations in B-ALL

Various genetic and molecular aberrations are associated with a distinct antigen expression pattern in ALL. Immunophenotyping may therefore rapidly direct further testing toward the suspected genetic lesion. Information from immunophenotyping can thus be used for selective screening instead of a broad genetic screening in case of limited time or resources.

Only a few individual markers are informative regarding a specific genetic subgroup. Examples for strong correlations of single markers with distinct genotypes include:

CD123 Overexpression of CD123, the interleukin-3 receptor alpha chain (IL-3Rα), alone is strongly associated with hyperdiploid pediatric B-ALL [19, 20, 53]. Sensitivity and specificity of CD123 expression for hyperdiploid genotype prediction have been reported to be 81.5% and 91.5%, respectively, with a positive predictive value of 78.6% [19]. A machine learning-based analysis of immunophenotypic data from 818 patients identified CD123 as the top ranked feature in hyperdiploidy prediction [54].

CD371 Strong expression of the surface antigen CD371 (CLL-1), encoded by *CLEC12A* is pathognomonic of *DUX4*-rearranged B-ALL [22, 55] and can be used as surrogate marker for this subtype in which genetic diagnosis is technically challenging and not yet broadly available. Notably, approximately 8% of all B-ALLs are CD371-positive and *DUX4r* B-ALL is thus the most frequent subtype with propensity to monocytoid shift during induction [21, 35].

CRLF2 Expression of the cytokine receptor like factor-2 (CRLF2; also known as thymic stromal lymphopoietin receptor, TSLPR) is characteristic for B-ALLs with a rearrangement of *CRLF2* [56–68]. *CRLF2r* arises mainly from reciprocal translocations either with the immunoglobulin heavy chain locus (*IGH*::*CRFL2*) or an interstitial deletion within PAR1 (*P2RY8*::*CRLF2*), both leading to overexpression of CRLF2 mRNA and protein [23]. Around 47% of *BCR-ABL1* like (Philadelphia chromosome-like) ALL harbor *CRLF2r* [59]. CRLF2 expression has also been associated with increased relapse risk in pediatric B-ALL patients harboring IKZF1 deletions [60].

NG2 The neuron/glial antigen 2 (NG2) is typically expressed in *KMT2A*-rearranged (*KMT2Ar*) B-ALL [61–64]. The monoclonal antibody (MoAb) 7.1 detecting aberrant NG2 is a highly specific and sensitive marker for leukemic cells harboring a *KMT2A* rearrangement [64]. Specificity and positive predictive value have been reported to be as high as 100% with all infants with ALL that are positive for NG2 having rearranged *KMT2A* [63]. However, some *KMT2Ar* cases cannot be identified using MoAb 7.1 alone [61, 63, 65], but marker expression patterns characteristic of *KMT2Ar* B-ALL exist [54].

In most cases expression patterns of multiple antigens need to be evaluated for genotype prediction rather than analyzing single markers [66]. In the following, common genetic B-ALL subtypes and their associated immunophenotypes are listed:

BCR::ABL1^{pos} ALL is characterized by overexpression of myeloid markers like CD13, CD33, and, in particular, CD66c; strong expression of CD10, CD34, CD45, CD52, CD99, and HLA-DR; as well as down-modulation of CD24 and CD38 [66–68].

BCR::ABL1-like ALL (which is not a homogeneous genetic group and includes *CRLF2*-rearranged ALL) shares gene expression signatures and immunophenotypic characteristics with *BCR::ABL1*^{pos}-ALL [69]: such cases usually present also as B-II with aberrant myeloid marker expression including CD66c, however, frequency and expression levels are lower. CD20 as well as CD99 are often highly expressed [70]. More than one third of cases express CD27 [70]. *CRLF2*-rearranged ALL in particular is uniquely characterized by single marker expression of TSLPR (CRLF2) in a B-II immunophenotype [56–58].

ETV6::RUNX1/t(12;21)(p13;q22): The immunophenotype of *ETV6::RUNX1* ALL is very characteristic and defined by CD27 positivity paired frequently but not always with absent or only partial CD44 expression [71, 72]. In addition, myeloid markers CD13 and/or CD33 are expressed in about one third of cases. Other features are strong expression of CD10, the presence of CD34 and low to negative CD20 and CD11a [66, 67, 70–74].

DUX4-rearranged ALL: strong CD371 expression is the hallmark of this subtype [22], in which

CD10 quite frequently is only weakly expressed or even negative [21]. In about half of cases CD2 is positive and less frequently also CD56 [21]. CD66c expression is frequent but mutually exclusive with CD2 [70]. CD20 and CD99 are rather negative or weakly expressed [70].

Hyperdiploidy: the immunophenotype of this subtype is characteristic and shows very weak or absent CD45 and aberrant positivity of CD123 [19, 20, 67]. In the majority of cases also CD10, CD66c, CD86 and CD99 are strongly expressed [67, 75–78].

KMT2A-rearranged ALL: *KMT2A::AFF1/t(4;11)(q21;q23)* cases commonly present as classical B-I ALL devoid of CD10 and CD20 expression as opposed to B-ALL with other KMT2A-rearrangements which may exhibit weak or partial CD10 expression [61–63, 67]. Also CD22 and CD24 are often only very weakly expressed or absent [79], whereas CD34, CD44, and CD45 are typically strongly positive. Expression of the myeloid antigens CD15 and CD65 is characteristic, as is NG2 antigen positivity [61–63, 70]. *KMT2A::MLLT1/t(11;19)(p23;p13.3)* cases exhibit similarity to the former but may lack CD34 and CD15/CD65 positivity. This subtype as well as *KMT2A::MLLT3/t(9;11)(p21;q23)* cases may also appear as B-III but with absent or weak/partial CD10 expression [80]. The latter may even occur with B-IV immunophenotype [81]. *KMT2A::MLLT3* cases usually do not express myeloid markers or the NG2 antigen. In case of B-IV, CD20 is usually only weakly expressed as opposed to classical (Burkitt-type) B-IV AL.

MEF2D-rearranged ALL: A distinctive antigen profile exists with CD5 positivity in more than half of cases, frequent cytoplasmic µ-chain positivity, low CD99 expression, and lack of aberrant myeloid markers [70, 82, 83]. CD10 expression correlates with fusion partner gene (*HNRNPUL1*) and outcome [82].

PAX5-aberrant ALLs are predominantly B-II and often express CD66c and CD20, whereas they lack expression of myeloid antigens [70]. Of note, PAX5-mutated and particularly those with PAX5-P80R mutation exhibit weak/negative CD10 and low CD58 [84].

TCF3::PBX1/t(1;19)(q23;p13): this subtype is usually a B-III with low/absent CD99 and also lacking expression of CD20, CD34 as well as of aberrant myeloid markers [67, 70, 74].

ZNF384-rearranged ALL usually exhibits only weak CD10 expression combined with strong positivity of myeloid antigens like CD33, in particular, and CD13, but not of CD66c [70, 79, 85]. In addition, also CD123 expression is typical. CD22 and CD34 are also strongly expressed [79].

5.4.2 Genotype–Immunophenotype Correlations in T-ALL

Unlike in B-ALL where single markers and marker expression patterns are well established predictors of distinct genetic subtypes, genotype–immunophenotype correlations in T-ALL are scarce. *SIL::TAL1*-positive patients often exhibit a more mature immunophenotype (EGIL T-IV) [67, 70].

References

1. Alaggio R, Amador C, Anagnostopoulos I, Attygalle AD, Araujo IBO, Berti E, et al. The 5th edition of the World Health Organization classification of Haematolymphoid Tumours: lymphoid neoplasms. Leukemia. 2022;36(7):1720–48.
2. Arber DA, Orazi A, Hasserjian R, Thiele J, Borowitz MJ, Le Beau MM, et al. The 2016 revision to the World Health Organization classification of myeloid neoplasms and acute leukemia. Blood. 2016;127(20):2391–405.
3. Wood BL, Arroz M, Barnett D, DiGiuseppe J, Greig B, Kussick SJ, et al. 2006 Bethesda international consensus recommendations on the immunophenotypic analysis of hematolymphoid neoplasia by flow cytometry: optimal reagents and reporting for the flow cytometric diagnosis of hematopoietic neoplasia. Cytometry B Clin Cytom. 2007;72(Suppl 1):S14–22.
4. Dworzak MN, Buldini B, Gaipa G, Ratei R, Hrusak O, Luria D, et al. AIEOP-BFM consensus guidelines 2016 for flow cytometric immunophenotyping of pediatric acute lymphoblastic leukemia. Cytometry B Clin Cytom. 2018;94(1):82–93.
5. Bene MC, Castoldi G, Knapp W, Ludwig WD, Matutes E, Orfao A, et al. Proposals for the immunological classification of acute leukemias. European

Group for the Immunological Characterization of Leukemias (EGIL). Leukemia. 1995;9(10):1783–6.

6. Hrusak O, de Haas V, Stancikova J, Vakrmanova B, Janotova I, Mejstrikova E, et al. International cooperative study identifies treatment strategy in childhood ambiguous lineage leukemia. Blood. 2018;132(3):264–76.
7. Coustan-Smith E, Mullighan CG, Onciu M, Behm FG, Raimondi SC, Pei D, et al. Early T-cell precursor leukaemia: a subtype of very high-risk acute lymphoblastic leukaemia. Lancet Oncol. 2009;10:147–56.
8. Bene MC, Nebe T, Bettelheim P, Buldini B, Bumbea H, Kern W, et al. Immunophenotyping of acute leukemia and lymphoproliferative disorders: a consensus proposal of the European LeukemiaNet work package 10. Leukemia. 2011;25(4):567–74.
9. Basso G, Veltroni M, Valsecchi MG, Dworzak MN, Ratei R, Silvestri D, et al. Risk of relapse of childhood acute lymphoblastic leukemia is predicted by flow cytometric measurement of residual disease on day 15 bone marrow. J Clin Oncol. 2009;27(31):5168–74.
10. Dworzak MN, Gaipa G, Ratei R, Veltroni M, Schumich A, Maglia O, et al. Standardization of flow cytometric minimal residual disease evaluation in acute lymphoblastic leukemia: multicentric assessment is feasible. Cytometry B Clin Cytom. 2008;74(6):331–40.
11. Maurer-Granofszky M, Schumich A, Buldini B, Gaipa G, Kappelmayer J, Mejstrikova E, et al. An extensive quality control and quality assurance (QC/QA) Program significantly improves inter-laboratory concordance rates of flow-cytometric minimal residual disease assessment in acute lymphoblastic leukemia: an I-BFM-FLOW-network report. Cancers (Basel). 2021;13(23):6148.
12. Theunissen P, Mejstrikova E, Sedek L, van der Sluijs-Gelling AJ, Gaipa G, Bartels M, et al. Standardized flow cytometry for highly sensitive MRD measurements in B-cell acute lymphoblastic leukemia. Blood. 2017;129(3):347–57.
13. Dworzak MN, Stolz F, Froschl G, Printz D, Henn T, Fischer S, et al. Detection of residual disease in pediatric B-cell precursor acute lymphoblastic leukemia by comparative phenotype mapping: a study of five cases controlled by genetic methods. Exp Hematol. 1999;27(4):673–81.
14. Tembhare PR, Subramanian Pg PG, Ghogale S, Chatterjee G, Patkar NV, Gupta A, et al. A high-sensitivity 10-color flow cytometric minimal residual disease assay in B-lymphoblastic leukemia/lymphoma can easily achieve the sensitivity of 2-in-10(6) and is superior to standard minimal residual disease assay: a study of 622 patients. Cytometry B Clin Cytom. 2020;98(1):57–67.
15. Bouriche L, Bernot D, Nivaggioni V, Arnoux I, Loosveld M. Detection of minimal residual disease in B cell acute lymphoblastic leukemia using an eight-color tube with dried antibody reagents. Cytometry B Clin Cytom. 2019;96(2):158–63.
16. Mikhailova E, Illarionova O, Komkov A, Zerkalenkova E, Mamedov I, Shelikhova L, et al. Reliable flow-cytometric approach for minimal residual disease monitoring in patients with B-cell precursor acute lymphoblastic leukemia after CD19-targeted therapy. Cancers (Basel). 2022;14(21):5445.
17. Karawajew L, Dworzak M, Ratei R, Rhein P, Gaipa G, Buldini B, et al. Minimal residual disease analysis by eight-color flow cytometry in relapsed childhood acute lymphoblastic leukemia. Haematologica. 2015;100(7):935–44.
18. Veltroni M, De Zen L, Sanzari MC, Maglia O, Dworzak MN, Ratei R, et al. Expression of CD58 in normal, regenerating and leukemic bone marrow B cells: implications for the detection of minimal residual disease in acute lymphocytic leukemia. Haematologica. 2003;88(11):1245–52.
19. Djokic M, Bjorklund E, Blennow E, Mazur J, Soderhall S, Porwit A. Overexpression of CD123 correlates with the hyperdiploid genotype in acute lymphoblastic leukemia. Haematologica. 2009;94(7):1016–9.
20. Bras AE, de Haas V, van Stigt A, Jongen-Lavrencic M, Beverloo HB, Te Marvelde JG, et al. CD123 expression levels in 846 acute leukemia patients based on standardized immunophenotyping. Cytometry B Clin Cytom. 2019;96(2):134–42.
21. Varotto E, Maurer-Granofszky M, Silvestri D, Scarparo P, Mejstrikova E, Brüggemann M, et al. Transient switch to myeloid lineage in acute lymphoblastic leukemia during induction therapy: the role of CD371 expression and implication for minimal residual disease detection. Blood. 2019;134(Supplement_1):377.
22. Schinnerl D, Mejstrikova E, Schumich A, Zaliova M, Fortschegger K, Nebral K, et al. CD371 cell surface expression: a unique feature of DUX4-rearranged acute lymphoblastic leukemia. Haematologica. 2019;104(8):e352–e5.
23. Russell L, Capasso M, Vater I, Akasaka T, Bernard OA, Calasanz MJ, et al. Deregulated expression of cytokine receptor gene, CRLF2, is involved in lymphoid transformation in B-cell precursor acute lymphoblastic leukemia. Blood. 2009;114(13):2688–98.
24. Campana D, Coustan-Smith E. Detection of minimal residual disease in acute leukemia by flow cytometry. Cytometry. 1999;38(4):139–52.
25. DiGiuseppe JA, Fuller SG, Borowitz MJ. Overexpression of CD49f in precursor B-cell acute lymphoblastic leukemia: potential usefulness in minimal residual disease detection. Cytometry B Clin Cytom. 2009;76(2):150–5.
26. Tembhare PR, Ghogale S, Ghatwai N, Badrinath Y, Kunder N, Patkar NV, et al. Evaluation of new markers for minimal residual disease monitoring in B-cell precursor acute lymphoblastic leukemia: CD73 and CD86 are the most relevant new markers to increase the efficacy of MRD 2016. Cytometry B Clin Cytom. 2018;94(1):100–11.
27. Sedek L, Theunissen P, Sobral da Costa E, van der Sluijs-Gelling A, Mejstrikova E, Gaipa G, et al. Differential expression of CD73, CD86 and CD304 in normal vs. leukemic B-cell precursors and their utility as stable minimal residual disease markers in child-

hood B-cell precursor acute lymphoblastic leukemia. J Immunol Methods. 2019;475:112429.
28. Muzzafar T, Medeiros LJ, Wang SA, Brahmandam A, Thomas DA, Jorgensen JL. Aberrant underexpression of CD81 in precursor B-cell acute lymphoblastic leukemia: utility in detection of minimal residual disease by flow cytometry. Am J Clin Pathol. 2009;132(5):692–8.
29. Dworzak MN, Froschl G, Printz D, Zen LD, Gaipa G, Ratei R, et al. CD99 expression in T-lineage ALL: implications for flow cytometric detection of minimal residual disease. Leukemia. 2004;18(4):703–8.
30. Roshal M, Fromm JR, Winter S, Dunsmore K, Wood BL. Immaturity associated antigens are lost during induction for T cell lymphoblastic leukemia: implications for minimal residual disease detection. Cytometry B Clin Cytom. 2010;78B:139–46.
31. Wood BL, Levin G, Wilson M, Winter SS, Dunsmore K, Loh ML, et al. High-throughput screening by flow cytometry identifies reduced expression of CD48 as a universal characteristic of T-ALL and a suitable target for minimal residual disease (MRD) detection. Blood. 2011;118(21):2547.
32. Gaipa G, Basso G, Maglia O, Leoni V, Faini A, Cazzaniga G, et al. Drug-induced immunophenotypic modulation in childhood ALL: implications for minimal residual disease detection. Leukemia. 2005;19(1):49–56.
33. Dworzak MN, Schumich A, Printz D, Potschger U, Husak Z, Attarbaschi A, et al. CD20 up-regulation in pediatric B-cell precursor acute lymphoblastic leukemia during induction treatment: setting the stage for anti-CD20 directed immunotherapy. Blood. 2008;112(10):3982–8.
34. Cherian S, Miller V, McCullouch V, Dougherty K, Fromm JR, Wood BL. A novel flow cytometric assay for detection of residual disease in patients with B-lymphoblastic leukemia/lymphoma post anti-CD19 therapy. Cytometry B Clin Cytom. 2018;94B:112–20.
35. Novakova M, Zaliova M, Fiser K, Vakrmanova B, Slamova L, Musilova A, et al. DUX4r, ZNF384r and PAX5-P80R mutated B-cell precursor acute lymphoblastic leukemia frequently undergo monocytic switch. Haematologica. 2021;106(8):2066–75.
36. Rossi JG, Bernasconi AR, Alonso CN, Rubio PL, Gallego MS, Carrara CA, et al. Lineage switch in childhood acute leukemia: an unusual event with poor outcome. Am J Hematol. 2012;87(9):890–7.
37. Hutter C, Attarbaschi A, Fischer S, Meyer C, Dworzak M, König M, et al. Acute monocytic leukaemia originating from MLL-MLLT3-positive pre-B cells. Br J Haematol. 2010;150(5):621–3.
38. Haddox CL, Mangaonkar AA, Chen D, Shi M, He R, Oliveira JL, et al. Blinatumomab-induced lineage switch of B-ALL with t(4:11)(q21;q23) KMT2A/AFF1 into an aggressive AML: pre- and post-switch phenotypic, cytogenetic and molecular analysis. Blood Cancer J. 2017;7(9):e607.
39. Asare JM, Rabik CA, Muller B, Brown PA, Cooper S. Investigational treatment options in phase I and phase II trials for relapsed or refractory acute lymphoblastic leukemia in pediatric patients. Expert Opin Investig Drugs. 2021;30(6):611–20.
40. Bride KL, Vincent TL, Im SY, Aplenc R, Barrett DM, Carroll WL, et al. Preclinical efficacy of daratumumab in T-cell acute lymphoblastic leukemia. Blood. 2018;131(9):995–9.
41. McMahon CM, Luger SM. Relapsed T cell ALL: current approaches and new directions. Curr Hematol Malig Rep. 2019;14(2):83–93.
42. Hogan LE, Bhatla T, Teachey DT, Sirvent FJB, Moppett J, Puyó PV, et al. Efficacy and safety of daratumumab (DARA) in pediatric and young adult patients (pts) with relapsed/refractory T-cell acute lymphoblastic leukemia (ALL) or lymphoblastic lymphoma (LL): results from the phase 2 DELPHINUS study. J Clin Oncol. 2022;40(16_suppl):10001.
43. Maude SL, Frey N, Shaw PA, Aplenc R, Barrett DM, Bunin NJ, et al. Chimeric antigen receptor T cells for sustained remissions in leukemia. N Engl J Med. 2014;371(16):1507–17.
44. Fry TJ, Shah NN, Orentas RJ, Stetler-Stevenson M, Yuan CM, Ramakrishna S, et al. CD22-targeted CAR T cells induce remission in B-ALL that is naive or resistant to CD19-targeted CAR immunotherapy. Nat Med. 2018;24(1):20–8.
45. Pan J, Niu Q, Deng B, Liu S, Wu T, Gao Z, et al. CD22 CAR T-cell therapy in refractory or relapsed B acute lymphoblastic leukemia. Leukemia. 2019;33(12):2854–66.
46. Riaz IB, Zahid U, Kamal MU, Husnain M, McBride A, Hua A, et al. Anti-CD 19 and anti-CD 20 CAR-modified T cells for B-cell malignancies: a systematic review and meta-analysis. Immunotherapy. 2017;9(12):979–93.
47. Qin H, Cho M, Haso W, Zhang L, Tasian SK, Oo HZ, et al. Eradication of B-ALL using chimeric antigen receptor-expressing T cells targeting the TSLPR oncoprotein. Blood. 2015;126(5):629–39.
48. Davies DM, Maher J. TSLPR: a new CAR in the showroom for B-ALL. Blood. 2015;126(5):567–9.
49. Ruella M, Barrett DM, Kenderian SS, Shestova O, Hofmann TJ, Perazzelli J, et al. Dual CD19 and CD123 targeting prevents antigen-loss relapses after CD19-directed immunotherapies. J Clin Invest. 2016;126(10):3814–26.
50. Png YT, Vinanica N, Kamiya T, Shimasaki N, Coustan-Smith E, Campana D. Blockade of CD7 expression in T cells for effective chimeric antigen receptor targeting of T-cell malignancies. Blood Adv. 2017;1(25):2348–60.
51. Libert D, Yuan CM, Masih KE, Galera P, Salem D, Shalabi H, et al. Serial evaluation of CD19 surface expression in pediatric B-cell malignancies following CD19-targeted therapy. Leukemia. 2020;34(11):3064–9.
52. Orlando EJ, Han X, Tribouley C, Wood PA, Leary RJ, Riester M, et al. Genetic mechanisms of target antigen loss in CAR19 therapy of acute lymphoblastic leukemia. Nat Med. 2018;24(10):1504–6.

53. Li Z, Chu X, Gao L, Ling J, Xiao P, Lu J, et al. High expression of Interleukin-3 receptor alpha chain (CD123) predicts favorable outcome in pediatric B-cell acute lymphoblastic leukemia lacking prognosis-defining genomic aberrations. Front Oncol. 2021;11:614420.
54. Kulis J, Wawrowski L, Sedek L, Wrobel L, Slota L, van der Velden VHJ, et al. Machine learning based analysis of relations between antigen expression and genetic aberrations in childhood B-cell precursor acute lymphoblastic Leukaemia. J Clin Med. 2022;11(9):2281.
55. Arber DA, Orazi A, Hasserjian RP, Borowitz MJ, Calvo KR, Kvasnicka HM, et al. International consensus classification of myeloid neoplasms and acute Leukemias: integrating morphologic, clinical, and genomic data. Blood. 2022;140(11):1200–28.
56. Konoplev S, Lu X, Konopleva M, Jain N, Ouyang J, Goswami M, et al. CRLF2-positive B-cell acute lymphoblastic leukemia in adult patients: a single-institution experience. Am J Clin Pathol. 2017;147(4):357–63.
57. Bugarin C, Sarno J, Palmi C, Savino AM, te Kronnie G, Dworzak M, et al. Fine tuning of surface CRLF2 expression and its associated signaling profile in childhood B-cell precursor acute lymphoblastic leukemia. Haematologica. 2015;100(6):e229–32.
58. Tasian SK, Doral MY, Borowitz MJ, Wood BL, Chen IM, Harvey RC, et al. Aberrant STAT5 and PI3K/mTOR pathway signaling occurs in human CRLF2-rearranged B-precursor acute lymphoblastic leukemia. Blood. 2012;120(4):833–42.
59. Roberts KG, Mullighan CG. Genomics in acute lymphoblastic leukaemia: insights and treatment implications. Nat Rev Clin Oncol. 2015;12(6):344–57.
60. Pastorczak A, Sedek L, Braun M, Madzio J, Sonsala A, Twardoch M, et al. Surface expression of cytokine receptor-like factor 2 increases risk of relapse in pediatric acute lymphoblastic leukemia patients harboring IKZF1 deletions. Oncotarget. 2018;9(40):25971–82.
61. Behm FG, Smith FO, Raimondi SC, Pui CH, Bernstein ID. Human homologue of the rat chondroitin sulfate proteoglycan, NG2, detected by monoclonal antibody 7.1, identifies childhood acute lymphoblastic leukemias with t(4;11)(q21;q23) or t(11;19)(q23;p13) and MLL gene rearrangements. Blood. 1996;87(3):1134–9.
62. Zangrando A, Intini F, te Kronnie G, Basso G. Validation of NG2 antigen in identifying BP-ALL patients with MLL rearrangements using qualitative and quantitative flow cytometry: a prospective study. Leukemia. 2008;22(4):858–61.
63. Borkhardt A, Wuchter C, Viehmann S, Pils S, Teigler-Schlegel A, Stanulla M, et al. Infant acute lymphoblastic leukemia – combined cytogenetic, immunophenotypical and molecular analysis of 77 cases. Leukemia. 2002;16(9):1685–90.
64. Smith FO, Rauch C, Williams DE, March CJ, Arthur D, Hilden J, et al. The human homologue of rat NG2, a chondroitin sulfate proteoglycan, is not expressed on the cell surface of normal hematopoietic cells but is expressed by acute myeloid leukemia blasts from poor-prognosis patients with abnormalities of chromosome band 11q23. Blood. 1996;87(3):1123–33.
65. Emerenciano M, Renaud G, Sant'Ana M, Barbieri C, Passetti F, Pombo-de-Oliveira MS, et al. Challenges in the use of NG2 antigen as a marker to predict MLL rearrangements in multi-center studies. Leuk Res. 2011;35(8):1001–7.
66. Kulis J, Sedek L, Slota L, Perkowski B, Szczepanski T. Commonly assessed markers in childhood BCP-ALL diagnostic panels and their association with genetic aberrations and outcome prediction. Genes (Basel). 2022;13(8):1374.
67. Hrusak O, Porwit-MacDonald A. Antigen expression patterns reflecting genotype of acute leukemias. Leukemia. 2002;16(7):1233–58.
68. Buldini B, Zangrando A, Michielotto B, Veltroni M, Giarin E, Tosato F, et al. Identification of immunophenotypic signatures by clustering analysis in pediatric patients with Philadelphia chromosome positive acute lymphoblastic leukemia. Am J Hematol. 2010;85(2):138–41.
69. Khoury JD, Solary E, Abla O, Akkari Y, Alaggio R, Apperley JF, et al. The 5th edition of the World Health Organization classification of Haematolymphoid Tumours: myeloid and histiocytic/dendritic neoplasms. Leukemia. 2022;36(7):1703–19.
70. Ohki K, Takahashi H, Fukushima T, Nanmoku T, Kusano S, Mori M, et al. Impact of immunophenotypic characteristics on genetic subgrouping in childhood acute lymphoblastic leukemia: Tokyo Children's cancer study group (TCCSG) study L04-16. Genes Chromosomes Cancer. 2020;59(10):551–61.
71. Vaskova M, Mejstrikova E, Kalina T, Martinkova P, Omelka M, Trka J, et al. Transfer of genomics information to flow cytometry: expression of CD27 and CD44 discriminates subtypes of acute lymphoblastic leukemia. Leukemia. 2005;19(5):876–8.
72. Zaliova M, Kotrova M, Bresolin S, Stuchly J, Stary J, Hrusak O, et al. ETV6/RUNX1-like acute lymphoblastic leukemia: a novel B-cell precursor leukemia subtype associated with the CD27/CD44 immunophenotype. Genes Chromosomes Cancer. 2017;56(8):608–16.
73. De Zen L, Orfao A, Cazzaniga G, Masiero L, Cocito MG, Spinelli M, et al. Quantitative multiparametric immunophenotyping in acute lymphoblastic leukemia: correlation with specific genotype. I. ETV6/AML1 ALLs identification. Leukemia. 2000;14(7):1225–31.
74. Tsagarakis NJ, Papadhimitriou SI, Pavlidis D, Marinakis T, Kostopoulos IV, Stiakaki E, et al. Flow cytometric predictive scoring systems for common fusions ETV6/RUNX1, BCR/ABL1, TCF3/PBX1 and rearrangements of the KMT2A gene, proposed for the initial cytogenetic approach in cases of B-acute lymphoblastic leukemia. Int J Lab Hematol. 2019;41(3):364–72.
75. Husak Z, Printz D, Schumich A, Pötschger U, Dworzak MN. Death induction by CD99 ligation

in TEL/AML1-positive acute lymphoblastic leukemia and normal B cell precursors. J Leukoc Biol. 2010;88(2):405–12.
76. Chen D, Camponeschi A, Wu Q, Gerasimcik N, Li H, Shen X, et al. CD99 expression is strongly associated with clinical outcome in children with B-cell precursor acute lymphoblastic leukaemia. Br J Haematol. 2019;184(3):418–23.
77. Coustan-Smith E, Song G, Clark C, Key L, Liu P, Mehrpooya M, et al. New markers for minimal residual disease detection in acute lymphoblastic leukemia. Blood. 2011;117(23):6267–76.
78. Pierzyna-Switala M, Sedek L, Kulis J, Mazur B, Muszynska-Roslan K, Koltan A, et al. Multicolor flow cytometry immunophenotyping and characterization of aneuploidy in pediatric B-cell precursor acute lymphoblastic leukemia. Cent Eur J Immunol. 2021;46(3):365–74.
79. Wang YZ, Qin YZ, Chang Y, Yuan XY, Chen WM, He LL, et al. Immunophenotypic characteristics of ZNF384 rearrangement compared with BCR-ABL1, KMT2A rearrangement, and other adult B-cell precursor acute lymphoblastic leukemia. Cytometry B Clin Cytom. 2022;102(5):360–9.
80. Attarbaschi A, Mann G, König M, Steiner M, Strehl S, Schreiberhuber A, et al. Mixed lineage leukemia -rearranged childhood pro-B and CD10-negative pre-B acute lymphoblastic leukemia constitute a distinct clinical entity. Clin Cancer Res. 2006;12(10):2988–94.
81. Blin N, Mechinaud F, Talmant P, Garand R, Boutard P, Dastugue N, et al. Mature B-cell lymphoblastic leukemia with MLL rearrangement: an uncommon and distinct subset of childhood acute leukemia. Leukemia. 2008;22:1056–9.
82. Ohki K, Butler ER, Kiyokawa N, Hirabayashi S, Bergmann AK, Moricke A, et al. Clinical characteristics and outcomes of B-cell precursor ALL with MEF2D rearrangements: a retrospective study by the Ponte di Legno childhood ALL working group. Leukemia. 2023;37(1):212–6.
83. Ohki K, Kiyokawa N, Saito Y, Hirabayashi S, Nakabayashi K, Ichikawa H, et al. Clinical and molecular characteristics of MEF2D fusion-positive B-cell precursor acute lymphoblastic leukemia in childhood, including a novel translocation resulting in MEF2D-HNRNPH1 gene fusion. Haematologica. 2019;104(1):128–37.
84. Li Y, Moriyama T, Yoshimura S, Zhao X, Li Z, Yang X, et al. PAX5 epigenetically orchestrates CD58 transcription and modulates blinatumomab response in acute lymphoblastic leukemia. Sci Adv. 2022;8(50):eadd6403.
85. Hirabayashi S, Ohki K, Nakabayashi K, Ichikawa H, Momozawa Y, Okamura K, et al. ZNF384-related fusion genes define a subgroup of childhood B-cell precursor acute lymphoblastic leukemia with a characteristic immunotype. Haematologica. 2017;102(1):118–29.

Minimal Residual Disease in Paediatric ALL: Significance and Methodological Approaches

6

Jan Trka, Michaela Reiterova, Giovanni Cazzaniga, and Eva Fronkova

6.1 Introduction

Minimal residual disease (MRD) is the amount of cancer cells undetectable by standard imaging or laboratory methods, which can be determined by special molecular genetic or immunological approaches. MRD monitoring has been used in clinical decision making in childhood acute leukaemia (ALL) for more than 20 years for both risk stratification, prognosis and relapse prediction. In the last decade, MRD monitoring has also been applied to monitor the efficacy of new targeted drugs. In this chapter, we discuss the advantages and pitfalls of different methods for MRD detection and their application in paediatric ALL (Table 6.1).

Virtually any feature that distinguishes a tumour cell from its physiological counterpart can be used for MRD monitoring. Of the molecular genetic methods, monitoring of transcripts of leukaemic fusion genes has the longest history, and monitoring of clonal-specific rearrangements of immunoglobulin (Ig) and T-cell receptor (TR) genes has great clinical relevance and versatility. The advent of new technologies such as next-generation sequencing (NGS) or so-called digital droplet PCR (DDPCR) in recent years has enormously expanded the possibilities for MRD monitoring. In addition to molecular genetic methods, flow cytometry (FCM) has become increasingly important in monitoring treatment response. The use of a particular method in practice is determined not only by the sensitivity and specificity of the test but also by the real-time feasibility, logistics, financial requirements of the method and the expertise of the investigating laboratory. The methods used have many technical and interpretive pitfalls and cannot be used in clinical decision-making without standardization and quality control of the tests performed.

J. Trka (✉) · M. Reiterova · E. Fronkova
Second Faculty of Medicine, Department of Paediatric Haematology and Oncology, Charles University, Prague, Czech Republic
e-mail: jan.trka@lfmotol.cuni.cz

G. Cazzaniga
Clinica Pediatrica, Università Di Milano, Milan, Italy

G. Escherich, V. Conter (eds.), *Acute Lymphoblastic Leukemia in Children and Adolescents*, Pediatric Oncology, https://doi.org/10.1007/978-3-031-71180-0_6

Table 6.1 MRD detection methods in paediatric ALL: advantages, disadvantages and applications

Method	Sensitivity	Advantages	Disadvantages	Applications
Gene fusion RNA level by qRT-PCR	10^{-4} to 10^{-5}	Easy to perform for recurrent fusions Fully standardized	mRNA handling Variable and changing expression Covers only a proportion of patients	BCR::ABL1 KMT2A fusions (if other methods unavailable)
Gene fusion DNA level by qPCR	10^{-4} to 10^{-5}	Exact quantification Same guidelines as for Ig/TR	Individual patients' systems NGS needed for breakpoint identification	BCR::ABL1 KMT2A fusions Any other gene fusion (alternate or complementary target)
Ig/TR by qPCR	Mostly 10^{-5a}	Exact quantification Fully standardized Applicable in 97% of patients	Demanding implementation Laborious and time consuming Ig/TR biology knowledge required Clonal evolution	All patients Front-line Post-relapse Pre- and post-SCT After immunotherapies
Ig/TR by NGS/qPCR (NGS for Ig/TR identification; qPCR for quantification)	Mostly 10^{-5a}	Exact quantification Fully standardized Applicable in 97% of patients Better selection of targets Better specificity	NGS needed for target identificationThroughput crucial Ig/TR biology knowledge required Clonal evolution	All patients Front-line Post-relapse Pre- and post-SCT After immunotherapies
Ig/TR by NGS	Mostly 10^{-5a}	Exact quantification Partly standardized Applicable in 97% of patients Excellent specificity Follows also clonal evolution	NGS needed Throughput crucial Ig/TR biology knowledge required	All patients Front-line Post-relapse Pre- and post-SCT After immunotherapies
Flow cytometry	10^{-4} to $10^{-5a,b}$	Fast turnaround Almost universally applicable Partly standardized	Sensitivity and specificity varies with BM regeneration Mostly "expert-based" Limited in immunotherapeutic setting	All patients (ideally very initial part of treatment) Front-line Post-relapse Pre- and post-SCT

[a]Sensitivity depends on the amount of analysed material, theoretical sensitivity up to 10^{-6}
[b]Depends on individual immunophenotype

6.2 Methods of Molecular Genetics

6.2.1 Monitoring of Fusion Genes

Detection of fusion transcripts is traditionally based on RNA. After reverse transcription into cDNA, the product is amplified using primers located in adjacent exons of specific genes in the fusion. The original two-round qualitative PCR has been replaced by quantitative reverse-transcriptase PCR (RT-qPCR), which has reduced the risk of cross-contamination of samples while providing data on transcript quantity. The method uses fluorescently labelled probes and quantification using a dilution series of a standard (usually a cloned plasmid). The advantage is that once established, the system can be used for all patients with the same type of fusion. The disadvantages remain the possibility of contamination of samples with, for example, plasmid standard and the possibility of RNA degradation during sample transport. Therefore, it is necessary to test the quality of RNA by parallel quantification of a control gene (e.g. *ABL1*, *GUS*). Due to its relative simplicity, this method was already put into practice in the late 1990s, especially in the case of the *BCR::ABL1* fusion gene in a proportion of ALL patients with this fusion gene. In the case of ALL, this method was also used for other fusion genes: *ETV6::RUNX1* (formerly *TEL::AML1*) [1], *TCF3::PBX1* (formerly *E2A::PBX1*), *KMT2A* (formerly *MLL*) fusion gene, especially *KMT2A::AFF1* (formerly *MLL::AF4*). However, with the exception of *BCR::ABL1*-positive ALL and *KMT2A::AFF1* gene fusion ALL, this method has given way to the more versatile method of quantifying Ig/TR rearrangements.

The quantification of these fusion transcripts has been standardized by the Europe Against Cancer consortium [2]. Thanks to the use of NGS RNA sequencing (RNA-seq) in recent years, a large number of new fusion genes have been discovered that can be used in an analogous manner if needed.

More technically robust is the quantification of fusion genes directly at the DNA level. This eliminates the risk of gene expression being affected by treatment or RNA degradation during transport. In addition, monitoring genomic fusion can avoid the influence of treatment-related changes in gene expression on quantification. However, fusion sites are often located deep within introns, and their identification by classical PCR-based methods has been very lengthy and laborious. Current NGS methods allow coverage of genomic fusions by probes and simplify the fusion-finding procedure. Therefore, quantification of fusion genes at the DNA level appears to be a very specific and sensitive method in the future. DNA-level fusion gene quantification is currently used, for example, for wide selection of various *KMT2A* gene fusions [3, 4] and its use in *BCR::ABL1*-positive ALL is developing, where it reveals distinct biological characteristics and thus clinical behaviour of subtypes of the disease (more below) [5].

6.2.2 Detection of Clonal-Specific Ig/TCR Rearrangements

This method, despite its undeniable methodological and interpretive challenges, has become the standard for MRD monitoring in lymphoid malignancies and specifically in paediatric ALL, with the exception of US treatment protocols. The principle is that lymphoid cells rearrange during their development the so-called V, D, J segments of genes that encode immunoglobulins in B lymphocytes or T-cell receptors in T lymphocytes. In B lymphocytes, these are immunoglobulin heavy chains (IGH), kappa light chains (IGK) and lambda (IGL) [6]. In T lymphocytes, these are TCR beta (TCRB), gamma (TCRG) and delta (TCRD), most of the TCR alpha rearrangements are not used in MRD monitoring [7–10]. Malignantly transformed clones then carry the same hypervariable CDR3 segment sequence that can be used for MRD monitoring. A phenomenon called lineage promiscuity can also be exploited, where lymphoblasts rearrange segments of a different type due to dysregulation of gene expression (e.g. TCR in B-precursor ALL, and vice versa) [11, 12]. A long-used and standardized procedure is the so-called ASO ("allele-specific oligonucleotides") method. The first step is the detection of clonality in the diagnostic sample [13], the clonal products arc sequenced, and patient-specific nucleotides are designed based on the sequence, which are then used to optimize the quantitative PCR system (qPCR at the DNA level). Because of the possibility of clonal evolution, it is recommended to use two independent targets for each patient [14]. The method has many pitfalls, yet it has been standardized within the EuroMRD consortium (www.euromrd.org) [15]. The greatest danger is the possibility of false positivities due to non-specific attachment of ASO primers to "healthy" sequences in lymphoid cells. Using the interpretation criteria, the individual sensitivity and quantification range (QR) for each patient must be determined based on the specific sample measurement outcome. This means that the final monitoring parameters may vary not only between patients and their two targets, but between individual patient-specific sampling over time. The accredited laboratory should report these data (sensitivity and QR) with every result. In practice, this means that, for example, a quantifiable result (expressed as the proportion of MRD relative to the diagnostic sample) may not mean a higher value than a sample with a "positive, non-quantifiable" value if the other sample has poorer measurement parameters and a lower QR. In specific cases with a large B-cell recovery, even the specificity criteria used are not sufficient. In the literature, we find proven cases (typically in ALL patients after allogeneic hematopoietic progenitor transplantation (SCT)) where a low positive MRD in the first 3 years after transplantation did not lead to a subsequent rise in MRD followed by disease relapse, without therapeutic intervention [16]. Direct demonstration of the non-specificity of MRD testing by ASO-qPCR in some specific situations was only brought about by a method based on next-generation sequencing [17].

6.2.3 NGS in MRD Monitoring

The availability of NGS, especially in the form of low-throughput sequencers, has greatly expanded the possibilities not only for diagnosis but also for monitoring MRD. Several groups have described approaches based on multiplex PCR amplification of Ig/TCR rearrangements and amplicon NGS, and have demonstrated the correlation of results obtained in this way with existing ASO-qPCR or flow cytometry methods in leukaemias [18–22]. Compared to qPCR, there is no need to design specific oligonucleotides and the result provides a comprehensive view of all rearrangements of a given type in the sample and thus also of the sequences of physiological lymphocytes. Using appropriate bioinformatics techniques, any clonal evolution caused by subsequent Ig/TR rearrangements can also be captured early. The sequencing library is generated using single- or double-round multiplex PCR. The primers for amplification of Ig/TR targets also include sequencing adaptors specific to the type of instrument used, as well as "barcodes", sequences of several nucleotides that help to identify a particular sample. This allows multiplexing of samples, which will reduce the cost of sequencing. The actual NGS is then performed at very high depth (up to 2 million reads per sample). The method has recently been widely promoted, mainly due to the involvement of the commercial sphere in the investigation (Adaptive Biotechnologies). Higher sensitivity than all existing methods (even e.g. 10^{-6} or one leukaemic cell among 1 million normal haematopoietic cells) is emphasized. However, it should be noted that the sensitivity of the method is not only determined by the number of reads per sample but mainly by the input amount of cells entering the reaction (which can be recalculated according to the DNA concentration). For the advertised sensitivity of 10^{-6}, more than 6 μg of DNA must be used in the reaction, which is technically very complicated and for some patients in periods of treatment with hypoplastic bone marrow, this amount of material is unattainable. The claimed higher sensitivity in the US studies is also due to the fact that the ASO-qPCR method was not used in the United States, and most of the historical clinical protocols whose data were used in these studies used less sensitive flow cytometry [23]. The method is currently being standardized within the EuroClonality-NGS and EuroMRD consortia. So far, a methodological approach for target detection for monitoring Ig/TR rearrangements using NGS [24] and bioinformatic analysis methods [25, 26] have been published. The MRD measurement itself is now being tested in a series of quality control experiments. Interim results show a very good correlation across more than 15 participating laboratories for both diagnostic screening by NGS. Regarding the MRD quantification itself, the normalization to the number of relevant cells needs to be addressed. In fact, the NGS method only quantifies in proportion to the total number of rearrangements of a given type (e.g. IgH). If the number of B cells is reduced due to targeted therapy (e.g. after treatment with the bispecific antibody or CAR-T cells), the quantification of total MRD using IgH rearrangements is overestimated. This can be addressed by parallel quantification of the internal control ("spike-in") [26]. A faster uptake of NGS for Ig/TR quantification in European laboratories is slowed down by the established and well standardized ASO-qPCR method. A concern is the cost of NGS, which can only compete with older methods if there is sufficient laboratory turnover and the ability to test multiple samples simultaneously.

Another (and in our estimation promising) future application of NGS is mutation monitoring. Here, however, the error rate of NGS reads is an obstacle that reduces sensitivity. The use of unique molecular identifiers (UMI) in the creation of sequencing libraries and other adaptations can circumvent this obstacle. At this time, the digital PCR method described below also seems to be promising for monitoring point mutations with high sensitivity.

6.2.4 Droplet Digital PCR

Droplet digital PCR (DDPCR) technology is based on qualitative PCR, but quantification is enabled by dispersing the template into a large number of droplets [27]. The method does not need a standard curve, but requires optimization to track a particular aberration in the same way as qPCR. A disadvantage is the diversity of platforms for the assay, which makes standardization difficult. Some studies have shown better quantification at lower levels and higher assay sensitivity than ASO-pPCR for Ig/TR [28]. Overall, however, DDPCR does not address the possibility of non-specific amplification of Ig/TR in healthy lymphocytes using ASO primers and thus does not provide a major difference in specificity compared to qPCR.

Clearly convincing results are provided by this method for monitoring point mutation, including ALL [29].

6.3 Flow Cytometry

The determination of MRD by flow cytometry is based on the differential expression of antigens by leukaemic cells from their non-malignant counterparts. Using fluorescently labelled antibodies against individual antigens, the presence of the features under investigation is quantitatively and qualitatively assessed. The set of all expressed markers then constitutes the so-called immunophenotype.

Traditionally, two approaches have been described in MRD analysis by flow cytometry, namely the search for leukaemia-associated immunophenotypes (LAIP) and the so-called difference from normal (DFN).

The LAIP approach exploits immunophenotypic abnormalities of malignant blasts that are not present in non-malignant cells [30]. The most common LAIPs are the expression of antigens of another cell lineage (e.g. expression of T-cell or myeloid features in B precursor leukaemia), asynchronous expression of antigens, atypically high/low antigen expression, etc. However, changes in the immunophenotype of blasts, which often occur to a greater or lesser extent in ALL during therapy [31–33], as well as changes in non-malignant cells (especially regenerating progenitors) during therapy, are becoming a problem [34, 35]. Significant changes in phenotype resulting in lineage switch, although rare, were described more frequently in distinct genetic subtypes of ALL. MRD assessment in these cases requires an individual approach [36, 37].

The DFN approach then carefully evaluates the immunophenotypic deviations of the cell line under analysis from normal developmental patterns and more closely follows the antigens expressed at each stage of development of the lineage. The presence of atypical cells can thus be commented on to some extent even without examination/knowledge of the diagnostic phenotype, but in most cases the sensitivity of such examination can be expected to be worse.

In practice, the two approaches are often combined, and in MRD analysis, both the presence of atypical cells of the diagnostic phenotype and the entire cell lineage and its deviations from normal are evaluated.

The undeniable advantage of flow cytometry is its speed: from sample preparation to data acquisition, the process takes 1–2 h. On the contrary, its lower sensitivity compared to molecular genetic methods has always been a disadvantage. Although, as with molecular methods, the total number of measured cells determines the sensitivity of the assay, whereas in Ig/TR detection a single cell with a specific rearrangement is theoretically sufficient for MRD determination, flow cytometry uses a limit of at least 10 [30] to 50 [38] cells forming a cluster to ensure sufficient specificity of the finding. This has led to efforts in recent years to increase the number of cells examined and to optimize the laboratory procedure. As we have shown in Theunissen et al. [39], when sufficient numbers of cells are acquired, the results of MRD assessment by flow cytometry and Ig/TR are then identical.

The sensitivity determined by the amount of cells measured refers to cases where the malignant cells are completely different from the non-malignant cells in the sample. Otherwise, however, the sensitivity is determined by the number of these non-malignant cells with an immunophenotype identical to the malignant blasts, since no reliable statement can be made as to the origin of these cells. This situation arises particularly when MRD is analysed in regenerating bone marrow samples at later stages of treatment.

In practice, the sensitivity of MRD examination by flow cytometry ranges from 10^{-3} to 10^{-5} depending on the immunophenotype of the cells and the time of sampling.

Another advantage of MRD detection by flow cytometry is its versatility: in ALL, where the use of cytometry is firmly established in individual treatment protocols, it can theoretically be used in all patients. What makes MRD detection by flow cytometry difficult to interpret in patients is the overlap with regenerating/non-malignant hematopoiesis at later stages of treatment. Here, as mentioned above, the sensitivity of the test then depends on the degree of specificity of the phenotype and distinction from non-malignant cells and thus varies between patients and diagnostic units.

Furthermore, with the advent of targeted therapies for haematological malignancies, the importance of flow cytometry has further increased. Although phenotypic changes that occur in patients (e.g. decreased CD19 expression with anti-CD19 therapy [40–42]) can complicate MRD testing by flow cytometry, analysis of the presence of a targetable molecule is also important for the actual indication (and possibly discontinuation or modification) of this therapy. Alternative gating strategy for malignant blast identification in these cases may lead to more reliable MRD analysis.

Technological advances have made it possible to increase the number of parameters measured simultaneously, further improving the specific identification of the blast population. The use of 6–12-parameter combinations is now the standard and the number of parameters measured is increasing. New technologies have also come into research use, namely mass cytometry, where antibodies are labelled with heavy metals instead of fluorochromes, and spectral cytometry, allowing for better differentiation of individual fluorochromes. Nevertheless, mass cytometry is mainly concerned with significant cell loss during processing and low measurement speed, which are two important aspects in MRD measurement.

The development also continues in the direction of standardization of the method, which increases the reproducibility of the data. Comparability of cytometric data is important in multicentre trials but also for the assessment of an individual patient over time [30, 38, 43, 44]. Within the European EuroFlow consortium, the principle of standardization of flow cytometry is being developed [45]. The current trend is now to develop dried reagent tubes or lyophilized antibody combinations, which, together with standardized instrument setups, guarantee maximum data comparability and contribute to correct interpretation. First approaches using automated MRD analysis are also emerging [46, 47], but so far data are very limited.

6.4 Practical Use of MRD and Clinical Implications in Paediatric ALL

The first studies of the relevance of MRD in ALL were in childhood leukaemia [48]. Already in 2000, the BFM group protocol successfully started to stratify patients into risk groups based on MRD at days 33 and 78 of treatment [49]. Comparison of the historical approach with the use of other prognostic parameters (morphological and clinical) showed the superiority of MRD-based stratification also in an international study on the ALL-IC 2002 protocol [50]. Today, stratification based on the rate of leukaemic cells elimination in the initial phases of treatment is part of all current treatment protocols for childhood ALL. Although the time points of investigation, the technologies used (virtually only flow cytometry and qPCR/NGS targeting Ig/TR rearrangements) and the cut-offs for clinical decisions differ, the key period is the induction phase of treatment. An excellent therapeutic response (corresponding to MRD negativity at the single cell detection level between 10,000 and 100,000 cells examined) at the end of induction is a sign of excellent patient prognosis. Similarly, persistent MRD levels after the start of consolidation therapy is a negative prognostic factor.

The current BFM group treatment protocol (AIEOP-BFM ALL 2017) uses a combination of multiple factors including MRD for treatment stratification. A high day 15 MRD (>10%) measured by flow cytometry places the patient at high risk, whereas a negative MRD measured by ASO-qPCR at day 33, assuming the absence of other risk factors, places the patient at low risk. Several additional endpoints are defined during the protocol, some of which are important for stratification and some of which are measured prospectively only. Other European treatment protocols for childhood ALL also use stratification by ASO-qPCR and/or FCM, and protocols in the United States introduce MRD detection by NGS from Adaptive Biotechnologies (https://www.adaptivebiotech.com/) in addition to FCM. The different response rates of the different subtypes have led to modifications in the tracking and response schemes—the slower T-ALL response is well known and reflected in many current protocols. This principle is more deeply elaborated in the current ALLTogether1 protocol for children and AYA, which elaborates stratification criteria for other, genetically defined BCP-ALL subtypes [51]. Flow cytometry also remains the standard method for MRD assessment in US protocols [34].

At the same time, MRD stratification was already used in MRD monitoring before and after SCT and in the treatment of relapse [52]. It was clearly shown that a positive MRD level before transplantation means an extreme risk of relapse after transplantation [53–55]. Monitoring of MRD after transplantation allows individualization of treatment (especially pre-emptive immunotherapy) and rapid response (within 1–2 days) to "molecular relapse" [56]. At certain time points after SCT (typically 180 days after SCT and beyond), MRD monitoring results can be significantly affected by the presence of regenerating lymphocytic cells, and the likelihood of false-positive results at very low MRD levels increases. In this specific situation, NGS with its higher specificity offers a clear advantage over conventional qPCR targeting Ig/TR rearrangements as well as flow cytometry [17].

Due to its versatility, ASO-qPCR targeting Ig/TR rearrangements can detect MRD in more than 95% of ALL patients, displacing the detection of fusion genes in the majority of patients. A specific group is ALL with the *BCR::ABL1* fusion gene. Two large studies examining the correlation of *BCR::ABL1* transcript quatification and later genomic DNA fusion levels with Ig/TR rearrangements in children with ALL have shown that MRD positivity defined by *BCR::ABL1* persists in a proportion of patients when MRD has already achieved negativity using lymphoid-specific Ig/TR rearrangements [57, 58]. These are patients with "CML-like" biology, in whom the underlying aberration is already in the stem cell and not in the lymphoid progenitor. BCR::ABL1 transcript monitoring, or optimally genomic fusion monitoring, in parallel with Ig/TR quantification is useful to identify "CML-like" patients, for whom biological and clinical behaviour as well as optimal treatment approach may be different from patients with “typical BCR::ABL1-positive ALL” [5].

Another exception is infantile ALL with frequent presence of *KMT2A* gene fusions, especially *KMT2A::AFF1*. Due to the immaturity of leukaemic blasts, these leukaemias are often oligoclonal and undergo subsequent rearrangements. Detection of *KMT2A* fusions at the DNA level is more reliable than ASO-qPCR for Ig/TR rearrangements in these leukaemias, and the use of NGS technology to identify the breakpoint at the DNA level has greatly facilitated this method. A similar approach is theoretically possible for any translocation and resulting DNA-level fusion.

MRD detection methods are also used in modern immunotherapies and cell therapies (treatment with (bi)specific antibodies and genetically modified T lymphocytes) and are considered the standard for evaluating their success. However, it is not possible to extrapolate the results of front-line treatment and the significance of MRD because the immunological situation after immunotherapies and cellular therapies is different from that during and after chemotherapy. An example is the relatively high percentage of CD19-negative relapses after CD19-directed therapy [40, 41]. Even in these situations, NGS, with its ability to overcome both immunophenotype change and Ig/TR rearrangement evolution, appears to be the most appropriate method.

6.4.1 Biological Material for the Determination of MRD Levels

Since it has long and repeatedly been demonstrated that peripheral blood MRD levels do not correspond to the leukaemic cell load in bone marrow (except for T-ALL), bone marrow is required as a standard biological material. Efforts to restrict bone marrow collection have led to discussions about whether the higher theoretical sensitivity of NGS and potentially multiparametric flow cytometry may aid in the replacement of bone marrow with peripheral blood. There is not yet sufficient evidence, and the high theoretical sensitivity of these procedures can only be exploited if a sufficient amount of material (DNA or cells) is available and examined.

MRD can also be determined in cerebrospinal fluid and this methodology has the chance to contribute to a new definition of CNS involvement and CNS relapse.

6.5 Conclusion

In summary, MRD detection methods are the cornerstone of stratifying paediatric ALL patients into risk groups with different treatment intensities, both in front-line therapy, relapse treatment and the use of novel cell therapies and immunotherapies. New approaches, particularly those based on NGS and multiparametric flow cytometry, increase the specificity and, in certain settings, the sensitivity of measurements and may thus contribute to the refinement of stratification criteria.

References

1. Fronkova E, Madzo J, Zuna J, Reznickova L, Muzikova K, Hrusak O, et al. TEL/AML 1 real-time quantitative reverse transcriptase PCR can complement minimal residual disease assessment in childhood ALL. Leukemia. 2005;19(7):1296–7.
2. Gabert J, Beillard E, van der Velden VH, Bi W, Grimwade D, Pallisgaard N, et al. Standardization and quality control studies of ‘real-time’ quantitative reverse transcriptase polymerase chain reaction of fusion gene transcripts for residual disease detection in leukemia – a Europe against cancer program. Leukemia. 2003;17(12):2318–57.
3. Meyer C, Larghero P, Almeida Lopes B, Burmeister T, Groger D, Sutton R, et al. The KMT2A recombinome of acute leukemias in 2023. Leukemia. 2023;37(5):988–1005. Pubmed Central PMCID: 10169636
4. Meyer C, Schneider B, Jakob S, Strehl S, Attarbaschi A, Schnittger S, et al. The MLL recombinome of acute leukemias. Leukemia. 2006;20(5):777–84.
5. Zuna J, Hovorkova L, Krotka J, Koehrmann A, Bardini M, Winkowska L, et al. Minimal residual disease in BCR::ABL1-positive acute lymphoblastic leukemia: different significance in typical ALL and in CML-like disease. Leukemia. 2022;36(12):2793–801.

6. Verhagen OJ, Willemse MJ, Breunis WB, Wijkhuijs AJ, Jacobs DC, Joosten SA, et al. Application of germline IGH probes in real-time quantitative PCR for the detection of minimal residual disease in acute lymphoblastic leukemia. Leukemia. 2000;14(8):1426–35.
7. Bruggemann M, van der Velden VH, Raff T, Droese J, Ritgen M, Pott C, et al. Rearranged T-cell receptor beta genes represent powerful targets for quantification of minimal residual disease in childhood and adult T-cell acute lymphoblastic leukemia. Leukemia. 2004;18(4):709–19.
8. van der Velden VH, Wijkhuijs JM, Jacobs DC, van Wering ER, van Dongen JJ. T cell receptor gamma gene rearrangements as targets for detection of minimal residual disease in acute lymphoblastic leukemia by real-time quantitative PCR analysis. Leukemia. 2002;16(7):1372–80.
9. van der Velden VH, Willemse MJ, van der Schoot CE, Hahlen K, van Wering ER, van Dongen JJ. Immunoglobulin kappa deleting element rearrangements in precursor-B acute lymphoblastic leukemia are stable targets for detection of minimal residual disease by real-time quantitative PCR. Leukemia. 2002;16(5):928–36.
10. Szczepanski T, van der Velden VH, Hoogeveen PG, de Bie M, Jacobs DC, van Wering ER, et al. Vdelta2-Jalpha rearrangements are frequent in precursor-B-acute lymphoblastic leukemia but rare in normal lymphoid cells. Blood. 2004;103(10):3798–804.
11. Szczepanski T, Beishuizen A, Pongers-Willemse MJ, Hahlen K, Van Wering ER, Wijkhuijs AJ, et al. Cross-lineage T cell receptor gene rearrangements occur in more than ninety percent of childhood precursor-B acute lymphoblastic leukemias: alternative PCR targets for detection of minimal residual disease. Leukemia. 1999;13(2):196–205.
12. Szczepanski T, Pongers-Willemse MJ, Langerak AW, Harts WA, Wijkhuijs AJ, van Wering ER, et al. Ig heavy chain gene rearrangements in T-cell acute lymphoblastic leukemia exhibit predominant DH6-19 and DH7-27 gene usage, can result in complete V-D-J rearrangements, and are rare in T-cell receptor alpha beta lineage. Blood. 1999;93(12):4079–85.
13. Pongers-Willemse MJ, Seriu T, Stolz F, d'Aniello E, Gameiro P, Pisa P, et al. Primers and protocols for standardized detection of minimal residual disease in acute lymphoblastic leukemia using immunoglobulin and T cell receptor gene rearrangements and TAL1 deletions as PCR targets: report of the BIOMED-1 CONCERTED ACTION: investigation of minimal residual disease in acute leukemia. Leukemia. 1999;13(1):110–8.
14. van der Velden VH, Panzer-Grumayer ER, Cazzaniga G, Flohr T, Sutton R, Schrauder A, et al. Optimization of PCR-based minimal residual disease diagnostics for childhood acute lymphoblastic leukemia in a multi-center setting. Leukemia. 2007;21(4):706–13.
15. van der Velden VH, Cazzaniga G, Schrauder A, Hancock J, Bader P, Panzer-Grumayer ER, et al. Analysis of minimal residual disease by Ig/TCR gene rearrangements: guidelines for interpretation of real-time quantitative PCR data. Leukemia. 2007;21(4):604–11.
16. Fronkova E, Muzikova K, Mejstrikova E, Kovac M, Formankova R, Sedlacek P, et al. B-cell reconstitution after allogeneic SCT impairs minimal residual disease monitoring in children with ALL. Bone Marrow Transplant. 2008;42(3):187–96.
17. Kotrova M, van der Velden VHJ, van Dongen JJM, Formankova R, Sedlacek P, Bruggemann M, et al. Next-generation sequencing indicates false-positive MRD results and better predicts prognosis after SCT in patients with childhood ALL. Bone Marrow Transplant. 2017;52(7):962–8.
18. Faham M, Zheng J, Moorhead M, Carlton VE, Stow P, Coustan-Smith E, et al. Deep-sequencing approach for minimal residual disease detection in acute lymphoblastic leukemia. Blood. 2012;120(26):5173–80. Pubmed Central PMCID: 3537310
19. Kotrova M, Muzikova K, Mejstrikova E, Novakova M, Bakardjieva-Mihaylova V, Fiser K, et al. The predictive strength of next-generation sequencing MRD detection for relapse compared with current methods in childhood ALL. Blood. 2015;126(8):1045–7. Pubmed Central PMCID: 4551355
20. Logan AC, Gao H, Wang C, Sahaf B, Jones CD, Marshall EL, et al. High-throughput VDJ sequencing for quantification of minimal residual disease in chronic lymphocytic leukemia and immune reconstitution assessment. Proc Natl Acad Sci USA. 2011;108(52):21194–9. Pubmed Central PMCID: 3248502
21. Theunissen PMJ, van Zessen D, Stubbs AP, Faham M, Zwaan CM, van Dongen JJM, et al. Antigen receptor sequencing of paired bone marrow samples shows homogeneous distribution of acute lymphoblastic leukemia subclones. Haematologica. 2017;102(11):1869–77. Pubmed Central PMCID: 5664391
22. Svaton M, Skotnicova A, Reznickova L, Rennerova A, Valova T, Kotrova M, et al. NGS better discriminates true MRD positivity for the risk stratification of childhood ALL treated on an MRD-based protocol. Blood. 2023;141(5):529–33.
23. Wood B, Wu D, Crossley B, Dai Y, Williamson D, Gawad C, et al. Measurable residual disease detection by high-throughput sequencing improves risk stratification for pediatric B-ALL. Blood. 2018;131(12):1350–9. Pubmed Central PMCID: 5865233 and royalties with Adaptive Biotechnologies. I.K., B.C., and D. Williamson have employment and equity ownership with Adaptive Biotechnologies. The remaining authors declare no competing financial interests.
24. Bruggemann M, Kotrova M, Knecht H, Bartram J, Boudjogrha M, Bystry V, et al. Standardized next-generation sequencing of immunoglobulin and T-cell receptor gene recombinations for MRD marker identification in acute lymphoblastic leukaemia; a

EuroClonality-NGS validation study. Leukemia. 2019;33(9):2241–53. Pubmed Central PMCID: 6756028
25. Duez M, Giraud M, Herbert R, Rocher T, Salson M, Thonier F. Vidjil: a web platform for analysis of high-throughput repertoire sequencing. PLoS One. 2016;11(11):e0166126. Pubmed Central PMCID: 5106020
26. Knecht H, Reigl T, Kotrova M, Appelt F, Stewart P, Bystry V, et al. Quality control and quantification in IG/TR next-generation sequencing marker identification: protocols and bioinformatic functionalities by EuroClonality-NGS. Leukemia. 2019;33(9):2254–65. Pubmed Central PMCID: 6756032
27. Huggett JF, Whale A. Digital PCR as a novel technology and its potential implications for molecular diagnostics. Clin Chem. 2013;59(12):1691–3.
28. Drandi D, Kubiczkova-Besse L, Ferrero S, Dani N, Passera R, Mantoan B, et al. Minimal residual disease detection by droplet digital PCR in multiple myeloma, mantle cell lymphoma, and follicular lymphoma: a comparison with real-time PCR. JMD. 2015;17(6):652–60.
29. Shirai R, Osumi T, Keino D, Nakabayashi K, Uchiyama T, Sekiguchi M, et al. Minimal residual disease detection by mutation-specific droplet digital PCR for leukemia/lymphoma. Int J Hematol. 2023;117(6):910–8. Pubmed Central PMCID: 10225364
30. Wood BL. Principles of minimal residual disease detection for hematopoietic neoplasms by flow cytometry. Cytometry B Clin Cytom. 2016;90(1):47–53.
31. Borowitz MJ, Pullen DJ, Winick N, Martin PL, Bowman WP, Camitta B. Comparison of diagnostic and relapse flow cytometry phenotypes in childhood acute lymphoblastic leukemia: implications for residual disease detection: a report from the children's oncology group. Cytometry B Clin Cytom. 2005;68(1):18–24.
32. Dworzak MN, Gaipa G, Schumich A, Maglia O, Ratei R, Veltroni M, et al. Modulation of antigen expression in B-cell precursor acute lymphoblastic leukemia during induction therapy is partly transient: evidence for a drug-induced regulatory phenomenon. Results of the AIEOP-BFM-ALL-FLOW-MRD-study group. Cytometry B Clin Cytom. 2010;78(3):147–53.
33. Gaipa G, Buracchi C, Biondi A. Flow cytometry for minimal residual disease testing in acute leukemia: opportunities and challenges. Expert Rev Mol Diagn. 2018;18(9):775–87.
34. Chen X, Wood BL. Monitoring minimal residual disease in acute leukemia: technical challenges and interpretive complexities. Blood Rev. 2017;31(2):63–75.
35. Theunissen PMJ, van den Branden A, Van Der Sluijs-Gelling A, De Haas V, Beishuizen A, van Dongen JJM, et al. Understanding the reconstitution of the B-cell compartment in bone marrow and blood after treatment for B-cell precursor acute lymphoblastic leukaemia. Br J Haematol. 2017;178(2):267–78.
36. Slamova L, Starkova J, Fronkova E, Zaliova M, Reznickova L, van Delft FW, et al. CD2-positive B-cell precursor acute lymphoblastic leukemia with an early switch to the monocytic lineage. Leukemia. 2014;28(3):609–20.
37. Novakova M, Zaliova M, Fiser K, Vakrmanova B, Slamova L, Musilova A, et al. DUX4r, ZNF384r and PAX5-P80R mutated B-cell precursor acute lymphoblastic leukemia frequently undergo monocytic switch. Haematologica. 2021;106(8):2066–75. Pubmed Central PMCID: 8327733
38. Rawstron AC, Bottcher S, Letestu R, Villamor N, Fazi C, Kartsios H, et al. Improving efficiency and sensitivity: European research initiative in CLL (ERIC) update on the international harmonised approach for flow cytometric residual disease monitoring in CLL. Leukemia. 2013;27(1):142–9.
39. Theunissen P, Mejstrikova E, Sedek L, van der Sluijs-Gelling AJ, Gaipa G, Bartels M, et al. Standardized flow cytometry for highly sensitive MRD measurements in B-cell acute lymphoblastic leukemia. Blood. 2017;129(3):347–57. Pubmed Central PMCID: 5291958
40. Libert D, Yuan CM, Masih KE, Galera P, Salem D, Shalabi H, et al. Serial evaluation of CD19 surface expression in pediatric B-cell malignancies following CD19-targeted therapy. Leukemia. 2020;34(11):3064–9. Pubmed Central PMCID: 8919057
41. Mejstrikova E, Hrusak O, Borowitz MJ, Whitlock JA, Brethon B, Trippett TM, et al. CD19-negative relapse of pediatric B-cell precursor acute lymphoblastic leukemia following blinatumomab treatment. Blood Cancer J. 2017;7(12):659. Pubmed Central PMCID: 5802535
42. Verbeek MWC, Buracchi C, Laqua A, Nierkens S, Sedek L, Flores-Montero J, et al. Flow cytometric minimal residual disease assessment in B-cell precursor acute lymphoblastic leukaemia patients treated with CD19-targeted therapies – a EuroFlow study. Br J Haematol. 2022;197(1):76–81. Pubmed Central PMCID: 9299641
43. Bjorklund E, Matinlauri I, Tierens A, Axelsson S, Forestier E, Jacobsson S, et al. Quality control of flow cytometry data analysis for evaluation of minimal residual disease in bone marrow from acute leukemia patients during treatment. J Pediatr Hematol Oncol. 2009;31(6):406–15.
44. Dworzak MN, Gaipa G, Ratei R, Veltroni M, Schumich A, Maglia O, et al. Standardization of flow cytometric minimal residual disease evaluation in acute lymphoblastic leukemia: multicentric assessment is feasible. Cytometry B Clin Cytom. 2008;74(6):331–40.
45. Kalina T, Flores-Montero J, van der Velden VH, Martin-Ayuso M, Bottcher S, Ritgen M, et al. EuroFlow standardization of flow cytometer instrument settings and immunophenotyping protocols. Leukemia. 2012;26(9):1986–2010. Pubmed Central PMCID: 3437409

46. Reiter M, Diem M, Schumich A, Maurer-Granofszky M, Karawajew L, Rossi JG, et al. Automated flow cytometric MRD assessment in childhood acute B-lymphoblastic leukemia using supervised machine learning. Cytometry Part A. 2019;95(9):966–75.
47. Nguyen PC, Nguyen V, Baldwin K, Kankanige Y, Blombery P, Came N, et al. Computational flow cytometry provides accurate assessment of measurable residual disease in chronic lymphocytic leukaemia. Br J Haematol. 2023;202(4):760–70.
48. van Dongen JJ, Seriu T, Panzer-Grumayer ER, Biondi A, Pongers-Willemse MJ, Corral L, et al. Prognostic value of minimal residual disease in acute lymphoblastic leukaemia in childhood. Lancet. 1998;352(9142):1731–8.
49. Conter V, Bartram CR, Valsecchi MG, Schrauder A, Panzer-Grumayer R, Moricke A, et al. Molecular response to treatment redefines all prognostic factors in children and adolescents with B-cell precursor acute lymphoblastic leukemia: results in 3184 patients of the AIEOP-BFM ALL 2000 study. Blood. 2010;115(16):3206–14.
50. Fronkova E, Mejstrikova E, Avigad S, Chik KW, Castillo L, Manor S, et al. Minimal residual disease (MRD) analysis in the non-MRD-based ALL IC-BFM 2002 protocol for childhood ALL: is it possible to avoid MRD testing? Leukemia. 2008;22(5):989–97.
51. EU Clinical Trials Register. ALLTogether Protocol_ Version 1.0. A treatment study protocol of the ALLTogether Consortium for children and young adults (1–45 years of age) with newly diagnosed acute lymphoblastic leukemia. EUDRACT number: 2018-001795-38.
52. Eckert C, Biondi A, Seeger K, Cazzaniga G, Hartmann R, Beyermann B, et al. Prognostic value of minimal residual disease in relapsed childhood acute lymphoblastic leukaemia. Lancet. 2001;358(9289):1239–41.
53. Bader P, Hancock J, Kreyenberg H, Goulden NJ, Niethammer D, Oakhill A, et al. Minimal residual disease (MRD) status prior to allogeneic stem cell transplantation is a powerful predictor for post-transplant outcome in children with ALL. Leukemia. 2002;16(9):1668–72.
54. Bader P, Kreyenberg H, Henze GH, Eckert C, Reising M, Willasch A, et al. Prognostic value of minimal residual disease quantification before allogeneic stem-cell transplantation in relapsed childhood acute lymphoblastic leukemia: the ALL-REZ BFM study group. J Clin Oncol. 2009;27(3):377–84.
55. Krejci O, van der Velden VH, Bader P, Kreyenberg H, Goulden N, Hancock J, et al. Level of minimal residual disease prior to haematopoietic stem cell transplantation predicts prognosis in paediatric patients with acute lymphoblastic leukaemia: a report of the pre-BMT MRD study group. Bone Marrow Transplant. 2003;32(8):849–51.
56. Bader P, Kreyenberg H, von Stackelberg A, Eckert C, Salzmann-Manrique E, Meisel R, et al. Monitoring of minimal residual disease after allogeneic stem-cell transplantation in relapsed childhood acute lymphoblastic leukemia allows for the identification of impending relapse: results of the ALL-BFM-SCT 2003 trial. J Clin Oncol. 2015;33(11):1275–84.
57. Hovorkova L, Zaliova M, Venn NC, Bleckmann K, Trkova M, Potuckova E, et al. Monitoring of childhood ALL using BCR-ABL1 genomic breakpoints identifies a subgroup with CML-like biology. Blood. 2017;129(20):2771–81.
58. Zaliova M, Fronkova E, Krejcikova K, Muzikova K, Mejstrikova E, Stary J, et al. Quantification of fusion transcript reveals a subgroup with distinct biological properties and predicts relapse in BCR/ABL-positive ALL: implications for residual disease monitoring. Leukemia. 2009;23(5):944–51.

Part III

Stratification and Treatment Considerations in ALL

7 Stratification and Treatment Considerations in B-Cell Precursor and T-Cell Acute Lymphoblastic Leukemia

Allison Barz Leahy, Francesco Ceppi, Stephen P. Hunger, and Valentino Conter

7.1 Introduction

Until the 1960s, ALL was uniformly fatal. Development of the first treatments in the 1950s gave rise to research consortium groups, which pioneered effective combination therapy approaches and have driven risk factor identification. Significant survival gains have been made through these groups, with the development of effective chemotherapy and combination strategies, treatment of occult central nervous system (CNS) leukemia, and treatment allocation based on host-, disease- and response-based prognostic factors.

A. B. Leahy (✉) · S. P. Hunger
Center for Childhood Cancer Research, Children's Hospital of Philadelphia, Philadelphia, PA, USA

Division of Oncology, Department of Pediatrics, Perelman School of Medicine, University of Pennsylvania, Philadelphia, PA, USA
e-mail: barza@chop.edu; hungers@chop.edu

F. Ceppi
Pediatric Hematology-Oncology Unit, Division of Pediatrics, Department Woman-Mother-Child, Lausanne University Hospital (CHUV) and University of Lausanne (UNIL), Lausanne, Switzerland
e-mail: francesco.ceppi@chuv.ch

V. Conter
Tettamanti Center, Fondazione IRCCS San Gerardo dei Tintori, Monza, Italy

7.1.1 Historical Perspective: ALL Stratification in the Children's Cancer Group, Pediatric Oncology Group, Children's Oncology Group, and the International Berlin–Frankfurt–Münster Study Group

Supported by the National Cancer Institute, the Children's Cancer Group (CCG) was formed in 1955 and the Pediatric Oncology Group (POG) in 1979—ultimately merging with two other consortia to become the Children's Oncology Group (COG) in 2000, which now includes over 225 centers across North America, Australia, New Zealand, and Europe. The Berlin–Frankfurt–Münster (BFM) study group, the largest European consortium focused exclusively on pediatric leukemia and lymphoma, was founded in 1975 following the West Berlin pilot study [1]. The BFM treatment strategy was gradually shared by several other cooperative groups that joined together as the BFM-Family in 1987, and now continues as the International BFM Study Group, including 28 study groups from 34 countries.

In the 1960s, all children with ALL were treated the same regardless of age or presenting features. This changed in the 1970s, when early trials demonstrated that certain subgroups had inferior outcomes [2, 3]. Subsequent studies stratified treatment based on identified high-risk

G. Escherich, V. Conter (eds.), *Acute Lymphoblastic Leukemia in Children and Adolescents*, Pediatric Oncology, https://doi.org/10.1007/978-3-031-71180-0_7

features: age, presenting white blood cell (WBC) count, CNS involvement, presence of extramedullary disease, erythrocyte rosetting (T-ALL), and treatment response at specific timepoints. CCG initially stratified only on WBC at diagnosis, [3] later incorporating age and marrow response on days 7 and 14. In the 1980s, the BFM further defined a "BFM risk factor," which used peripheral blast count and liver and spleen size to delineate four risk groups. Simultaneously, it also became clear that immunophenotype and certain chromosomal aberrations were important prognostic factors. Early treatment response was extensively investigated in the 1990s, including the significance of minimal residual disease (MRD) at end-of-induction (EOI) measured by multiparameter flow cytometry or polymerase chain reaction (PCR) at different timepoints. In the last two decades, MRD and leukemia genetics have become the most relevant stratification factors in high-income countries. Clinical risk factors remain valuable in resource-limited settings.

7.1.2 Immunophenotypic Classification

The majority (80–85%) of pediatric ALL cases express cell surface or cytoplasmic proteins that indicate origin from an early B-cell progenitor, formally referred to as B-cell precursor ALL, now simply termed B-ALL, [4] with T-ALL making up most of the remainder (approximately 15%), and mixed phenotype acute leukemia (MPAL) being comparatively rare (1.5%) [5].

Early T-cell precursor (ETP) ALL, a subtype of potential prognostic significance, accounts for 10–15% of pediatric T-ALL cases [6–8] and is defined [4] by a characteristic immunophenotype of positive intracytoplasmic CD3 and CD7 expression, CD1a/CD8-negative, along with negative or dim expression of CD5 and positive for at least one stem cell or myeloid antigen [9].

MPAL is distinguished by an aberrant expression of more than one hematopoietic lineage paired with an absence of a recognizable predominant lineage, requiring demonstration of myeloid differentiation plus a lymphoid phenotype by flow cytometry [4]. The majority (approximately 60%) present as B-lymphoid/myeloid, with T-lymphoid/myeloid immunophenotype being the second most common. In rare cases, a B + T-lymphoid immunotype is identified [10].

7.2 Stratification

7.2.1 General Stratification Strategies

Risk stratification is central to the management of B-ALL, ensuring intensification of therapy for patients at high risk of relapse with the goal of limiting treatment toxicity for those curable with less intensive regimens. Current treatment regimens require evaluation of clinical, immunophenotypic, cytogenetic, and molecular markers, detailed below, to determine appropriate treatment intensity. In T-ALL, there have been no reproducibly prognostic variables on which to stratify treatment [11–15] aside from MRD [16–18]. Risk stratification in MPAL is limited, resting primarily on the definition of treatment failure following intense chemotherapy [19–21].

7.2.2 Presenting Characteristics

7.2.2.1 Age, Leukocyte Count

Patient age and WBC at diagnosis are easily determined and remain powerful independent prognostic indicators for B-ALL, despite improvement in outcomes for specific subgroups and overall intensification of therapy. To standardize risk classification and collection of prognostic factor information for children with ALL, the NCI facilitated a consensus definition of standard and high risk based on WBC and age, now known as the NCI Rome Criteria [22]. The relationship between initial WBC and outcome in B-ALL is continuous—with higher WBC counts portending a poorer prognosis, a relationship not observed in T-ALL. Older age at presentation demonstrates the same linear relationship. Based on examination of outcome data of children

(>12 months old), the thresholds of WBC ≥50,000/μL or age ≥ 10 years were defined as high risk. Standard risk (SR) patients were defined by an age between 1 and 9 years with a presenting WBC count of <50,000/uL [22].

7.2.2.2 Extramedullary Disease

Overt central nervous system involvement (CNS3) at diagnosis is rare, affecting 1.5% of patients with B-ALL [23] and 7.5% with T-ALL, [24] and confers a worse outcome when compared to CNS1 status; thus, modern approaches intensify therapy in response to this risk factor. Previously it was thought that poor outcomes associated with low levels of CNS involvement were mitigated by contemporary CNS-directed therapies; however, recent data demonstrate that in B-ALL even low levels of CNS leukemia predict inferior outcome and higher risk of CNS relapse [23].

7.2.3 Molecular Genomics

Chromosomal aberration and gene rearrangements are strong prognostic factors, both favorable and unfavorable, in B-ALL. The most significant genetic alterations are described below. While there have been numerous chromosomal rearrangements and point mutations identified in T-ALL [25] none have clear prognostic value and do not guide treatment. Similarly, there are no specific chromosomal or genetic abnormalities exclusively associated with MPAL.

Favorable

- Hyperdiploidy: Chromosome number, or ploidy, is a highly significant prognostic factor in childhood B-ALL [26]. A hyperdiploid karyotype, defined as more than 50 chromosomes, can be detected in up to 25% of children presenting with B-ALL and is associated with favorable outcome, [27–31] and cases with higher chromosome numbers (>57) demonstrate the most favorable outcomes [32]. DNA index, a ratio of flow-cytometry-determined DNA content of leukemia cells to that of normal diploid cells, can also be used to determine ploidy, with a DNA index of >1.0 indicating hyperdiploidy, and > 1.16 predictive of a favorable prognosis [33]. The presence of specific trisomies has also been shown to be favorable [30]. Although it is unknown why high hyperdiploidy is associated with a good prognosis, hyperdiploid ALL cells are more sensitive in vitro to methotrexate, mercaptopurine, and L-asparaginase [27, 34, 35].
- *ETV6::RUNX1*: *ETV6::RUNX1* fusion results from the often cryptic t(12;21)(p12;q22), detected in approximately 25% of B-ALL [36–41]. This translocation typically occurs in patients between 1 and 10 years with a low WBC count and without hyperdiploidy, [39, 40] is frequently seen in CD10-positive cases, [42] and is associated with favorable outcome [43, 44]. Relapses in t(12;21) ALL occur late, but typically retain their chemosensitivity and have a high probability of cure with second-line therapies [39].

Unfavorable

- Hypodiploidy*:* Hypodiploid ALL, defined by fewer than 44 chromosomes or a DNA index of <1.0, is characterized by multiple whole-chromosomal losses and extremely poor outcomes [45–48]. Distinct genetic subtypes include near-haploid ALL (24–31 chromosomes), low-hypodiploid ALL (32–39 chromosomes) and, less commonly, high-hypodiploid ALL (40–43 chromosomes) [49]. "Masked hypodiploidy," occurs when the hypodiploid clone is doubled, and can be mistaken for hyperdiploidy, [50] although outcomes remain dismal [46]. Near-diploid cases with 44–45 chromosomes commonly harbor dicentric chromosomes or other known chromosomal rearrangements (for example, *ETV6::RUNX1*) [51] and do not share the poor outcomes of hypodiploid ALL [46, 47, 52]. *TP53* mutations occur in approximately 90% of low-hypodiploid ALL cases, and are present in the germline in half [49]. Patients with 44 chromosomes had significantly better EFS than those with fewer, but a linear relationship between chromosome number and outcome otherwise has not been shown [47]. In a retrospective study assessing 306 cases of pediatric hypodiploid ALL enrolled on 16 cooperative group studies between 1997 and 2013, 5-year event-free survival (EFS) was 55.1% and overall survival (OS) was 61.2% [53]. No improvement in outcomes has been achieved with hematopoietic stem cell transplant (HSCT) [53, 54].

- *KMT2A*-rearrangements (*KMT2A*-R): More than 100 partner genes have been identified, but seven partners account for nearly 90% of *KMT2A*-R, [55] with alterations in 5% of all pediatric ALL cases, [56] in most topoisomerase II inhibitor treatment-related leukemias, and in 70–80% of infant ALL [57] (Chap. X). Associated leukemias are often chemorefractory and have the potential for lineage switch to a myeloid phenotype [58, 59]. The t(4;11) with *KMT2A*::*AFF1* fusion is the most frequent *KMT2A*-R detected in children older than 12 months (1–2%) [55] and frequently exhibits myeloid marker co-expression [60]. A recent large international study of non-infant *KMT2A*-R childhood ALL found end-of-induction remission rates of greater than 90%, but a 69% 5-year EFS [61]. Compared to historical data, the prognosis of non-infant *KMT2A*-R ALL has improved, [61] but treatment outcomes are inferior to ALLs without rearrangements with no evidence of benefit from HSCT.
- *TCF3*::*HLF:* A rare translocation, t(17;19) encodes the oncogenic fusion transcription factor *TCF3::HLF*, with affected patients commonly suffering treatment failure and high fatality rates, despite intensive chemotherapy and HSCT [62]
- iAMP21: Intrachromosomal amplification of chromosome 21, found in approximately 2% of childhood ALL, [63] is associated with poor prognosis and has a high risk of relapse when treated with less aggressive chemotherapy [64, 65]. Patients are typically older (median age 9 years), but present with lower WBC counts [66]
- *IKZF1*^{plus}: The AIEOP-BFM ALL 2000 trial identified *IKZF1* deletions co-occurring with deletions in *CDKN2A*/*CDKN2B*, *PAX5*, or PAR1 in the absence of *ERG* deletion in 6% of patients. This *IKZF1*^{plus} subset was associated with poor outcome, with a 5-year EFS of 53% versus 77% in *IKZF1*-deletion (but not *IKZF1*^{plus}) and 87% in patients without *IKZF1* aberration ($p < 0.0001$) [67]. Further stratified on EOI MRD, 5-year EFS for MRD-negative *IKZF1*^{plus} patients was 94% compared to 40% in MRD-intermediate- and 30% in MRD-high-risk *IKZF1*^{plus} patients ($p < 0.0001$) [67]
- Ph-positive and ABL-class fusions: See specific Chapter.

7.2.4 Treatment Response

7.2.4.1 Prednisone Response in the BFM

Prednisone Poor Response (PPR) is defined by morphological detection of ≥1000 lymphoblasts/μL peripheral blood after a 7-day prednisone window (combined with one intrathecal injection of methotrexate on day 1) [68–70]. About 10% of patients have a PPR, which confers an increased risk of relapse, although treatment of PPR patients in the high-risk arm has led to significant outcome improvements [71]. Following implementation of PCR-MRD and MFC-MRD on day 15 for risk stratification in BFM studies, PPR has become less important as a high-risk criterion in B-ALL but retains independent prognostic value in T-ALL [71]. Because PPR as the only HR criterion in AIEOP-BFM ALL 2009 was observed in only 2.3% of B-ALL patients who had a cumulative relapse incidence of only 10%, [72] it is no longer used to stratify B-ALL patients in BFM studies.

7.2.4.2 Day 7 and 14 Bone Marrow Response in CCG/COG Studies

Early bone marrow response during multi-agent induction therapy was prognostic of remission and overall survival in American trials in the 1970s, [3, 73, 74] with subsequent trials replicating its importance on induction days 7 and 14 [75–78]. Early marrow response then became a key aspect of risk stratification in both CCG and

COG ALL trials [79–84] with slow early response (SER), defined by an M2/M3 bone marrow, triggering treatment intensification. Morphologic evaluation at these time points has been supplanted by MRD and is no longer used.

7.2.4.3 MRD: Multicolor Flow Cytometry (MFC)

ALL cells have patterns of cell surface antigen expression by MFC that distinguish them from normal cells and can be used as a marker of the malignant clone to detect MRD. MFC can be used to measure MRD in almost all cases with a sensitivity of 10^{-4} (one leukemic cell among 10,000 normal cells). Improving technologies allow analysis of up to 18 markers in a single cell [85]. The EuroFlow consortium developed a standardized eight-color antibody panel and laboratory procedure to measure MRD in B-ALL with a sensitivity of $\leq 1 \times 10^{-5}$, comparable to RQ-PCR-based antigen-receptor rearrangement detection MRD [86]. Currently, MFC panels comprising six to eight monoclonal antibodies combinations are the most used. Some COG trials now use day 8 peripheral blood MFC MRD to stratify treatment, whereas AIEOP-BFM ALL and ALL-IC studies stratify treatment using day 15 MFC marrow MRD [87]. The COG also found that NCI HR B-ALL patients that remained MRD-positive at the end of consolidation (EOC) had a very poor outcome, meriting alternative therapies, while the small number of EOC MRD-positive NCI SR patients had more favorable outcomes [20, 88].

7.2.4.4 MRD Detection by Real-Time Quantitative PCR of IG/TR Gene Rearrangements

High-sensitivity PCR analysis of patient-specific *IG* and *TR* gene rearrangements to measure MRD in ALL patients were developed in the 1990s. The EORTC Childhood Leukaemia Group [89] reported that MRD $\geq 10^{-2}$ at the end of induction, or $\geq 10^{-3}$ at later time points was associated with high risk of relapse [89]. The BFM consortium reported that EOC (timepoint 2, TP2) MRD $\geq 10^{-3}$ was associated with a threefold higher relapse rate compared to patients with MRD $\leq 10^{-4}$, while patients with negative MRD at end of induction (TP1) had excellent outcomes [90]. Based on these results, MRD-based risk stratification was implemented in AIEOP-BFM ALL 2000, stratifying patients into three MRD risk groups: standard risk (MRD-SR): MRD-negative at TP1 and TP2 with at least two markers demonstrating sensitivities of $\leq 10^{-4}$; medium risk (MRD-MR): MRD-positive at TP1 or TP2, but MRD $< 10^{-3}$ at TP2 with at least two markers; and high risk (MRD-HR): MRD $\geq 10^{-3}$ at TP2 (one marker sufficient) [16, 91]. Among 3184 B-ALL patients, patients with MRD SR (42%), IR (52%), and HR (6%) had a 5-year EFS of 92.3%, 77.6%, and 50.1%, respectively [16, 91]. For 464 T-ALL patients, MRD SR (16%), IR (63%), and HR (21%) had a 7-year EFS of 91.1%, 80.6%, and 49.8% respectively. Interestingly, patients who converted to MRD-negative at TP2 (32%) had a favorable outcome [16].

7.2.4.5 Induction Failure

Induction failure (failure to achieve morphologic CR after 4–6 weeks of induction chemotherapy) is rare, occurring in about 1% of B-ALL and 5% of T-ALL patients [92–95] and confers an unfavorable outcome. Of approximately 44,000 newly diagnosed pediatric ALL patients treated by 14 cooperative study groups between 1985 and 2000, 2.4% had induction failure with a subsequent 10-year OS of 32% (median follow-up 8.3 years, range 1.5–22.1). Older age, T-cell phenotype, *KMT2A*-R, and an EOI M3 marrow were associated with particularly poor outcome [95]. Results from retrospective studies from UKALL2003 [96] and the COG supported the expansion of induction failure definitions to include MRD assessment [97], subsequently implemented in risk stratification by many groups [98].

7.2.5 Current ALL Stratification in Major Consortia Trials

See Table 7.1. Of note, patients with Ph + leukemia are categorized and treated separately (see Chap. X).

Table 7.1 High-risk features resulting in intensification of therapy on current treatment protocols

	COG	DFCI	St. Jude	AIEOP-BFM	ALLIC-BFM	ALLTogether
Age (in years)	<1 or ≥ 10	≥15	<1 or ≥ 10	<1	<6 months	>10 and > 16
WBC	≥50,000 cells/μL	≥50,000 cells/μL	≥50,000 cells/μL	N/A	N/A	≥50,000 cells/μL[a]
CNS	CNS3	CNS3	CNS3	N/A	N/A	CNS3
Immunophenotype	T cell treated on a different protocol, stratified by disease response at the end of induction and consolidation.	T-ALL	T-ALL	T-ALL	T-ALL	T-ALL
Genetics	iAMP21, *KMT2A*-R, *TCF3*::*HLF*, or hypodiploid (<44 chromosomes, DNA index <0.81, or other clear evidence of hypodiploid clone)	iAMP21, *KMT2A*-R, *TCF3*::*HLF*, IKZF1 deletion, or low hypodiploid (≤40 chromosomes)	iAMP21, t(1;9), *KMT2A*-R, hypodiploid (<44 chromosomes, DNA index <0.95, or genome-wide DNA copy-number alterations and gene expression), *MEF2D* fusion	Any *KMT2A*-R (if <1 year), *KMT2A*-*AFF1*, *TCF3*::*HLF*, *IKZF1*^{plus} or hypodiploid (<45 chromosomes)	Any *KMT2A*-R (if <6 months), *KMT2A*-*AFF1*, *TCF3*::*HLF*, *IKZF1*^{plus} or hypodiploid (<44 chromosomes)	iAMP21, *KMT2A*-R, *TCF3*::*HLF*, low hypodiploidy
Extramedullary	N/A	N/A	Ultrasound-proven testicular disease	N/A	N/A	Mediastinal mass, other extramedullary disease[b]
Disease response	MRD-positive at end induction	MRD-positive at end-induction (assessed at two time points for high-risk patients)	≥1% on D15 or ≥ 0.01% on end of induction (immunologic or molecular methods), rising MRD, other time points	MRD-positivity at day 15 (by MFC), TP1 or TP2 (by PCR) Prednisone poor response in T-ALL only.	MRD positivity by MFC at day 15, TP1 or TP2 Prednisone poor response in T-ALL only.	MRD positive at TP1 or TP2
Other	Steroid pretreatment	N/A	N/A	N/A	N/A	N/A

[a]If MRD at TP2 (EOC) ≥0.01%
[b]If not in CR1 at TP2 (EOC)

7.2.5.1 North America

COG risk stratification for B-ALL is based on age, WBC, leukemia genetics, and early MRD response. Favorable genetics are *ETV6::RUNX1* and double trisomies of chromosomes 4 and 10. There are two main risk categories: standard risk (favorable, average, and high) and high risk (favorable and all others). T-ALL is stratified into standard, intermediate, and very high-risk categories based on EOI and EOC MFC-MRD.

Dana-Farber Cancer Institute Consortium (DFCI) risk stratification is initially determined before induction day 11 based on age, WBC, leukemia genetics, CNS status, and immunophenotype (initial risk group assignments: low risk, high risk, and very high risk). Final risk group is determined at the end of induction 1a (TP1) and 1b (TP2) and relies on next-generation sequencing (NGS) MRD with patients stratified into four categories: final low risk, final intermediate, final high, and final very high risk.

St. Jude Children's Research Hospital (SJCRH) categorizes patients into one of three categories (low, standard, or high risk) based on age, WBC, leukemia genetics, presence of extramedullary disease (CNS and testicular), immunophenotype, and early response measured by immunologic or molecular methods on day 15 and EOI. *ETV6::RUNX1* defines favorable genetics.

7.2.5.2 Europe

There are three main European pediatric oncology clinical trial ALL consortia: the Associazione Italiana Ematologia Oncologia Pediatrica and BFM (AIEOP-BFM); the Intercontinental BFM (IC-BFM); and the ALLTogether Consortium, which includes pediatric oncology groups of Belgium (BSPHO), France (SFCE), Germany (CoALL), the Netherlands (DCOG), Nordic Society of Pediatric Hematology and Oncology (NOPHO), Portugal (SHOP), Spain (SEHOP), and the United Kingdom (UKALL). The AIEOP-BFM and IC-BFM consortia, which include other European and also non-European groups, use the same treatment strategies and run parallel complementary studies; they differ in the specific randomization questions asked within the protocols, with higher level of resources required within AIEOP-BFM. Each consortium has specific treatment recommendations for patients with Down syndrome.

In AIEOP-BFM ALL studies, B-ALL stratification (standard, medium, and high risk) is based on leukemia genetics as well as bone marrow MRD response on Induction day 15 by MFC, and at EOI and EOC by Ig/TR PCR. Approximately 30% of patients are considered standard risk, 50% medium risk, and 20% high risk. T-ALL is considered HR if the patient is a PPR, does not achieve a CR at EOI, or has high MRD ($\geq 5 \times 10^{-4}$) at EOC.

The ALL IC-BFM consortium stratifies patients into standard, intermediate, and high risk based on leukemia genetics and bone marrow MFC-MRD response. High risk is defined as MRD $\geq$10% on induction day 15 or $\geq$ 0.05% at EOI only for B-ALL or $\geq$ 0.05% at EOC for both B and T ALL. Favorable genetics are considered *ETV6::RUNX1* or hyperdiploidy. Patients who do not fit the criteria for standard or high risk are classified as intermediate risk. Infants <6 months old are stratified separately. T-ALL is stratified as in AIEOP-BFM, with prednisone response and MRD measured by MFC at all timepoints.

ALLTogether initially categorizes patients based on NCI risk criteria and immunophenotype. After Induction therapy B-ALL cases are stratified into standard risk versus intermediate risk–low and intermediate risk–high, with a novel approach based on different MRD cutoffs for different genetic parameters and CNS status. A small fraction of patients are classified as high risk based on very high MRD at EOI (>5%) or possession of t(17;19) and may qualify for alternate therapies as described below.

7.3 Treatment

Although individual consortia vary in their approach to specific risk groups, most ALL regimens are divided into specific blocks: remission induction (BFM IA), consolidation (BFM IB) and CNS prevention, interim maintenance (IM; BFM Protocol M), delayed intensification (DI;

BFM IIA and IIB), and maintenance or continuation. The most intensive treatment occurs in the first 6–9 months, with 2–3 years of total therapy.

7.3.1 COG Treatment Approach

7.3.1.1 B-ALL Induction

Risk-adjusted therapy is delivered based on NCI-risk group, leukemia genetics, and treatment response. Broadly, lower-risk patients receive a three-drug induction, composed of vincristine, glucocorticoid, and pegaspargase, and high-risk patients receive a four-drug induction with an anthracycline. A dexamethasone-based induction has been adopted in young children given its efficacy in achieving a marrow remission while also providing CNS treatment [99]. However, the benefits to dexamethasone are balanced against increased toxicity, [100, 101] and COG AALL0232 demonstrated no benefit and higher toxicity (osteonecrosis) for B-ALL patients 10 years or older, compared to a prednisone-based induction [101].

7.3.1.2 Post-induction Therapy

Consolidative regimens follow induction and reinforce remission in both the marrow and CNS. Weekly intrathecal treatments or high-dose systemic chemotherapy are used to specifically target the CNS and are followed by periods of intensified therapy with multiple agents to minimize the development of chemotherapy resistance. Consolidation therapy differs based on risk group, with SR patients receiving 4 weeks of daily oral 6-mercaptopurine (6-MP) with weekly intrathecal methotrexate (ITM), and HR patients receiving an 8-week augmented BFM IB phase including cyclophosphamide, low-dose cytarabine, 6-MP, vincristine, and pegaspargase with weekly ITM during the first 4 weeks. Agents in IM and DI generally include vincristine, methotrexate, pegaspargase, dexamethasone, an anthracycline, cyclophosphamide, low-dose cytarabine, 6-MP or 6-thioguanine (6-TG), and periodic ITM. For high-risk patients, these periods of treatment intensification are particularly important, with data demonstrating that stronger regimens improve outcomes, [81] although further intensification of cytotoxics has not been uniformly successful [102] and highlights the need for molecularly targeted approaches. This intensive treatment period typically lasts for the first 6–8 months, followed by protracted use of lower-dose agents in maintenance, the goal of which is to use low-intensity chemotherapy to eliminate residual leukemic clones and to prevent the emergence of new ones. This is accomplished by the administration of daily oral 6-MP, a purine analogue, in tandem with low dose oral methotrexate—a strategy that has been shown to be critical in prolonging remission [103]. Exposure to 6-MP can be measured by patient leukocyte count, with decreased WBC and absolute neutrophil count during maintenance associated with higher levels of 6-MP/MTX levels and a lower relapse rate [104]. Thus, adherence to this oral regimen is important and has a significant impact on outcomes—with a mean adherence rate of <95% conferring an almost threefold increased risk of relapse [105]. The addition of intermittent vincristine and glucocorticoid pulses during maintenance has been associated with a prolonged remission duration, [106] but other data have suggested that these pulses can be less frequent, [107] or even eliminated for some groups [108].

7.3.1.3 CNS-Directed Therapy

Patients at high risk for CNS relapse are those who have CNS disease [109] or hyperleukocytosis at diagnosis, T-cell immunophenotype, high-risk genetic abnormalities, [110] or t(1;19) [111]. CNS treatment and prophylaxis is accomplished using intrathecal chemotherapy, high-dose systemic agents that cross the blood-brain barrier (e.g., methotrexate and cytarabine), or cranial radiotherapy (CRT). Treatment course intensity is stratified by relapse risk. Current COG trials administer 1800 cGy to high-risk patients with CNS3 disease at diagnosis, whereas SJCRH and

DFCI intensifies their CNS treatments by adding intrathecal and systemic therapies without prophylactic cranial radiation.

7.3.1.4 T-ALL

While there have been numerous chromosomal rearrangements and point mutations identified specific to T-ALL, [25] none are prognostic or used to guide treatment currently. Similarly, age and WBC count at diagnosis are not associated with the overall outcome. Rather, treatment response is a more important prognostic determinant than clinical or laboratory features—with EOC response more meaningful than EOI [16]. Induction for all age groups is dexamethasone-based, given the striking survival advantage [112] and acceptable rates of toxicity [113] seen in prior trials. Nelarabine, a purine nucleoside analog, which demonstrated a high response rate as monotherapy in the relapsed setting, [114] also improved disease-free survival when added to augmented BFM chemotherapy in COG AALL0434 [115].

With intensification of therapy, outcomes for T-ALL now rival those of high-risk B-ALL [116]; however, relapsed disease remains difficult to salvage and has a dismal prognosis [117] Further, T-ALL patients have higher rates of CNS relapse and a shorter median time to relapse compared to B-ALL [118]. Current trials have focused on relapse prevention as well as eliminating CRT for those who are not at highest risk. As such, the recently completed COG AALL1231 trial incorporated bortezomib, [119] a proteasome inhibitor that has been shown to help overcome chemotherapy resistance in other malignancies, [120–122] and limits CRT to very high-risk patients and to CNS3 intermediate-risk patients [119]. Evaluation of consecutive COG trials, AALL0434 and AALL1231, demonstrated that CNS1 and CNS2 subjects had similar survival outcomes regardless of CRT use, and that CNS3 patients treated with nelarabine had similar OS to CNS1 and CNS2 patients, supporting the use of nelarabine as standard of care [123]. Other consortium groups have intensified intrathecal chemotherapy administration and eliminated cranial radiation entirely.

7.3.2 European Treatment Approach

7.3.2.1 Induction

All patients on AIEOP-BFM and IC-BFM protocols receive a four-drug phase IA with steroids, vincristine, daunomycin, and an asparaginase preparation, with SR patients receiving only two doses of daunomycin and T-ALL PPR receiving cyclophosphamide in addition. Most patients on AIEOP-BFM receive prednisone, except those with T-ALL who are prednisone good responders (PGR) who then receive dexamethasone. ALLTogether uses dexamethasone, vincristine, and L-asparaginase for B-ALL patients and for those who are NCI-SR, while high-risk patients receive a four-drug induction with daunomycin. In IC-BFM protocols, non-SR patients with CD20+ B-ALL are randomized to receive rituximab, a humanized chimeric anti-CD20 monoclonal antibody, during induction and thereafter, versus the standard backbone.

7.3.2.2 Consolidation

In AIEOP-BFM, B-ALL patients receive a 4-week phase IB, except for those considered early HR (approximately 20%), who receive a hemi-augmented phase IB with 6 weeks of therapy and randomization for treatment with bortezomib. SR T-ALL patients similarly receive the standard 4-week phase IB, whereas non-SR patients are randomized to receive a prolonged phase IB (6 weeks) versus the standard (4 weeks). In IC-BFM protocols, all patients receive a standard phase IB, but non-SR patients (both B- and T-ALL, approximately 75%) are randomized to receive pegylated-L-asparaginase versus not. In ALLTogether, all patients receive the standard phase IB except SR patients who receive a shortened and modified phase with 6-MP, asparaginase and low-dose cytarabine for 2 weeks.

7.3.2.3 Post-consolidation

Patients on the ALL AIEOP-BFM and IC-BFM protocols receive high-dose methotrexate (HD-MTX) prior to protocol II, but MR patients in AIEOP-BFM undergo randomization for a cycle of blinatumomab at the start of Maintenance, whereas HR patients are randomized to receive three blocks of non-cross-resistant drugs (the BFM "high risk" blocks) versus one high risk block paired with two courses of blinatumomab. HR patients in the IC-BFM protocol receive six BFM high-risk blocks. Treatment in both protocols then includes one reinduction phase (protocol II) and maintenance therapy until 2 years from the date of diagnosis.

In ALLTogether, SR and IR-low patients receive two courses of HD-MTX followed by a reinduction phase randomized for treatment with or without anthracyclines. SR patients then move on to 2 years of maintenance therapy, whereas IR-low patients receive two additional cycles of HD-MTX and maintenance randomized to treatment with or without vincristine and dexamethasone pulses. IR-high-risk patients receive reinduction with anthracycline, two cycles of HD-MTX and eight doses of asparaginase, followed by two courses of HD-MTX and a maintenance randomization of three arms: (1) dexamethasone pulses alone, (2) treatment with inotuzumab followed by dexamethasone pulses, and (3) treatment with dexamethasone pulses and 6-thioguanine concurrently. Patients on ALLTogether with very high-risk features and B-ALL are eligible for treatment with CAR T cell therapy (see Chapter) or HSCT. Those with T-ALL, or for whom CAR T cells are not available, are treated with intensive chemotherapy followed by HSCT, or intensive chemotherapy blocks, HD-MTX, reinduction and maintenance to complete 2 years of treatment.

7.3.3 Novel Agents

Inotuzumab, a CD22-directed monoclonal antibody conjugated to the potent cytotoxin calicheamicin, has demonstrated that it is effective and well tolerated in heavily pretreated children with relapsed/refractory B-ALL [124] and is now being tested in the frontline treatment of HR B-ALL patients as part of COG AALL1732 (NCT03959085) and in the ALLTogether protocols (NCT04307576). Blinatumomab, a bispecific CD19-directed CD3 T-cell engager, demonstrates a favorable efficacy and toxicity profile in the relapsed/refractory population, [125–127] and so has been introduced as a randomized question for the upfront treatment of SR patients, including those with Down syndrome, in COG AALL1731 (NCT03914625), as well as in AIEOP-BFM (NCT03643276) for patients with chemo-refractory disease or those at intermediate risk of relapse. AIEOP-BFM protocols have also incorporated bortezomib to overcome chemotherapy resistance in those with B-ALL and slow induction response. CAR T-cell therapy is used in the ALLTogether protocols for patients with very high-risk features and is being studied in a subset of very high risk B-ALL patients in COG AALL1721 (NCT03876769).

7.3.4 Treatment Considerations for Specific ALL Subtypes

Based on Immunophenotype

- *ETP*: Historically associated with worse prognosis compared to non-ETP T-ALL, characterized by a higher likelihood of high end of induction MRD or frank induction failure, but recent trial results demonstrate similar EFS and OS rates, [7, 8] and treatment consolidation with HSCT is based on treatment response, similar to non-ETP ALLs.
- *MPAL*: There is not a chromosomal or genetic abnormality exclusively associated with MPAL and the current consensus is that MPAL is initially treated as B-ALL, with subsequent treatment based on response [21, 128]. Both COG and BFM studies suggest that initiating treatment with ALL therapy results in similar or greater OS than starting with AML regimens [21, 129]. For MPAL patients who are CD19-negative with no other lymphoid features, the BFM recommends starting with AML-type therapy, [129] whereas the ongo-

ing COG frontline AALL1732 trial initiates ALL therapy for all patients with MPAL, regardless of phenotype or blast population [21]. No clear benefit for HSCT in CR1 has been identified, [21, 129] but HSCT should be considered for refractory disease [129]

Based on Molecular Genomics

Treatment is intensified in most modern ALL protocols for iAMP21, *KMT2A*-R, *TCF3*::*HLF*, and hypodiploidy, with some consortium protocols intensifying therapy for *IKZF1*-deletion or *IKZF1*^{Plus} (see Table 7.1).

7.3.5 Duration of Therapy

Most regimens treat patients for approximately 2–3 years, with no optimal length of maintenance therapy yet identified [130]. Historically, COG provided a longer duration of maintenance therapy for males, but this practice was abandoned based on data from SJCRH, DFCI, NOPHO, and BFM trials demonstrating similar outcomes using sex-neutral durations of therapy, [131, 132] and a slight EFS advantage, but absence of difference in OS based on sex in prior COG trials.

7.4 Concluding Remarks

Despite the differences in stratification and treatment of childhood ALL described in this chapter, results achieved by different groups in high income countries are quite similar worldwide, with recent studies showing that further intensification of chemotherapy is unlikely to provide better outcomes. Clinical research aims thus to investigate if the same or better results can be obtained with reduced toxicity. The approaches are based on the personalized characterization of the disease and treatment response, and on the investigation of benefits of novel treatments such as targeted therapies and or immunotherapy.

References

1. Riehm H, Gadner H, Welte K. The west-berlin therapy study of acute lymphoblastic leukemia in childhood – report after 6 years (author's transl). Klin Padiatr. 1977;189:89–102.
2. Riehm H, Feickert HJ, Schrappe M, et al. Therapy results in five ALL-BFM studies since 1970: implications of risk factors for prognosis. Haematol Blood Transfus. 1987;30:139–46.
3. Miller DR, Leikin S, Albo V, et al. Prognostic factors and therapy in acute lymphoblastic leukemia of childhood: CCG-141: a report from childrens cancer study group. Cancer. 1983;51:1041–9.
4. Swerdlow S, editor. WHO classification of tumours of haematopoietic and lymphoid tissues. 4th ed. World Health Organization; 2017.
5. Weinberg OK, Arber DA. Mixed-phenotype acute leukemia: historical overview and a new definition. Leukemia. 2010;24:1844–51.
6. Coustan-Smith E, Mullighan CG, Onciu M, et al. Early T-cell precursor leukaemia: a subtype of very high-risk acute lymphoblastic leukaemia. Lancet Oncol. 2009;10:147–56.
7. Wood BL, Winter SS, Dunsmore KP, et al. T-lymphoblastic leukemia (T-ALL) shows excellent outcome, lack of significance of the early thymic precursor (ETP) immunophenotype, and validation of the prognostic value of end-induction minimal residual disease (MRD) in children's oncology group (COG) study AALL0434. Blood. 2014;124:1–1.
8. Conter V, Valsecchi MG, Buldini B, et al. Early T-cell precursor acute lymphoblastic leukaemia in children treated in AIEOP centres with AIEOP-BFM protocols: a retrospective analysis. Lancet Haematol. 2015;3:e80–6.
9. Arber DA, Orazi A, Hasserjian R, et al. The 2016 revision to the World Health Organization classification of myeloid neoplasms and acute leukemia. Blood. 2016;127:2391–405.
10. Matutes E, Pickl WF, Veer MV, et al. Mixed-phenotype acute leukemia: clinical and laboratory features and outcome in 100 patients defined according to the WHO 2008 classification. Blood. 2011;117:3163–71.
11. Jenkinson S, Kirkwood AA, Goulden N, et al. Impact of PTEN abnormalities on outcome in pediatric patients with T-cell acute lymphoblastic leukemia treated on the MRC UKALL2003 trial. Leukemia. 2016;30:39–47.
12. Paganin M, Grillo MF, Silvestri D, et al. The presence of mutated and deleted PTEN is associated with an increased risk of relapse in childhood T cell acute lymphoblastic leukaemia treated with AIEOP-BFM ALL protocols. Br J Haematol. 2018;182:705–11.
13. Petit A, Trinquand A, Chevret S, et al. Oncogenetic mutations combined with MRD improve outcome prediction in pediatric T-cell acute lymphoblastic leukemia. Blood. 2018;131:289–300.

14. Teachey DT, Pui C-H. Comparative features and outcomes between paediatric T-cell and B-cell acute lymphoblastic leukaemia. Lancet Oncol. 2019;20:e142–54.
15. Raetz EA, Teachey DT. T-cell acute lymphoblastic leukemia. Hematology. 2016;2016:580–8.
16. Schrappe M, Valsecchi MG, Bartram CR, et al. Late MRD response determines relapse risk overall and in subsets of childhood T-cell ALL: results of the AIEOP-BFM-ALL 2000 study. Blood. 2011;118:2077–84.
17. Pui C-H, Pei D, Raimondi SC, et al. Clinical impact of minimal residual disease in children with different subtypes of acute lymphoblastic leukemia treated with response-adapted therapy. Leukemia. 2017;31:333–9.
18. Parekh C, Gaynon PS, Abdel-Azim H. End of induction minimal residual disease alone is not a useful determinant for risk stratified therapy in pediatric T-cell acute lymphoblastic leukemia. Pediatr Blood Cancer. 2015;62:2040–3.
19. Maruffi M, Sposto R, Oberley MJ, et al. Therapy for children and adults with mixed phenotype acute leukemia: a systematic review and meta-analysis. Leukemia. 2018;32:1515–28.
20. Borowitz MJ, Wood BL, Devidas M, et al. Prognostic significance of minimal residual disease in high risk B-ALL: a report from children's oncology group study AALL0232. Blood. 2015;126:964–71.
21. Orgel E, Alexander TB, Wood BL, et al. Mixed-phenotype acute leukemia: a cohort and consensus research strategy from the children's oncology group acute leukemia of ambiguous lineage task force. Cancer. 2020;126:593–601.
22. Smith M, Arthur D, Camitta B, et al. Uniform approach to risk classification and treatment assignment for children with acute lymphoblastic leukemia. J Clin Oncol. 1996;14:18–24.
23. Winick N, Devidas M, Chen S, et al. Impact of initial CSF findings on outcome among patients with National Cancer Institute standard- and high-risk B-cell acute lymphoblastic leukemia: a report from the children's oncology group. J Clin Oncol. 2017;35:2527–34.
24. Dunsmore KP, Winter S, Devidas M, et al. COG AALL0434: a randomized trial testing nelarabine in newly diagnosed t-cell malignancy. J Clin Oncol. 2018;36:10500.
25. Liu Y, Easton J, Shao Y, et al. The genomic landscape of pediatric and young adult T-lineage acute lymphoblastic leukemia. Nat Genet. 2017;49:1211–8.
26. Secker-Walker LM, Lawler SD, Hardisty RM. Prognostic implications of chromosomal findings in acute lymphoblastic leukaemia at diagnosis. Br Med J. 1978;2:1529.
27. Moorman AV, Richards SM, Martineau M, et al. Outcome heterogeneity in childhood high-hyperdiploid acute lymphoblastic leukemia. Blood. 2003;102:2756–62.
28. Heerema NA, Sather HN, Sensel MG, et al. Prognostic impact of trisomies of chromosomes 10, 17, and 5 among children with acute lymphoblastic leukemia and high hyperdiploidy (> 50 chromosomes). J Clin Oncol. 2000;18:1876–87.
29. Hann I, Vora A, Harrison G, et al. Determinants of outcome after intensified therapy of childhood lymphoblastic leukaemia: results from Medical Research Council United Kingdom acute lymphoblastic leukaemia XI protocol. Br J Haematol. 2001;113:103–14.
30. Sutcliffe MJ, Shuster JJ, Sather HN, et al. High concordance from independent studies by the children's cancer group (CCG) and pediatric oncology group (POG) associating favorable prognosis with combined trisomies 4, 10, and 17 in children with NCI standard-risk B-precursor acute lymphoblastic leukemia: a children's oncology group (COG) initiative. Leukemia. 2005;19:734–40.
31. Schrappe M. Evolution of BFM trials for childhood ALL. Ann Hematol. 2004;83(Suppl 1):S121–3.
32. Dastugue N, Suciu S, Plat G, et al. Hyperdiploidy with 58-66 chromosomes in childhood B-acute lymphoblastic leukemia is highly curable: 58951 CLG-EORTC results. Blood. 2013;121:2415–23.
33. Trueworthy R, Shuster J, Look T, et al. Ploidy of lymphoblasts is the strongest predictor of treatment outcome in B-progenitor cell acute lymphoblastic leukemia of childhood: a pediatric oncology group study. J Clin Oncol. 1992;10:606–13.
34. Kaspers GJ, Smets LA, Pieters R, et al. Favorable prognosis of hyperdiploid common acute lymphoblastic leukemia may be explained by sensitivity to antimetabolites and other drugs: results of an in vitro study. Blood. 1995;85:751–6.
35. Synold TW, Relling MV, Boyett JM, et al. Blast cell methotrexate-polyglutamate accumulation in vivo differs by lineage, ploidy, and methotrexate dose in acute lymphoblastic leukemia. J Clin Invest. 1994;94:1996–2001.
36. Aldrich MC, Zhang L, Wiemels JL, et al. Cytogenetics of Hispanic and white children with acute lymphoblastic leukemia in California. Cancer Epidemiol Prev Biomarkers. 2006;15:578–81.
37. Romana SP, Mauchauffé M, Coniat ML, et al. The t(12;21) of acute lymphoblastic leukemia results in a tel-AML1 gene fusion. Blood. 1995;85:3662–70.
38. Pui C-H, Carroll WL, Meshinchi S, et al. Biology, risk stratification, and therapy of pediatric acute Leukemias: an update. J Clin Oncol. 2011;29:551–65.
39. Shurtleff SA, Buijs A, Behm FG, et al. TEL/AML1 fusion resulting from a cryptic t(12;21) is the most common genetic lesion in pediatric ALL and defines a subgroup of patients with an excellent prognosis. Leukemia. 1995;9:1985–9.
40. Borkhardt A, Cazzaniga G, Viehmann S, et al. Incidence and clinical relevance of TEL/AML1 fusion genes in children with acute lymphoblastic

leukemia enrolled in the German and Italian multicenter therapy trials. Blood. 1997;90:571–7.
41. Loh ML, Silverman LB, Young ML, et al. Incidence of TEL/AML1 fusion in children with relapsed acute lymphoblastic leukemia. Blood. 1998;92:4792–7.
42. Loh ML, Rubnitz JE. TEL/AML1-positive pediatric leukemia: prognostic significance and therapeutic approaches. Curr Opin Hematol. 2002;9:345–52.
43. Loh ML, Goldwasser MA, Silverman LB, et al. Prospective analysis of TEL/AML1-positive patients treated on Dana-Farber Cancer Institute consortium protocol 95-01. Blood. 2006;107:4508–13.
44. Rubnitz JE, Wichlan D, Devidas M, et al. Prospective analysis of TEL gene rearrangements in childhood acute lymphoblastic leukemia: a children's oncology group study. J Clin Oncol. 2008;26: 2186–91.
45. Harrison CJ, Moorman AV, Broadfield ZJ, et al. Three distinct subgroups of hypodiploidy in acute lymphoblastic leukaemia. Br J Haematol. 2004;125:552–9.
46. Heerema NA, Nachman JB, Sather HN, et al. Hypodiploidy with less than 45 chromosomes confers adverse risk in childhood acute lymphoblastic leukemia: a report from the children's cancer group. Blood. 1999;94:4036–45.
47. Nachman JB, Heerema NA, Sather H, et al. Outcome of treatment in children with hypodiploid acute lymphoblastic leukemia. Blood. 2007;110:1112–5.
48. Pui CH, Carroll AJ, Raimondi SC, et al. Clinical presentation, karyotypic characterization, and treatment outcome of childhood acute lymphoblastic leukemia with a near-haploid or hypodiploid less than 45 line. Blood. 1990;75:1170–7.
49. Holmfeldt L, Wei L, Diaz-Flores E, et al. The genomic landscape of hypodiploid acute lymphoblastic leukemia. Nat Genet. 2013;45:242–52.
50. Carroll AJ, Shago M, Mikhail FM, et al. Masked hypodiploidy: hypodiploid acute lymphoblastic leukemia (ALL) mimicking hyperdiploid ALL in children: a report from the children's oncology group. Cancer Genet. 2019;238:62–8.
51. Raimondi SC, Zhou Y, Mathew S, et al. Reassessment of the prognostic significance of hypodiploidy in pediatric patients with acute lymphoblastic leukemia. Cancer. 2003;98:2715–22.
52. Pui C, Carroll A, Raimondi S, et al. Clinical presentation, karyotypic characterization, and treatment outcome of childhood acute lymphoblastic leukemia with a near-haploid or hypodiploid less than 45 line. Blood. 1990;75:1170–7.
53. Pui C-H, Rebora P, Schrappe M, et al. Outcome of children with hypodiploid acute lymphoblastic leukemia: a retrospective multinational study. J Clin Oncol. 2019;37:770.
54. McNeer JL, Devidas M, Dai Y, et al. Hematopoietic stem cell transplantation does not improve the poor outcome of children with hypodiploid acute lymphoblastic leukemia: a report from children's oncology group. J Clin Oncol. 2019;37:780.
55. Meyer C, Hofmann J, Burmeister T, et al. The MLL recombinome of acute leukemias in 2013. Leukemia. 2013;27:2165–76.
56. Raimondi SC, Peiper SC, Kitchingman GR, et al. Childhood acute lymphoblastic leukemia with chromosomal breakpoints at 11q23. Blood. 1989;73:1627–34.
57. Meyer C, Burmeister T, Gröger D, et al. The MLL recombinome of acute leukemias in 2017. Leukemia. 2018;32:273–84.
58. Rossi JG, Bernasconi AR, Alonso CN, et al. Lineage switch in childhood acute leukemia: an unusual event with poor outcome. Am J Hematol. 2012;87:890–7.
59. Tirtakusuma R, Szoltysek K, Milne P, et al. Epigenetic regulator genes direct lineage switching in MLL/AF4 leukemia. Blood. 2022;140:1875–90.
60. Alexander TB, Gu Z, Iacobucci I, et al. The genetic basis and cell of origin of mixed phenotype acute leukaemia. Nature. 2018;562:373–9.
61. Attarbaschi A, Möricke A, Harrison CJ, et al. Outcomes of childhood noninfant acute lymphoblastic leukemia with 11q23/ KMT2A rearrangements in a modern therapy era: a retrospective international study. J Clin Oncol. 2023;41:1404–22.
62. Fischer U, Forster M, Rinaldi A, et al. Genomics and drug profiling of fatal TCF3-HLF−positive acute lymphoblastic leukemia identifies recurrent mutation patterns and therapeutic options. Nat Genet. 2015;47:1020–9.
63. Harrison CJ. Blood spotlight on iAMP21 acute lymphoblastic leukemia (ALL), a high-risk pediatric disease. Blood. 2015;125:1383–6.
64. Moorman AV, Robinson H, Schwab C, et al. Risk-directed treatment intensification significantly reduces the risk of relapse among children and adolescents with acute lymphoblastic leukemia and Intrachromosomal amplification of chromosome 21: a comparison of the MRC ALL97/99 and UKALL2003 trials. J Clin Oncol. 2013;31:3389–96.
65. Heerema NA, Carroll AJ, Devidas M, et al. Intrachromosomal amplification of chromosome 21 is associated with inferior outcomes in children with acute lymphoblastic leukemia treated in contemporary standard-risk children's oncology group studies: a report from the children's oncology group. J Clin Oncol. 2013;31:3397–402.
66. Harrison CJ, Moorman AV, Schwab C, et al. An international study of intrachromosomal amplification of chromosome 21 (iAMP21): cytogenetic characterization and outcome. Leukemia. 2014;28:1015–21.
67. Stanulla M, Dagdan E, Zaliova M, et al. IKZF1 plus defines a new minimal residual disease–dependent very-poor prognostic profile in pediatric B-cell precursor acute lymphoblastic leukemia. J Clin Oncol. 2018;36:1240–9.
68. Konrad M, Metzler M, Panzer S, et al. Late relapses evolve from slow-responding subclones in t(12;21)-positive acute lymphoblastic leukemia: evidence for the persistence of a preleukemic clone. Blood. 2003;101:3635–40.

69. Reiter A, Schrappe M, Ludwig WD, et al. Chemotherapy in 998 unselected childhood acute lymphoblastic leukemia patients. Results and conclusions of the multicenter trial ALL-BFM 86. Blood. 1994;84:3122–33.
70. Dördelmann M, Reiter A, Borkhardt A, et al. Prednisone response is the strongest predictor of treatment outcome in infant acute lymphoblastic leukemia. Blood. 1999;94:1209–17.
71. Marshall GM, Pozza LD, Sutton R, et al. High-risk childhood acute lymphoblastic leukemia in first remission treated with novel intensive chemotherapy and allogeneic transplantation. Leukemia. 2013;27:1497–503.
72. Personal communication from M. Schrappe and V. Conter.
73. Gaynon PS, Bleyer WA, Steinherz PG, et al. Day 7 marrow response and outcome for children with acute lymphoblastic leukemia and unfavorable presenting features. Med Pediatr Oncol. 1990;18:273–9.
74. Miller DR, Leikin S, Albo V, et al. Use of prognostic factors in improving the design and efficiency of clinical trials in childhood leukemia: children's cancer study group report. Cancer Treat Rep. 1980;64:381–92.
75. Gaynon PS, Desai AA, Bostrom BC, et al. Early response to therapy and outcome in childhood acute lymphoblastic leukemia. Cancer. 1997;80:1717–26.
76. Gaynon PS. Prognostic factors in acute lymphoblastic leukemia. J Pediatr Hematol Oncol. 2000;22:403–4.
77. Schultz KR, Pullen DJ, Sather HN, et al. Risk- and response-based classification of childhood B-precursor acute lymphoblastic leukemia: a combined analysis of prognostic markers from the pediatric oncology group (POG) and children's cancer group (CCG). Blood. 2006;109:926–35.
78. Steinherz PG, Gaynon PS, Breneman JC, et al. Cytoreduction and prognosis in acute lymphoblastic leukemia – the importance of early marrow response: report from the Childrens Cancer Group. J Clin Oncol. 1996;14:389–98.
79. Matloub Y, Bostrom BC, Hunger SP, et al. Escalating intravenous methotrexate improves event-free survival in children with standard-risk acute lymphoblastic leukemia: a report from the children's oncology group. Blood. 2011;118:243–51.
80. Nachman J, Sather HN, Gaynon PS, et al. Augmented Berlin-Frankfurt-Munster therapy abrogates the adverse prognostic significance of slow early response to induction chemotherapy for children and adolescents with acute lymphoblastic leukemia and unfavorable presenting features: a report from the children's cancer group. J Clin Oncol. 1997;15:2222–30.
81. Seibel NL, Steinherz PG, Sather HN, et al. Early postinduction intensification therapy improves survival for children and adolescents with high-risk acute lymphoblastic leukemia: a report from the children's oncology group. Blood. 2007;111:2548–55.
82. Bowman WP, Larsen EL, Devidas M, et al. Augmented therapy improves outcome for pediatric high risk acute lymphocytic leukemia: results of children's oncology group trial P9906. Pediatr Blood Cancer. 2011;57:569–77.
83. Lange BJ, Bostrom BC, Cherlow JM, et al. Double-delayed intensification improves event-free survival for children with intermediate-risk acute lymphoblastic leukemia: a report from the children's cancer group. Blood. 2002;99:825–33.
84. Matloub Y, Lindemulder S, Gaynon PS, et al. Intrathecal triple therapy decreases central nervous system relapse but fails to improve event-free survival when compared with intrathecal methotrexate: results of the children's cancer group (CCG) 1952 study for standard-risk acute lymphoblastic leukemia, reported by the children's oncology group. Blood. 2006;108:1165–73.
85. Chattopadhyay PK, Price DA, Harper TF, et al. Quantum dot semiconductor nanocrystals for immunophenotyping by polychromatic flow cytometry. Nat Med. 2006;12:972–7.
86. Theunissen P, Mejstrikova E, Sedek L, et al. Standardized flow cytometry for highly sensitive MRD measurements in B-cell acute lymphoblastic leukemia. Blood. 2017;129:347–57.
87. Basso G, Veltroni M, Valsecchi MG, et al. Risk of relapse of childhood acute lymphoblastic leukemia is predicted by flow cytometric measurement of residual disease on day 15 bone marrow. J Clin Oncol. 2009;27:5168–74.
88. Rau RE, Dai Y, Devidas M, et al. Prognostic impact of minimal residual disease at the end of consolidation in NCI standard-risk B-lymphoblastic leukemia: a report from the children's oncology group. Pediatr Blood Cancer. 2021;68:e28929.
89. Cavé H, van der Werff Ten Bosch J, Suciu S, Guidal C, Waterkeyn C, Otten J, Bakkus M, Thielemans K, Grandchamp B, Vilmer E, Nelken B. Clinical significance of minimal residual disease in childhood acute lymphoblastic leukemia. New Engl J Med. 1998;339:591–8.
90. van Dongen JJ, Seriu T, Panzer-Grümayer ER, et al. Prognostic value of minimal residual disease in acute lymphoblastic leukaemia in childhood. Lancet. 1998;352:1731–8.
91. Conter V, Bartram CR, Valsecchi MG, et al. Molecular response to treatment redefines all prognostic factors in children and adolescents with B-cell precursor acute lymphoblastic leukemia: results in 3184 patients of the AIEOP-BFM ALL 2000 study. Blood. 2010;115:3206–14.
92. Janka-Schaub GE, Stührk H, Kortüm B, et al. Initial response to therapy as an important prognostic factor in acute lymphoblastic leukemia in childhood. COALL study group. Klin Padiatr. 1991;203:231–5.

93. Silverman LB, Gelber RD, Young ML, et al. Induction failure in acute lymphoblastic leukemia of childhood. Cancer. 1999;85:1395–404.
94. Oudot C, Auclerc M-F, Levy V, et al. Prognostic factors for leukemic induction failure in children with acute lymphoblastic leukemia and outcome after salvage therapy: the FRALLE 93 study. J Clin Oncol. 2008;26:1496–503.
95. Schrappe M, Hunger SP, Pui CH, Saha V, Gaynon PS, Baruchel A, Conter V, Otten J, Ohara A, Versluys AB, Escherich G. Outcomes after induction failure in childhood acute lymphoblastic leukemia. New Engl J Med. 2012;366:1371–81.
96. O'Connor D, Moorman AV, Wade R, et al. Use of minimal residual disease assessment to redefine induction failure in pediatric acute lymphoblastic leukemia. J Clin Oncol. 2017;35:660–7.
97. Gupta S, Devidas M, Loh ML, et al. Flow-cytometric vs. -morphologic assessment of remission in childhood acute lymphoblastic leukemia: a report from the Children's oncology group (COG). Leukemia. 2018;32:1370–9.
98. Buchmann S, Schrappe M, Baruchel A, et al. Remission, treatment failure, and relapse in pediatric ALL: an international consensus of the Ponte-di-Legno consortium. Blood. 2021;139:1785–93.
99. Teuffel O, Kuster SP, Hunger SP, et al. Dexamethasone versus prednisone for induction therapy in childhood acute lymphoblastic leukemia: a systematic review and meta-analysis. Leukemia. 2011;25:1232–8.
100. Möricke A, Zimmermann M, Valsecchi MG, et al. Dexamethasone vs prednisone in induction treatment of pediatric ALL: results of the randomized trial AIEOP-BFM ALL 2000. Blood. 2016;127:2101–12.
101. Larsen EC, Devidas M, Chen S, et al. Dexamethasone and high-dose methotrexate improve outcome for children and young adults with high-risk B-acute lymphoblastic leukemia: a report from children's oncology group study AALL0232. J Clin Oncol. 2016;34:2380–8.
102. Burke MJ, Salzer WL, Devidas M, et al. Replacing cyclophosphamide/cytarabine/mercaptopurine with cyclophosphamide/etoposide during consolidation/delayed intensification does not improve outcome for pediatric B-cell acute lymphoblastic leukemia: a report from the COG. Haematologica. 2019;104:986–92.
103. Toksvang LN, Lee SHR, Yang JJ, et al. Maintenance therapy for acute lymphoblastic leukemia: basic science and clinical translations. Leukemia. 2022;36:1749–58.
104. Schmiegelow K, Nersting J, Nielsen SN, et al. Maintenance therapy of childhood acute lymphoblastic leukemia revisited – should drug doses be adjusted by white blood cell, neutrophil, or lymphocyte counts? Pediatr Blood Cancer. 2016;63:2104–11.
105. Bhatia S, Landier W, Hageman L, et al. Systemic exposure to thiopurines and risk of relapse in children with acute lymphoblastic leukemia: a children's oncology group study. JAMA Oncol. 2015;1:287–95.
106. Bleyer WA, Sather HN, Nickerson HJ, et al. Monthly pulses of vincristine and prednisone prevent bone marrow and testicular relapse in low-risk childhood acute lymphoblastic leukemia: a report of the CCG-161 study by the childrens cancer study group. J Clin Oncol. 1991;9:1012–21.
107. Angiolillo AL, Schore RJ, Kairalla JA, et al. Excellent outcomes with reduced frequency of vincristine and dexamethasone pulses in standard-risk B-lymphoblastic leukemia: results from children's oncology group AALL0932. J Clin Oncol. 2021;39:1437–47.
108. Conter V, Valsecchi MG, Silvestri D, et al. Pulses of vincristine and dexamethasone in addition to intensive chemotherapy for children with intermediate-risk acute lymphoblastic leukaemia: a multicentre randomised trial. Lancet. 2007;369:123–31.
109. Pui C-H. Toward optimal central nervous system–directed treatment in childhood acute lymphoblastic leukemia. J Clin Oncol. 2003;21:179–81.
110. Pui C-H, Howard SC. Current management and challenges of malignant disease in the CNS in paediatric leukaemia. Lancet Oncol. 2008;9:257–68.
111. Jeha S, Pei D, Raimondi SC, et al. Increased risk for CNS relapse in pre-B cell leukemia with the t(1;19)/TCF3-PBX1. Leukemia. 2009;23:1406–9.
112. Vrooman LM, Stevenson KE, Supko JG, et al. Postinduction dexamethasone and individualized dosing of Escherichia Coli L-Asparaginase each improve outcome of children and adolescents with newly diagnosed acute lymphoblastic leukemia: results from a randomized study – Dana-Farber Cancer Institute ALL consortium protocol 00-01. J Clin Oncol. 2013;31:1202–10.
113. Vora A, Goulden N, Mitchell C, et al. Augmented post-remission therapy for a minimal residual disease-defined high-risk subgroup of children and young people with clinical standard-risk and intermediate-risk acute lymphoblastic leukaemia (UKALL 2003): a randomised controlled trial. Lancet Oncol. 2014;15:809–18.
114. Kurtzberg J, Ernst TJ, Keating MJ, et al. Phase I study of 506U78 administered on a consecutive 5-day schedule in children and adults with refractory hematologic malignancies. J Clin Oncol. 2005;23:3396–403.
115. Dunsmore KP, Winter SS, Devidas M, et al. Children's oncology group AALL0434: a phase III randomized clinical trial testing Nelarabine in newly diagnosed T-cell acute lymphoblastic leukemia. J Clin Oncol. 2020;38:3282–93.
116. Winter SS, Dunsmore KP, Devidas M, et al. Improved survival for children and young adults with T-lineage acute lymphoblastic leukemia: results from the children's oncology group AALL0434 methotrexate randomization. J Clin Oncol. 2018;36:2926–34.
117. Raetz EA, Borowitz MJ, Devidas M, et al. Reinduction platform for children with first mar-

row relapse of acute lymphoblastic leukemia: a children's oncology group study. J Clin Oncol. 2008;26:3971–8.
118. Goldberg JM, Silverman LB, Levy DE, et al. Childhood T-cell acute lymphoblastic leukemia: the Dana-Farber Cancer Institute acute lymphoblastic leukemia consortium experience. J Clin Oncol. 2003;21:3616–22.
119. Teachey DT, Devidas M, Wood BL, et al. Children's oncology group trial AALL1231: a phase III clinical trial testing Bortezomib in newly diagnosed T-cell acute lymphoblastic leukemia and lymphoma. J Clin Oncol. 2022;40:2106–18.
120. Mitsiades N, Mitsiades CS, Richardson PG, et al. The proteasome inhibitor PS-341 potentiates sensitivity of multiple myeloma cells to conventional chemotherapeutic agents: therapeutic applications. Blood. 2003;101:2377–80.
121. Ma MH, Yang HH, Parker K, et al. The proteasome inhibitor PS-341 markedly enhances sensitivity of multiple myeloma tumor cells to chemotherapeutic agents. Clin Cancer Res. 2003;9:1136–44.
122. An J, Sun Y, Fisher M, et al. Antitumor effects of bortezomib (PS-341) on primary effusion lymphomas. Leukemia. 2004;18:1699–704.
123. Gossai NP, Devidas M, Chen Z, et al. Central nervous system status is prognostic in T-cell acute lymphoblastic leukemia: a children's oncology group report. Blood. 2023;141:1802.
124. O'Brien MM, Ji L, Shah NN, et al. Phase II trial of Inotuzumab Ozogamicin in children and adolescents with relapsed or refractory B-cell acute lymphoblastic leukemia: children's oncology group protocol AALL1621. J Clin Oncol. 2022;40:956–67.
125. von Stackelberg A, Locatelli F, Zugmaier G, et al. Phase I/phase II study of Blinatumomab in pediatric patients with relapsed/refractory acute lymphoblastic leukemia. J Clin Oncol. 2016;34:4381–9.
126. Gore L, Locatelli F, Zugmaier G, et al. Survival after blinatumomab treatment in pediatric patients with relapsed/refractory B-cell precursor acute lymphoblastic leukemia. Blood Cancer J. 2018;8:80.
127. Brown PA, Ji L, Xu X, et al. Effect of postreinduction therapy consolidation with blinatumomab vs chemotherapy on disease-free survival in children, adolescents, and young adults with first relapse of B-cell acute lymphoblastic leukemia. JAMA. 2021;325:833–42.
128. Rasekh EO, Osman R, Ibraheem D, et al. Acute lymphoblastic leukemia–like treatment regimen provides better response in mixed phenotype acute leukemia: a comparative study between adults and pediatric MPAL patients. Ann Hematol. 2021;100:699–707.
129. Hrusak O, de Haas V, Stancikova J, et al. International cooperative study identifies treatment strategy in childhood ambiguous lineage leukemia. Blood. 2018;132:264–76.
130. Teachey DT, Hunger SP, Loh ML. Optimizing therapy in the modern age: differences in length of maintenance therapy in acute lymphoblastic leukemia. Blood. 2021;137:168–77.
131. Möricke A, Zimmermann M, Reiter A, et al. Long-term results of five consecutive trials in childhood acute lymphoblastic leukemia performed by the ALL-BFM study group from 1981 to 2000. Leukemia. 2010;24:265–84.
132. Pui C-H, Boyett JM, Relling MV, et al. Sex differences in prognosis for children with acute lymphoblastic leukemia. J Clin Oncol. 1999; 17:818.

Stratification and Treatment of Adolescents and Young Adults with Acute Lymphoblastic Leukaemia

8

Rachael Hough, Anthony Moorman, and Helene Hallbook

8.1 Retrospective Studies Comparing Outcomes of AYA Patients Treated on Paediatric or Adult Protocols for Philadelphia Chromosome-Negative ALL

Historically, adolescents were treated on either paediatric or adult ALL protocols, depending on whether they were referred to paediatric or adult trained haematologists. In the mid-2000s it was therefore possible to compare outcomes depending on the type of protocol used (Table 8.1). All international consortia reported the same observation that outcomes were superior in those treated with paediatric protocols. Event-free survival (EFS) rates were improved by 7–45% and overall survival rates by 7–41%. Given the complexity of ALL protocols it is difficult to ascertain the precise reasons for this difference. However, it is clear that, compared to the adult approach, paediatric protocols use more lymphodepleting drugs such as asparaginase, vincristine and steroids, less myelosuppressive drugs, less allogeneic haematopoietic stem cell transplantation and more CNS directed therapy such as intrathecal chemotherapy.

R. Hough (✉)
University College London Hospital's NHS Foundation Trust, London, UK
e-mail: rachaelhough@nhs.net

A. Moorman
Wolfson Childhood Cancer Research Centre, Newcastle University Centre for Cancer, Newcastle upon Tyne, UK

H. Hallbook
Akademiska sjukhuset, Uppsala, Sweden

G. Escherich, V. Conter (eds.), *Acute Lymphoblastic Leukemia in Children and Adolescents*, Pediatric Oncology, https://doi.org/10.1007/978-3-031-71180-0_8

Table 8.1 Retrospective studies comparing AYA ALL outcomes with paediatric or adult protocols

Protocols	No. of patients	Age range (years)	EFS (%)	DFS	OS	References
ALL97/99 (paediatric) UKALL XII/E2993 (adult)	61 67	15–17 15–17	65 at 5 years 49 at 5 years	–	71 at 5 years 56 at 5 years	[26]
NOPHO ALL92/ALL2000/BFM-83/ Nalle-90 (paediatric) ALL-90/–94/–2000 (adult)	128 97	10–17 15–25	67 at 5 years 60 at 5 years	–	77 at 5 years 70 at 5 years	[27]
DCOG ALL6–9 (paediatric) HOVON ALL-5/–18 (adult)	47 44	15–18 15–18	69 at 5 years 34 at 5 years	71 at 5 years 37 at 5 years	79 at 5 years 38 at 5 years	[28]
CCG 1882/1901 (paediatric) CALGB 8811/9111/9311/9511/19802 (adult)	197 124	16–20 16–20	63 at 7 years 34 at 7 years	–	67 at 7 years 46 at 7 years	[29]
NOPHO ALL1992 (paediatric) SVALL ABCDV (adult)	36 23	15–18 15–20	74 at 5 years 39 at 5 years	–	–	[30]
FRALLE-93 (paediatric) LALA-94 (adult)	77 100	15–20 15–20	67 at 5 years 41 at 5 years	72 at 5 years 49 at 5 years	78 at 5 years 45 at 5 years	[31]
AIEOP ALL95/2000 (paediatric) GIMEMA ALL0496/2000 (adult)	150 95	14–18 14–18	–	–	80 at 2 years 71 at 2 years	[32]
JALSG ALL202-U (paediatric) JALSG ALL97-U (adult)	139 104	15–24 15–24	–	67 at 5 years 44 at 5 years	73 at 5 years 45 at 5 years	[33]

8.2 Prospective Studies of Paediatric and Paediatric-Inspired Protocols for Philadelphia Chromosome Negative ALL in AYA Patients

In response to the findings of the retrospective studies discussed above, study groups around the world have either increased the upper age limit of their paediatric protocols or adapted their adult protocols to include more 'paediatric' elements (paediatric-inspired protocols).

In the UK, the upper age limit of the paediatric UKALL2003 protocol was sequentially increased to the 25th birthday. The 5-year OS was 76% and the haematopoietic stem cell transplantation (HSCT) rate 6% for the 229 AYA patients aged 16–24, but a notable higher relapse risk was observed compared with younger patients [1]. The Nordic-Baltic NOPHO ALL 2008 study included patients between 1 and 45 years. The frequency of high-risk patients increased with higher age, as did the relapse risk in the standard and intermediate risk groups. The 5-year overall survival was 78% for the 221 patients aged 18–45 years, with an HSCT frequency of 16% [2].

Table 8.2 provides a summary of publications focusing on the outcomes of AYA ALL patients treated in prospective clinical trials. Overall current event free and overall survival rates in this age group are between 59%–74% and 65%–78%, respectively, with HSCT frequencies of 10–43%. The proportion of patients relapsing on first line

Table 8.2 Prospective paediatric or paediatric-inspired trials in AYA ALL

Protocol	No. of patients	Age range (years)	EFS (%)	OS (%)	Relapse (%)	References
UKALL2003	229	16–24	72 at 5 years	76 at 5 years	8.8 at 5 years	[1]
NOPHO ALL2008	221	18–45	74 at 5 years	78 at 5 years	19 at 5 years	[2]
CCG 1961	262	16–21	72 at 5 years	78 at 5 years	18 at 5 years	[4]
FRALLE93	40	16–45	70 at 3 years	70 at 3 years	30 at 3 years	[5]
PETHEMA ALL-96	81	15–30	61 at 6 years	69 at 6 years	28 at 6 years	[6]
GMALL 05/93, 07/03	1529	15–35	–	65 at 5 years	–	[34]
CALGB 10403	295	17–39	59 at 3 years	73 at 3 years	31 at 3 years	[35]
HOVON 70 (FRALLE 93)	54	17–40	66 at 2 years	74 at 2 years	–	[36]
GRAALL-2005[a]	200	18–24	60 at 5 years	68 at 5 years	32 at 5 years	[3]

[a]Original study included patients 18–59 years, data given for the 18–24 year subset

therapy is around 9–31% and varies across reports depending on protocol used and the age range of patients recruited.

The age range used to define the 'AYA' population varies across different countries. This is reflected in the published data on AYA ALL outcomes as seen in Table 8.2. At the current time, it is not known if there is an upper age limit for these protocols, above which the benefits of using paediatric or paediatric-inspired ALL protocols is offset by increasing toxicity. However, the French GRAALL-2005 study, which included patients aged 18–59 years, suggests that this upper age limit may be around 55 years [3].

8.3 Epidemiology and Biology

The incidence of ALL in the AYA population is one to two cases per 100,000 which is much lower than among children <10 years old. Childhood ALL is driven by genetic lesions that arise in utero generating a pre-leukaemic clone which persists in early childhood. The acquisition of additional genetic events causes the development of frank leukaemia. This is unlikely to be the causal mechanism for the majority of AYAs with ALL. A distinct aetiology for AYA ALL is supported by GWAS identifying a strong influence for a specific inherited GATA3 variant. Further evidence comes from biological and genetics studies showing that the AYA ALL population is highly heterogeneous. The frequency of T-cell disease is higher than among both younger children and older adults (~25–30% vs. 10–15%). Genomic studies of BCP-ALL have shown that classic paediatric-type chromosomal abnormalities (e.g. *ETV6::RUNX1* and high hyperdiploidy) are rarer than among young children. However, classic adult-type chromosomal abnormalities (e.g. *BCR::ABL1*, low hypodiploidy and *KMT2A* fusions) are also less common among the AYA population compared to older adults (Fig. 8.1). A similar picture is emerging in AYA patients with T-cell disease where the frequency of many genomic abnormalities sits in between that observed in younger children and older adults. For example the frequency of *SIL::TAL1* fusions decreases with age whilst genomic abnormalities linked to ETP-ALL increase with age. Whilst there are no genetic abnormalities that are unique to the AYA population, in BCP-ALL the frequency of chromosomal translocations involving the *IGH* locus is higher compared to both young children and older adults. *IGH* translocations result in the juxtaposi-

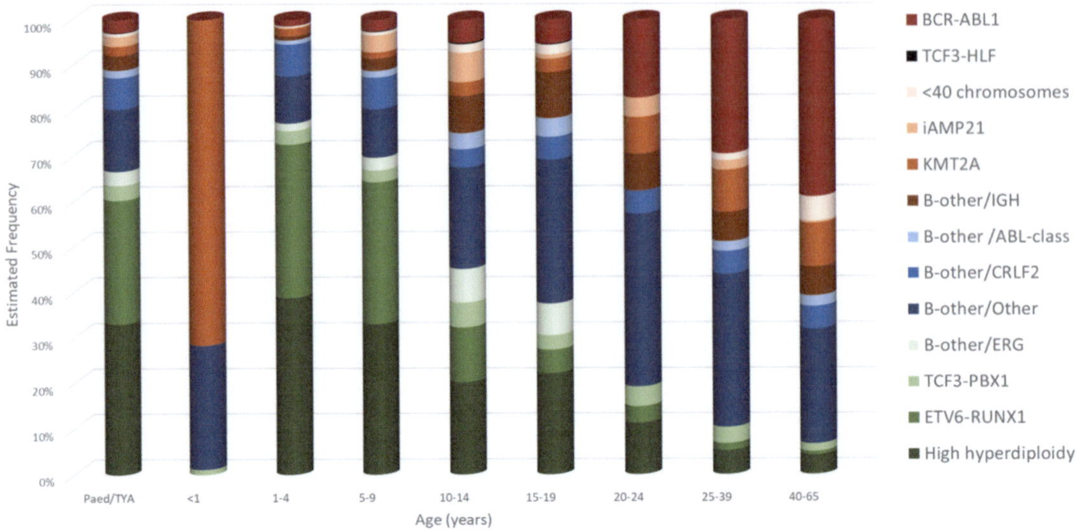

Fig. 8.1 Estimated age-specific frequencies of key genetic abnormalities in B-cell precursor ALL

tion of an oncogene (e.g. *CRLF2*, *ID4*, *CEBPB*, *CEBPE* and *CEBPA*) to the *IGH* enhancer driving its over-expression.

8.4 Risk Stratification

An accurate assessment of an individual patient's risk of relapse is essential in allocating a treatment approach such that excess toxicity is avoided in those at very low risk of relapse and treatment intensity can be increased in those with a greater risk. This risk stratification in ALL is based on clinical features at presentation and an assessment of early response to therapy.

Both retrospective and prospective studies in AYA ALL have demonstrated that, compared to children, AYA patients have a higher likelihood of poor prognostic factors at presentation such as T-cell immunophenotype and deleterious genetic profiles [1, 2, 4–6]. Compared with younger children the frequency of good risk genetics (high hyperdiploidy, *ETV6::RUNX1*) is lower whilst the frequency of high risk genetics (low hypodiploidy, *BCR::ABL1*, *KMT2A* fusions) is higher as described above. In addition, AYA patients are more likely to have a poorer early response to chemotherapy with higher minimal residual disease (MRD) levels at key time points, such as the end of induction [1, 2]. Importantly, age has no impact on the relative contribution of each of these prognostic factors (clinical and MRD) to the risk of relapse and thus the same stratification can accurately predict lower/higher relapse rates within specific age groups [7].

8.5 Current Challenges in Improving Outcomes in AYA ALL

The use of paediatric or paediatric-inspired protocols has led to the improved event free and overall survival rates in AYA ALL shown in Table 8.2. There remain two key reasons for treatment failure: relapse and toxicity.

As a result of the more aggressive disease biology in AYA ALL described above, the risk of relapse is higher in this age group compared to children [1, 2]. Relapse tends to occur early after diagnosis and the outcome with further conventional chemotherapy is dismal. In the UK, AYA patients relapsing after first line therapy with UKALL2003, had an overall survival of only 20% with mortality resulting from disease progression or toxicity in equal proportions [8]. Prevention of relapse, with better risk stratification and novel protocols for those at highest risk, and improvement in the treatment of relapse (discussed later) will be key in improving overall outcomes.

AYA patients also have an increased risk of toxicity with conventional chemotherapy. Different study groups around the world have consistently shown that these patients have a higher risk of induction death, death in remission, serious adverse events and an increased likelihood of treatment delays [1, 2, 4, 6, 9]. Interestingly, age does not impact specific toxicities equally. There are some toxicities where age appears to have no impact, such as line related thrombosis and infection and vincristine neurotoxicity where there may be other dominant risk factors such as the presence of a central venous catheter or genetic polymorphisms respectively. Other toxicities such as infection, steroid-induced psychosis and thrombosis seem to increase in frequency with increasing age. Interestingly, avascular necrosis appears to primarily affect teenagers and appears to be less common in children younger than 10 years or adults aged 20 years or older. The reasons for this increased toxicity are poorly understood but may be a reflection of some of the physiological changes specific to this age group which are summarised in Table 8.3.

8.6 Treatment of Relapse

Historically, the treatment strategy of AYA patients following relapse has relied upon intensive chemotherapy (such as FLA-Ida) to cytoreduce the disease to an MRD less than 0.01% followed by consolidation with an allogeneic haematopoietic stem cell transplant in second complete remission.

However, significant advances have been more recently made in the use of immunotherapy in this setting, in which novel therapies target specific antigens expressed on the leukaemic blasts (primarily CD19 and CD22).

In a randomised phase 3 study, blinatumomab (CD19 directed) was compared to conventional salvage chemotherapy for Philadelphia chromosome negative and positive B-ALL patients in relapse [10]. The complete remission rate was significantly higher in the blinatumomab group, as well as MRD negativity, and 6-month OS and EFS both in the first and the later relapse. Similarly, inotuzumab ozogamicin (CD22 directed) was compared to standard chemotherapy for B-ALL [11]. Inotuzumab ozogamicin was associated with higher complete remission rates, MRD negativity, PFS and OS. Importantly, a higher proportion of patients were able to proceed to allogeneic HSCT but the incidence of veno-occlusive disease was noted to be higher in those receiving Inotuzumab. The results of the

Table 8.3 Physiological changes in the AYA population which can result in subtherapeutic dosing or increased toxicity [37–39]

Adolescence is a period of rapid growth and development
Change in body composition (increase fat mass—Females, increase muscle mass—Males)—May affect volume of distribution/plasma drug concentrations
Increasing and pulsatile growth hormone levels during puberty—May affect metabolism of chemotherapy drugs
Maturation of sex steroid pathway—Affects drug-metabolising enzymes, e.g. decreased CYP1A2, CYP2B6, CYP2C19
Increased consumption of alcohol, tobacco, recreational drugs, anabolic steroids—Interaction with cytochrome p450
Increased risk of dietary exploration and eating disorders—Substantial impact on hepatic metabolism
Increased use of oral contraceptive pills—Inhibition of CYP2B6 and CYP2C19
PK studies generally not AYA-specific
Dexamethasone/methotrexate oral clearance half that of children

phase 2 BLAST study have been more recently reported where MRD-positive B-ALL received blinatumomab [12]. A high frequency of MRD negativity was achieved, and, in this setting, some longtime survivors were observed without proceeding to HSCT.

There is also a rapidly expanding literature on the role of chimeric antigen receptor (CAR) T cells in the management of refractory or relapsed B-ALL. Two products are currently licensed for treatment in this setting; tisagenlecleucel for patients aged up to 25 years [13] and KTE-X19 (brexucabtagene autoleucel) in adults [14]. These novel therapies can be curative in patients who have failed multiple lines of conventional chemotherapy and HSCT. At present around 30–40% of children and young people receiving tisagenlecleucel will require no further therapy. The key reasons for treatment failure are lack of CAR T cell persistence or antigen negative escape and other CAR T products are already in ongoing clinical trials to address these problems. Whilst the value of CAR T cell therapy in the refractory and relapsed setting is already established, it may be that this technology could benefit high risk patients receiving front-line therapy.

At present there is a paucity of novel therapies approved for the treatment of refractory or relapsed T-ALL. However, new agents such as daratumumab and CAR T-cell strategies are already in early phase trials.

8.7 Philadelphia Chromosome (*BCR::ABL1*)-Positive ALL

Before the introduction of TKI, the long-time prognosis was dismal in Ph-positive ALL regardless of the patients age. After the introduction of imatinib as addition to induction chemotherapy, the CR rates improved reaching 92–100%, giving the opportunity especially for younger adults to proceed to an allogeneic haematopoietic stem cell transplantation. Several adult studies (including patients up to 65 years) have been published regarding treatment with imatinib and standard chemotherapy with an 4 or 5 year OS between 38% and 52% [15–19].

Despite publication of several studies with dasatinib, nilotinib or ponatinib together with chemotherapy as upfront treatment, no randomised study comparing imatinib with second or third generation TKI is published for adult patients, even if retrospective comparisons have been made. A propensity score analysis by Sasaki et al. found longer OS and EFS when hyper-CVAD was combined with ponatinib than with dasatinib [20].

HSCT has, until recently, been the undisputable standard of care for young adult Ph-positive patients with an identified donor. The GMALL group conducted a study comparing MRD triggered versus upfront imatinib post HSCT [21]. The upfront arm had a lower incidence of molecular reappearance of *BCR-ABL1,* but the 5-year OS in both groups was high and the authors conclude that both strategies result in excellent long-term outcomes. No adult randomised trials have been conducted comparing first-, second- and third-generation TKI post HSCT.

Recently, 'chemotherapy free' treatment has evolved and the GIMEMA group have treated adult patients (aged 24–82 years) with an induction of dasatinib and glucocorticoids followed by blinatumomab, resulting in excellent results (18 months OS 95%) [22]. Post-consolidation was left open and HSCT was allowed. Studies including ponatinib and blinatumomab are ongoing in the GIMEMA-group and at MDAnderson. The latter has presented early results with promising 2 year OS at 93% [23]. Due to the encouraging results from emerging upfront therapies, the role of HSCT is not any longer obvious neither for AYA nor older adult Ph-positive patients and further studies, including data regarding risk grouping within the Ph-positive cohort, is needed.

Genomic studies have identified a genetic subgroup of ALL called ABL-class fusions which are also sensitive to treatment with a TKI. This heterogeneous group of rearrangements results in the fusion of *ABL1*, *ABL2*, *PDGFRB* and *CSF1R* with a variety of partners genes (e.g. *EBF1*, *ETV6*). ABL-class fusions occur in both BCP-ALL and T-ALL and some studies have shown a higher frequency among AYA patients. The most common fusion is *EBF1-PDGFRB* which, like other ABL-class fusions, has been linked with a very poor outcome when treated without a TKI. The majority of treatment protocols advocate adjuvant therapy with a TKI for these patients. The new international Ph-positive trial for patients <18 years old will include patients with an ABL-class fusion.

8.8 Specific Holistic Considerations for AYA Patients

The AYA group represents a distinct entity and young people should be considered to be neither large children nor small adults. In addition to the distinct ALL biology, host physiology and susceptibility to toxicity with chemotherapy described above, young people are also in a significant psychosocial transition from being a dependent child focused on the present to a future orientated adult who is aware of others around them. Table 8.4 summarises the key psychosocial factors requiring transition during adolescence and young adulthood. Being diagnosed with ALL and receiving treatment for it can substantially impact on normal psychosocial development as young people need to face their potential mortality, receive therapy which affects their physical appearance, become increasingly dependent (financially and emotionally) on their parents and caregivers and often become isolated from friends and their education. These challenges can lead to psychological morbidity and adherence difficulties. Compliance is a complicated issue that may impact on taking medication, responding to toxicities (e.g. sepsis) and physicians ensuring that young people receive the treatment schedule on time.

Table 8.4 Psychosocial transitions during adolescence and young adulthood

Acquisition of a future-orientated outlook
Gradual separation from parents
Moving out of family home
Establishment of financial and emotional independence
Formation of mature relationships and concern for the welfare of others
Development of self-confidence, individuality, sexual identity

In response to these specific AYA needs, the first adolescent cancer service was established at the Middlesex Hospital in London in 1990. Since then, AYA services have developed in centres across the world. These units are able to focus on the holistic needs of young people, providing extensive multidisciplinary support, opportunities for peer to peer support, education and employment support and providing age specific information and consent processes. Such services may improve patient experience and recruitment to clinical trials [24, 25].

8.9 Conclusion

There have been significant advances made in the management and outcomes of treatment for ALL in adolescents and young adults over the last 15 years. The use of paediatric or paediatric-inspired protocols is now associated with an expected EFS of 70–80%. The two key challenges to improving outcomes further are to reduce toxicity and prevent relapse. Given that treatment failure is generally due in equal part to disease progression/relapse and toxicity, modification of conventional strategies is unlikely to achieve significant improvement given that any benefits achieved with an increase in dose intensity to reduce relapse is likely to be offset by an increase in toxicity and vice versa. The advent of immunotherapy and other targeted therapies present an exciting opportunity to achieve this by incorporating these agents into front line therapy and also in improving relapse outcomes. Young people also face age-specific issues which must also be addressed to maximise the short and long term quality of survival following treatment for ALL.

References

1. Hough R, Rowntree C, Goulden N, et al. Efficacy and toxicity of a paediatric protocol in teenagers and young adults with Philadelphia chromosome negative acute lymphoblastic leukaemia: results from UKALL 2003. Br J Haematol. 2016;172(3):439–51. https://doi.org/10.1111/bjh.13847.
2. Toft N, Birgens H, Abrahamsson J, et al. Results of NOPHO ALL2008 treatment for patients aged 1-45 years with acute lymphoblastic leukemia. Leukemia. 2018;32(3):606–15. https://doi.org/10.1038/leu.2017.265.
3. Huguet F, Chevret S, Leguay T, et al. Intensified therapy of acute lymphoblastic leukemia in adults: report of the randomized GRAALL-2005 clinical trial. J Clin Oncol. 2018;36(24):2514–23. https://doi.org/10.1200/JCO.2017.76.8192.
4. Nachman JB, La MK, Hunger SP, et al. Young adults with acute lymphoblastic leukemia have an excellent outcome with chemotherapy alone and benefit from intensive postinduction treatment: a report from the children's oncology group. J Clin Oncol. 2009;27(31):5189–94. https://doi.org/10.1200/JCO.2008.20.8959.
5. Hocking J, Schwarer AP, Gasiorowski R, et al. Excellent outcomes for adolescents and adults with acute lymphoblastic leukemia and lymphoma without allogeneic stem cell transplant: the FRALLE-93 pediatric protocol. Leuk Lymphoma. 2014;55(12):2801–7. https://doi.org/10.3109/10428194.2014.894191.
6. Ribera JM, Oriol A, Sanz MA, et al. Comparison of the results of the treatment of adolescents and young adults with standard-risk acute lymphoblastic leukemia with the Programa Espanol de Tratamiento en Hematologia pediatric-based protocol ALL-96. J Clin Oncol. 2008;26(11):1843–9. https://doi.org/10.1200/JCO.2007.13.7265.
7. Enshaei A, O'Connor D, Bartram J, et al. A validated novel continuous prognostic index to deliver stratified medicine in pediatric acute lymphoblastic leukemia. Blood. 2020;135(17):1438–46. https://doi.org/10.1182/blood.2019003191.
8. Sellar RS, Rowntree C, Vora AJ, et al. Relapse in teenage and young adult patients treated on a paediatric minimal residual disease stratified ALL treatment protocol is associated with a poor outcome: results from UKALL2003. Br J Haematol. 2018;181(4):515–22. https://doi.org/10.1111/bjh.15208.
9. Toft N, Birgens H, Abrahamsson J, et al. Toxicity profile and treatment delays in NOPHO ALL2008-comparing adults and children with Philadelphia chromosome-negative acute lymphoblastic leukemia. Eur J Haematol. 2016;96(2):160–9. https://doi.org/10.1111/ejh.12562.
10. Dombret H, Topp MS, Schuh AC, et al. Blinatumomab versus chemotherapy in first salvage or in later salvage for B-cell precursor acute lymphoblastic leukemia. Leuk Lymphoma. 2019;60(9):2214–22. https://doi.org/10.1080/10428194.2019.1576872.
11. Kantarjian HM, DeAngelo DJ, Stelljes M, et al. Inotuzumab ozogamicin versus standard of care in relapsed or refractory acute lymphoblastic leukemia: final report and long-term survival follow-up from the randomized, phase 3 INO-VATE study. Cancer. 2019;125(14):2474–87. https://doi.org/10.1002/cncr.32116.
12. Gokbuget N, Zugmaier G, Dombret H, et al. Curative outcomes following blinatumomab in adults with minimal residual disease B-cell precursor acute lymphoblastic leukemia. Leuk Lymphoma. 2020;61(11):2665–73. https://doi.org/10.1080/10428194.2020.1780583.
13. Maude SL, Laetsch TW, Buechner J, et al. Tisagenlecleucel in children and young adults with B-cell lymphoblastic leukemia. N Engl J Med. 2018;378(5):439–48. https://doi.org/10.1056/NEJMoa1709866.
14. Shah BD, Ghobadi A, Oluwole OO, et al. KTE-X19 for relapsed or refractory adult B-cell acute lymphoblastic leukaemia: phase 2 results of the single-arm, open-label, multicentre ZUMA-3 study. Lancet. 2021;398(10299):491–502. https://doi.org/10.1016/S0140-6736(21)01222-8.
15. Wassmann B, Pfeifer H, Goekbuget N, et al. Alternating versus concurrent schedules of imatinib and chemotherapy as front-line therapy for Philadelphia-positive acute lymphoblastic leukemia (Ph+ ALL). Blood. 2006;108(5):1469–77. https://doi.org/10.1182/blood-2005-11-4386.
16. Tanguy-Schmidt A, Rousselot P, Chalandon Y, et al. Long-term follow-up of the imatinib GRAAPH-2003 study in newly diagnosed patients with de novo Philadelphia chromosome-positive acute lymphoblastic leukemia: a GRAALL study. Biol Blood Marrow Transplant. 2013;19(1):150–5. https://doi.org/10.1016/j.bbmt.2012.08.021.
17. Hatta Y, Mizuta S, Matsuo K, et al. Final analysis of the JALSG Ph+ALL202 study: tyrosine kinase inhibitor-combined chemotherapy for Ph+ALL. Ann Hematol. 2018;97(9):1535–45. https://doi.org/10.1007/s00277-018-3323-8.
18. Fielding AK, Rowe JM, Buck G, et al. UKALLXII/ECOG2993: addition of imatinib to a standard treatment regimen enhances long-term outcomes in Philadelphia positive acute lymphoblastic leukemia. Blood. 2014;123(6):843–50. https://doi.org/10.1182/blood-2013-09-529008.
19. Ribera JM, Garcia O, Montesinos P, et al. Treatment of young patients with Philadelphia chromosome-positive acute lymphoblastic leukaemia using increased dose of imatinib and deintensified chemotherapy before allogeneic stem cell transplantation. Br J Haematol. 2012;159(1):78–81. https://doi.org/10.1111/j.1365-2141.2012.09240.x.
20. Sasaki K, Jabbour EJ, Ravandi F, et al. Hyper-CVAD plus ponatinib versus hyper-CVAD plus

dasatinib as frontline therapy for patients with Philadelphia chromosome-positive acute lymphoblastic leukemia: a propensity score analysis. Cancer. 2016;122(23):3650–6. https://doi.org/10.1002/cncr.30231.
21. Pfeifer H, Wassmann B, Bethge W, et al. Randomized comparison of prophylactic and minimal residual disease-triggered imatinib after allogeneic stem cell transplantation for BCR-ABL1-positive acute lymphoblastic leukemia. Leukemia. 2013;27(6):1254–62. https://doi.org/10.1038/leu.2012.352.
22. Foa R, Bassan R, Vitale A, et al. Dasatinib-Blinatumomab for Ph-positive acute lymphoblastic leukemia in adults. N Engl J Med. 2020;383(17):1613–23. https://doi.org/10.1056/NEJMoa2016272.
23. Short N. Ponatinib and blinatumomab for patients with Philadelphia chromosome-positive acute lymphoblastic leukemia: updated results from a phase II study. HemaSphere. 2022;6:15–6. https://doi.org/10.1097/01.HS9.0000843352.55138.40.
24. Hough R, Sandhu S, Khan M, et al. Are survival and mortality rates associated with recruitment to clinical trials in teenage and young adult patients with acute lymphoblastic leukaemia? A retrospective observational analysis in England. BMJ Open. 2017;7(10):e017052. https://doi.org/10.1136/bmjopen-2017-017052.
25. Furness CL, Smith L, Morris E, Brocklehurst C, Daly S, Hough RE. Cancer patient experience in the teenage young adult population- key issues and trends over time: an analysis of the United Kingdom National Cancer Patient Experience Surveys 2010-2014. J Adolesc Young Adult Oncol. 2017;6(3):450–8. https://doi.org/10.1089/jayao.2016.0058.
26. Ramanujachar R, Richards S, Hann I, et al. Adolescents with acute lymphoblastic leukaemia: outcome on UK national paediatric (ALL97) and adult (UKALLXII/E2993) trials. Pediatr Blood Cancer. 2007;48(3):254–61. https://doi.org/10.1002/pbc.20749.
27. Usvasalo A, Raty R, Knuutila S, et al. Acute lymphoblastic leukemia in adolescents and young adults in Finland. Haematologica. 2008;93(8):1161–8. https://doi.org/10.3324/haematol.12466.
28. De Bont JM, Van Der Holt B, Dekker AW, Sonneveld P, Pieters R. Significant difference in outcome for adolescents with acute lymphoblastic leukemia treated on pediatric vs adult protocols in The Netherlands. Leukemia. 2004;18(12):2032–5. https://doi.org/10.1038/sj.leu.2403538.
29. Stock W, La M, Sanford B, et al. What determines the outcomes for adolescents and young adults with acute lymphoblastic leukemia treated on cooperative group protocols? A comparison of children's cancer group and cancer and leukemia group B studies. Blood. 2008;112(5):1646–54. https://doi.org/10.1182/blood-2008-01-130237.
30. Hallbook H, Gustafsson G, Smedmyr B, et al. Treatment outcome in young adults and children >10 years of age with acute lymphoblastic leukemia in Sweden: a comparison between a pediatric protocol and an adult protocol. Cancer. 2006;107(7):1551–61. https://doi.org/10.1002/cncr.22189.
31. Boissel N, Auclerc MF, Lheritier V, et al. Should adolescents with acute lymphoblastic leukemia be treated as old children or young adults? Comparison of the French FRALLE-93 and LALA-94 trials. J Clin Oncol. 2003;21(5):774–80. https://doi.org/10.1200/JCO.2003.02.053.
32. Testi AM. Difference in outcome of adolescents with acute lymphoblastic leukemia (ALL) enrolled in pediatric (AIEOP) and adult (GIMEMA) protocols. Blood. 2004;104(11)
33. Hayakawa F, Sakura T, Yujiri T, et al. Markedly improved outcomes and acceptable toxicity in adolescents and young adults with acute lymphoblastic leukemia following treatment with a pediatric protocol: a phase II study by the Japan adult leukemia study group. *Blood*. Cancer J. 2014;4(10):e252. https://doi.org/10.1038/bcj.2014.72.
34. Gökbuget N. Significant improvement of outcome in adolescents and young adults (AYAs) aged 15-35 years with acute lymphoblastic leukemia (ALL) with a pediatric derived adult ALL protocol; results of 1529 AYAs in 2 consecutive trials of the German multicenter study group for adult ALL (GMALL). Blood. 2013;122(21):839.
35. Stock W, Luger SM, Advani AS, et al. A pediatric regimen for older adolescents and young adults with acute lymphoblastic leukemia: results of CALGB 10403. Blood. 2019;133(14):1548–59. https://doi.org/10.1182/blood-2018-10-881961.
36. Rijneveld AW, van der Holt B, Daenen SM, et al. Intensified chemotherapy inspired by a pediatric regimen combined with allogeneic transplantation in adult patients with acute lymphoblastic leukemia up to the age of 40. Leukemia. 2011;25(11):1697–703. https://doi.org/10.1038/leu.2011.141.
37. Veal GJ, Hartford CM, Stewart CF. Clinical pharmacology in the adolescent oncology patient. J Clin Oncol. 2010;28(32):4790–9. https://doi.org/10.1200/JCO.2010.28.3473.
38. McCance-Katz EF, Sullivan LE, Nallani S. Drug interactions of clinical importance among the opioids, methadone and buprenorphine, and other frequently prescribed medications: a review. Am J Addict. 2010;19(1):4–16. https://doi.org/10.1111/j.1521-0391.2009.00005.x.
39. Hukkanen J, Jacob P 3rd, Peng M, Dempsey D, Benowitz NL. Effect of nicotine on cytochrome P450 1A2 activity. Br J Clin Pharmacol. 2011;72(5):836–8. https://doi.org/10.1111/j.1365-2125.2011.04023.x.

9 Central Nervous System-Directed Therapy

Nikolai Gajic, Jan Stary, and Christina Halsey

9.1 Introduction

Involvement of the central nervous system (CNS) in acute lymphoblastic leukaemia (ALL) remains a major clinical challenge. Overt CNS leukaemia, when identified through standard of care diagnostics, is present in 3–5% of patients at initial diagnosis and 30–40% at relapse [1–4]. However, an assortment of literature suggest this is likely an underestimate. It is therefore paramount to consider CNS directed therapy when striving to achieve curative treatment in paediatric ALL.

CNS leukaemia is almost always a disease of the leptomeninges with parenchymal involvement only observed at very late stages. Entry of leukaemic cells into the CNS occurs via the circulation. In vivo studies have revealed that cells likely gain access to the meninges via the blood leptomeningeal barrier or the blood CSF barrier [5–7]. Furthermore, ALL cells have been observed to track bridging veins transversing the bone marrow and subarachnoid space, offering alternate means of entry [8]. No study has demonstrated exclusivity to a particular route and therefore it is conceivable that ALL cells invade the CNS through several independent avenues simultaneously. Involvement of the brain parenchyma is thought to result from extension through the pia–glial membrane or via interference with local perfusion secondary to constriction of vessels by perivascular arachnoid leukaemia [9].

The CNS, being a pharmacological and immunological sanctuary, may also serve as a reservoir for leukaemic cells seeding to the bone marrow at the time of relapse, although direct evidence for this is lacking.

9.2 Historical Perspective

As clinical strategies and approaches to childhood ALL advanced, children had steadily improved response rates [10–12]. However, early chemotherapy protocols struggled to maintain remission and as such relapse, often presenting with CNS involvement, became a prominent clinical challenge. Between 1948 and 1960 the incidence of overt CNS leukaemia increased from 3% to 40%, coinciding with a threefold increase in median survival of patients suffering with the disease [13] Moreover, clinicians observed the phenomenon of 'isolated CNS relapse' wherein children would present with signs and symptoms of meningeal infiltration in the absence of bone

N. Gajic · C. Halsey (✉)
Wolfson Wohl Cancer Research Centre, School of Cancer Sciences, College of Medical Veterinary and Life Sciences, University of Glasgow, Glasgow, UK
e-mail: Chris.Halsey@glasgow.ac.uk

J. Stary
Second Faculty of Medicine, Department of Pediatric Hematology and Oncology, Charles University and University Hospital Motol, Prague, Czech Republic

G. Escherich, V. Conter (eds.), *Acute Lymphoblastic Leukemia in Children and Adolescents*, Pediatric Oncology, https://doi.org/10.1007/978-3-031-71180-0_9

marrow involvement [14, 15]. This was thought to be due to inadequate penetration of anti-leukaemia drugs, administered systemically, into the CNS compartment, gaining the CNS a reputation as a 'sanctuary site' for ALL cells [16].

Despite attempts to eradicate CNS disease through intensification of systemic chemotherapy, CNS relapses remained a problem. Moreover, several autopsy studies revealed patients commonly harboured CNS disease despite no evidence of CNS leukaemia on microscopy of cerebrospinal fluid (CSF). Price and Johnson observed that among the 126 ALL cases, 60% demonstrated CNS involvement [9]. Similarly, Evans et al. and Moore et al. found that 75% and 70% of their ALL post-mortem case studies, respectively, showed CNS infiltration despite most being treated as CNS-negative patients [17, 18]. There was a categorical need for CNS-directed ALL therapy.

Introduction of CNS-directed therapy led to one of the greatest steps forward in the improvement of childhood ALL survival rates [19]. Initial attempts at incorporating CNS-directed therapy into ALL treatment did so through prophylactic craniospinal irradiation and cranial irradiation (CRT) [20–22] The first study to report apparent control of CNS disease was Pinkel in 1970. Pinkel combined CRT dosed between 20 and 24 Gy with chemotherapeutic agents. Fifty percent of children enrolled in the study were relapse free for at least 5 years [22]. A breakthrough in the treatment of the disease. The 'Total Therapy trials at St Jude's Children's Research Hospital in Tennessee, USA and the 'Sanctuary Trial' carried out by the Southwest Oncology Group, consolidated this finding as their application of CRT produced substantial improvements to treatment outcomes among paediatric ALL patients [19, 23, 24]. The significance of this advance was well portrayed in 'Total Therapy VI' wherein administration of 24 Gy CRT alongside intrathecal (IT) methotrexate (MTX) reduced the incidence of CNS relapse from 65% to 10% [24–26]. In accordance with this evidence, pre-symptomatic CRT became the standard of care.

However, follow up of children who had received CRT revealed an extremely toxic side effect profile, particularly among patients below 5 years [27, 28]. Prevalence of CRT neurotoxic sequelae was observed to increase in a dose and length dependant manner [29]. Neurotoxicities included secondary brain tumours [30–32], intellectual impairment [33–35], reduced growth and final height [36–38], neuropsychological dysfunction [39, 40] and hormone dysfunction [41].

The side-effects of CRT resulted in attempts to wholly, or partially, replace it with IT chemotherapy. As evidence emerged radiation became limited to the brain, dosages were reduced and ultimately CRT became reserved for cases of high-risk disease or when blast cells were identifiable within the CSF at diagnosis. In 2003, a meta-analysis of 43 randomized controlled trials concluded that CRT could be replaced by long-term IT therapy and that high-dose intravenous (IV) methotrexate (MTX) could improve treatment outcomes (defined as event free survival (EFS), CNS relapses, non-CNS relapses, death in remission and isolated CNS relapse) [42]. It is worth noting that when radiation is omitted there is an apparent increased dependence upon systemic chemotherapy to maintain treatment outcome. The CCG-105 trial found that when radiation was excluded, EFS was significantly diminished among those receiving IT chemotherapy with only minimal standard systemic therapy. However, when more intensive systemic treatment was administered the disparity was resolved [43].

9.3 Diagnosis

9.3.1 Clinical Evaluation

Most children with CNS ALL harbour no neurological symptoms and as such bedside clinical evaluation is often not an accurate reflection of the presence or extent of CNS disease among patients. However, symptoms that have been associated with CNS ALL include headaches (17% of cases), nausea/vomiting (14% of cases), lethargy and irritability [44]. Symptoms are more common among patients with CNS3 and/or neurological signs on examination [45]. Neurological signs may include nuchal rigidity and/or papilledema. Cranial nerve involvement is rare, however, when present has been known to most commonly impact the facial nerve (CN VII) presenting with facial palsy, followed by CN III, IV and VI [46].

9.3.2 CSF Analysis

Cell counting and microscopic examination of CSF constitute current methods used in clinical practice for classifying CNS disease. Microscopic evaluation involves centrifugation of the patient CSF sample and morphological assessment through microscopy (cytospin). The results of which allow patients to be classified into one of three risk groups based on the number of leukocytes, the presence of leukaemic blasts in the CSF and further subclassified by the presence or absence of red cells (Table 9.1).

Reported frequencies of CNS involvement at diagnosis range from 8% to 13%, with approximately 4% of patients harbouring a CNS 3 classification [44, 47–49]. However, it is believed that reported CNS frequencies are an underestimate of true disease prevalence. Evidence in support of this includes observations of ex vivo leukocyte decay in CSF, a lack of blast cell presence in CSF and autopsy findings of CNS infiltration in patients who had previously been considered to have bone marrow disease only [17, 18, 50]. As such, several novel detection modalities have been considered as potential alternatives in clinical practice. These include flow cytometric analysis, MRI and clone specific PCR.

Clinical data indicate that flow cytometry may provide superior means of detection than cytospin analysis. Bromberg found that among 219 patients, flow cytometry was able to detect blast cells in 44/219 (20.1%) of cases at diagnosis compared to 19/219 (8.7%) by cytospin [51]. Similarly, Thastrup found that among 673 patients, flow cytometry detected CNS involvement in 171 cases (25.4%) whereas traditional cytospin only 13.4% [52]. Moreover, several studies have found flow cytometry to have greater clinical accuracy than current methods when seeking to predict relapse risk among CNS 1/2 patients [53].

However, flow cytometry is expensive and requires stringent protocol; for example, the technique demands that samples be collected in specialized TransFix/EDTA tubes, which must be analysed within 72 h [54]. Additionally, there remains controversy regarding the threshold event detection that constitutes a positive result and the associated prognostic significance with which a CNS-positive diagnosis is associated [55]. Not all patients who are CNS-positive at diagnosis will relapse, however, and given the known toxicity of CNS-directed therapy the risk-benefit of treatment intensification is unclear. Furthermore, there is little evidence to direct the reduction or omission of CNS-directed therapy among patients who are flow cytometry negative at diagnosis. Larger prospective studies are needed to better define very high-risk and very low-risk groups.

9.3.3 Neuroradiology

Neuroradiological options for CNS ALL include cranial CT and MRI. MRI is more sensitive than CT and thus is the preferred radiological means of detecting CNS ALL [56]. MRI is not indicated as a stand-alone diagnostic tool as CSF

Table 9.1 Classification of cytospin findings in CNS ALL

Category	Definition
CNS 1	≤5 WBC/μL without blasts
CNS 2	≤ 5 WBC/μL CSF with identifiable blasts
CNS 3	>5 WBC/μL CSF with identifiable blasts or cranial nerve palsies or cerebral mass
Traumatic lumbar puncture +	≥10 erythrocytes/μL CSF with blasts
Traumatic lumbar puncture –	≥10 erythrocytes/μL without blasts

analysis provides superior means of disease detection and MRI harbours a high false negative rate [57]. However, in the small cohort of patients with clinical evidence of cranial nerve involvement at diagnosis, MRI has been found to be a useful tool to distinguish involvement of the CNS, particularly when patients present with negative CSF findings [44, 58, 59]. Notwithstanding, positive CNS involvement on MRI at diagnosis has been associated with poorer overall disease outcomes [60].

9.4 Risk Stratification

As with other facets of ALL therapy, accurate assessment and prognosis of CNS status is central to management and treatment decisions. Several large international study groups have attempted to ascertain the prognostic significance of the presence and/or extent of CNS involvement at time of diagnosis and endeavour to incorporate this insight into clinical management strategies.

Several clinical trials have found that the presence of blast cells in the CSF, i.e. CNS 2 or 3 status, is an independent negative predictive factor for EFS [47, 49, 61]. Furthermore, it was observed in a trial conducted by the Nordic Society for Paediatric Haematology/Oncology (NOPHO) that the presence of leukaemia cells in the CSF, detected by flow cytometry or cytospin at diagnosis is associated with increased relapse, including bone marrow relapse [52]. Recent clinical trials conducted in the US emphasized the significance of CNS involvement, with CNS 3 predicting a significantly worse EFS and relapse rate than CNS 2, which consecutively showed significantly worse outcomes than those with CNS 1 status at diagnosis. As such, augmentation of CNS directed treatment is recommended in all patients with CNS 2 status [49]. However, other trials have failed to show a prognostic significance associated with CNS 2 status and this may reflect diagnostic uncertainty when evaluating low levels of blasts and/or differences in treatment intensity [62]. CNS 3 patients, on most modern protocols, will receive weekly or twice weekly IT during induction, which is typically sufficient to diminish leukaemic cells to an undetectable level [47, 49]. However, in approximately one in ten cases, blast cells remain detectable in the CSF after 15 days; the prognostic significance of this finding has not yet been ascertained [52].

A subgroup that has proven particularly difficult to risk stratify and therefore ascribe the most appropriate treatment are CNS2/TLP-positive patients. Several studies have observed that TLP positive patients have significantly worse clinical outcomes than TLP-negative patients with comparable CNS disease burden at diagnosis [31, 47, 52, 63]. This was observed in the ALL-BFM95 trial wherein the 5-year EFS among TLP-positive patients was 73 ± 4.0% in comparison to the approximately 80% in TLP-negative cases [47]. There have been several hypotheses attempting to establish the reason for worse outcomes among TLP-positive patients. First, there is the possibility that LP injury introduces blast cells into the CSF which therefore causes iatrogenic advancement of disease, although given the mounting evidence that the majority patients have subclinical CNS involvement this is unlikely. Second, subgroup analysis of patients with CNS2/TLP-positive status compared to those of CNS 1/CNS 2 have significantly higher WBC counts, higher incidence of T cell disease and higher NCI-HR status at diagnosis. However, when CNS2/TLP-positive patients are compared to CNS 3 these characteristics are congruent. It has therefore been posited that the traumatic event of TLP obscures the true level of blast cells at diagnosis and thus this cohort harbours CNS3 disease. It is also conceivable that TLP positive patients do not receive sufficient IT chemotherapy because the needle was not in the appropriate position, or the subsequent haematoma impairs IT medication circulation within the CNS space. Clinical trials have attempted to include additional doses of IT chemotherapy among this subcohort of patients; however, this intensification failed to improve their comparatively inferior outcomes [47, 64]. Interestingly, the COG-1991/1961 protocols found that the prognostic significance of CNS2/TP positive status could be ameliorated by intensifying IT chemo at the start of therapy and including dexamethasone [65].

9.5 Treatment of Newly Diagnosed Patients

All modern CNS prophylaxis protocols employ a combination of systemic and IT therapy, with radiotherapy reserved for a select cohort of high-risk patients in some study groups and omitted altogether in others. Research has demonstrated that the restricted application of radiation and omission from most modern protocol does not impact the risk of CNS relapse nor the overall survival. The main agents employed for their significant CNS efficacy are glucocorticoids, methotrexate (MTX), cytarabine (AraC) and asparaginase with the first three available for intrathecal (IT) administration as well as systemic. Many clinical studies have, and continue to, investigate optimal protocols with research objectives seeking to identify (i) the most appropriate glucocorticoid, (ii) the optimal use of systemic MTX, (iii) the relative benefits of single versus triple IT therapy and (iv) the role of cranial irradiation in modern practice. Generally, outcomes such as overall survival (OS), event free survival (EFS), incidence of relapse (both BM and CNS) and associated neurotoxicities are drawn upon to engender comparison between treatment arms. A summary of the overall treatment options is shown in Fig. 9.1.

9.5.1 Glucocorticoids

Glucocorticoids penetrate the CNS and are used to treat a range of neurological disorders, such as cerebral oedema, haemorrhage and meningitis [66]. In the context of CNS prophylaxis, glucocorticoids are employed for their cytotoxic as well as their anti-inflammatory properties, working synergistically with MTX and AraC to mitigate against inflammatory side effects associated with these agents [67, 68]. Data from several large randomized controlled trials have demonstrated that when dexamethasone, rather than

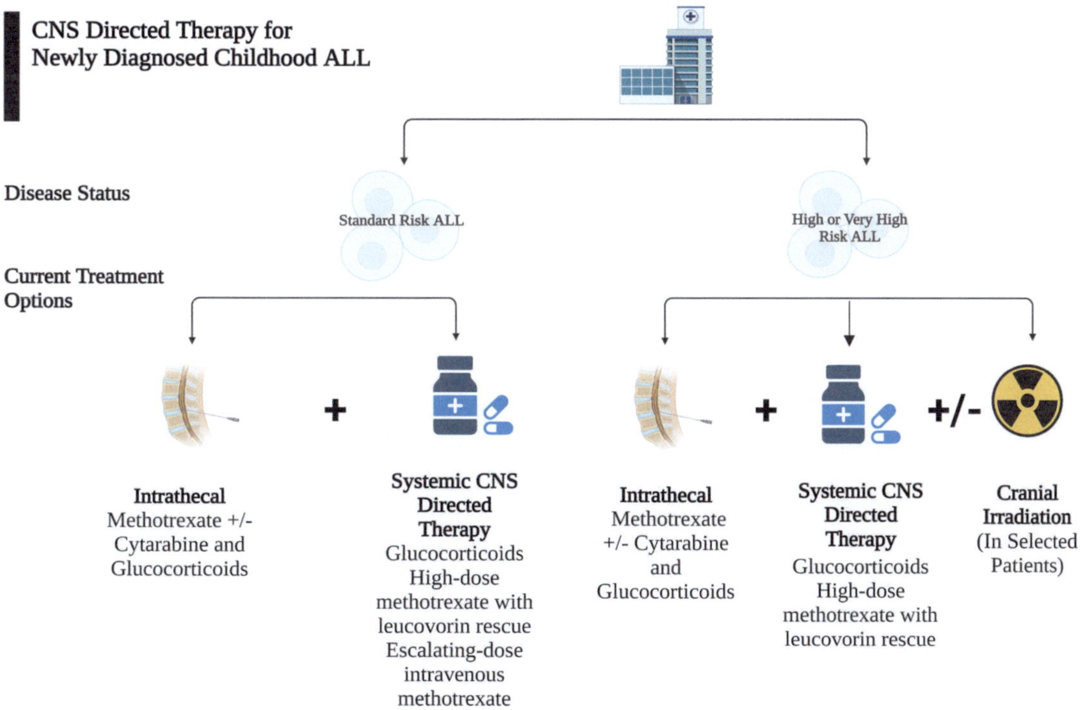

Fig. 9.1 CNS-directed treatment regimens for newly diagnosed childhood ALL. (Figure created from Biorender.com)

prednisone, was incorporated into CNS-directed therapy patients had significantly superior EFS and lower rates of CNS relapse, however equivalent overall survival (OS) [69]. It has been postulated that this may be the consequence of prednisone's shorter half-life and reduced penetration in the CNS [70]. However, further studies found that when the dose ratio between prednisone and dexamethasone was adjusted EFS and rates of relapse became equivalent, implying that the relative efficacy of prednisone and dexamethasone could be dose dependent [71]. Glucocorticoids have been known to be associated with toxicities such as osteopenia, osteonecrosis, infection and myopathy. Among published literature toxicity is more commonly associated with dexamethasone [3, 72, 73]. However, toxicities have been observed to differ according to the concomitant chemotherapies used [74, 75]. Therefore, selection of type and dosage of glucocorticoid should be based on treatment phase, risk of relapse and other chemotherapeutics incorporated into treatment regimen.

9.5.2 Systemic Methotrexate (MTX)

MTX may be considered the mainstay of CNS prophylaxis. MTX binds and inhibits dihydrofolate reductase with a greater than 1000-fold affinity over folate and thus competitively inhibits the conversion of dihydrofolate into tetrahydrofolate [76]. Tetrahydrofolate is required for DNA synthesis and therefore reduced production directly targets the proliferative ability of leukaemic cells. MTX can be administered systemically or intrathecally.

Systemic MTX administration may be incorporated into CNS prophylaxis because of MTX's capacity to penetrate the BBB and achieve therapeutic doses in the CNS [77]. However, achieving therapeutic concentrations in the CNS demands a high-dose IV regimen (defined as >500 mg/m^2) and thus has several important treatment considerations. High-dose regimens require a 2–3-day period of multiple leucovorin (folinic acid) doses to terminate MTX's toxic effect on normal tissues (termed leucovorin 'rescue') alongside close monitoring of hydration status, renal function and MTX plasma concentrations [78–80]. Several clinical studies have attempted to identify the optimal mode of systemic MTX administration among ALL patients. The Children's Oncology Group (COG) AALL0232 compared the effectiveness of contrasting methods of systemic MTX administration among 3154 high-risk B-ALL patients aged between 1 and 30 years [81]. Patients were randomized to receive high dose MTX or Capizzi style regimen. The Capizzi regimen incorporates escalating doses of IV MTX starting at 100 mg/m^2 during the maintenance phase [82]. The study found that the high-dose protocol produced an improved 5-year EFS associated with a non-significantly reduced rate of CNS relapse, without excess toxicity. However, when studied in T-ALL in COG AALL0434, the Capizzi regimen was superior to high-dose MTX for both 5-year EFS and OS [83]. It is worth noting that the AALL0434 trial was designed to include CRT for all intermediate and high-risk patients. In the Capizzi arm patients received CRT during the second month of therapy, whereas, in part to reduce neurotoxicities associated with CRT prior to high-dose MTX, patients in the high-dose arm received CRT in the seventh month of therapy. It is conceivable that earlier CRT administration may have prevented T cell trafficking to medullary and sanctuary sites and as such may have affected the differences observed in EFS and OS.

9.5.3 Intrathecal Methotrexate

The mainstay of CNS-directed therapy is intrathecal MTX which can be administered in isolation or as part of so-called intrathecal triple therapy (ITT) alongside cytarabine and a glucocorticoid. IT administration attempts to maximize CNS-ALL drug exposure in the CSF while reducing systemic drug toxicity [84]. Clinical research has sought to compare the efficacy of isolated MTX with ITT. The COG AALL1131 compared ITT combining MTX, AraC and hydrocortisone with single IT MTX among 1734 B-ALL classified as high risk, although CNS3 patients were excluded

[85]. However, failure to reach markers of significance saw the trial cross the futility boundary and was halted early. Data from the study showed a non-significant trend towards reduced CNS relapse in the ITT arm but was balanced by an opposite trend towards isolated BM relapses. This paradigm has been observed in several trials wherein intensification of CNS-directed therapy can be successful in reducing rates of CNS relapse but increasing rates of late BM relapse, ultimately resulting in overall similar EFS/OS and sometimes even worse OS. These trends underpin the need for novel therapeutic strategies that are better equipped to target ALL cells in cases that are more prone to relapse.

9.5.4 Cytarabine

Cytarabine (AraC) is an anti-metabolite that inhibits DNA replication and repair in rapidly dividing cells such as those seen in ALL [86]. High-dose systemic AraC has in the past been used successfully as part of CNS prophylaxis; however, in current practice, it is most commonly incorporated as part of ITT [87]. IT AraC is seldom used in isolation as it has been considered inferior to MTX due to its shorter half-life and diminished capacity to penetrate deeper CNS structures [88].

9.5.5 Radiotherapy

On account of the significant neurotoxicity associated with CRT, several clinical trials have attempted to wholly omit CRT from CNS prophylaxis. CRT can successfully be removed from most patients‘ treatment protocol without impacting EFS, CNS relapse and OS [89–91]. Radiation is still incorporated for some high-risk groups namely those with CNS 3 status and/or high-risk features for relapse or as part of conditioning before haemopoietic stem cell transplantation (HSCT). In 2016 an international meta-analysis followed the treatment course of over 16,000 children, aged between 1 and 18 from 10 different centres [92]. The study concluded that cranial irradiation did not impact CNS relapse in the era of modern treatment protocols. However, subgroup analysis of CNS3 patients revealed that omission of radiotherapy increased the risk of isolated and/or combined CNS relapse, this was found to have no impact on EFS or OS.

9.5.6 T-ALL Considerations

T-ALL is biologically distinct from B-ALL. The risk of CNS involvement and CNS relapse is higher in T-ALL reflected in the intensified systemic and CNS directed therapies recommended for T-ALL patients [93]. Accordingly, CRT is more commonly applied among T-ALL patients particularly in those with high-risk features [94]. However, as with B-ALL, several trial groups have attempted to reduce and/or omit radiotherapy from treatment protocols and when doing so have achieved positive results [95].

The agent Nelarabine has been assessed as a frontline therapy in the treatment of T-ALL. Nelarabine is a prodrug of arabinosylguanine nucleotide triphosphate (ara-GTP), a purine nucleoside analogue, that is specifically cytotoxic to T-lymphocytes and T-lymphoblastoid cells [96]. Nelarabine is converted to ara-GTP, then enters T cells and competitively binds to DNA, inhibiting synthesis and eliciting cytotoxicity [97]. While ara-GTP also accumulates in B cells, its half-life is significantly longer among T cells resulting in a more profound cytotoxic effect [98, 99]. Nelarabine was incorporated as a frontline systemic agent in the COG AALL0434 trial. The study enrolled 1562 T-ALL patients all of whom received an augmented BFM backbone [83]. Intermediate- and high-risk patients were randomly assigned, after induction, to receive or not six 5-day courses of nelarabine. The 5-year EFS among patients with T-ALL randomly assigned to nelarabine (n = 323) and no nelarabine (n = 336) were 88.2% ± 2.4% (p = 0.029) and 82.1% ± 2.7% (p = 0.029), respectively. Nelarabine was also associated with a significant decrease in rates of CNS relapses, with 5-year CNS relapses of 1.3% compared to 6.9% (p = 0.0001) in patients who did not receive nelarabine [83]. However, no difference in OS was observed between treatment arms. Moreover, incongruent dosage of systemic chemotherapy and timing of CRT, as previously discussed, between the two treatment arms are important to consider when assessing the outcomes of the trial.

9.5.7 Ph-Positive ALL Considerations

The Philadelphia (Ph) chromosome is a reciprocal translocation between chromosome 9 and 22 [t(9;22)(q34:q11)] that results in the expression of the BCR-ABL fusion gene [100]. Around 3–5% of paediatric cases are said to be Ph positive with increasing incidence among adolescent and adult patients [101]. Compared to Ph-negative patients, Ph-positive patients report high rates of CNS involvement at diagnosis and an increased frequency of CNS relapse [102, 103]. Tyrosine kinase inhibitors (TKI) have significantly improved the OS among Ph positive patients. However, the first-generation TKI Imatinib, has poor CNS penetration and therefore did little to ameliorate CNS disease [104]. The second-generation TKI Dasatinib demonstrated efficacy against CNS disease in pre-clinical models and case series prompting further investigation in clinical trial. However, data arising from these studies have been inconclusive for determining the definite efficacy of dasatinib for CNS ALL [105–108]. Further research is required to assess the optimal use of TKIs in CNS-directed treatment.

9.6 Side Effects of CNS-Directed Therapy

The neurotoxic sequelae of CRT are well established, and these have prompted modern protocols, where possible, to omit radiation from treatment regimens. However, even in the absence of radiation, neurotoxicity remains a significant complication associated with CNS prophylaxis and must be taken into consideration when making treatment decisions. The incidence of acute symptomatic neurotoxicity or neurotoxic serious adverse events (SAE) arising from frontline ALL therapy ranges between 10% and 12% [109, 110]. Toxicities include seizures, cerebral sinus venous thrombosis, stroke like syndrome (SLS) and posterior reversible encephalopathy syndrome [111]. Moreover, among long term survivors of childhood ALL who received chemotherapy-only CNS prophylaxis approximately 16.8% experience impaired processing speeds, 15.9% executive function, 14.5% attention, 13.1% memory and 9.3% severe intellectual impairment. There is a loose relationship between IV/IT MTX and dexamethasone dose-intensity and neurocognitive outcomes, and it is likely that additional environmental and genetic risk-factors ultimately determine individual risk [112]. Long-term follow up of survivors of childhood ALL has shown evidence of diminished white matter integrity on MRI scanning which indicates a potential reduction in cognitive reserve. Theoretically this raises concerns about increased rates of dementia, although this is unproven [113–115].

MTX neurotoxicity may be defined as symptomatic neurotoxicity +/− leucoencepalopathy linked with the administration of IV or IT MTX, where other causes have been ruled out [116]. MTX neurotoxicity occurs in 3–7% of children treated for ALL [117–119]. Presentations characteristically include seizures, encephalopathy, and SLS. SLS is a rare well-described neurotoxicity associated with MTX. SLS is characterized by a waxing and waning symptomatic onset within 3–21 days of MTX administration. Symptoms used to define SLS include any one of new-onset paralysis, movement disorder, bilateral weakness, aphasia and/or altered mental status, and there may be associated seizures. These are accompanied by, often transient, oval-shaped lesions of the subcortical white matter observable on diffuse-weighted MRI but absent on CT, although imaging may be normal especially if delayed. SLS as with other MTX neurotoxicities is typically transient in nature, with resolution occurring between 1 and 7 days [111, 118–120].

During a neurotoxic episode management generally comprises supportive care, guided by frequent neurological examinations. Anticonvulsants may be considered in the event of prolonged or repeated seizures. The mechanism of MTX neurotoxicity was initially believed to be the result of homeostatic alterations to CNS folate metabolism; however, several alternative hypotheses have been proposed within the literature, and these are discussed at length in the following studies [121–123]. Grounded from this mechanistic insight, two agents have been proposed as secondary preventative measures for use within the acute setting. The first is aminophylline, a competitive inhibitor of adenosine targeting vasodilation—which may be most useful for acute presentations (less than 24 h post methotrexate) with nausea, vomiting, headache and drowsiness [124]. The second is dextromethorphan, an N-methyl-D-aspartate (NMDA) antagonist proposed to combat the excitatory effects of homocysteine on NMDA receptors, which has been used in small case series for patients with classical SLS [118]. However, evidence in support of both agents is limited due to a lack of controls and difficulty demonstrating efficacy owing to the transient nature of neurotoxic episodes.

Following an initial MTX-associated neurotoxic incident clinical literature recommends the reinstatement of MTX into therapeutic regimen; this is referred to as MTX rechallenge. Omission of MTX following an initial neurotoxic episode is associated with an increased risk of CNS relapse [119]. Several studies have endorsed MTX rechallenge through validation of its safety, demonstrating that between 82% and 92% of patients do not experience a second symptomatic episode [117–119]. However, it is recommended that MTX rechallenge be delayed until the child has made a full neurological recovery. This may mean omitting MTX for up to 14 days, in such cases MTX may be substituted by AraC +/− hydrocortisone for one to two doses aiming to resume IT MTX as soon as possible thereafter. Following resumption of MTX, leucovorin rescue may be considered to minimize the risk of a repeated neurological episode.

9.7 Treatment of CNS Relapse

CNS relapse is defined as CNS3 status emerging after complete remission (CR). Patients with emergence of CNS2 status after CR typically require repeated investigation within 1–4 weeks. If CNS2 status is identified on repeated examination and confirmed by FCM and/or FISH it can be defined as CNS relapse [125].

CNS prophylaxis has successfully reduced the incidence of CNS relapse to less than 5% overall. However, the CNS is involved in more than 30% of relapse cases. Relapses can be confined to the CNS, so called isolated CNS relapse, or combined with overt bone marrow involvement. Several clinical risk factors for CNS relapse have been identified, these include but are not limited to: T-cell immunophenotype, presence of BCR-ABL1, KMT2A rearrangement, TCF3-PBX1 fusion, hyperleukocytosis and overt CNS leukaemia at diagnosis. However, the majority of patients harbouring these risk factors do not relapse in the CNS and most CNS relapses occur in non-high-risk patients [4]. CRT is considered standard treatment for relapse in CNS. There are high rates of subclinical BM involvement, even in apparent isolated CNS relapses and it is well established that systemic therapy is also required for long-term cure [126].

Management of relapsed CNS disease remains less than satisfactory. In the UK ALL R3 relapse trial, isolated and combined CNS relapses occurred significantly earlier than those with isolated BM relapses [127]. First remission duration has been identified as an important prognostic variable in isolated extramedullary relapse. Univariate analysis found that OS was significantly better when relapse occurred after 36 months than before this time (80.8%, 95% CI: 66.9–97.5% versus 31.2%, 95% CI: 15.1–64.6%, respectively; $P = 0.0008$) [128]. Furthermore, 5-year OS among those with combined CNS and isolated CNS relapse were 40.9% and 50.8%, respectively. 68% of secondary relapses were observed to have occurred in the CNS and of these two out of three relapses had occurred despite the patient having received CRT without HSCT [64, 129].

Given the poor salvage rate after a second relapse, one approach may be to offer an allogeneic haematopoietic stem cell transplantation (HSCT) to all CNS relapses with the exception of those with a late isolated CNS recurrence [129]. Late isolated CNS relapses may be curable with chemo-radiotherapy [130]. Late combined relapses with high end-of-induction minimal residual disease (MRD) were indicated for HSCT in the ALL-REZ BFM 2002 relapsed study. This regimen significantly improved patient outcomes when compared to earlier BFM relapse protocol (EFS 18% in ALL-REZ BFMP95/96 vs. 64% in ALL-REZ BFM2002) [131, 132]. Among the small cohort of patients who experience early and very early isolated CNS relapse, nonsignificant trends favouring HSCT over chemotherapy and CRT have also been observed. However, the optimal therapeutic regimen for children with isolated CNS relapse remains undetermined [64, 129, 133]. Importantly the outcomes of CNS relapses may depend on the front-line chemotherapy regimen. Historically children relapsing following less intensive front-line protocols may have been easier to salvage than those who relapse following intensive use of dexamethasone and methotrexate used in modern protocols. In an attempt to reduce reliance upon CRT attempts have been made to use immunotherapy to treat CNS relapse with mixed results (see below).

9.8 Immunotherapy for CNS-ALL

Under physiological conditions immune cell inhabitants of human CSF consist of memory T cells (90%), B cells (5%) and monocytes (5%) with absolute absence of granulocytes and NK cells. Several immunotherapeutic strategies have sought to exploit this immune presence, particularly the T-cell cohort, in novel CNS-directed therapies.

Blinatumomab is a bispecific monoclonal antibody construct that enables CD3-positive T cells to recognize and eliminate CD19-positive cells. Current data for blinatumomab provide evidence of limited efficacy in CNS ALL. In the phase I/II trial of paediatric patients with relapsed/refractory ALL, CNS prophylaxis was administered concurrently with blinatumomab without additional CNS toxicity, suggesting it is feasible and tolerated [134]. However, recent data published from a COG phase III RCT found that among patients with an isolated extramedullary relapse the post-reinduction use of blinatumomab did not result in a statistically significance difference in disease-free survival compared with standard chemotherapy [135].

Chimeric antigen receptor T cells (CAR T cells) are genetically modified T cells re-engineered to recognise and eliminate cells expressing a specific target antigen. CARs consist of four main components: (i) an extracellular target antigen-binding domain, (ii) a hinge region, (iii) a transmembrane domain and (iv) cytoplasmic activator and co-stimulatory domains. CAR specificity comes from their extracellular domain, for example, CD19 and CD22, while the cytoplasmic domain attempts to recapitulate the normal series of events by which T cells are activated and incorporates co-stimulatory domains, such as CD28 or 4-1BB (CD137), to facilitate CAR T-cell survival and proliferation. CAR T-cell therapy may be considered when initial response to reinduction is suboptimal, HSCT is not feasible, and/or the patient is very young with increased risk of long-term toxicity following CRT [136]. There has been promising evidence in support of CAR-T activity within the CNS; however, this is not absolute. CAR T-cell presence have been observed in the CSF of ALL CAR-T treated patients, a finding that corroborates with multiple case reports describing the clearance of CNS leukaemia with CAR T-cell therapy [137–139]. Furthermore, the Pediatric Real World CAR Consortium where they reported CD19 CAR T-cell therapy outcomes and toxicities for patients with CNS positivity were similar to those with isolated BM involvement [140]. However, a retrospective analysis reported six out of eight cases of isolated CNS relapse treated with CD19 CAR T-cell therapy developed subsequent CNS relapse [141]. There has also been ambiguity regarding the longevity of response. It has been posited that the microenvironment may cause anergy or exhaustion of CAR T cells within the CNS compartment, resulting in antigen-positive relapse despite CAR T-cell persistence in the CSF [142]. Moreover, significant neurotoxic sequelae have been also been observed among patients with high leukaemic CNS burden; however, this may be diminished to an acceptable degree under intensive management schedules [140, 141, 143, 144].

9.9 Future Directions

Current clinical practice lacks the ability to sensitively and specifically risk stratify patients based on their CNS disease burden. The current one size fits all approach may result in patients harbouring low-risk features being exposed to avoidable toxicity and consequential neurological sequelae, whereas patients with markedly high-risk features may be undertreated. Moreover, the inability to accurately measure CNS disease burden and response to interventions impinges upon the development and testing of novel therapeutics. Current strategies employed cannot accurately monitor the effectiveness of new agents, particularly when treating patients with subclinical disease.

As previously discussed, flow cytometry has been advocated as more sensitive method for CSF analysis; however, further work is needed to refine CNS-relapse risk based on flow cytometry results combined with other risk factors. Moreover, leukaemic cells in the CNS are known to be adherent to the stroma making CSF analysis suboptimal when seeking to truly evaluate the extent of CNS infiltration. It is conceivable that measuring a CSF biomarker, released, or up taken by leukaemic cells, may provide a more accurate indication of disease burden. Indirect biomarker candidates include CSF glucose, B2 microglobulin and LDH [145–147]. LDH is relatively non-specific but has been used to good effect as a biomarker for CNS lymphoma [148]. Contemporary methods, utilizing modern analytic techniques, have characterized the CSF proteome and/or metabolome in attempt to detect blast presence more accurately. These include but are not limited to aberrant catalase levels and upregulated serine proteases. Both these changes reflect the adaptations acquired by leukaemic cells as they strive to survive within the CNS microenvironment [149, 150]. cfDNA and miRNA detection within the CSF have also been considered; however, evidence supporting their utility as a clinically useful biomarker is currently lacking [151–153].

Current chemotherapeutic agents are considerably constrained by neurotoxicity. Replacing current treatment options with novel therapeutics, is essential in advancing the landscape of ALL therapy. The CSF provides a nutrient-poor microenvironment characterized by a low oxygen, lipid and micronutrient supply [154]. As such, cells have been observed to adapt their physiology to facilitate survival within this new environment. Targeting these survival mechanisms such as altered metabolism, cell cycle regulation and apoptosis may provide novel therapeutic targets [6, 155–157].

Finally, It has been hypothesized that leukaemic cells enter the CNS by crossing the blood-leptomeningeal barrier via meningeal microvasculature. Several preclinical trials have endeavoured to exploit this hypothesis by altering the molecular archetype of microvasculature and ligand binding capacity of lymphoblasts [8, 158]. Use of P13K inhibitors reduced the integrin expression among BCP-ALL cells in vitro, and successfully lowered CNS burden in BCP-ALL xenograft models. A second mode of targeting CNS invasion is through hinderance of chemokine signalling. It has been well established that under physiological conditions lymphocytes express chemokines (e.g. CXCR3, CXCR4, CCR7) that prompt migration to the CNS by virtue of corresponding ligands on brain endothelium and choroid plexus epithelium [159]. This phenomenon has also been observed in ALL wherein in T-ALL CXCR4 expression was associated with CNS involvement and was subsequently utilized as a therapeutic target through means of the CXCR4 inhibitor—plerixafor (AMD-3100). This successfully reduced CNS infiltration in T-ALL xenograft models [160,

161]. It should be noted, however, that at the time of original diagnosis or relapse the leukaemic cells are already present in the CNS and therefore targeting cell entry is unlikely to be successful.

9.10 Conclusion

CNS-directed therapy in patients with ALL is essential for cure. The introduction of CNS prophylaxis in the 1960s contributed to vast improvements to overall survival; however, the employment of CRT within these early treatment regimens harboured a significant neurotoxic burden. Advancements in our understanding of systemic and intrathecal chemotherapeutics has allowed CRT to be almost entirely omitted from most modern protocols, while maintaining rates of OS, EFS and relapse. Despite these successes, significant challenges remain—current CNS active agents are neurotoxic and the lack of accurate predictive biomarkers for CNS relapse impedes the development of risk-adapted CNS therapy.

References

1. Lange BJ, Bostrom BC, Cherlow JM, Sensel MG, La MK, Rackoff W, et al. Double-delayed intensification improves event-free survival for children with intermediate-risk acute lymphoblastic leukemia: a report from the children's cancer group. Blood. 2002;99(3):825–33.
2. Hutchinson RJ, Gaynon PS, Sather H, Bertolone SJ, Cooper HA, Tannous R, et al. Intensification of therapy for children with lower-risk acute lymphoblastic leukemia: long-term follow-up of patients treated on children's cancer group trial 1881. J Clin Oncol. 2003;21(9):1790–7.
3. Bostrom BC, Sensel MR, Sather HN, Gaynon PS, La MK, Johnston K, et al. Dexamethasone versus prednisone and daily oral versus weekly intravenous mercaptopurine for patients with standard-risk acute lymphoblastic leukemia: a report from the children's cancer group. Blood. 2003;101(10):3809–17.
4. Frishman-Levy L, Izraeli S. Advances in understanding the pathogenesis of CNS acute lymphoblastic leukaemia and potential for therapy. Br J Haematol. 2017;176(2):157–67.
5. Frishman-Levy L, Shemesh A, Bar-Sinai A, Ma C, Ni Z, Frenkel S, et al. Central nervous system acute lymphoblastic leukemia: role of natural killer cells. Blood, J Am Soc Hematol. 2015;125(22):3420–31.
6. Münch V, Trentin L, Herzig J, Demir S, Seyfried F, Kraus JM, et al. Central nervous system involvement in acute lymphoblastic leukemia is mediated by vascular endothelial growth factor. Blood, J Am Soc Hematol. 2017;130(5):643–54.
7. Williams MT, Yousafzai YM, Elder A, Rehe K, Bomken S, Frishman-Levy L, et al. The ability to cross the blood–cerebrospinal fluid barrier is a generic property of acute lymphoblastic leukemia blasts. Blood, J Am Soc Hematol. 2016;127(16):1998–2006.
8. Yao H, Price TT, Cantelli G, Ngo B, Warner MJ, Olivere L, et al. Leukaemia hijacks a neural mechanism to invade the central nervous system. Nature. 2018;560(7716):55–60.
9. Price RA, Johnson WW. The central nervous system in childhood leukemia. I The arachnoid. Cancer. 1973;31(3):520–33.
10. Farber S, Diamond LK. Temporary remissions in acute leukemia in children produced by folic acid antagonist, 4-aminopteroyl-glutamic acid. N Engl J Med. 1948;238(23):787–93.
11. Sutow WW, Garcia F, Starling KA, Williams TE, Lane DM, Gehan EA. L-asparaginase therapy in children with advanced leukemia. The southwest cancer chemotherapy study group. Cancer. 1971;28(4):819–24.
12. Burchenal JH, Murphy ML, Ellison RR, Sykes MP, Tan TC, Leone LA, et al. Clinical evaluation of a new antimetabolite, 6-mercaptopurine, in the treatment of leukemia and allied diseases. Blood. 1953;8(11):965–99.
13. Evans AE. Central nervous system involvement in children with acute Leukemia; a study of 921 patients. Cancer. 1964;17:256–8.
14. Nies BA, Bodey GP, Thomas LB, Brecher G, Freireich EJ. The persistence of extramedullary leukemic infiltrates during bone marrow remission of acute leukemia. Blood. 1965;26(2):133–41.
15. Schwarzenberg L, Mathé G, Schneider M, Amiel JL, Cattan A, Schlumberger JR. Attempted adoptive immunotherapy of acute leukaemia by leucocyte transfusions. Lancet. 1966;2(7459):365–8.
16. Thomas LB. Pathology of leukemia in the brain and meninges: postmortem studies of patients with acute leukemia and of mice given inoculations of L1210 leukemia. Cancer Res. 1965;25(9):1555–71.
17. Evans AE, Gilbert ES, Zandstra R. The increasing incidence of central nervous system leukemia in children. (children's cancer study group a). Cancer. 1970;26(2):404–9.
18. Moore EW, Thomas LB, Shaw RK, Freireich EJ. The central nervous system in acute leukemia: a postmortem study of 117 consecutive cases, with particular reference to hemorrhages, leukemic infiltrations, and the syndrome of meningeal leukemia. Arch Intern Med. 1960;105:451–68.

19. Pinkel D, Simone J, Hustu HO, Aur RJ. Nine years' experience with "total therapy" of childhood acute lymphocytic leukemia. Pediatrics. 1972;50(2):246–51.
20. Aur RJ, Simone JV, Hustu HO, Verzosa MS. A comparative study of central nervous system irradiation and intensive chemotherapy early in remission of childhood acute lymphocytic leukemia. Cancer. 1972;29(2):381–91.
21. Ortega JA, Nesbit ME, Sather HN, Robison LL, D'Angio GJ, Hammond GD. Long-term evaluation of a CNS prophylaxis trial – treatment comparisons and outcome after CNS relapse in childhood ALL: a report from the Childrens Cancer Study Group. J Clin Oncol. 1987;5(10):1646–54.
22. Pinkel D. Treatment of childhood acute lymphocytic leukemia. J Pediatr. 1970;77(6):1089–91.
23. Nesbit ME, Sather H, Robison LL, Donaldson M, Littman P, Ortega JA, et al. Sanctuary therapy: a randomized trial of 724 children with previously untreated acute lymphoblastic leukemia: a report from children's cancer study group. Cancer Res. 1982;42(2):674–80.
24. Omar AA, Basiouny L, Elnoby AS, Zaki A, Abouzid M. St. Jude total therapy studies from I to XVII for childhood acute lymphoblastic leukemia: a brief review. J Egypt Natl Canc Inst. 2022;34(1):25.
25. Rivera GK, Pinkel D, Simone JV, Hancock ML, Crist WM. Treatment of acute lymphoblastic leukemia – 30 years' experience at St. Jude Children's Research Hospital. N Engl J Med. 1993;329(18):1289–95.
26. Simone JV. A history of St Jude Children's Research Hospital. Br J Haematol. 2003;120(4):549–55.
27. Eiser C, Lansdown R. Retrospective study of intellectual development in children treated for acute lymphoblastic leukaemia. Arch Dis Child. 1977;52(7):525.
28. Neglia JP, Meadows AT, Robison LL, Kim TH, Newton WA, Ruymann FB, et al. Second neoplasms after acute lymphoblastic leukemia in childhood. N Engl J Med. 1991;325(19):1330–6.
29. Chemaitilly W, Li Z, Huang S, Ness KK, Clark KL, Green DM, et al. Anterior hypopituitarism in adult survivors of childhood cancers treated with cranial radiotherapy: a report from the St Jude lifetime cohort study. J Clin Oncol. 2015;33(5):492–500.
30. Relling MV, Rubnitz JE, Rivera GK, Boyett JM, Hancock ML, Felix CA, et al. High incidence of secondary brain tumours after radiotherapy and antimetabolites. Lancet. 1999;354(9172):34–9.
31. Möricke A, Reiter A, Zimmermann M, Gadner H, Stanulla M, Dördelmann M, et al. Risk-adjusted therapy of acute lymphoblastic leukemia can decrease treatment burden and improve survival: treatment results of 2169 unselected pediatric and adolescent patients enrolled in the trial ALL-BFM 95. Blood. 2008;111(9):4477–89.
32. Schmiegelow K, Levinsen MF, Attarbaschi A, Baruchel A, Devidas M, Escherich G, et al. Second malignant neoplasms after treatment of childhood acute lymphoblastic leukemia. J Clin Oncol. 2013;31(19):2469–76.
33. Brown RT, Madan-Swain A, Walco GA, Cherrick I, Ievers CE, Conte PM, et al. Cognitive and academic late effects among children previously treated for acute lymphocytic leukemia receiving chemotherapy as CNS prophylaxis. J Pediatr Psychol. 1998;23(5):333–40.
34. Jankovic M, Masera G, Brouwers P, Valsecchi MG, Veldhuizen AV, Kingma A, et al. Association of 1800 cGy cranial irradiation with intellectual function in children with acute lymphoblastic leukaemia. Lancet. 1994;344(8917):224–7.
35. Meadows AT, Gordon J, Massari DJ, Littman P, Fergusson J, Moss K. Declines in IQ scores and cognitive dysfunctions in children with acute lymphocytic leukaemia treated with cranial irradiation. Lancet. 1981;2(8254):1015–8.
36. Hokken-Koelega ACS, Van Doorn JWD, Hählen K, Stijnen T, De Muinck K-SSMPF, Drop SLS. Long-term effects of treatment for acute lymphoblastic Leukemia with and without cranial irradiation on growth and puberty: a comparative study. Pediatr Res. 1993;33(6):577–82.
37. Sklar C, Mertens A, Walter A, Mitchell D, Nesbit M, O'Leary M, et al. Final height after treatment for childhood acute lymphoblastic leukemia: comparison of no cranial irradiation with 1800 and 2400 centigrays of cranial irradiation. J Pediatr. 1993;123(1):59–64.
38. Vandecruys E, Dhooge C, Craen M, Benoit Y, De Schepper J. Longitudinal linear growth and final height is impaired in childhood acute lymphoblastic leukemia survivors after treatment without cranial irradiation. J Pediatr. 2013;163(1):268–73.
39. Moleski M. Neuropsychological, neuroanatomical, and neurophysiological consequences of CNS chemotherapy for acute lymphoblastic leukemia. Arch Clin Neuropsychol. 2000;15(7):603–30.
40. Said JA, Waters BG, Cousens P, Stevens MM. Neuropsychological sequelae of central nervous system prophylaxis in survivors of childhood acute lymphoblastic leukemia. J Consult Clin Psychol. 1989;57(2):251–6.
41. Follin C, Erfurth EM. Long-term effect of cranial radiotherapy on pituitary-hypothalamus area in childhood acute lymphoblastic Leukemia survivors. Curr Treat Options Oncol. 2016;17(9):50.
42. Clarke M, Gaynon P, Hann I, Harrison G, Masera G, Peto R, Richards S. CNS-directed therapy for childhood acute lymphoblastic leukemia: Childhood ALL Collaborative Group overview of 43 randomized trials. J Clin Oncol. 2003;21(9):1798–809.
43. Tubergen DG, Gilchrist GS, O'Brien RT, Coccia PF, Sather HN, Waskerwitz MJ, et al. Prevention of CNS disease in intermediate-risk acute lymphoblastic leukemia: comparison of cranial radiation and intrathecal methotrexate and the importance of systemic therapy: a children's cancer group report. J Clin Oncol. 1993;11(3):520–6.

44. Levinsen M, Taskinen M, Abrahamsson J, Forestier E, Frandsen TL, Harila-Saari A, et al. Clinical features and early treatment response of central nervous system involvement in childhood acute lymphoblastic leukemia. Pediatr Blood Cancer. 2014;61(8):1416–21.
45. Hanmantgad S, Khakoo Y. 133 – system cancer and the central nervous system involvement. In: Swaiman KF, Ashwal S, Ferriero DM, Schor NF, Finkel RS, Gropman AL, et al., editors. Swaiman's pediatric neurology. 6th ed. Elsevier; 2017. p. 1017–20.
46. Paryani SB, Donaldson SS, Amylon MD, Link MP. Cranial nerve involvement in children with leukemia and lymphoma. J Clin Oncol. 1983;1(9):542–5.
47. Burger B, Zimmermann M, Mann G, Kuhl J, Loning L, Riehm H, et al. Diagnostic cerebrospinal fluid examination in children with acute lymphoblastic leukemia: significance of low leukocyte counts with blasts or traumatic lumbar puncture. J Clin Oncol. 2003;21(2):184–8.
48. Schultz KR, Pullen DJ, Sather HN, Shuster JJ, Devidas M, Borowitz MJ, et al. Risk-and response-based classification of childhood B-precursor acute lymphoblastic leukemia: a combined analysis of prognostic markers from the Pediatric oncology group (POG) and children's cancer group (CCG). Blood. 2007;109(3):926–35.
49. Winick N, Devidas M, Chen S, Maloney K, Larsen E, Mattano L, et al. Impact of initial CSF findings on outcome among patients with National Cancer Institute standard-and high-risk B-cell acute lymphoblastic leukemia: a report from the children's oncology group. J Clin Oncol. 2017;35(22):2527.
50. Thastrup M, Marquart HV, Schmiegelow K. Flow cytometric detection of malignant blasts in cerebrospinal fluid: a biomarker of central nervous system involvement in childhood acute lymphoblastic Leukemia. Biomol Ther. 2022;12(6)
51. Bromberg JEC, Breems DA, Kraan J, Bikker G, van der Holt B, Smitt PS, et al. CSF flow cytometry greatly improves diagnostic accuracy in CNS hematologic malignancies. Neurology. 2007;68(20):1674.
52. Thastrup M, Marquart HV, Levinsen M, Grell K, Abrahamsson J, Albertsen BK, et al. Flow cytometric detection of leukemic blasts in cerebrospinal fluid predicts risk of relapse in childhood acute lymphoblastic leukemia: a Nordic Society of Pediatric Hematology and Oncology study. Leukemia. 2020;34(2):336–46.
53. de Haas V, Pieters R, van der Sluijs-Gelling AJ, Zwaan CM, de Groot-Kruseman HA, Sonneveld E, et al. Flowcytometric evaluation of cerebrospinal fluid in childhood ALL identifies CNS involvement better then conventional cytomorphology. Leukemia. 2021;35(6):1773–6.
54. Johansson U, Bloxham D, Couzens S, Jesson J, Morilla R, Erber W, et al. Guidelines on the use of multicolour flow cytometry in the diagnosis of haematological neoplasms. Br J Haematol. 2014;165(4):455–88.
55. Craig FE, Ohori NP, Gorrill TS, Swerdlow SH. Flow cytometric immunophenotyping of cerebrospinal fluid specimens. Am J Clin Pathol. 2011;135(1):22–34.
56. Kalın S, Koral K. Imaging of central nervous system involvement in Pediatric hematologic disorders. Turk Arch Pediatr. 2022;57(3):267–81.
57. Lauer M, Kernen E, Schwabe D, Lehrnbecher T, Porto L. The role of magnetic resonance imaging in the diagnosis of central nervous system involvement in children with acute lymphoblastic leukemia. Pediatr Blood Cancer. 2020;67(10):e28294.
58. Ranta S, Palomäki M, Levinsen M, Taskinen M, Abrahamsson J, Mellgren K, et al. Role of neuroimaging in children with acute lymphoblastic leukemia and central nervous system involvement at diagnosis. Pediatr Blood Cancer. 2017;64(1):64–70.
59. Ranta S, Nilsson F, Harila-Saari A, Saft L, Tani E, Söderhäll S, et al. Detection of central nervous system involvement in childhood acute lymphoblastic leukemia by cytomorphology and flow cytometry of the cerebrospinal fluid. Pediatr Blood Cancer. 2015;62(6):951–6.
60. Guenette JP, Tirumani SH, Keraliya AR, Shinagare AB, Ramaiya NH, Jagannathan JP. MRI findings in patients with Leukemia and positive CSF cytology: a single-institution 5-year experience. Am J Roentgenol. 2016;207(6):1278–82.
61. Mahmoud HH, Rivera GK, Hancock ML, Krance RA, Kun LE, Behm FG, et al. Low leukocyte counts with blast cells in cerebrospinal fluid of children with newly diagnosed acute lymphoblastic leukemia. N Engl J Med. 1993;329(5):314–9.
62. Thastrup M, Duguid A, Mirian C, Schmiegelow K, Halsey C. Central nervous system involvement in childhood acute lymphoblastic leukemia: challenges and solutions. Leukemia. 2022;
63. Gajjar A, Harrison PL, Sandlund JT, Rivera GK, Ribeiro RC, Rubnitz JE, et al. Traumatic lumbar puncture at diagnosis adversely affects outcome in childhood acute lymphoblastic leukemia. Blood, J Am Soc Hematol. 2000;96(10):3381–4.
64. Pui CH, Campana D, Pei D, Bowman WP, Sandlund JT, Kaste SC, et al. Treating childhood acute lymphoblastic leukemia without cranial irradiation. N Engl J Med. 2009;360(26):2730–41.
65. Jastaniah W, Elimam N, Abdalla K, Khattab TM, Felimban S, Abrar MB. Does the early intensification of intrathecal therapy improve outcomes in pediatric acute lymphoblastic leukemia patients with CNS2/TLP+ status at diagnosis? Hematology. 2015;20(10):561–6.
66. Eadie M, Brophy T, Ohlrich G, Tyrer J. Dexamethasone: pharmacokinetics in neurological patients. Clin Exp Neurol. 1984;20:107–18.
67. Inaba H, Pui CH. Glucocorticoid use in acute lymphoblastic leukaemia. Lancet Oncol. 2010;11(11):1096–106.

68. Möricke A, Zimmermann M, Valsecchi MG, Stanulla M, Biondi A, Mann G, et al. Dexamethasone vs prednisone in induction treatment of pediatric ALL: results of the randomized trial AIEOP-BFM ALL 2000. Blood. 2016;127(17):2101–12.
69. Mitchell C, Richards S, Harrison C, Eden T. Long-term follow-up of the United Kingdom Medical Research Council protocols for childhood acute lymphoblastic leukaemia, 1980–2001. Leukemia. 2009;24:406–18.
70. Balis FM, Lester C, Chrousos G, Heideman R, Poplack D. Differences in cerebrospinal fluid penetration of corticosteroids: possible relationship to the prevention of meningeal leukemia. J Clin Oncol. 1987;5(2):202–7.
71. Domenech C, Suciu S, De Moerloose B, Mazingue F, Plat G, Ferster A, et al. Dexamethasone (6 mg/m2/day) and prednisolone (60 mg/m2/day) were equally effective as induction therapy for childhood acute lymphoblastic leukemia in the EORTC CLG 58951 randomized trial. Haematologica. 2014;99(7):1220–7.
72. Mitchell CD, Richards SM, Kinsey SE, Lilleyman J, Vora A, Eden TO, et al. Benefit of dexamethasone compared with prednisolone for childhood acute lymphoblastic leukaemia: results of the UK Medical Research Council ALL97 randomized trial. Br J Haematol. 2005;129(6):734–45.
73. Vrooman LM, Neuberg DS, Stevenson KE, Supko JG, Sallan SE, Silverman LB. Dexamethasone and individualized Asparaginase dosing are each associated with superior event-free survival in childhood acute lymphoblastic Leukemia: results from DFCI-ALL consortium protocol 00-01. Blood. 2009;114(22):321.
74. Belgaumi AF, Al-Bakrah M, Al-Mahr M, Al-Jefri A, Al-Musa A, Saleh M, et al. Dexamethasone-associated toxicity during induction chemotherapy for childhood acute lymphoblastic leukemia is augmented by concurrent use of daunomycin. Cancer: interdisciplinary international journal of the American cancer. Society. 2003;97(11):2898–903.
75. Yang L, Panetta JC, Cai X, Yang W, Pei D, Cheng C, et al. Asparaginase may influence dexamethasone pharmacokinetics in acute lymphoblastic leukemia. J Clin Oncol. 2008;26(12):1932–9.
76. Wojtuszkiewicz A, Peters GJ, van Woerden NL, Dubbelman B, Escherich G, Schmiegelow K, et al. Methotrexate resistance in relation to treatment outcome in childhood acute lymphoblastic leukemia. J Hematol Oncol. 2015;8(1):61.
77. Glantz MJ, Cole BF, Recht L, Akerley W, Mills P, Saris S, et al. High-dose intravenous methotrexate for patients with nonleukemic leptomeningeal cancer: is intrathecal chemotherapy necessary? J Clin Oncol. 1998;16(4):1561–7.
78. Ackland SP, Schilsky RL. High-dose methotrexate: a critical reappraisal. J Clin Oncol. 1987;5(12):2017–31.
79. Balis FM, Poplack DG. Central nervous system pharmacology of antileukemic drugs. Am J Pediatr Hematol Oncol. 1989;11(1):74–86.
80. Bostrom BC, Erdmann GR, Kamen BA. Systemic methotrexate exposure is greater after intrathecal than after oral administration. J Pediatr Hematol Oncol. 2003;25(2):114–7.
81. Larsen EC, Devidas M, Chen S, Salzer WL, Raetz EA, Loh ML, et al. Dexamethasone and high-dose methotrexate improve outcome for children and young adults with high-risk B-acute lymphoblastic Leukemia: a report from children's oncology group study AALL0232. J Clin Oncol. 2016;34(20):2380–8.
82. Pinkerton CR, Mills S, Chessells JM. Modified Capizzi maintenance regimen in children with relapsed acute lymphoblastic leukaemia. Med Pediatr Oncol. 1986;14(2):69–72.
83. Dunsmore KP, Winter SS, Devidas M, Wood BL, Esiashvili N, Chen Z, et al. Children's oncology group AALL0434: a phase III randomized clinical trial testing Nelarabine in newly diagnosed T-cell acute lymphoblastic Leukemia. J Clin Oncol. 2020;38(28):3282–93.
84. Kerr JZ, Berg S, Blaney SM. Intrathecal chemotherapy. Crit Rev Oncol Hematol. 2001;37(3):227–36.
85. Salzer WL, Burke MJ, Devidas M, Dai Y, Hardy KK, Kairalla JA, et al. Impact of intrathecal triple therapy versus intrathecal methotrexate on disease-free survival for high-risk B-lymphoblastic Leukemia: children's oncology group study AALL1131. J Clin Oncol. 2020;38(23):2628–38.
86. Faruqi A, Tadi P. Cytarabine. StatPearls Publishing, Treasure Island; 2021.
87. Jurczak W, Kroll-Balcerzak R, Giebel S, Machaczka M, Giza A, Ogórka T, et al. Liposomal cytarabine in the prophylaxis and treatment of CNS lymphoma: toxicity analysis in a retrospective case series study conducted at polish lymphoma research group Centers. Med Oncol. 2015;32(4):90.
88. Blasberg RG, Patlak C, Fenstermacher JD. Intrathecal chemotherapy: brain tissue profiles after ventriculocisternal perfusion. J Pharmacol Exp Ther. 1975;195(1):73–83.
89. Schmiegelow K, Forestier E, Hellebostad M, Heyman M, Kristinsson J, Söderhäll S, et al. Long-term results of NOPHO ALL-92 and ALL-2000 studies of childhood acute lymphoblastic leukemia. Leukemia. 2010;24(2):345–54.
90. Liu HC, Yeh TC, Hou JY, Chen KH, Huang TH, Chang CY, et al. Triple intrathecal therapy alone with omission of cranial radiation in children with acute lymphoblastic leukemia. J Clin Oncol. 2014;32(17):1825–9.
91. Möricke A, Zimmermann M, Reiter A, Henze G, Schrauder A, Gadner H, et al. Long-term results of five consecutive trials in childhood acute lymphoblastic leukemia performed by the ALL-BFM study group from 1981 to 2000. Leukemia. 2010;24(2):265–84.

92. Vora A, Andreano A, Pui CH, Hunger SP, Schrappe M, Moericke A, et al. Influence of cranial radiotherapy on outcome in children with acute lymphoblastic Leukemia treated with contemporary therapy. J Clin Oncol. 2016;34(9):919–26.
93. Pullen J, Shuster J, Link M, Borowitz M, Amylon M, Carroll A, et al. Significance of commonly used prognostic factors differs for children with T cell acute lymphocytic leukemia (ALL), as compared to those with B-precursor ALL. A Pediatric oncology group (POG) study. Leukemia. 1999;13(11):1696–707.
94. Kelly MJ, Trikalinos TA, Dahabreh IJ, Gianferante M, Parsons SK. Cranial radiation for pediatric T-lineage acute lymphoblastic leukemia: a systematic review and meta-analysis. Am J Hematol. 2014;89(10):992–7.
95. Hofmans M, Suciu S, Ferster A, Van Vlierberghe P, Mazingue F, Sirvent N, et al. Results of successive EORTC-CLG 58 881 and 58 951 trials in paediatric T-cell acute lymphoblastic leukaemia (ALL). Br J Haematol. 2019;186(5):741–53.
96. Cohen MH, Johnson JR, Justice R, Pazdur R. FDA drug approval summary: Nelarabine (Arranon®) for the treatment of T-cell lymphoblastic leukemia/lymphoma. Oncologist. 2008;13(6):709–14.
97. Gandhi V, Keating MJ, Bate G, Kirkpatrick P. Nelarabine. Nat Rev Drug Discov. 2006;5:17.
98. Scharenberg J, Spaapen L, Rijkers G, Wadman S, Staal G, Zegers B. Mechanisms of deoxyguanosine toxicity for human T and B lymphocytes. Purine and pyrimidine metabolism in Man V. Springer; 1986. p. 191–9.
99. Gandhi V, Plunkett W, Rodriguez CO Jr, Nowak BJ, Du M, Ayres M, et al. Compound GW506U78 in refractory hematologic malignancies: relationship between cellular pharmacokinetics and clinical response. J Clin Oncol. 1998;16(11):3607–15.
100. Kang ZJ, Liu YF, Xu LZ, Long ZJ, Huang D, Yang Y, et al. The Philadelphia chromosome in leukemogenesis. Chin J Cancer. 2016;35:48.
101. Kaczmarska A, Śliwa P, Zawitkowska J, Lejman M. Genomic analyses of Pediatric acute lymphoblastic Leukemia Ph+ and Ph-like-recent Progress in treatment. Int J Mol Sci. 2021;22(12)
102. Aricò M, Valsecchi MG, Camitta B, Schrappe M, Chessells J, Baruchel A, et al. Outcome of treatment in children with Philadelphia chromosome–positive acute lymphoblastic leukemia. N Engl J Med. 2000;342(14):998–1006.
103. Sanchez R, Ayala R, Alonso RA, Martínez MP, Ribera J, García O, et al. Clinical characteristics of patients with central nervous system relapse in BCR-ABL1-positive acute lymphoblastic leukemia: the importance of characterizing ABL1 mutations in cerebrospinal fluid. Ann Hematol. 2017;96(7):1069–75.
104. Takayama N, Sato N, O'Brien SG, Ikeda Y, Si O. Imatinib mesylate has limited activity against the central nervous system involvement of Philadelphia chromosome-positive acute lymphoblastic leukaemia due to poor penetration into cerebrospinal fluid. Br J Haematol. 2002;119(1):106–8.
105. Porkka K, Koskenvesa P, Lundán T, Rimpiläinen J, Mustjoki S, Smykla R, et al. Dasatinib crosses the blood-brain barrier and is an efficient therapy for central nervous system Philadelphia chromosome–positive leukemia. Blood, J Am Soc Hematol. 2008;112(4):1005–12.
106. Slayton WB, Schultz KR, Kairalla JA, Devidas M, Mi X, Pulsipher MA, et al. Dasatinib plus intensive chemotherapy in children, adolescents, and young adults with Philadelphia chromosome–positive acute lymphoblastic leukemia: results of Children's oncology group trial AALL0622. J Clin Oncol. 2018;36(22):2306.
107. Shen S, Chen X, Cai J, Yu J, Gao J, Hu S, et al. Effect of dasatinib vs imatinib in the treatment of pediatric Philadelphia chromosome–positive acute lymphoblastic leukemia: a randomized clinical trial. JAMA Oncol. 2020;6(3):358–66.
108. Schultz K, Carroll A, Heerema N, Bowman W, Aledo A, Slayton W, et al. Long-term follow-up of imatinib in pediatric Philadelphia chromosome-positive acute lymphoblastic leukemia: children's oncology group study AALL0031. Leukemia. 2014;28(7):1467–71.
109. Parasole R, Petruzziello F, Menna G, Mangione A, Cianciulli E, Buffardi S, et al. Central nervous system complications during treatment of acute lymphoblastic leukemia in a single pediatric institution. Leuk Lymphoma. 2010;51(6):1063–71.
110. Banerjee J, Niinimäki R, Lähteenmäki P, Hed Myrberg I, Arola M, Riikonen P, et al. The spectrum of acute central nervous system symptoms during the treatment of childhood acute lymphoblastic leukaemia. Pediatr Blood Cancer. 2020;67(2):e27999.
111. Schmiegelow K, Attarbaschi A, Barzilai S, Escherich G, Frandsen TL, Halsey C, et al. Consensus definitions of 14 severe acute toxic effects for childhood lymphoblastic leukaemia treatment: a Delphi consensus. Lancet Oncol. 2016;17(6):e231–e9.
112. Krull KR, Brinkman TM, Li C, Armstrong GT, Ness KK, Srivastava DK, et al. Neurocognitive outcomes decades after treatment for childhood acute lymphoblastic leukemia: a report from the St Jude lifetime cohort study. J Clin Oncol. 2013;31(35):4407.
113. Zeller B, Tamnes CK, Kanellopoulos A, Amlien IK, Andersson S, Due-Tønnessen P, et al. Reduced neuroanatomic volumes in long-term survivors of childhood acute lymphoblastic leukemia. J Clin Oncol. 2013;31(17):2078–85.
114. Waber DP. Central nervous system late effects: a new frontier? Pediatr Blood Cancer. 2011;57(3):355–6.
115. Armstrong FD. Implications of 25-year follow-up of white matter integrity and neurocognitive function of childhood leukemia survivors: a wake-up call. J Clin Oncol. 2013;31(27):3309–11.
116. Śliwa-Tytko P, Kaczmarska A, Lejman M, Zawitkowska J. Neurotoxicity associated with treatment of acute lymphoblastic Leukemia che-

motherapy and immunotherapy. Int J Mol Sci. 2022;23(10):5515.
117. Badke C, Fleming A, Iqbal A, Khilji O, Parhas S, Weinstein J, et al. Rechallenging with intrathecal methotrexate after developing subacute neurotoxicity in children with hematologic malignancies. Pediatr Blood Cancer. 2016;63(4):723–6.
118. Bhojwani D, Sabin ND, Pei D, Yang JJ, Khan RB, Panetta JC, et al. Methotrexate-induced neurotoxicity and leukoencephalopathy in childhood acute lymphoblastic leukemia. J Clin Oncol. 2014;32(9):949.
119. Mateos MK, Marshall GM, Barbaro PM, Quinn MCJ, George C, Mayoh C, et al. Methotrexate-related central neurotoxicity: clinical characteristics, risk factors and genome-wide association study in children treated for acute lymphoblastic leukemia. Haematologica. 2022;107(3):635
120. Bond J, Hough R, Moppett J, Vora A, Mitchell C, Goulden N. 'Stroke-like syndrome'caused by intrathecal methotrexate in patients treated during the UKALL 2003 trial. Leukemia. 2013;27(4):954–6.
121. Franca R, Rebora P, Bertorello N, Fagioli F, Conter V, Biondi A, et al. Pharmacogenetics and induction/consolidation therapy toxicities in acute lymphoblastic leukemia patients treated with AIEOP-BFM ALL 2000 protocol. Pharmacogenomics J. 2017;17(1):4–10.
122. Si T, Yanagimachi M, Tanoshima R, Urayama KY, Tanaka F, Aida N, et al. Influence of ADORA2A gene polymorphism on leukoencephalopathy risk in MTX-treated pediatric patients affected by hematological malignancies. Pediatr Blood Cancer. 2016;63(11):1983–9.
123. Ramalingam R, Kaur H, Scott JX, Sneha LM, Arunkumar G, Srinivasan A, et al. Evaluation of cytogenetic and molecular markers with MTX-mediated toxicity in pediatric acute lymphoblastic leukemia patients. Cancer Chemother Pharmacol. 2022;89(3):393–400.
124. Razi W, Haque AU, Sadiq H, Ullah R, Jabbar N, Mirza S. Safety and efficacy of aminophylline in intrathecal methotrexate-related neurological toxicity in large Pediatric oncology Centre. Age (Years). 2021;8:3–91.
125. Buchmann S, Schrappe M, Baruchel A, Biondi A, Borowitz M, Campbell M, et al. Remission, treatment failure, and relapse in pediatric ALL: an international consensus of the Ponte-di-Legno consortium. Blood. 2022;139(12):1785–93.
126. Hagedorn N, Acquaviva C, Fronkova E, Von Stackelberg A, Barth A, zur Stadt U, et al. Submicroscopic bone marrow involvement in isolated extramedullary relapses in childhood acute lymphoblastic leukemia: a more precise definition of "isolated" and its possible clinical implications, a collaborative study of the resistant disease Committee of the International BFM study group. Blood, the journal of the American society of. Hematology. 2007;110(12):4022–9.
127. Parker C, Krishnan S, Hamadeh L, Irving JAE, Kuiper RP, Révész T, et al. Outcomes of patients with childhood B-cell precursor acute lymphoblastic leukaemia with late bone marrow relapses: long-term follow-up of the ALLR3 open-label randomised trial. Lancet Haematol. 2019;6(4):e204–e16.
128. Gandemer V, Chevret S, Petit A, Vermylen C, Leblanc T, Michel G, et al. Excellent prognosis of late relapses of ETV6/RUNX1-positive childhood acute lymphoblastic leukemia: lessons from the FRALLE 93 protocol. Haematologica. 2012;97(11):1743–50.
129. Masurekar AN, Parker CA, Shanyinde M, Moorman AV, Hancock JP, Sutton R, et al. Outcome of central nervous system relapses in childhood acute lymphoblastic leukaemia–prospective open cohort analyses of the ALLR3 trial. PLoS One. 2014;9(10):e108107.
130. Barredo JC, Devidas M, Lauer SJ, Billett A, Marymont M, Pullen J, et al. Isolated CNS relapse of acute lymphoblastic leukemia treated with intensive systemic chemotherapy and delayed CNS radiation: a pediatric oncology group study. J Clin Oncol. 2006;24(19):3142–9.
131. Eckert C, Henze G, Seeger K, Hagedorn N, Mann G, Panzer-Grumayer R, et al. Use of allogeneic hematopoietic stem-cell transplantation based on minimal residual disease response improves outcomes for children with relapsed acute lymphoblastic leukemia in the intermediate-risk group. J Clin Oncol. 2013;31(21):2736–42.
132. Eckert C, Groeneveld-Krentz S, Kirschner-Schwabe R, Hagedorn N, Chen-Santel C, Bader P, et al. Improving stratification for children with late bone marrow B-cell acute lymphoblastic leukemia relapses with refined response classification and integration of genetics. J Clin Oncol. 2019;37(36):3493.
133. Jeha S, Pei D, Choi J, Cheng C, Sandlund JT, Coustan-Smith E, et al. Improved CNS control of childhood acute lymphoblastic leukemia without cranial irradiation: St Jude total therapy study 16. J Clin Oncol. 2019;37(35):3377.
134. von Stackelberg A, Locatelli F, Zugmaier G, Handgretinger R, Trippett TM, Rizzari C, et al. Phase I/phase II study of blinatumomab in pediatric patients with relapsed/refractory acute lymphoblastic leukemia. J Clin Oncol. 2016;34(36):4381–9.
135. Brown PA, Ji L, Xu X, Devidas M, Hogan LE, Borowitz MJ, et al. Effect of Postreinduction therapy consolidation with Blinatumomab vs chemotherapy on disease-free survival in children, adolescents, and young adults with first relapse of B-cell acute lymphoblastic Leukemia: a randomized clinical trial. JAMA. 2021;325(9):833–42.
136. Hunger SP, Raetz EA. How I treat relapsed acute lymphoblastic leukemia in the pediatric population. Blood. 2020;136(16):1803–12.
137. Grupp SA, Kalos M, Barrett D, Aplenc R, Porter DL, Rheingold SR, et al. Chimeric antigen receptor-modified T cells for acute lymphoid leukemia. N Engl J Med. 2013;368(16):1509–18.

138. He X, Xiao X, Li Q, Jiang Y, Cao Y, Sun R, et al. Anti-CD19 CAR-T as a feasible and safe treatment against central nervous system leukemia after intrathecal chemotherapy in adults with relapsed or refractory B-ALL. Leukemia. 2019;33(8):2102–4.
139. Htun KT, Gong Q, Ma L, Wang P, Tan Y, Wu G, et al. Successful treatment of refractory and relapsed CNS acute lymphoblastic Leukemia with CD-19 CAR-T immunotherapy: a case report. Front Oncol. 2021;11:699946.
140. Fabrizio VA, Phillips CL, Lane A, Baggott C, Prabhu S, Egeler E, et al. Tisagenlecleucel outcomes in relapsed/refractory extramedullary ALL: a Pediatric real world CAR consortium report. Blood Adv. 2022;6(2):600–10.
141. Jacoby E, Ghorashian S, Vormoor B, De Moerloose B, Bodmer N, Molostova O, et al. CD19 CAR T-cells for pediatric relapsed acute lymphoblastic leukemia with active CNS involvement: a retrospective international study. Leukemia. 2022;36(6):1525–32.
142. Li T, Zhao L, Zhang Y, Xiao Y, Wang D, Huang L, et al. CAR T-cell therapy is effective but not long-lasting in B-cell lymphoma of the brain. Front Oncol. 2020:10.
143. Qi Y, Zhao M, Hu Y, Wang Y, Li P, Cao J, et al. Efficacy and safety of CD19-specific CAR T cell–based therapy in B-cell acute lymphoblastic leukemia patients with CNSL. Blood, J Am Soc Hematol. 2022;139(23):3376–86.
144. Maude SL, Teachey DT, Porter DL, Grupp SA. CD19-targeted chimeric antigen receptor T-cell therapy for acute lymphoblastic leukemia. Blood, J Am Soc Hematol. 2015;125(26):4017–23.
145. Warrier IA, Ravindranath Y, Bedros A, Cejka J, Inoue S. Significance of elevated B2 Microglobulin (B2m) in the cerebrospinal fluid (CSF) of children with acute leukemia (AL). Pediatr Res. 1981;15(4):579.
146. Vicente V. Cerebrospinal fluid levels beta2 microglobulin and ferritin in lymphoproliferative disorders. 1982.
147. Evans D, O'Rourke C, Jones PM. The cerebrospinal fluid in acute leukaemia of childhood: studies with the Cytocentrifuge. J Clin Pathol. 1974;27(3):226–30.
148. Rao D, Ghalaut VS, Ghalaut P, Rao S. Case series: CSF LDH, proteins and electrolyte levels in patients of acute lymphocytic leukemia. Clin Chim Acta. 2012;413(13–14):1045–8.
149. Priola GM, Foster MW, Deal AM, Richardson BM, Thompson JW, Blatt J. Cerebrospinal fluid proteomics in children during induction for acute lymphoblastic leukemia: a pilot study. Pediatr Blood Cancer. 2015;62(7):1190–4.
150. Mo F, Ma X, Liu X, Zhou R, Zhao Y, Zhou H. Altered CSF proteomic profiling of paediatric acute lymphocytic leukemia patients with CNS infiltration. J Oncol. 2019;2019:3283629.
151. Zhang H, Luo X-Q, Zhang P, Huang L-B, Zheng Y-S, Wu J, et al. MicroRNA patterns associated with clinical prognostic parameters and CNS relapse prediction in pediatric acute leukemia. PLoS One. 2009;4(11):e7826.
152. Egyed B, Kutszegi N, Sági JC, Gézsi A, Rzepiel A, Visnovitz T, et al. MicroRNA-181a as novel liquid biopsy marker of central nervous system involvement in pediatric acute lymphoblastic leukemia. J Transl Med. 2020;18(1):1–12.
153. Wang Y, Springer S, Zhang M, McMahon KW, Kinde I, Dobbyn L, et al. Detection of tumor-derived DNA in cerebrospinal fluid of patients with primary tumors of the brain and spinal cord. Proc Natl Acad Sci. 2015;112(31):9704–9.
154. Plaks V, Kong N, Werb Z. The cancer stem cell niche: how essential is the niche in regulating stemness of tumor cells? Cell Stem Cell. 2015;16(3):225–38.
155. Chen X, Huang J, Xu N, Fan Z, Nie D, Huang F, et al. A phase 2 study of sorafenib combined with conventional therapies in refractory central nervous system leukemia. Cancer. 2022;
156. Shi Y, Beckett MC, Blair HJ, Tirtakusuma R, Nakjang S, Enshaei A, et al. Phase II-like murine trial identifies synergy between dexamethasone and dasatinib in T-cell acute lymphoblastic leukemia. Haematologica. 2021;106(4):1056.
157. Kato I, Nishinaka Y, Nakamura M, Akarca AU, Niwa A, Ozawa H, et al. Hypoxic adaptation of leukemic cells infiltrating the CNS affords a therapeutic strategy targeting VEGFA. Blood, J Am Soc Hematol. 2017;129(23):3126–9.
158. Ridge SM, Whiteley AE, Yao H, Price TT, Brockman ML, Murray AS, et al. Pan-PI3Ki targets multiple B-ALL microenvironment interactions that fuel systemic and CNS relapse. Leuk Lymphoma. 2021;62(11):2690–702.
159. Ransohoff RM, Engelhardt B. The anatomical and cellular basis of immune surveillance in the central nervous system. Nat Rev Immunol. 2012;12(9):623–35.
160. Alsadeq A, Fedders H, Vokuhl C, Belau NM, Zimmermann M, Wirbelauer T, et al. The role of ZAP70 kinase in acute lymphoblastic leukemia infiltration into the central nervous system. Haematologica. 2017;102(2):346.
161. Jost TR, Borga C, Radaelli E, Romagnani A, Perruzza L, Omodho L, et al. Role of CXCR4-mediated bone marrow colonization in CNS infiltration by T cell acute lymphoblastic leukemia. J Leukoc Biol. 2016;99(6):1077–87.

An Overview of the Genetics and Treatment of Down Syndrome ALL

10

Anthony Moorman and Sujith Samarasinghe

10.1 Introduction

Children with Down syndrome (DS) are at an increased risk of developing acute lymphoblastic leukaemia (ALL). However, it is a rare cohort and is characterised by unique clinical features and poorer outcomes. There is a decreased prevalence of favourable cytogenetics (*ETV6::RUNX1*, high hyperdiploid), a decreased prevalence of unfavourable chromosomal abnormalities (*BCR::ABL1*, *KMT2A::AFF1*) but overexpression of *CRLF2* and JAK-STAT activation is common. Whilst it is unclear if JAK inhibitors are beneficial, preliminary data with targeted therapy such as CAR T cells suggest, that novel agents may hold promise.

10.2 Epidemiology

Individuals with Down syndrome have a significantly increased risk of developing B-cell precursor ALL (30–40 fold) and acute megakaryocyte-erythroid leukaemia (150 fold). DS-ALL is a rare cohort, accounting for around 2–3% of all childhood ALL. It is almost exclusively precursor B-ALL, with less than 1% of DS ALL cases being T-ALL. In contrast to transient abnormal myelopoiesis (TAM), DS-ALL is rare in infants. Whilst myeloid leukaemia of Down syndrome (ML-DS) is rare after the age of 4, the average of presentation of DS-ALL is 5 years, with cases presenting into adolescence [1].

10.3 Genetics

Trisomy or partial trisomy of chromosome 21, the hallmark of DS, perturbs foetal and neonatal haematopoiesis disrupting the development of B lymphocytes, erythrocytes and myelocytes. This altered bone marrow microenvironment provides a setting that facilitates the development and maintenance of leukaemia cells. Genome-wide association studies (GWAS) have found that the top four single-nucleotide polymorphisms (SNP) linked with ALL development target the same genes in DS and non-DS patients; namely *ARID5B*, *IKZF1*, *CDKN2A* and *GATA3*. However, there is evidence for increased occurrence of the *CDKN2A*-associated SNP in DS-ALL. Thus, trisomy 21 itself appears to be the major factor responsible for the increased risk of BCP-ALL. Interestingly, acquired trisomy 21 occurs in approximately half of non-DS-ALL patients.

A. Moorman
Leukaemia Research Cytogenetics Group, Translational and Clinical Research Institute, Newcastle University, Newcastle upon Tyne, UK
e-mail: anthony.moorman@newcastle.ac.uk

S. Samarasinghe (✉)
Department of Haematology, Great Ormond Street Hospital, London, UK
e-mail: Sujith.Samarasinghe@gosh.nhs.uk

G. Escherich, V. Conter (eds.), *Acute Lymphoblastic Leukemia in Children and Adolescents*, Pediatric Oncology, https://doi.org/10.1007/978-3-031-71180-0_10

Despite this connection, the landscape of somatic cytogenetic and genomic abnormalities in DS-ALL is distinct from that observed in non-DS patients.

ETV6::RUNX1 and high hyperdiploidy (51–67 chromosomes) occur in more than half of non-DS-ALL patients but less than a quarter of DS-ALL patients. Classic high-risk chromosomal abnormalities (e.g. *BCR::ABL1*, *KMT2A* fusions, iAMP21, *TCF3::HLF*, near-haploidy and low hypodiploidy) are extremely rare in DS-ALL accounting for less than 2% cases compared with around 10% of non-DS BCP-ALL cases. Similarly, the frequency of *TCF3::PBX1* is lower amongst DS versus non-DS ALL patients (<1% v 5%) [1].

In contrast, more than 50% of DS-ALL patients harbour a genetic abnormality that deregulates the *CRLF2* gene located in the pseudo-autosomal region 1 (PAR1) of chromosome X/Y resulting in its over-expression. This compares to ~5% in non-DS patients with ALL. The principal genetic abnormalities driving *CRLF2* over-expression are *P2RY8::CRLF2* and *IGH::CRLF2* fusion. A *P2RY8::CRLF2* fusion is generated from an interstitial deletion within the PAR1 region. This results in the loss of *CSF2RA*, *IL3RA*, and the 3′ portion of *P2RY8* and the juxtaposition of the *CRLF2* gene to the promoter region of *P2RY8*. *IGH::CRLF2* arises from one of two chromosomal translocations—t(X;14)(p22;q32) or t(Y;14)(p11;q32)—both of which result in the juxtaposition of the *CRLF2* gene to the *IGH* enhancer. More rarely, *CRLF2* activating mutations (e.g. F232C) can drive *CRLF2* over-expression. Whilst *CRLF2* over-expression activates JAK-STAT pro-survival signalling, it alone is not sufficient to drive leukaemogenesis. In the majority of *CRLF2*-r cases, additional mutations and genetic abnormalities are found that also activate the JAK-STAT pathway. The most common are *JAK2* R683G/S activating mutations but *JAK1*, *JAK3* and *IL7R* mutations have also been reported. Not all *CRLF2*-r cases will have concomitant JAK mutations and in such cases *NRAS* and *KRAS* mutations are often observed [2].

Activation of the JAK-STAT pathway is one of the defining features of the *BCR::ABL1*/Philadelphia-like gene expression profile and therefore the vast majority of *CRLF2*-r cases will be categorised into this subtype. However, unlike cases with an ABL-class fusion (gene fusions involving *ABL1*, *ABL2*, *PDGFRB* and *CSF1R*), *CRLF2*-r cases are not sensitive to tyrosine-kinase inhibitors and are therefore clinically distinct. Although there is in vitro evidence that cells harbouring a *CRLF2*-r are sensitive to JAK2 inhibitors (e.g. ruxolitinib) there is no evidence currently that JAK2 inhibitors are effective clinically.

The second DS associated chromosomal abnormality in ALL is the t(8;14)(q11;q32) translocation that results in over-expression of the *CEBPD* gene via its juxtaposition to the IGH enhancer. The frequency of this translocation is approximately 3%. Although not common it is significantly higher than amongst non-DS cases where it is observed is less than 0.3% cases. In fact, approximately 50% of all *IGH::CEBPD* cases with ALL have DS. This abnormality belongs to a wider group of abnormalities that over-express members of *CEBP* gene family (*CEBPA*, *CEBPB*, *CEBPE*, etc.) via juxtaposition of the gene to an immunoglobulin enhancer element. However, only *IGH::CEBPD* is associated with DS.

The spectrum of other secondary genetic abnormalities particularly copy number alterations and mutations is broadly similar in DS and non-DS ALL. However, the frequency of some abnormalities can vary due to the differing frequencies of primary abnormalities. The major difference observed in DS-ALL is the frequency of *IKZF1* deletions which at 30% is around twice that seen in non-DS-ALL. *IKZF1* deletions are known to associate with *CRLF2*-r, so this increase is expected.

10.4 Outcomes and Risk Stratification

DS-ALL patients have worse outcomes compared to non-DS-ALL patients and thus represent a high-risk cohort. However, outcome heterogeneity within DS-ALL has been reported in relation to both age, white cell count, genetics and treatment response. A retrospective analysis of 653 DS-ALL cases treated on 16 international trials between 1995 and 2005 compared to a large non-DS-ALL cohort showed a higher 8-year cumulative incidence of relapse (26% vs. 15%, respectively) and 2-year treatment-related mortality (7% vs. 2%, respectively) [1]. As a result, there was a lower 8-year event-free survival (EFS) (64% vs. 81% respectively) and 10-year overall survival (OS) (70% vs. 88% respectively). This study also demonstrated that patients who were < 6 years old, had a white cell count of <10 × 10^9/L, *ETV6::RUNX1* positive or had high hyperdiploidy had significantly improved outcomes. Further genetic analysis of this cohort revealed no prognostic effect for *CRLF2*-r abnormalities but a significantly adverse effect of *IKZF1* deletions. Patients with an *IKZF1* deletion had at least a twofold increased risk of relapse (Table 10.1).

An updated analysis amongst eight cooperative groups comparing DS-ALL patients (*n* = 136) with matched non-DS-ALL controls (*n* = 407) between 2002 and 2018 continued to show worse outcomes for the DS-ALL patients. There were higher rates of induction TRM (6% vs. 0.8%, respectively) and post induction TRM (12.2% vs. 2.7%, respectively). Crucially rates of minimal residual disease (MRD) clearance in the DS-ALL cohort were similar to the non-DS ALL cohort suggesting that for most DS-ALL patients, the worse EFS is not due to initial chemo-resistance. Analysing the effect of *IKZF1* deletions within this case-control study suggests an interplay between DS-ALL and *IKZF1* deletions. *IKZF1* deletions were associated with a higher risk of relapse amongst both DS and non-DS-ALL patients. However, DS-ALL patients with an *IKZF1* deletion had a 5-year risk of relapse of 37% (17–57%) yielding a hazard ratio of 8.1 (3.3 to 20.1) compared with DS-ALL patients without an *IKZF1* deletion. In contrast, amongst non-DS-ALL patients the effect of *IKZF1* deletion was more modest with a hazard ratio of 1.9 (0.9–3.9).

Table 10.1 Biological and clinical features

Biological and clinical features
Nearly always precursor B-ALL phenotype
High rate of relapse with IKZF1 deletions
CRLF2 aberrant expression in over 50% of cases
Decreased prevalence of favourable chromosomal abnormalities (*ETV6::RUNX1*, high hyperdiploid)
Decreased prevalence of unfavourable chromosomal abnormalities (*BCR::ABL1*, *KMT2A* fusions)
High rate of treatment-related mortality throughout all phases

Risk stratification in DS-ALL specific protocols is restricted by the relatively small number of patients. The excess of TRM observed amongst these patients prevents any further intensification of therapy. The traditional risk factors of younger age and lower white cell count do apply in DS-ALL but their role in actively risk-stratifying patients is limited. The same is true for good risk cytogenetic abnormalities such as *ETV6::RUNX1* and high hyperdiploidy. The very high incidence of abnormalities deregulating the JAK-STAT pathway makes DS-ALL an attractive cohort for targeted therapy with *JAK2* inhibitors and, in time, this may prove an important risk-stratifying predictive biomarker. However, there is no evidence that the presence of a *CRLF2*-r has a major prognostic effect with standard chemotherapy. Hence it is not currently a risk-stratifying feature in DS-ALL. In contrast, *IKZF1* deletions are present in one-third of DS-ALL and have been linked with a very high risk of relapse.

In the ALLTogether 01 trial, risk stratification and treatment is different to non DS-ALL patients (Tables 10.2 and 10.3). Based on an analysis of DS-ALL outcomes on four different trials (UKALL, COALL, NOPHO and DCOG), the key prognostic features were the presence of end induction MRD and *IKZF1* deletions. Based on this evidence, stratification of the DS-ALL patients in the ALLTogether1 protocol will be into three groups: standard risk (SR), intermediate risk (IR) and high risk (HR). Stratification will be based on clinical features, genetics and MRD as for other patients, but in addition, deletion of the *IKZF1*-gene will be specifically stratifying for Down syndrome patients.

Table 10.2 Outcomes of 88 DS children from the ALLTogether consortium (UKALL and DCOG) with or without *IKZF1* deletion

	IKZF1 deletion			
	No	Yes	Total	*P*
N	68 (77)	20 (23)	88 (100)	
RR	9.6 (4.1–21.5)	49.4 (27.3–76.7)	17.6 (10.4–29.0)	<0.0001
EFS	71.6 (59.1–80.9)	35.0 (15.7–55.2)	63.2 (52.1–72.4)	0.0001
OS	86.2 (64.1–84.7)	44.4 (22.5–64.4)	69.0 (58.1–77.6)	0.0009

RR relapse risk, *EFS* event free survival, *OS* overall survival

Table 10.3 Outcomes of 164 children with DS-ALL from the ALLTogether consortium (UKALL, DCOG, CoALL and NOPHO) depending on end of induction MRD

	MRD-driven risk groups				
	True negative	Detectable ≤5%	> 5%	Total	*P*
N	42 (26)	113 (69)	9 (5)	164 (100)	
RR	5.4 (1.4–19.9)	16.4 (10.2–25.8)	48.6 (18.7–88.2)	15.0 (9.9–22.4)	<0.0001
EFS	87.8 (73.2–94.8)	71.8 (62.2–79.4)	33.3 (7.8–62.3)	73.5 (65.7–79.8)	0.0001
OS	87.5 (72.4–94.6)	75.7 (66.3–82.8)	33.3 (7.8–62.3)	76.0 (68.4–82.1)	0.0009

10.5 Current Treatment Approaches

10.5.1 Measures to Reduce TRM and Toxicity

DS-ALL patients have an increased risk of TRM compared to non-DS-ALL patients. On the UKALL 2003 trial (2003–2011) there was a 21.6% TRM in the 86 DS patients. In comparison the TRM for non DS-ALL patients was 3.3%, odds ratio = 209.7 (65.3–673.4), $P < 0.00005$]. The excess TRM was primarily due to infection, especially respiratory tract infections. Infection related mortality was 12 times more common in DS-ALL patients than non-DS-ALL cases with most cases occurring during maintenance therapy. A combination of bacterial, viral and fungal infections was responsible for infection related mortality. The causes of the increased risk of infection are multifactorial and include an increased risk of chemotherapy induced mucositis, immunodeficiency, congenital cardiac defects, gastrointestinal reflux and tracheomalacia. In addition to an increased risk of TRM, DS-ALL patients are also more likely to develop specific chemotherapy-induced toxicities such as mucositis, steroid toxicity, seizures and non-CNS thrombosis. In part, this is due to increased cellular/tissue uptake of drugs such as methotrexate.

Due to the high TRM seen in the DS-ALL cohorts on the UK trial UKALL 2003, several modifications were introduced to the successor study UKALL 2011. This included avoiding giving anthracyclines in induction except to those with a slow morphological response (≥25% blasts) on day 15, use of a single delayed intensification and 2 years maintenance for boys and girls. End of induction MRD was found to be highly discriminant for future relapse. As such, post induction therapy was stratified based on end of induction MRD enabling treatment de-escalation in the MRD low risk with no pulses in maintenance. There was enhanced supportive care with antibiotic prophylaxis during periods of neutropenia, clinical review three times per week and intensive treatment of febrile neutropenia. Since these measures, there has been an improvement in TRM. Preliminary analysis of UKALL 2011, post these measures, showed a 6.7% TRM for the trial overall-(unpublished data). As such, whilst these measures have improved TRM, it continues to remain higher than the non-DS ALL population. Whilst dexamethasone was used in induction in UKALL protocols, The Children's

Oncology Group (COG) restricts dexamethasone in induction to those under the age of 10, using prednisolone for those aged ten and over. Due to the heightened methotrexate sensitivity, The AIEOP BFM ALL groups limit exposure to high doses of intravenous MTX by adopting a dose capping (starting dose 500 mg/m^2 with folinic acid rescue) and if tolerated, then adopting a cautious dose escalation strategy.

The role of prophylactic antibiotics is controversial—ciprofloxacin prophylaxis is recommended during intensive phases in the UK but not by all other consortia. There is currently no evidence for routine antifungal prophylaxis or immunoglobulin replacement. Despite these differences, there is no difference in outcomes between the different DS-ALL treatment protocols.

10.5.2 Measures to Reduce Relapse

DS ALL patients are rare and beside the above-mentioned multinational overviews not many trial groups have published the results of DS ALL patients. Treatment intention historically on the part of physicians may also have been different to that of non-DS-ALL patients due to the increased toxicity of the DS-ALL cohort. In support of this, a Nordic study showed that DS-ALL patients received 25% lower doses of 6 MP and methotrexate in maintenance, suggesting that physicians are reluctant to dose escalate due to concerns over-toxicity. It is therefore possible that the increased relapse rates seen in DS-ALL have been in part due to under-dosing. In contrast, the Dana Faber consortium does not dose adjust or make modifications to chemotherapy for the DS-ALL patients. They showed in two successive trials using this approach, that similar outcomes could be achieved to that of non-DS children.

Both UKALL 2003 and CCLG 1991 trials did not show any benefit for two delayed intensifications compared to one which included standard risk DS-ALL patients. CCLG 1991 also compared escalating IV methotrexate without leucovorin rescue post induction compared to standard interim maintenance with oral methotrexate. Whilst not statistically significant there was a trend in favour of escalating IV methotrexate compared to standard interim maintenance in DS-ALL (EFS 94% vs. 81%, respectively). As such in the current ALLTogether1 protocol, all DS-ALL patients receive an induction without anthracyclines, with one delayed intensification and escalating IV methotrexate without leucovorin rescue reserved for patients with detectable MRD.

10.6 Novel Agents

Novel agents are required to improve relapse and reduce TRM in DS-ALL. One such agent is blinatumomab. Blinatumomab is a CD19/CD3-bispecific T-cell receptor-engaging (BiTE) antibody that is designed to link CD19+ B cells with CD3+ T cells, resulting in a cytotoxic T-cell response against CD19+ leukaemia/lymphoma. Recent studies have demonstrated that blinatumomab is more effective and less toxic than intensive chemotherapy in children and young persons (CYP) with relapsed B-ALL. Furthermore, blinatumomab is standard of care in adults with persistent MRD during first line therapy based on the BLAST study. The ALL Together consortium is therefore conducting a prospective, single-arm, international multicentre study conducted to determine the feasibility of replacing two consolidation blocks with two cycles of blinatumomab in DS-ALL patients who are MRD detectable at end of induction) (ALLTogether1 trial). It is hypothesised that replacing consolidation with blinatumomab will lead to an enhanced rate of MRD negativity and be safer.

The COG (AALL1731) is also examining the use of blinatumomab in high-risk DS-ALL and standard-risk DS-ALL with an end of induction MRD $\geq$ 0.01%. Three cycles of blinatumomab will be administered, one each after consolidation, interim maintenance and one in place of the second half of delayed intensification. The COG has reported a high rate of seizures in the NCI risk patients on this study with blinatumomab

(24% rate of seizures in NCI risk patients) and now use levetiracetam prophylaxis in all DS-ALL patients receiving blinatumomab. Most seizures occurred in cycle one and in some cases blinatumomab was successfully resumed. There has not been an increased rate of seizures seen in those aged under ten. The AIEOP-BFM 2017 protocol is randomly allocating all patients at medium risk, including DS patients, a single cycle of blinatumomab after protocol II prior to maintenance therapy. In the high-risk group, DS-ALL patients will receive two cycles of blinatumomab rather than two high-risk chemotherapy blocks.

Table 10.4 Strategies to reduce relapse and toxicity

Measures to reduce relapse
Blinatumomab replacing blocks of chemotherapy
Tisagenlecleucel for high-risk patients
Treatment intensification in *IKZF1*-deleted and/or MRD-positive patients
Maintain dose intensity during maintenance
Measures to reduce toxicity
Treatment de-escalation in patients with low risk/ undetectable MRD
Omission of second delayed intensification
Omission of anthracycline during induction
Aggressive treatment of suspected infection
Antibiotic prophylaxis during intensive periods

10.7 Relapse

A review of DS-ALL relapses between 1983 and 2000, with matched controls suggested that DS-ALL relapse outcomes were significantly worse compared to matched non-DS-ALL controls due to the high rate of TRM (5-year OS 17% vs. 51%, respectively). Between 2000 and 2012 there was a reduction in DS-ALL TRM but outcomes remain lower than non-DS patients (5-year OS 31% vs. 53% respectively). In part this may be due to physician reluctance to escalate treatment intensity due to concerns regarding toxicity, such as with stem cell transplant. Nevertheless, a study of 27 DS children who underwent a HSCT showed disease relapse was more of a risk (3-year relapse risk 54%) than TRM (3-year risk 22%) in the modern era.

One novel agent that holds promise in relapsed/refractory DS-ALL is chimeric antigen receptor therapy. Tisagenlecleucel is a CD19-directed, genetically modified, autologous T-cell immunotherapy that modifies targeted leukemic cells and is approved for patients up to 25 years old with relapsed or refractory (r/r) B-cell ALL. A review of 16 relapsed/refractory DS-ALL treated with Tisagenlecleucel showed that outcomes and toxicities were similar to the non-DS ALL population. 88% achieved a complete remission and 86% of these were MRD negative [3]. Toxicity was also similar with 44% experiencing grade 3/4 cytokine release syndrome and grade 3/4 prolonged cytopenias, whilst 13% had grade 3/4 neurological events. Crucially no grade 3/4 infections were seen. The 12-month relapse free survival was 57.3% and overall survival was 85.9%. These outcomes suggest that Tisagenlecleucel could be considered as a treatment option for first line DS-ALL relapse (Table 10.4).

10.8 Conclusion

DS-ALL remains a high-risk cohort especially for those patients with an *IKZF1* deletion. There have been improvements in outcome more recently brought about through a reduction in TRM and using MRD risk stratified therapy. Further improvements will require the exploration of use of novel agents such a blinatumomab and chimeric antigen receptor therapy.

References

1. Buitenkamp TD, Izraeli S, Zimmermann M, Forestier E, Heerema NA, van den Heuvel-Eibrink MM, Pieters R, Korbijn CM, Silverman LB, Schmiegelow K, Liang DC, Horibe K, Arico M, Biondi A, Basso G, Rabin KR, Schrappe M, Cario G, Mann G, Morak M, Panzer-Grümayer R, Mondelaers V, Lammens T, Cavé H, Stark B, Ganmore I, Moorman AV, Vora A, Hunger SP, Pui CH, Mullighan CG, Manabe A, Escherich G,

Kowalczyk JR, Whitlock JA, Zwaan CM. Acute lymphoblastic leukemia in children with down syndrome: a retrospective analysis from the Ponte di Legno study group. Blood. 2014;123(1):70–7.
2. Lee P, Bhansali R, Izraeli S, Hijiya N, Crispino JD. The biology, pathogenesis and clinical aspects of acute lymphoblastic leukemia in children with down syndrome. Leukemia. 2016;30(9):1816–23.
3. Laetsch TW, Maude SL, Balduzzi A, Rives S, Bittencourt H, Boyer MW, Buechner J, De Moerloose B, Qayed M, Phillips CL, Pulsipher MA, Hiramatsu H, Tiwari R, Grupp SA. Tisagenlecleucel in pediatric and young adult patients with down syndrome-associated relapsed/refractory acute lymphoblastic leukemia. Leukemia. 2022;36(6):1508–15.

Stratification and Treatment of Infants

11

Daisuke Tomizawa and Rob Pieters

11.1 Introduction

ALL in infants (<1 year old) accounts for less than 5% of childhood ALL. Infant ALL comprises two distinct subtypes; ALL with rearrangements of *histone lysine methyltransferase 2A* gene (*KMT2A*, previously known as *mixed lineage leukemia* [*MLL*] gene) which accounts for approximately 70–80% of infant ALL, and ALL with germline *KMT2A* gene [1]. *KMT2A* gene rearrangement occurs as a result of balanced chromosomal translocations involving chromosome 11q23 locus, which results in fusion of the N terminus of the *KMT2A* gene with the C terminus of one of over 90 known partner genes [2]. Among those, *AFF1* (*AF4*) comprises approximately 40–50% of the infant *KMT2A*-rearranged (KMT2A-r) ALL cases followed by *MLLT1* (*ENL*) and *MLLT2* (*AF9*).

Infants with KMT2A-r ALL often present as a very aggressive leukemia with hyperleukocytosis and frequent involvement of extramedullary sites such as central nervous system (CNS), liver, spleen, and/or skin (leukemia cutis). Majority of KMT2A-r ALL has an immature CD10-negative B-cell precursor phenotype frequently co-expressed with myeloid-specific antigens (e.g., CD117, CD13, CD33, CD65, CD15), suggesting that infant KMT2A-r ALL originates from very immature lymphoid progenitors. In fact, KMT2A-r leukemia in infants could present as a mixed phenotype acute leukemia (MPAL), and occasionally, a myeloid "lineage switch" (usually to acute monocytic leukemia) is observed [3].

Prognosis of infants with KMT2A-r ALL is extremely poor, with <40% event-free survival (EFS) rate in the majority of the published clinical trials worldwide (Table 11.1, Fig. 11.1b, c) [4, 5]. On the other hand, EFS rate of infants with germline *KMT2A* (KMT2A-g) ALL is in the range of 70–90%, almost similar to that of ALL in children 1 year old or older (Table 11.1, Fig. 11.1a, b) [5–7].

D. Tomizawa (✉)
Division of Leukemia and Lymphoma, Children's Cancer Center, National Center for Child Health and Development, Tokyo, Japan
e-mail: tomizawa-d@ncchd.go.jp

R. Pieters
Princess Máxima Center for Pediatric Oncology, Utrecht, The Netherlands
e-mail: R.Pieters@prinsesmaximacentrum.nl

G. Escherich, V. Conter (eds.), *Acute Lymphoblastic Leukemia in Children and Adolescents*, Pediatric Oncology, https://doi.org/10.1007/978-3-031-71180-0_11

Table 11.1 Outline and results of recently completed major clinical trials for infant ALL

		JPLSG-MLL-10	Interfant-06	COG AALL0631
Patient accrual period		2011–2014	2006–2016	2008–2014
Patient number		LR: $n = 15$ IR: $n = 19$ HR: $n = 56$	LR: $n = 167$ MR: $n = 320$ HR: $n = 164$	LR: $n = 64$ IR: $n = 111$ HR: $n = 35$
Risk group definition	LR	*KMT2A* germline	*KMT2A* germline	*KMT2A* germline
	IR/MR	Other KMT2A-r	Other KMT2A-r	Other KMT2A-r
	HR	KMT2A-r Age < 6 months old, or CNS-3	KMT2A-r and Age < 6 months old PRED poor responder, or WBC ≥300,000/μL	KMT2A-r Age < 3 months old
Induction therapy		Interfant-based	Interfant-based	Interfant-based
Post-induction randomization for KMT2A-r cases		None (single arm)	IB (ALL-like) vs. ADE/MAE (AML-like) consolidation	± lestaurtinib (FLT3 inhibitor)
HSCT indication		All HR	All HR and MR with positive MRD at EOC	None
Patients actually transplanted among patients achieving CR1		52% of all patients 64% of KMT2A-r patients	18% of all patients 25% of KMT2A-r patients	None
EFS rate (year)		Overall: 70.9% (3) KMT2A-g (LR): 93.3% (3) KMT2A-r (IR + HR): 66.2% (3) IR 94.4% (3) HR 56.6% (3)	Overall: 46.1% (6) KMT2A-g (LR): 73.9% (6) KMT2A-r (MR + HR): 36.4% (6) MR 44.5% (6) HR 20.9% (6)	Overall: Not reported KMT2A-g (LR): 87.3% (5) KMT2A-r (IR + HR): 34% (5) IR 40% (5) HR 17% (5)

COG Children's Oncology Group, *JPLSG* Japanese Pediatric Leukemia/Lymphoma Study Group, *ADE* combination of cytarabine, daunorubicin, and etoposide, *ALL* acute lymphoblastic leukemia, *AML* acute myeloid leukemia, *CNS* central nervous system, *EFS* event-free survival, *EOC* end of consolidation, *FLT3* fms-related tyrosine kinase 3, *HR* high risk, *HSCT* hematopoietic stem cell transplantation, *IR* intermediate risk, *KMT2A-g* germline *KMT2A* gene, *KMT2A-r* rearranged *KMT2A* gene, *LR* low risk, *MAE* mitoxantrone, cytarabine, and etoposide, *MR* medium risk, *MRD* minimal residual disease, *PRED* prednisone, *WBC* white blood cells

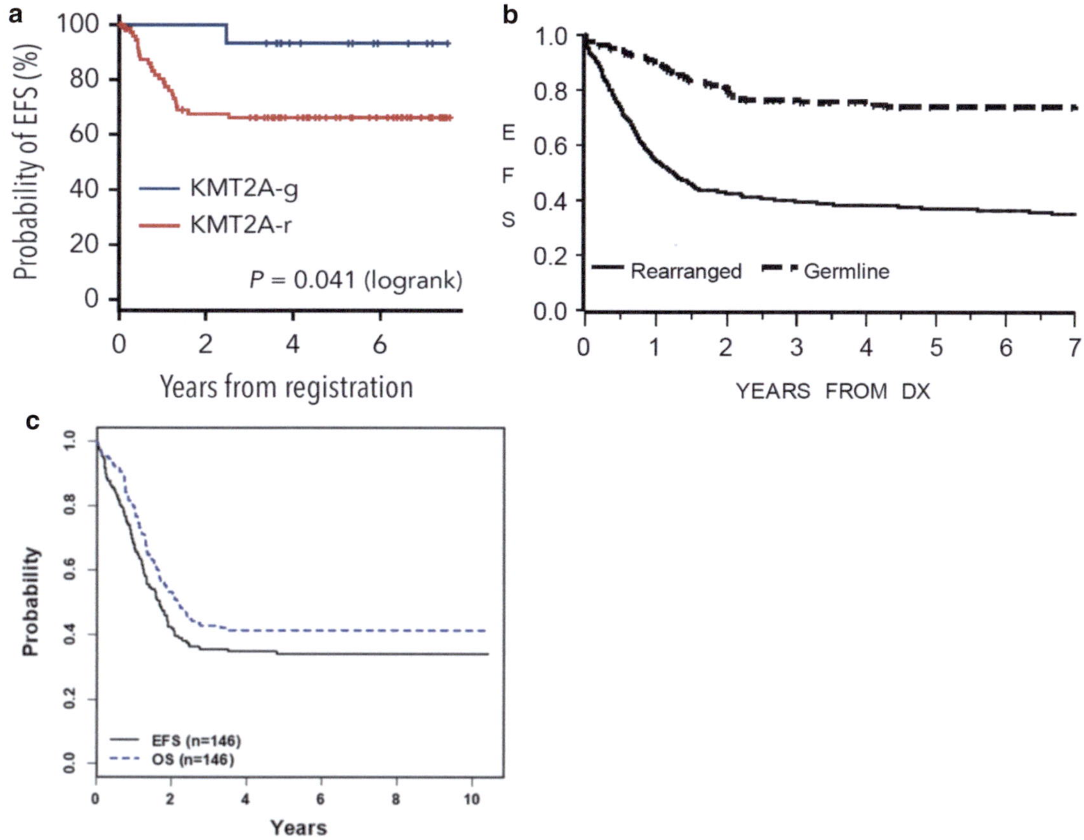

Fig. 11.1 Outcome of infants with ALL according to the *KMT2A* gene status in the recent studies by the JPLSG, Interfant, and COG. (**a**) EFS in JPLSG MLL-10 (Tomizawa et al. [7]); (**b**) EFS in Interfant-06 (Pieters et al. [11]); and (**c**) EFS and OS of infants with KMT2A-r ALL in COG AALL0631 (Brown et al. [1])

11.2 Risk Stratifications in Infant ALL

Risk stratifications used in the recently completed infant ALL clinical trials conducted by three major cooperative study groups, Interfant (mainly consisting of European countries), Children's Oncology Group (COG, mainly consisting of North American centers), and the Japan Children's Cancer Group (JCCG; formerly, the Japanese Pediatric Leukemia/Lymphoma Study Group [JPLSG]), are shown in Table 11.1 [8].

Presence of *KMT2A* rearrangement is the most significant poor prognostic factor in infant ALL; therefore, all three groups consider KMT2A-g ALL as low-risk (LR) group and KMT2A-r ALL as either high-risk (HR) or intermediate-risk (IR) group according to the other additional prognostic factors. Among the infants with KMT2A-r ALL, young age at diagnosis is significantly associated with poor prognosis, although cutoff age used is somewhat different. Clinical features such as high white blood cell count (WBC) or CNS disease at diagnosis are also associated with poor prognosis, but these are at the same time more or less associated with young age at presentation [9–11].

Similar to ALL in older children, treatment response is highly prognostic in infant ALL. "Prednisone response" evaluating residual leukemic blasts in peripheral blood following 7-day prednisone monotherapy and a single intrathecal methotrexate injection, is widely used for risk stratification in pediatric ALL protocols. Nearly 30% of the infants with ALL fall into prednisone poor responders (≥1000 blasts/μL), while it is less than 10% in older children with B-lineage ALL [12, 13]. In recent years, measurement of minimal (or measurable) residual disease (MRD) at early phases of therapy (e.g., at end of induction [EOI] and/or at end of early consolidation [EOC]) has become a major stratification tool in pediatric ALL protocols [14]. Flow cytometric MRD detecting aberrant combinations of leukemic cell-surface antigen or PCR amplification targeting leukemic clone specific rearrangement of immunoglobulin (Ig) or T-cell receptor (TCR) genes are the two major techniques that could detect submicroscopic levels of residual leukemia with sensitivity of 0.01% and 0.01–0.001%, respectively. MRD is highly predictive of relapse risk also in infant ALL, therefore, is used in risk stratifications in currently ongoing trials. However, there are several cautions especially when using Ig/TCR PCR-MRD in infant KMT2A-r ALL. It has been reported that only half of the Ig/TCR targets in infant ALL cases reached a quantitative range of at least 10^{-4} and that approximately 10% of infant ALL samples resulted in underestimation of actual MRD load [15]. This phenomenon is due to a lower frequency of Ig/TCR rearrangements and oligoclonality of infant KMT2A-r ALL cells [16]. In that sense, use of *KMT2A* genomic breakpoint as a PCR target, as utilized in Interfant-06, might be preferable because it should be present in total leukemic clones.

However, currently used risk-stratification is still not predictive enough to segregate infants with ALL into truly appropriate risk groups. Use of more sensitive MRD assays by next generation sequencing (NGS) has shown to reliably detect leukemic blasts at levels of $\leq 10^{-6}$ cells, which may be helpful to identify infants with ALL at very low risk of relapse [17]. Recently, the Japanese group have identified that multi-omics approach by combining RNA sequencing, methylation array analysis, whole exome and targeted sequencing can segregate infants with KMT2A-r ALL into five integrative clusters [18]. Among these five clusters, infants with significant expression of IRX transcription factors and immature B-cell differentiation signatures ("IRX-undifferentiated" cluster) possessed 100% frequency and the heaviest burden of RAS pathway mutations, and moreover a distinct poor prognosis compared to the other four groups. These novel techniques may refine risk stratifications in infant ALL in the future.

11.3 Treatment of Infant KMT2A-r ALL

11.3.1 Chemotherapy

As with ALL in older children, conventional chemotherapy is still a mainstay of treating infants with ALL. A "hybrid chemotherapy" incorporating acute myeloid leukemia (AML)-like drugs (e.g., cytarabine) to ALL chemotherapy backbone is generally used to treat infants with ALL based on in vitro drug sensitivity assays of infant ALL cells demonstrating high sensitivity to cytarabine while showing high resistance against major key ALL drugs such as prednisone and asparaginase [19]. The greater cytarabine sensitivity of infant ALL blasts is explained by the high expression of human equilibrative nucleoside transporter 1 (hENT1), which cytarabine mainly depends on to permeate the cell membrane [20]. Currently, all the major study groups adopt an identical induction therapy based on Interfant-99/Interfant-06, adding cytarabine to typical four-drug pediatric ALL induction, which enables more than 90% of the patients to obtain complete remission (CR) (Fig. 11.2a) [5, 11].

One of the issues of infant ALL chemotherapy rather lies in the post-induction phase because nearly half of the patients in remission eventually relapse in the relatively early phase of the treatment (usually 4–5 months after achieving CR). A failure of improving the outcome of infants with ALL by intensifying delayed intensification phase with "VIMARAM (combination of high-dose cytarabine, high-dose methotrexate, and others)" in the Interfant-99 study lead the Interfant group to intensify early intensification phase with two courses of AML-like chemotherapy (ADE [cytarabine, daunorubicin, and etoposide] followed by MAE [cytarabine, mitoxantrone, and etoposide]) comparing with a single course

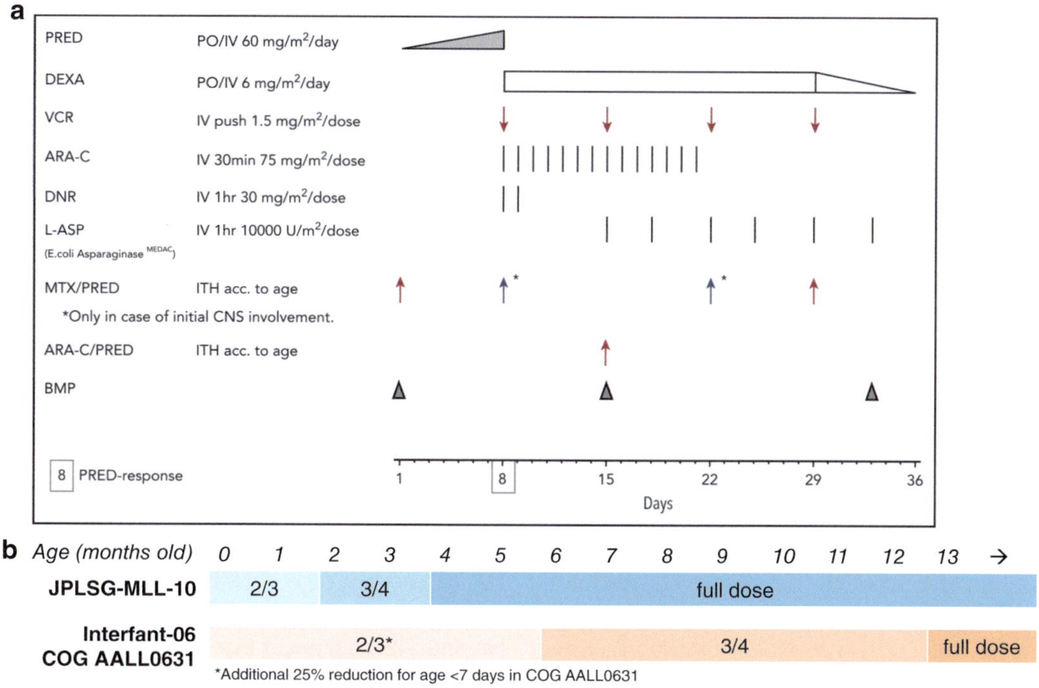

Fig. 11.2 (**a**) Interfant induction (Brown et al. [1]) and (**b**) age-related dose modification criteria in three major study groups (Interfant, COG, JPLSG) (authors' original work). *ARA-C* cytarabine, *BMP* bone marrow procedure, *DEXA* dexamethasone, *DNR* daunorubicin, *ITH* intrathecal, *L-ASP*, L-asparaginase, *MTX* methotrexate, *PRED* prednisone, *VCR* vincristine

of ALL-like chemotherapy "IB (cyclophosphamide, 6-mercaptopurine, and cytarabine)" in the Interfant-06 study [5, 11]. Although the 6-year disease-free survival (DFS) was not different between the two approaches as a whole (39.3% vs. 36.8%, $P = 0.47$), patients with negative PCR-based MRD at EOI showed a significantly better DFS with ALL-like consolidation, while those with high EOI-MRD showed a better DFS with AML-like consolidations [21]. Thus, levels of MRD following the Interfant-based induction might be useful to select appropriate consolidation chemotherapies for infants with KMT2A-r ALL. The JCCG is testing clofarabine/high-dose cytarabine combination in early and delayed consolidation phases in their currently ongoing MLL-17 study (jrct.niph.go.jp, jRCTs041190043). Clofarabine is a second-generation purine nucleoside analog and have shown highest in vitro activity among all the nucleoside analogs as well as synergistic cytotoxicity in combination with cytarabine to infant KMT2A-r ALL cells [22]. Additionally, clofarabine induces demethylation of the promoter region of a tumor suppressor gene *FHIT (fragile histidine triad)* which is often hypermethylated in infant KMT2A-r ALL. Anyhow, role of early consolidation to achieve negative MRD state at EOC seems to be extremely important to improve the outcome of infants with KMT2A-r ALL: 60.2% DFS rate was achieved in patients with negative EOC-MRD in Interfant-06, and this is also supported by the JPLSG study MLL-10 showing 66.7% EFS rate in patients with positive EOI-MRD (flow cytometry-based) but successfully achieving negative EOC-MRD [5, 7].

Another issue on chemotherapy for infant ALL is that pharmacokinetic (PK) and pharmacodynamic (PD) data for most of the chemotherapeutic drugs currently used are lacking or very limited in this age group [23–27]. PK in infants is influenced by many age-specific factors: higher percentage of total and extracellular body water content than older children or adults, higher unbound active fraction of drugs because of lower affinity of drugs to serum protein, lower P450 enzyme activity, lower tubular and glomerular function, and lower bodyweight-to-body surface area ratio [28]. Currently, each cooperative study group is adjusting the dose according to age of the patients based on anecdotal evidence; however, these doses are generally based on tolerability rather than on therapeutic effect (Fig. 11.2b). Recently, 3-year EFS rate of 66.2% in infants with KMT2A-r ALL was reported in the JPLSG-MLL-10 study, and one of the factors for its extraordinary favorable outcome is speculated as a result of adopting less stringent age-related dose modification compared to the Interfant or COG studies, thus enabled to achieve a rapid MRD clearance at EOI [7]. Therefore, this Japanese schedule for dose modification is used in the new Interfant-21 study (clinicaltrials.gov, NCT05327894) in which the Interfant and JCCG joined forces.

11.3.2 Hematopoietic Stem Cell Transplantation

There is a controversy over the role of allogeneic hematopoietic stem cell transplantation (HSCT) as a curative option for infants with ALL. A retrospective analysis of children and young adults with KMT2A-r ALL treated by 11 cooperative groups and single institutions in the United States and Europe did not demonstrate improved DFS and overall survival (OS) in infants with t(4;11) ALL who underwent any HSCT compared to those who underwent chemotherapy alone [29]. Combined analysis of the studies Children's Cancer Group (CCG) 1953 and Pediatric Oncology Group (POG) 9407 showed a 5-year EFS rate of 48.8% in infants who received HSCT vs. 48.7% in infants who received chemotherapy alone ($P = 0.60$) [30]. Given these negative results on benefit of HSCT, the recent COG infant ALL studies have eliminated an indication of HSCT for infants with ALL in the first CR (Table 11.1). On the other hand, analysis of the Interfant-99 study demonstrated a benefit of HSCT in the small (20% of all infant ALL) high-risk subset of infants with KMT2A-r ALL (age < 6 months old at diagnosis with either prednisone poor responder or WBC ≥300,000/μL) in terms of DFS (59.0% vs. 22.7%, $P = 0.01$) and OS (66.0% vs. 19.3%, $P = 0.001$) rates [31]. Therefore, indication of HSCT was restricted to infants with HR group in the Interfant-06 study [5]. Although only 76 out of the 143 HR patients who reached CR received HSCT due to an early event before HSCT could be performed, their 4-year DFS after HSCT was 44.0% (the 6-year EFS of all 164 HR patients was 20.9%). However, considering that the 4-year DFS of the medium-risk group infants with MRD $\geq 10^{-4}$ who had received HSCT was only 18.8%, the role of HSCT seems to be limited for infants with positive MRD. In the JPLSG-MLL-10, HSCT was also restricted to the HR cases only (age < 180 days at diagnosis or presence of CNS leukemia). Among the 56 HR patients, 43 underwent HSCT in the first CR and 29 patients were in continuous CR (the 3-year EFS of all 56 HR patients was 56.8%) [32].

A retrospective study on 132 infants with KMT2A-r ALL using nationwide registry data in Japan has demonstrated no difference in relapse, non-relapse mortality, and OS regarding donor type and conditioning [33]. Considering the risk of late effects, myeloablative conditioning without total body irradiation (e.g., busulfan/etoposide/cyclophosphamide used in JPLSG-MLL-10 or fludarabine/treosulfan (or busulfan)/thiotepa used in Interfant-06) would be a preferred choice for transplanting infants with KMT2A-r ALL [34]. However, cautions are needed because busulfan-based conditioning is associated with risk of sinusoidal obstruction syndrome and/or pulmonary complications, which could be life-threatening. The MLL-10 data show that these complications may occur even if the target AUC of busulfan has been set properly by therapeutic drug monitoring (TDM) [32].

According to the Interfant-06 and the JPLSG-MLL-10 data, HSCT seems to offer a durable remission in 40–50% of the infants with high-risk features. Therefore, HSCT should remain as a therapeutic option for selected patients at the current moment. However, considering its limited efficacy for truly unfavorable patients (e.g.,

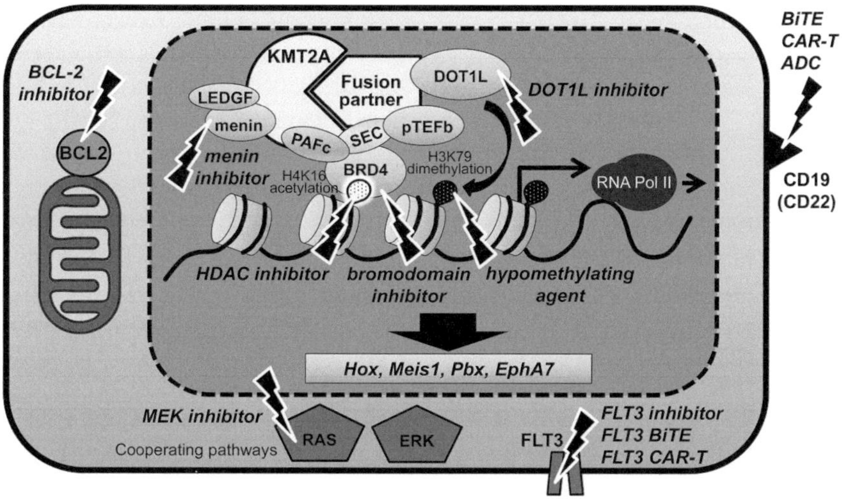

Fig. 11.3 Potential targets and targeted therapy for infants with KMT2A-rearranged ALL (Tomizawa et al. [7]). *ADC* antibody-drug conjugate, *BiTE* bispecific T-cell engager, *CAR-T* chimeric antigen receptor T cell

MRD-positive cases) and its potential risk of both acute and late toxicities, HSCT should be replaced by promising novel therapies in the future.

11.3.3 Novel Therapies

It is obvious that further improvement in the outcome of infant KMT2A-r ALL is unlikely to be achieved by conventional chemotherapy with or without HSCT. Outcome of relapsed/refractory infant ALL is even poorer with approximately 20% OS rate and there is no standardized approach for these patients [35, 36]. Therefore, novel therapeutic options should be explored and introduced to contemporary therapy for infant ALL (Fig. 11.3). Additionally, international collaboration is important given the rarity of the disease. Development of several novel therapies with effort on international collaboration among the Interfant, COG, and JCCG is currently underway.

11.3.3.1 Immunotherapies

Immunotherapies targeting CD19 and/or CD22 are emerging as attractive therapeutic options especially for relapsed/refractory B-lineage ALL. Blinatumomab, a CD19/CD3 bispecific T-cell engaging antibody, has shown a promising effect and safety for 11 patients with relapsed/refractory KMT2A-r ALL who had been initially diagnosed during infancy in the United Kingdom and Ireland: nine patients became MRD negative and two patients had a > 1-log reduction in MRD, and all patients proceeded to HSCT without intervening therapy (3-year post-transplant EFS and OS was 47% and 81%, respectively) [37]. There is a concern on risk of CD19-negative ALL relapse and/or myeloid lineage switch when CD19-targeted immunotherapy is administered especially to KMT2A-r ALL cases [38]; however, only one AML lineage switched case was observed in this series. Interfant group conducted a single-arm pilot phase II study testing the feasibility, safety, and efficacy of blinatumomab combining with the Interfant-06 chemotherapy backbone [39]. A single course of blinatumomab was given after initial induction chemotherapy followed by the Interfant-06 schedule. Among the 30 infants with newly diagnosed KMT2A-r ALL, 28 patients (93%) became MRD negative or not quantifiable (<0.05%) post-blinatumomab course and 2-year DFS rate was 81.6%. Given the promising result of the pilot study, blinatumomab-combined therapy will be evaluated in a larger number of patients in the next international non-randomized phase 3 study Interfant-21.

Inotuzumab ozogamicin, a CD22-targeted antibody conjugated with calicheamicin, is also drawing attention as a promising agent for B-lineage ALL, but low levels of CD22 expression in KMT2A-r ALL might be a limitation for its use in infants with KMT2A-r ALL. An international retrospective analysis on 12 infants and three young children (<3 years old) with relapsed/refractory ALL treated with inotuzumab are reported: seven patients (46%) achieved CR and one MRD-positive patient turned MRD negative (<0.01%), and five patients had no response [40].

Finally, chimeric antigen receptor (CAR) T-cell therapy is expected as a curative option for infant ALL. According to the retrospective analysis from the Pediatric Real-World CAR Consortium in the United States, 14 infants with relapsed/refractory B-ALL (12 KMT2A-r, one KMT2A-g, and one unknown) who had received tisagenlecleucel were identified [41]. Nine patients (64%) achieved MRD-negative CR and seven of these patients (50%) remained in CR at the last follow-up with only one patient undergoing HSCT after CAR-T. Disease status at CAR-T infusion is one of the most important factors to predict post-CAR-T relapse, and all nine responders were in morphological CR, while all five refractory patients had high disease burden (>5% bone marrow blasts) before CAR-T infusion. There is a controversy whether prior blinatumomab exposure would affect CAR-T outcome, but all three patients with previous history of blinatumomab use had responded. This is in line with the recent paper showing that only patients not responding to blinatumomab have a poorer response to CAR-T cell therapy [42]. Myeloid lineage switch was observed in four patients (one responder and three nonresponders to CAR-T). Overall, tisagenlecleucel was tolerable in these patients with only three patients experiencing ≥grade 3 cytokine release syndrome and no neurotoxicity was observed. A recent European study on tisagenlecleucel use in young KMT2A-r relapsed children showed comparable responses but no lineage switches [43]. Also, autologous CAR-T cells were successfully generated in these small children. Thus, CAR-T seems to be a promising therapeutic option for infants, although the data are still limited. Others have reported that generating autologous CAR-T cells in infants may be challenging because of small patient size, high leukemia burden, and heavily pretreated status which would result in impaired host T-cell function and expansion. Recently, two successful infant cases with relapsed KMT2A-r ALL who received third-party CD19 CAR-T cells were reported [44]. This "off-the-shelf" allogeneic CAR-T was manufactured by disrupting TCR alpha and CD52 to avoid rejection and graft-versus-host disease (GVHD) by a gene-editing technique. Unlike autologous CAR-T, response duration of allogeneic CAR-T seems shorter [45]; thus, allogeneic CAR-T will need subsequent HSCT after CAR-T. Despite such limitations, allogeneic CAR-T would offer an important therapeutic option for those who failed T-cell apheresis or further CAR-T manufacturing process.

11.3.3.2 FLT3 Inhibitors

Gene-expression profile studies have shown a unique pattern of infant KMT2A-r ALL. One of the highly expressed is *fms-related tyrosine kinase 3* (*FLT3*) gene, which was associated with poor prognosis [46]. COG has evaluated in their AALL0631 study whether the FLT3 inhibitor lestaurtinib improves EFS for infants with newly diagnosed KMT2A-r ALL in combination with post-induction chemotherapy [4]. Overall, no significant difference in 3-year EFS was observed (36% in lestaurtinib arm vs. 39% in chemotherapy arm, $P = 0.67$), but the patients who had shown both inhibition of FLT3-activated cell line by lestaurtinib-treated patient plasma (FLT3 inhibitor PD assay) and ex vivo sensitivity of patient diagnostic blasts to lestaurtinib (FLT3 inhibitor ex vivo assay) demonstrated 88% EFS rate. Unlike the conventional cytotoxic drugs, selection of appropriate patients who would benefit from the drug by individualized approach might be necessary to truly enhance the effect of certain molecularly targeted agents.

11.3.3.3 Epigenetic Agents

Recent genomic studies have revealed that infant KMT2A-r leukemia cells are characterized by aberrant methylated genomic state with very few cooperating gene alterations [47]. Its leukemogenesis is driven by leukemia-specific histone modifications such as H3K79 dimethylation induced via DOT1L recruitment by KMT2A fusion proteins, which leads to site-specific hypermethylation and to aberrant transcription of leukemogenic genes [48, 49]. Thus, epigenetic modifiers such as hypomethylating agents (e.g., azacytidine, decitabine) and/or histone deacetylase inhibitors (e.g., vorinostat, panobinostat) are attractive targeting agents for infant KMT2A-r ALL [50–52]. A pilot study testing azacytidine in combination with Interfant-backbone chemotherapy was conducted in the COG AALL15P1 study, however, EFS was similar to the previous infant ALL studies [53]. In the early clinical trial testing single-agent DOT1L inhibitor pinometostat for adults and children with KMT2A-r leukemia, clinical activity was unfortunately modest [54].

11.3.3.4 BCL-2 Inhibitors

BCL-2 family proteins regulate the intrinsic apoptosis pathway by integrating diverse prosurvival or proapoptotic intracellular signals. Recent studies revealed that *KMT2A* rearrangement directly induces BCL-2 overexpression in ALL cells by promoting DOT1L-mediated H3K79 methylation at the *BCL2* locus [55]. BCL-2 inhibitor venetoclax has shown potent in vitro and in vivo single-agent activity against KMT2A-r ALL and synergized with standard ALL induction chemotherapy in a xenograft model. A study plan incorporating venetoclax/azacytidine therapy in blinatumomab-combined chemotherapy is currently underway by the COG.

11.3.3.5 Menin Inhibitors

Menin is a product of *MEN1* tumor suppressor gene which binds to the rearranged KMT2A complex and leads to the upregulation of leukemogenic genes such as *HOX* and *MEIS1*, and thus to subsequent development of acute leukemia [56, 57]. Menin inhibitors bind to the KMT2A pocket on menin and block the interaction between menin and KMT2A, and rapidly suppress KMT2A target gene expression and remodel chromatin-associated complexes. Menin inhibitors have shown selective, profound single agent activity in KMT2A-r PDX models. Phase 1/2 clinical trials testing menin inhibitors for relapsed/refractory acute leukemia are already underway and have demonstrated promising results [58].

11.4 Treatment of Infant KMT2A-g ALL

KMT2A-g ALL accounts for 20–30% of infant ALL and confers distinct characteristics and prognosis to KMT2A-r ALL [5–7]. Ninety percent of the KMT2A-g ALL cases present as B-lymphoblastic (majority are CD10-positive) and 4–10% as T-lymphoblastic leukemia. Clinically, infants with KMT2A-g ALL are diagnosed at older age (majority are over 6 months old) and with lower WBC count. Biologically, frequency of cytogenetic abnormalities commonly seen in pediatric ALL, such as *ETV6::RUNX1* or high hyperdiploidy, are rarely seen and have distinct gene expression pattern that is both different from infant KMT2A-r ALL and pediatric non-infant B-ALL [59]. Recently, fusions of *NUTM1* located at chromosome 15q14 were identified in 20–30% of the infants with KMT2A-g ALL [60]. Infants with *NUTM1*-rearranged ALL were relatively young (54% were < 6 months old at diagnosis) and showed excellent response at EOI (91% had MRD <0.05%), and excellent outcome (100% EFS and OS in 4 years). In addition, rearrangement of *PAX5* gene have been detected in 20% of the infants with KMT2A-g ALL, and in contrast to the *NUTM1*-rearranged cases, patients were older and had unfavorable outcome (3-year EFS rate of 25%) [61]. In addition to leukemia biology, MRD ≥0.05% at EOI was significantly associated with poor outcome among infants with KMT2A-g ALL in the Interfant-06 study [62]. Majority of infants with KMT2A-g ALL could be cured with a uniform conventional chemotherapy specifically designed for infants, and EFS rate of the recently completed clinical trials range from 73.9% to 93.3% (Table 11.1, Fig. 11.1a, b) [5–7].

Given the recent discovery on biological backgrounds on infant KMT2A-g ALL, it might be appropriate to treat these patients with risk-stratified therapy based on cytogenetic abnormalities and MRD in the same context with pediatric non-infant ALL.

11.5 Toxicities and Supportive Care on Infant ALL Treatment

Given the vulnerability of infants to cytotoxic agents, toxicity management is extremely important. Particularly during the remission induction phase, infants are at high risk of tumor lysis syndrome and intracranial hemorrhage because of the high leukemic burden in KMT2A-r ALL. To prevent severe tumor lysis syndrome, use of rasburicase is strongly recommended in cases with high WBC and, although controversies exist, exchange transfusion or leukapheresis should be considered for patients presenting with very high WBC (e.g., ≥500,000/μL) [63]. Infectious management is also critical when treating infants with ALL: broad-spectrum intravenous antibiotics for fever and neutropenia; consideration of antifungal prophylaxis in addition to empiric antifungal therapy for persistent or recurrent fever after 3–5 days of broad-spectrum antibiotics; prophylaxis against *Pneumocystis jirovecii.* Other measures that may be considered although their use has not been proven are prophylaxis against respiratory syncytial virus with palivizumab; intravenous immunoglobulin (IVIG) therapy for infants with IgG levels <500 mg/dL; prophylactic use of granulocyte colony stimulating factor; and full hospitalization (at least during induction) until evidence of marrow recovery [7, 64, 65].

Infants are also at high risk of developing late toxicities. In the French study evaluating 113 patients with infant leukemia (55 were ALL) with a median follow-up period of 11.7 years, at least one complication was observed in 84 (74.3%) patients. The most frequent late effect was growth failure (47.8%), followed by overweight (22.1%), low weight (21.2%), gonadal dysfunction (13.8%), hypothyroidism (10.6%), cardiac dysfunction (8%), CNS complication (5.3%), hyperferritinemia (5.1%), cataract (4.4%), and secondary tumor (4.4%) [66]. In particular, infant ALL survivors those who underwent HSCT are at highest risk, and various late effects are observed in the Japanese MLL96 and MLL98 cohort such as chronic GVHD, hypothyroidism, skin abnormalities, ophthalmologic complications, pulmonary complications, dental abnormalities, and neurocognitive problems [10]. In addition, there have been a case series report on fatal secondary T-cell immunodeficiency soon after the completion of chemotherapy [67]. It is not clear whether this phenomenon is derived from age-related, therapy-related, or disease-related factors. According to the retrospective survey among the JPLSG-MLL-10 cohort, severe chemotherapy-induced immunodeficiency in infants with ALL appears to be rare [68]. But close monitoring on immune function should be considered for follow-up of infant ALL patients.

References

1. Brown P, Pieters R, Biondi A. How I treat infant leukemia. Blood. 2019;133(3):205–14.
2. Meyer C, Larghero P, Almeida Lopes B, Burmeister T, Groger D, Sutton R, et al. The KMT2A recombinome of acute leukemias in 2023. Leukemia. 2023;37(5):988–1005.
3. Sakaki H, Kanegane H, Nomura K, Goi K, Sugita K, Miura M, et al. Early lineage switch in an infant acute lymphoblastic leukemia. Int J Hematol. 2009;90(5):653–5.
4. Brown PA, Kairalla JA, Hilden JM, Dreyer ZE, Carroll AJ, Heerema NA, et al. FLT3 inhibitor lestaurtinib plus chemotherapy for newly diagnosed KMT2A-rearranged infant acute lymphoblastic leukemia: children's oncology group trial AALL0631. Leukemia. 2021;35(5):1279–90.
5. Pieters R, De Lorenzo P, Ancliffe P, Aversa LA, Brethon B, Biondi A, et al. Outcome of infants younger than 1 year with acute lymphoblastic leukemia treated with the Interfant-06 protocol: results from an international phase III randomized study. J Clin Oncol. 2019;37(25):2246–56.
6. Guest EM, Kairalla JA, Hilden JM, Dreyer ZE, Carroll AJ, Heerema NA, et al. Outstanding outcomes in infants with KMT2A-germline acute lymphoblastic leukemia treated with chemotherapy alone: results of the children's oncology group AALL0631 trial. Haematologica. 2022;107(5):1205–8.
7. Tomizawa D, Miyamura T, Imamura T, Watanabe T, Moriya Saito A, Ogawa A, et al. A risk-stratified

therapy for infants with acute lymphoblastic leukemia: a report from the JPLSG MLL-10 trial. Blood. 2020;136(16):1813–23.
8. Kotecha RS, Gottardo NG, Kees UR, Cole CH. The evolution of clinical trials for infant acute lymphoblastic leukemia. Blood Cancer J. 2014;4(4):e200.
9. Hilden JM, Dinndorf PA, Meerbaum SO, Sather H, Villaluna D, Heerema NA, et al. Analysis of prognostic factors of acute lymphoblastic leukemia in infants: report on CCG 1953 from the children's oncology group. Blood. 2006;108(2):441–51.
10. Tomizawa D, Koh K, Sato T, Kinukawa N, Morimoto A, Isoyama K, et al. Outcome of risk-based therapy for infant acute lymphoblastic leukemia with or without an MLL gene rearrangement, with emphasis on late effects: a final report of two consecutive studies, MLL96 and MLL98, of the Japan infant leukemia study group. Leukemia. 2007;21(11):2258–63.
11. Pieters R, Schrappe M, De Lorenzo P, Hann I, De Rossi G, Felice M, et al. A treatment protocol for infants younger than 1 year with acute lymphoblastic leukaemia (Interfant-99): an observational study and a multicentre randomised trial. Lancet. 2007;370(9583):240–50.
12. Reiter A, Schrappe M, Ludwig WD, Hiddemann W, Sauter S, Henze G, et al. Chemotherapy in 998 unselected childhood acute lymphoblastic leukemia patients. Results and conclusions of the multicenter trial ALL-BFM 86. Blood. 1994;84(9):3122–33.
13. Dordelmann M, Reiter A, Borkhardt A, Ludwig WD, Gotz N, Viehmann S, et al. Prednisone response is the strongest predictor of treatment outcome in infant acute lymphoblastic leukemia. Blood. 1999;94(4):1209–17.
14. Campana D, Pui CH. Minimal residual disease-guided therapy in childhood acute lymphoblastic leukemia. Blood. 2017;129(14):1913–8.
15. Van der Velden VH, Corral L, Valsecchi MG, Jansen MW, De Lorenzo P, Cazzaniga G, et al. Prognostic significance of minimal residual disease in infants with acute lymphoblastic leukemia treated within the Interfant-99 protocol. Leukemia. 2009;23(6):1073–9.
16. Jansen MW, Corral L, van der Velden VH, Panzer-Grumayer R, Schrappe M, Schrauder A, et al. Immunobiological diversity in infant acute lymphoblastic leukemia is related to the occurrence and type of MLL gene rearrangement. Leukemia. 2007;21(4):633–41.
17. Faham M, Zheng J, Moorhead M, Carlton VE, Stow P, Coustan-Smith E, et al. Deep-sequencing approach for minimal residual disease detection in acute lymphoblastic leukemia. Blood. 2012;120(26):5173–80.
18. Isobe T, Takagi M, Sato-Otsubo A, Nishimura A, Nagae G, Yamagishi C, et al. Multi-omics analysis defines highly refractory RAS burdened immature subgroup of infant acute lymphoblastic leukemia. Nat Commun. 2022;13(1):4501.
19. Pieters R, den Boer ML, Durian M, Janka G, Schmiegelow K, Kaspers GJ, et al. Relation between age, immunophenotype and in vitro drug resistance in 395 children with acute lymphoblastic leukemia – implications for treatment of infants. Leukemia. 1998;12(9):1344–8.
20. Stam RW, den Boer ML, Meijerink JP, Ebus ME, Peters GJ, Noordhuis P, et al. Differential mRNA expression of Ara-C-metabolizing enzymes explains Ara-C sensitivity in MLL gene-rearranged infant acute lymphoblastic leukemia. Blood. 2003;101(4):1270–6.
21. Stutterheim J, van der Sluis IM, de Lorenzo P, Alten J, Ancliffe P, Attarbaschi A, et al. Clinical implications of minimal residual disease detection in infants with KMT2A-rearranged acute lymphoblastic leukemia treated on the Interfant-06 protocol. J Clin Oncol. 2021;39(6):652–62.
22. Stumpel DJ, Schneider P, Pieters R, Stam RW. The potential of clofarabine in MLL-rearranged infant acute lymphoblastic leukaemia. Eur J Cancer. 2015;51(14):2008–21.
23. Thompson PA, Murry DJ, Rosner GL, Lunagomez S, Blaney SM, Berg SL, et al. Methotrexate pharmacokinetics in infants with acute lymphoblastic leukemia. Cancer Chemother Pharmacol. 2007;59(6):847–53.
24. Lonnerholm G, Valsecchi MG, De Lorenzo P, Schrappe M, Hovi L, Campbell M, et al. Pharmacokinetics of high-dose methotrexate in infants treated for acute lymphoblastic leukemia. Pediatr Blood Cancer. 2009;52(5):596–601.
25. Albertsen BK, Harila-Saari A, Jahnukainen K, Lahteenmaki P, Riikonen P, Mottonen M, et al. Asparaginase treatment in infants with acute lymphoblastic leukemia; pharmacokinetics and asparaginase hypersensitivity in Interfant-06. Leuk Lymphoma. 2019;60(6):1469–75.
26. Takachi T, Arakawa Y, Nakamura H, Watanabe T, Aoki Y, Ohshima J, et al. Personalized pharmacokinetic targeting with busulfan in allogeneic hematopoietic stem cell transplantation in infants with acute lymphoblastic leukemia. Int J Hematol. 2019;110(3):355–63.
27. Barnett S, Hellmann F, Parke E, Makin G, Tweddle DA, Osborne C, et al. Vincristine dosing, drug exposure and therapeutic drug monitoring in neonate and infant cancer patients. Eur J Cancer. 2022;164:127–36.
28. Kearns GL, Abdel-Rahman SM, Alander SW, Blowey DL, Leeder JS, Kauffman RE. Developmental pharmacology – drug disposition, action, and therapy in infants and children. N Engl J Med. 2003;349(12):1157–67.
29. Pui CH, Gaynon PS, Boyett JM, Chessells JM, Baruchel A, Kamps W, et al. Outcome of treatment in childhood acute lymphoblastic leukaemia with rearrangements of the 11q23 chromosomal region. Lancet. 2002;359(9321):1909–15.
30. Dreyer ZE, Dinndorf PA, Camitta B, Sather H, La MK, Devidas M, et al. Analysis of the role of hematopoietic stem-cell transplantation in infants with acute lymphoblastic leukemia in first remission and MLL gene rearrangements: a report from the children's oncology group. J Clin Oncol. 2011;29(2):214–22.
31. Mann G, Attarbaschi A, Schrappe M, De Lorenzo P, Peters C, Hann I, et al. Improved outcome with

hematopoietic stem cell transplantation in a poor prognostic subgroup of infants with mixed-lineage-leukemia (MLL)-rearranged acute lymphoblastic leukemia: results from the Interfant-99 study. Blood. 2010;116(15):2644–50.

32. Takachi T, Watanabe T, Miyamura T, Moriya Saito A, Deguchi T, Hori T, et al. Hematopoietic stem cell transplantation for infants with high-risk KMT2A gene-rearranged acute lymphoblastic leukemia. Blood Adv. 2021;5(19):3891–9.
33. Kato M, Hasegawa D, Koh K, Kato K, Takita J, Inagaki J, et al. Allogeneic haematopoietic stem cell transplantation for infant acute lymphoblastic leukaemia with KMT2A (MLL) rearrangements: a retrospective study from the paediatric acute lymphoblastic leukaemia working group of the Japan Society for Haematopoietic Cell Transplantation. Br J Haematol. 2015;168(4):564–70.
34. Balduzzi A, Buechner J, Ifversen M, Dalle JH, Colita AM, Bierings M. Acute lymphoblastic Leukaemia in the youngest: Haematopoietic stem cell transplantation and beyond. Front Pediatr. 2022;10:807992.
35. Tomizawa D, Koh K, Hirayama M, Miyamura T, Hatanaka M, Saikawa Y, et al. Outcome of recurrent or refractory acute lymphoblastic leukemia in infants with MLL gene rearrangements: a report from the Japan infant leukemia study group. Pediatr Blood Cancer. 2009;52(7):808–13.
36. Driessen EM, de Lorenzo P, Campbell M, Felice M, Ferster A, Hann I, et al. Outcome of relapsed infant acute lymphoblastic leukemia treated on the interfant-99 protocol. Leukemia. 2016;30(5):1184–7.
37. Clesham K, Rao V, Bartram J, Ancliff P, Ghorashian S, O'Connor D, et al. Blinatumomab for infant acute lymphoblastic leukemia. Blood. 2020;135(17):1501–4.
38. Wolfl M, Rasche M, Eyrich M, Schmid R, Reinhardt D, Schlegel PG. Spontaneous reversion of a lineage switch following an initial blinatumomab-induced ALL-to-AML switch in MLL-rearranged infant ALL. Blood Adv. 2018;2(12):1382–5.
39. van der Sluis IM, de Lorenzo P, Kotecha RS, Attarbaschi A, Escherich G, Nysom K, et al. Blinatumomab added to chemotherapy in infant lymphoblastic leukemia. N Engl J Med. 2023;388(17):1572–81.
40. Brivio E, Chantrain CF, Gruber TA, Thano A, Rialland F, Contet A, et al. Inotuzumab ozogamicin in infants and young children with relapsed or refractory acute lymphoblastic leukaemia: a case series*. Br J Haematol. 2021;193(6):1172–7.
41. Moskop A, Pommert L, Baggott C, Prabhu S, Pacenta HL, Phillips CL, et al. Real-world use of tisagenlecleucel in infant acute lymphoblastic leukemia. Blood Adv. 2022;6(14):4251–5.
42. Myers RM, Taraseviciute A, Steinberg SM, Lamble AJ, Sheppard J, Yates B, et al. Blinatumomab nonresponse and high-disease burden are associated with inferior outcomes after CD19-CAR for B-ALL. J Clin Oncol. 2022;40(9):932–44.
43. Ghorashian S, Jacoby E, De Moerloose B, Rives S, Bonney D, Shenton G, et al. Tisagenlecleucel therapy for relapsed or refractory B-cell acute lymphoblastic leukaemia in infants and children younger than 3 years of age at screening: an international, multicentre, retrospective cohort study. Lancet Haematol. 2022;9(10):e766–e75.
44. Qasim W, Zhan H, Samarasinghe S, Adams S, Amrolia P, Stafford S, et al. Molecular remission of infant B-ALL after infusion of universal TALEN gene-edited CAR T cells. Sci Transl Med. 2017;9(374):eaaj2013.
45. Benjamin R, Graham C, Yallop D, Jozwik A, Mirci-Danicar OC, Lucchini G, et al. Genome-edited, donor-derived allogeneic anti-CD19 chimeric antigen receptor T cells in paediatric and adult B-cell acute lymphoblastic leukaemia: results of two phase 1 studies. Lancet. 2020;396(10266):1885–94.
46. Armstrong SA, Staunton JE, Silverman LB, Pieters R, den Boer ML, Minden MD, et al. MLL translocations specify a distinct gene expression profile that distinguishes a unique leukemia. Nat Genet. 2002;30(1):41–7.
47. Andersson AK, Ma J, Wang J, Chen X, Gedman AL, Dang J, et al. The landscape of somatic mutations in infant MLL-rearranged acute lymphoblastic leukemias. Nat Genet. 2015;47(4):330–7.
48. Krivtsov AV, Armstrong SA. MLL translocations, histone modifications and leukaemia stem-cell development. Nat Rev Cancer. 2007;7(11):823–33.
49. Stumpel DJ, Schotte D, Lange-Turenhout EA, Schneider P, Seslija L, de Menezes RX, et al. Hypermethylation of specific microRNA genes in MLL-rearranged infant acute lymphoblastic leukemia: major matters at a micro scale. Leukemia. 2011;25(3):429–39.
50. Stumpel DJ, Schneider P, van Roon EH, Boer JM, de Lorenzo P, Valsecchi MG, et al. Specific promoter methylation identifies different subgroups of MLL-rearranged infant acute lymphoblastic leukemia, influences clinical outcome, and provides therapeutic options. Blood. 2009;114(27):5490–8.
51. Stumpel DJ, Schneider P, Seslija L, Osaki H, Williams O, Pieters R, et al. Connectivity mapping identifies HDAC inhibitors for the treatment of t(4;11)-positive infant acute lymphoblastic leukemia. Leukemia. 2012;26(4):682–92.
52. Garrido Castro P, van Roon EHJ, Pinhancos SS, Trentin L, Schneider P, Kerstjens M, et al. The HDAC inhibitor panobinostat (LBH589) exerts in vivo anti-leukaemic activity against MLL-rearranged acute lymphoblastic leukaemia and involves the RNF20/RNF40/WAC-H2B ubiquitination axis. Leukemia. 2018;32(2):323–31.
53. Guest EM, Kairalla JA, Devidas M, Hibbitts E, Carroll AJ, et al. Azacitidine as epigenetic priming for chemotherapy is safe and well-tolerated in infants with newly diagnosed KMT2A-rearranged acute lymphoblastic leukemia: Children's Oncology Group trial AALL15P1. Haematologica. 2024 [Epub ahead of print] https://doi.org/10.3324/haematol.2024.285158.

54. Stein EM, Garcia-Manero G, Rizzieri DA, Tibes R, Berdeja JG, Savona MR, et al. The DOT1L inhibitor pinometostat reduces H3K79 methylation and has modest clinical activity in adult acute leukemia. Blood. 2018;131(24):2661–9.
55. Benito JM, Godfrey L, Kojima K, Hogdal L, Wunderlich M, Geng H, et al. MLL-rearranged acute lymphoblastic Leukemias activate BCL-2 through H3K79 methylation and are sensitive to the BCL-2-specific antagonist ABT-199. Cell Rep. 2015;13(12):2715–27.
56. Yokoyama A, Somervaille TC, Smith KS, Rozenblatt-Rosen O, Meyerson M, Cleary ML. The menin tumor suppressor protein is an essential oncogenic cofactor for MLL-associated leukemogenesis. Cell. 2005;123(2):207–18.
57. Krivtsov AV, Evans K, Gadrey JY, Eschle BK, Hatton C, Uckelmann HJ, et al. A Menin-MLL inhibitor induces specific chromatin changes and eradicates disease in models of MLL-rearranged leukemia. Cancer Cell. 2019;36(6):660–73 e11.
58. Issa GC, Aldoss I, DiPersio J, Cuglievan B, Stone R, Arellano M, et al. The menin inhibitor revumenib in KMT2A-rearranged or NPM1-mutant leukaemia. Nature. 2023;615(7954):920–4.
59. Stam RW, Schneider P, Hagelstein JA, van der Linden MH, Stumpel DJ, de Menezes RX, et al. Gene expression profiling-based dissection of MLL translocated and MLL germline acute lymphoblastic leukemia in infants. Blood. 2010;115(14):2835–44.
60. Boer JM, Valsecchi MG, Hormann FM, Antic Z, Zaliova M, Schwab C, et al. Favorable outcome of NUTM1-rearranged infant and pediatric B cell precursor acute lymphoblastic leukemia in a collaborative international study. Leukemia. 2021;35(10):2978–82.
61. Fazio G, Bardini M, De Lorenzo P, Grioni A, Quadri M, Pedace L, et al. Recurrent genetic fusions redefine MLL germ line acute lymphoblastic leukemia in infants. Blood. 2021;137(14):1980–4.
62. Stutterheim J, de Lorenzo P, van der Sluis IM, Alten J, Ancliffe P, Attarbaschi A, et al. Minimal residual disease and outcome characteristics in infant KMT2A-germline acute lymphoblastic leukaemia treated on the Interfant-06 protocol. Eur J Cancer. 2022;160:72–9.
63. Nguyen R, Jeha S, Zhou Y, Cao X, Cheng C, Bhojwani D, et al. The role of Leukapheresis in the current management of hyperleukocytosis in newly diagnosed childhood acute lymphoblastic leukemia. Pediatr Blood Cancer. 2016;63(9):1546–51.
64. Salzer W, Dinndorf P, Dreyer Z, Hilden J, Reaman GH. Analysis of infectious complications in infants with acute lymphoblastic leukemia treated on the children's cancer group protocol 1953: a report from the children's oncology group. J Pediatr Hematol Oncol. 2009;31(6):398–405.
65. Salzer WL, Jones TL, Devidas M, Dreyer ZE, Gore L, Winick NJ, et al. Decreased induction morbidity and mortality following modification to induction therapy in infants with acute lymphoblastic leukemia enrolled on AALL0631: a report from the children's oncology group. Pediatr Blood Cancer. 2015;62(3):414–8.
66. Gandemer V, Bonneau J, Oudin C, Berbis J, Bertrand Y, Tabone MD, et al. Late effects in survivors of infantile acute leukemia: a study of the L.E.A program. Blood Cancer J. 2017;7(1):e518.
67. Geerlinks AV, Issekutz T, Wahlstrom JT, Sullivan KE, Cowan MJ, Dvorak CC, et al. Severe, persistent, and fatal T-cell immunodeficiency following therapy for infantile leukemia. Pediatr Blood Cancer. 2016;63(11):2046–9.
68. Arakawa Y, Hasegawa D, Miyamura T, Ohshima J, Kimura S, Imamura T, et al. Postchemotherapy immune status in infants with acute lymphoblastic leukemia: a report from the JPLSG MLL-10 trial. Pediatr Blood Cancer. 2022;69(10):e29772.

12 Clinical Management of Philadelphia Chromosome-Positive and ABL-Class Fusion-Positive Acute Lymphoblastic Leukemia

Thai Hoa Tran, Veronica Leoni, Nicolò Peccatori, Lewis B. Silverman, and Andrea Biondi

12.1 Introduction

Philadelphia chromosome-positive (Ph^+) acute lymphoblastic leukemia (ALL) is an ALL subtype defined by the canonical t(9;22)(q34;q11.2) translocation, which leads to the production of the constitutively active BCR::ABL1 oncoprotein. Historically, patients with Ph^+ ALL had unfavorable outcomes despite hematopoietic stem cell transplantation (HSCT) in first complete remission (CR1) [1, 2]. The development of molecularly targeted therapy with ABL-directed tyrosine kinase inhibitors (TKIs) such as imatinib, dasatinib, or ponatinib has dramatically improved the outcome of Ph^+ ALL. With this therapeutic advance, a high percentage of both pediatric and adult Ph^+ ALL patients can be cured with the combination of cytotoxic chemotherapy and TKI (without HSCT), establishing the first paradigm of successful molecularly targeted therapy in acute leukemias. Nevertheless, the outcome of Ph^+ ALL remains inferior compared to that of other ALL subtypes even in the TKI era [3–13].

Over the past two decades, advances in genomics have deepened our understanding of ALL biology and unraveled novel genomically defined subtypes with distinct prognostic and therapeutic significance. In 2009, a new subtype of B-ALL was identified by two independent groups under the name of Philadelphia chromosome-like (Ph-like) or *BCR::ABL1*-like ALL [14, 15]. Ph-like ALL occurs in approximately 15% of pediatric B-ALL (higher in those with high-risk features) and shares a similar gene expression profile with Ph^+ ALL despite the absence of the *BCR::ABL1* fusion. Ph-like ALL is characterized by a heterogeneous spectrum of kinase-activating alterations, including a ABL-

Authors Thai Hoa Tran and Veronica Leoni contributed equally as co-first authors.

T. H. Tran (✉)
Division of Pediatric Hematology-Oncology, Charles-Bruneau Cancer Center, CHU Sainte-Justine, Montreal, QC, Canada
e-mail: thai.hoa.tran@umontreal.ca

V. Leoni (✉)
Pediatrics, Fondazione IRCCS San Gerardo Dei Tintori, Monza, Italy

N. Peccatori
Tettamanti Center, Fondazione IRCCS San Gerardo dei Tintori, Monza, Italy

L. B. Silverman
Pediatric Hematology Oncology and Stem Cell Transplant, Columbia University Irving Medical Center, New York, NY, USA
e-mail: ls4119@cumc.columbia.edu

A. Biondi
Pediatrics, Fondazione IRCCS San Gerardo Dei Tintori, Monza, Italy

Tettamanti Center, Fondazione IRCCS San Gerardo dei Tintori, Monza, Italy

School of Medicine and Surgery, University of Milano-Bicocca, Monza, Italy

G. Escherich, V. Conter (eds.), *Acute Lymphoblastic Leukemia in Children and Adolescents*, Pediatric Oncology, https://doi.org/10.1007/978-3-031-71180-0_12

class gene rearrangements in approximately 15% of Ph-like cases, henceforth referred to as ABL-class Ph-like ALL or ABL-class fusion-positive ALL. Although Ph$^+$ and ABL-class Ph-like ALLs are now recognized by the WHO as two separate ALL entities, both exhibit similar biological and clinical features in terms of epidemiology, prognosis, and sensitivity to TKIs [16–24]. For these reasons, children and adults diagnosed with ABL-class fusion-positive ALL are currently eligible to be included jointly within Ph$^+$ ALL clinical trials.

In this chapter, the biology, epidemiology, and clinical features of pediatric Ph$^+$ ALL and ABL-class fusions-positive ALL will be reviewed. Subsequently, an overview of past, current, and future treatment strategies for these two ALL subtypes will be discussed.

12.2 Biology of Ph$^+$ ALL and ABL-Class Fusion-Positive ALL

The Philadelphia chromosome was first discovered by Nowell and Hungerford in 1960 in the city that it was named after and became the first genetic abnormality identified in human cancer [25]. Dr. Janet Rowley demonstrated in 1973 that the Philadelphia chromosome resulted from the reciprocal t(9;22)(q34;q11.2) translocation, which encoded the chimeric BCR::ABL1 oncoprotein [26]. The *BCR::ABL1* fusion gene joins the entire coding region of *ABL1* (exons 2–11) of chromosome 9 to the *BCR* gene on chromosome 22. There are two major regions within the *BCR* gene where breakpoints typically occur; the major breakpoint cluster region (M-BCR) lies between exons 12 and 16, and the minor breakpoint cluster region (m-BCR) encompasses the first two exons 1 and 2. Translocations involving the M-BCR generate the larger p210 BCR::ABL1 fusion protein which accounts for the majority of chronic myeloid leukemia (CML) cases, whereas translocations within the m-BCR region encode for the smaller p190 BCR::ABL1 transcript protein that arises in approximately 90% of pediatric Ph$^+$ ALL [4]. The molecular consequence of the *BCR::ABL1* oncogene derives from the constitutive ABL1 kinase activity and aberrant phosphorylation of downstream pathways, as a result of lack of autoinhibition from the loss of the N-terminal regulatory domain of ABL1 and homodimerization and autophosphorylation of the oncoprotein [4]. *BCR::ABL1* fusion gene acts as a leukemia-initiating driver alteration as several preclinical studies have demonstrated its transforming capacity within cell lines and murine models of CML and ALL [4, 27].

In addition to the oncogenic *BCR::ABL1* fusion gene, Ph$^+$ ALL is characterized by additional genomic abnormalities, notably deletions in genes critical in lymphoid development. *IKZF1* alterations, a biomarker of HR ALL, occur in about 70% of Ph$^+$ ALL compared with approximately 15% of Ph-negative ALL [28]. Intragenic deletions of *IKZF1* represent the most common alterations, predominantly deletions of exons 4–7 of *IKZF1,* which encode for the DNA-binding domains and give rise to the dominant-negative IKZF1 isoform (IK6) [28]. Preclinical studies demonstrated that *IKZF1* alterations induce a stem cell-like phenotype, promote aberrant adhesion, and decrease responsiveness to TKI in *BCR::ABL1*-positive murine models [29, 30]. Other B-cell transcription factors are also frequently altered in Ph$^+$ ALL, such as *CDKN2A/B*, *PAX5*, and/or *EBF1* [29]. Recent studies also reported on the prevalence of *IKZF1^{plus}* in Ph$^+$ ALL, which is defined by the co-deletion of *IKZF1* with additional lymphoid transcription factor genes (i.e., *CDKN2A/B* and/or *PAX5*), in 24–46% of Ph$^+$ ALL and is associated with inferior outcome [31, 32].

Gene expression profiling and next-generation sequencing studies have expanded the discovery of novel ABL-class fusions other than *BCR::ABL1* in B-ALL. These ABL-class fusions are almost exclusively found among patients who display a kinase-activated transcriptional signature similar to Ph$^+$ ALL, enriched in *IKZF1* deletions and harbor a heterogeneous spectrum of ABL-class fusions that are sensitive to ABL-directed TKIs [33]. Collectively, ABL-class fusion-positive ALL comprises approximately 3% of B-ALL or 15% of Ph-like ALL. The four most common ABL-class gene rearrangements are those involving *ABL1*, *ABL2*, *CSF1R* and *PDGFRB* with various 5′ partner genes [23]. Rarely, *PDGFRA* and *KIT* fusions have also been reported within ABL-class Ph-like B-ALL [34]. Similar to *BCR::ABL1*, all ABL-class fusions are in-frame, retain an intact tyrosine kinase domain, and the 5′ partner provides a dimerization domain for autophosphorylation and leads to constitutive kinase activation. A vast body of preclinical work from engineered cell lines, murine models and *ex vivo* data showed that these ABL-class fusions demonstrated exquisite sensitivity to either imatinib, dasatinib, or ponatinib. Several anecdotal cases and small series have reported favorable clinical responses and short-term outcomes of patients with ABL-class fusion-positive ALL treated with combination of TKI and chemotherapy, further supporting that these patients may benefit from treatment strategies similar to those for Ph^+ ALL. Nevertheless, in contrast to the *BCR::ABL1* fusion gene, which has been routinely integrated in the diagnostic workup of *de novo* ALL, the diverse spectrum of ABL-class fusions contributes to its diagnostic challenge. Several pediatric oncology consortia are now using targeted fusion panels or RNA-sequencing to identify these fusions at diagnosis. Rapid turnaround time can be achieved with commercial FISH probes for initial screening with subsequent molecular confirmatory testing [35].

12.3 Epidemiology, Clinical Features and Outcomes of Ph^+ ALL and ABL-Class Fusion-Positive ALL in the Pre-TKI Era

Ph^+ ALL is an uncommon childhood ALL subtype and its incidence increases with age. Ph^+ ALL occurs in approximately 3–5% of pediatric ALL, but its prevalence rises to 5–15% among adolescents, and it accounts for 25–30% of adult ALL cases. The prevalence of Ph-like ALL is almost three times more common than Ph^+ ALL, comprising around 15% of pediatric B-ALL. Its frequency also increases with age, with a prevalence ranging from 12% in children to 21% in adolescents to 27% in young adults. Among Ph-like ALL patients, ABL-class fusions have been identified in approximately 15% of cases, corresponding to 2–3% of childhood B-ALL. Hence, Ph^+ ALL and ABL-class fusion-positive ALLs constitute collectively 5–8% of pediatric B-ALL [18–20]. Boys are more often affected than girls in both Ph^+ and Ph-like ALL patients. Children with Ph^+ and ABL-class Ph-like ALLs often present with higher risk disease, including a higher frequency of hyperleukocytosis (white blood cell (WBC) $\geq 100 \times 10^9/L$) at diagnosis and worse initial treatment response marked by higher rates of poor prednisone responders, induction failure and higher end-induction and end-consolidation minimal residual disease (MRD) levels compared to other B-ALL subsets [19–24].

The outcomes of children with Ph^+ ALL in the pre-TKI era were dismal, and Ph^+ ALL was regarded as the ALL subtype associated with the worst prognosis in both children and adults. Historically, conventional chemotherapy treatment yielded very poor results with event-free survival (EFS) less than 30% and HSCT in CR1 represented the best curative option for patients with available donors. As reported by a large international retrospective study of 610 pediatric Ph^+ ALL patients treated between 1995 and 2005, the prognosis of children with Ph^+ ALL remained unfavorable despite the use of HSCT in CR1 [1]. The 7-year EFS and overall survival (OS) were 32% and 45%, respectively, for the entire cohort. For those who were transplanted in CR1, the outcomes remained unsatisfactory with 5-year disease-free survival (DFS) and OS of 44% and 54%, due to high rates of relapse and transplant-related mortality (TRM) [2].

The clinical characteristics and outcomes of ABL-class fusion-positive ALL cases treated in the pre-TKI era have also been described. Cario et al. reported the results of 46 ABL-class fusion-positive ALL patients treated according to two AIEOP-BFM protocols from 2000 to 2018. This retrospective study demonstrated an unfavorable outcome of these patients, with 5-year EFS, OS, and cumulative incidence of relapse (CIR) at 49%, 70%, and 26%, respectively. Compared to other ALL patients treated on the AIEOP-BFM 2000 trial, ABL-class fusion-positive ALL patients had a higher rate of prednisone poor response (50.0% vs. 5.6%; $p < 0.0001$), end-of-induction (EOI) MRD $\geq$ 5% (47.8% vs. 2.2%; $p < 0.0001$), high-risk patients based on persistent MRD on day 78 (78.3% vs. 11.1%; $p < 0.0001$) and HSCT in first remission (54.3% vs. 4.9%; $p < 0.0001$). Of interest, the clinical features, such as age distribution and rate of presenting hyperleukocytosis, and the overall outcomes of these patients were very similar to those of Ph⁺ ALL patients treated according to the AIEOP-BFM ALL 2000 protocol in the pre-TKI era [36]. In 2021, an international retrospective study by the Ponte di Legno group established the baseline characteristics and outcome of 122 children with ABL-class fusion-positive ALL in the pre-TKI era, demonstrating that the outcome of these children was unfavorable with an overall 5-year CIR, EFS, and OS of 31%, 59%, and 76%, respectively [21]. This report, representing the largest cohort of ABL-class fusion-positive ALL, also highlighted the variability in MRD response and clinical outcomes depending on the specific fusion subtype. For instance, children with *PDGFRB* and *ABL2* fusions were more likely to have post-induction MRD levels $\geq$ 1% compared to those harboring *ABL1* or *CSF1R* rearrangements. Consequently, there was a differential outcome with inferior 5-year OS for *PDGFRB* (74.8%) and *ABL2* fusions (37.5%) compared to *ABL1* (82.9%) or *CSF1R* fusions (90.0%) (log-rank $p = 0.0030$).

12.4 Treatment of Ph⁺ ALL and ABL-Class Fusion-Positive ALL: The Revolution of TKIs

In the last 20 years, two large cooperative groups, the North American Children's Oncology Group (COG) and the multinational European-based Ph⁺ ALL group (EsPhALL), have conducted consecutive clinical trials combining TKIs with chemotherapy with the goal of improving the outcome of pediatric Ph⁺ ALL. Importantly, the results of these trials also demonstrated that HSCT in CR1 may not be a necessary component of treatment in the TKI era, especially for patients who achieved early response following the first 8–10 weeks of induction chemotherapy and TKI (Table 12.1).

The COG group first assessed the combination of post-induction imatinib with an intensive chemotherapy backbone in the pilot COG AALL0031 trial (NCT00022737), whose early results were published in 2009 [6]. In this study, which accrued patients between 2002 and 2006, exposure to imatinib was increased progressively in five patient cohorts and it was clearly demonstrated that continuous imatinib exposure at 340 mg/m^2 daily (cohort 5) resulted in a significant 3-year EFS improvement compared to historical controls treated without imatinib (80 ± 11% vs. 35 ± 4%; $p < 0.0001$). No significant increase in toxicity was observed with the addition of imatinib to this intensive chemotherapy regimen compared to the control group. In this study, all patients who had an HLA-identical family donor ($n = 21$) were allocated to HSCT in CR1 with imatinib given for 6 months following HSCT; even though it was not called for in the protocol, several patients ($n = 11$) were taken to unrelated HSCT in CR1. With longer follow-up, the 5-year DFS for cohort 5 patients treated with chemotherapy plus imatinib (without HSCT in CR1) was 70 ± 12%, not significantly different than patients who received related-donor HSCT (65 ± 11%) or unrelated-donor HSCT in CR1 (59 ± 15%; $p = 0.60$) [7].

Between 2004 and 2009, the EsPhALL group conducted a randomized controlled study EsPhALL2004 (EudraCT 2004–001647-30/ NCT00287105) investigating post-induction imatinib therapy (300 mg/m^2) combined with a Berlin–Frankfurt–Munster (BFM)-based intensive chemotherapy backbone (different than the backbone used in the COG AALL0031 trial) in children and adolescents with Ph⁺ ALL. In this trial, imatinib was discontinuously administered. Patients were stratified according to early prednisone response and complete remission at the end of induction as good or poor risk. Good-risk patients were randomized to receive chemotherapy plus imatinib or chemotherapy alone, while

Table 12.1 Treatment and outcome of pediatric Ph^+ ALL and ABL-class fusion-positive ALL among different study groups

Studies	COG AALL0031	EsPhALL 2004	EsPhALL 2010	COG AALL0622	COG AALL1122	CCCG-ALL-2015	PdL cohort	AIEOP-BFM cohort	French cohort	UKALL2011 cohort
Patients	Ph^+ ALL (cohort 5)	Ph^+ ALL	Ph^+ ALL	Ph^+ ALL	Ph^+ ALL	Ph^+ ALL	ABL-class fusion-positive ALL	ABL-class fusion-positive ALL	ABL-class fusion-positive ALL	ABl-class fusion-positive ALL
Phase	3	2	2	2	2	3	Retrospective	Retrospective	Retrospective	Case series
TKI	Imatinib 340 mg/m^2	Imatinib 300 mg/m^2	Imatinib 300 mg/m^2	Dasatinib 60 mg/m^2	Dasatinib 60 mg/m^2	Imatinib 300 mg/m^2 vs Dasatinib 80 mg/m^2	No TKI	Imatinib ($n = 8$) Dasatinib ($n = 5$)	Imatinib ($n = 12$) Dasatinib ($n = 6$) Ponatinib ($n = 1$)	Imatinib
Years	2002–2006	2004–2009	2010–2014	2008–2012	2012–2014	2015–2018	2000–2018	2011–2018	N/A	N/A
Patients (n)	49	178	155	60	106	97 (imatinib) 92 (dasatinib)	122	13	19	13
HSCT in CR1	41%	81%	38%	32%	14%	2%	37%	69%	47%	69%
5-year EFS	68%	60%	57%	60%	55%	39% (imatinib) 60% (dasatinib)	59%	63%	3-year: 55%	4-year: 84%
5-year OS	81%	72%	72%	86%	82%	72% (imatinib) 74% (dasatinib)	76%	76%	3-year: 77%	4-year: 84%

AIEOP-BFM Associazione Italiana di Ematologica e Oncologio Pediatrica-Berlin-Frankfurt-Munster, *CCCG* Chinese Children's Cancer Group, *COG* Children's Oncology Group, *CR1* complete first remission, *EFS* event-free survival, *EsPhALL* European Ph^+ ALL working group, *HSCT* hematopoietic stem cell transplantation (allogeneic), *OS* overall survival, *PdL* Ponte di Legno, *TKI* tyrosine kinase inhibitor all poor-risk patients were assigned to receive chemotherapy plus imatinib. All poor-risk patients were allocated to HSCT in CR1; additionally, good-risk patients with any HLA-matched donor (related or unrelated) were also allocated to HSCT in CR1. The results of the EsPhALL2004 trial reported a 4-year disease-free survival (DFS) of 72.9% for good-risk patients who received chemotherapy plus imatinib and 61.7% for those who did not receive imatinib [8]. The poor-risk group had a 4-year EFS of 53.5%, supporting the historical evidence that poor-prednisone response (PPR) remains a significant negative prognostic factor in Ph^+ ALL. Of note, because of the high rate of CR1 HSCT in the EsPhALL2004 cohort (80% overall and 77% in good-risk patients), it was not possible to assess whether HSCT could be safely omitted without adversely impacting outcome in any subgroup of TKI-treated patients.

Due to the results of the COG AALL0031 study, which demonstrated the advantage of continuous imatinib exposure, the EsPhALL trial was amended in 2010 to include imatinib dosed in this way beginning at day 15 of induction. Additionally, from 2012, indication of CR1 HSCT was restricted to poor responders only defined by end of induction 1B MRD $\geq 5 \times 10^{-4}$ or MRD positivity at any detectable level following the three HR Consolidation blocks, based on the hypothesis that good responders may not need HSCT if treated with TKI. The aim of the EsPhALL2010 (EudraCT 2004–001647-30/NCT00287105) study was to investigate whether early and protracted exposure to imatinib could further improve outcome compared to EsPhALL2004 while limiting CR1 HSCT to poor responders only. The overall results of the EsPhALL2010 trial were similar to those obtained in EsPhALL2004 with a 5-year EFS and OS of 57% and 72%, respectively, although CR1 HSCT was reduced by half (80% vs. 38% of patients) [9]. These data, together with the previous COG AALL0031 study results, re-defined the standard-of-care in pediatric Ph^+ ALL patients in the TKI era, limiting CR1 HSCT indication only to high-risk patients based on MRD response. However, even with the omission of HSCT, treatment on the EsPhALL2010 trial was associated with a high rate of toxicities, especially infectious complications, and there was a higher rate of treatment-related mortality on that trial compared with the high-risk arm of AEIOP-BFM trials using similar chemotherapy backbone without TKI in Ph-negative ALL patients.

From 2008 to 2012, the COG group conducted AALL0622 (NCT00720109), a phase 2 trial in newly diagnosed children with Ph^+ ALL, assessing the safety and feasibility of combining the second-generation dual ABL/SRC kinase inhibitor, dasatinib, with the identical chemotherapy backbone of AALL0031. In this trial, patients received dasatinib at 60 mg/m^2 continuously starting on day 15 of induction. The rationale for testing dasatinib was its superior *in vitro* efficacy in blocking the ABL-kinase activity (>300 times more potent than imatinib) and its ability to cross the blood–brain barrier more effectively than imatinib. Therefore, in contrast to the previous studies where all Ph^+ ALL patients received cranial irradiation (CRT), CRT in AALL022 was limited to patients who were CNS-3 (CSF with 5 or more WBC per high power field, with positive blasts on cytospin) at diagnosis. The results of the AALL0622 trial were published in 2018 by Slayton et al., reporting similar outcomes compared to the predecessor COG AALL0031 trial with imatinib, with an overall 5-year EFS and OS of 60% and 86%, respectively. Dasatinib plus intensive chemotherapy was well tolerated and induced better early response rates (98% of EOI complete remission, 59% EOI MRD <0.01% and 89% end-of-consolidation (EOC) MRD <0.01%) compared with AALL0031, on which TKI was not started until completion of the induction phase. However, the improved early response rate compared with AALL0031 did not translate to improved EFS. This can be partially explained by the increased rate of isolated central nervous system (CNS) relapse (15%) compared with AALL0031 (6%) on which all patients received CRT, suggesting that dasatinib, despite its superior CNS penetration compared with imatinib, was not as effective as cranial radiation in preventing CNS relapses. On AALL0622, HSCT was recommended for high-risk patients based on EOI MRD ≥ 1% and/or MRD≥ 0.01% at the end-of-consolidation 2 response and for all patients with available matched sibling donor (MSD), irrespective of MRD response. HSCT in CR1 was performed in 32% of the enrolled patients (nine standard-risk (SR), eight HR, and two not risk-classified because of missing MRD) and no difference in 5-year EFS was found between the transplanted and the non-transplanted group (61 ± 13% vs. 60 ± 8%; $p = 0.84$), thus providing additional evidence that non-high-risk patients (i.e., those with favorable early response) could be successfully treated without HSCT in CR1 [11].

In 2012, the first transatlantic Ph$^+$ ALL trial AALL1122/CA180–372 (EudraCT 2011–001123-20/NCT01460160) was jointly conducted by COG and EsPhALL. In this phase 2 international trial, the treatment strategies from the COG AAAL0622 and the European EsPhALL2010 were merged, and continuous daily dasatinib at 60 mg/m^2 was administered from day 15 of induction in combination with the EsPhALL chemotherapy backbone. CR1 HSCT was indicated only for HR patients defined by end 1B-MRD ≥ 0.05% or persistent MRD positivity after 3 HR consolidation blocks, and cranial irradiation was limited to patients with overt CNS leukemia (CNS-3 at diagnosis). The 5-year EFS and OS were 55% and 82%, respectively, with only 14% of patients undergoing HSCT in CR1 and 15% receiving CRT either as part of HSCT conditioning regimens or with chemotherapy due to CNS-3 status at diagnosis. The toxicity data of AALL1122/CA180–372 confirmed the previous observation from EsPhALL2010, with treatment-related mortality of about 9%, almost entirely due to fatal infections [37]. Nevertheless, with the implementation of aggressive supportive care measures and the decreased frequency of CR1 HSCT, there was a trend toward improved 5-year OS when comparing AALL1122 with EsPhALL2010 trial results.

Recently, the first randomized clinical trial comparing imatinib versus dasatinib in *de novo* pediatric Ph$^+$ ALL, CCCG-ALL-2015 (ChiCTR-IPR-14005706), was conducted by the Chinese Children's Cancer Group from 2015 to 2018. Patients were randomly assigned to receive daily dasatinib (80 mg/m^2) vs. imatinib (300 mg/m^2) in association with the modified St. Jude Total XV/XVI chemotherapy backbone. Shen et al. reported a significantly better outcome in the dasatinib arm, with 4-year EFS of 71.0% vs. 48.9%; $p = 0.005$, 4-year OS of 88.4% vs. 69.2%; $p = 0.04$ and 4-year CIR 19.8% vs. 34.4%; $p = 0.01$ between dasatinib- and imatinib-treated groups, respectively. Of note, the follow-up was short, the outcomes of patients treated with dasatinib resemble the early outcomes of AALL0622 (3-year EFS of 84.6% for SR patients) and AALL1122 (3-year EFS of 65.5%), and the outcome of the imatinib arm was strikingly inferior compared to those reported by COG and EsPhALL studies with imatinib [38, 39]. This outcome difference between dasatinib vs. imatinib could potentially be contributed by the different TKI dosage used in CCCG-ALL-2015 and previous COG/EsPhALL trials (higher dasatinib and lower imatinib dosing).

The evidence from all these consecutive prospective clinical trials has led to an international consensus that early and continuous administration of TKI in combination with chemotherapy represents the standard-of-care for newly diagnosed children with Ph$^+$ ALL, with CR1 HSCT reserved to slow-responding/high-risk patients. The data from all of these trials suggests that both imatinib and dasatinib are efficacious first-line TKI options with comparable outcomes in newly diagnosed children with Ph$^+$ ALL [40].

Due to the rarity of pediatric Ph$^+$ ALL, international collaboration is essential to design a randomized controlled trial to further improve the outcome and define the new standard-of-care treatment for children with Ph$^+$ ALL. The ongoing EsPhALL2017/AALL1631 (NCT03007147) trial is an international collaborative study conducted jointly by COG and EsPhALL with the primary objective of reducing treatment-related mortality and morbidity without adversely impacting DFS in SR Ph$^+$ ALL patients. It is a phase 3 randomized trial with a non-inferiority design, comparing the DFS, OS and toxicity of SR patients treated with imatinib combined with either the EsPhALL chemotherapy backbone or a less intensive chemotherapy regimen similar to those administered to Ph-negative HR B-ALL on COG trials. For high-risk patients (as previously defined in AALL1122/EsPhALL2010 trials), the trial is investigating the feasibility of administering imatinib maintenance post-HSCT. Furthermore, taking into consideration the similar biological and clinical characteristics of ABL-class fusion-positive ALL and Ph$^+$ ALL, the EsPhALL2017/AALL1631 trial was amended in 2021 to also include patients with ABL-class fusions other than *BCR::ABL1*. This trial will be the largest international prospective trial ever conducted in pediatric ABL-class fusion-positive ALL including *BCR::ABL1* and its results could establish a new, less toxic chemotherapy backbone on which novel targeted agents and/or immunotherapy can be tested in future trials.

12.5 Prognostic Factors in Ph$^+$ ALL

Unlike the rest of childhood ALL, in which such factors as age and presenting WBC have been shown to significantly predict outcome, very few prognostic factors have been identified in pediatric Ph$^+$ ALL. In the EsPhALL2004 trial, presenting WBC $\geq 100 \times 10^9$/L was the only independent risk factor associated with poor prognosis in multivariable analysis (HR: 5.26; 95% CI: 2.37–11.70; $p < 0.0001$) [10]; however, this finding has not been validated in other trials. Early response to therapy has emerged as the only factor used for risk stratification in pediatric Ph$^+$ ALL, although the evidence of its prognostic significance is not as robust as it is in other ALL subtypes.

There are conflicting data regarding the prognostic significance of MRD in the pediatric Ph$^+$ ALL population. In a post hoc analysis of 90 patients enrolled on the EsPhALL2004 trial with available MRD results [41], MRD at both end of induction IA (TP1) and end of induction IB (TP2) appeared to be correlated with long-term outcome. Using real-time quantitative polymerase chain reaction (RQ-PCR) of rearranged immunoglobulin/T-cell receptor (Ig/TCR) genes for MRD assessment, 9 of 90 patients had negative MRD (defined as $<1 \times 10^{-4}$ at EOI/timepoint 1 [TP1]) and none relapsed. Eleven patients with TP1 MRD $< 5 \times 10^{-4}$ (low-positive) and 70 patients with TP1 MRD $\geq 5 \times 10^{-4}$ (high-positive) had comparable 5-year CIR of 36.4% and 35.2%, respectively. Patients with prior detectable MRD who converted to MRD negativity at the end of induction 1B (TP2) had a lower risk of relapse compared to that of patients who achieved MRD negativity at later timepoints (5-year CIR 14.3% vs. 36.4%) [41]. Conversely, results from other pediatric Ph$^+$ ALL trials, including AALL0031, AALL0622 and AALL1122, did not demonstrate that MRD was prognostically significant [7, 11, 38]. This discrepancy might be explained by the fact that MRD was being used to risk-stratify treatment in some of these trials (such as AALL0622 and AALL1122); thus, patients with high levels of MRD received more intensive therapy, such as HSCT, which could have abrogated prognostic significance.

Interpretation of the prognostic significance of early response in pediatric Ph$^+$ ALL is complicated by the fact that different assays have been used to assess MRD, including the Ig/TCR PCR MRD assay, flow cytometry and *BCR::ABL1* RQ-PCR, and these assays often yield different results. In the AALL1122 trial, MRD was assessed by all three assays, although treatment decisions were based upon Ig/TCR PCR MRD results. The highest concordance rate in MRD assessment at different timepoints was between Ig/TCR PCR and flow cytometry (97.7%), followed by Ig/TCR vs. *BCR::ABL1* RQ-PCR (90.1%) and the lowest between *BCR::ABL1* RQ-PCR and flow cytometry (82.3%) [37]. The kinetics of MRD clearance also differed between MRD assays, while nearly 90% of patients achieved MRD negativity by Ig/TCR PCR or flow cytometry after the three high-risk consolidation blocks, only 32% of patients achieved MRD negativity by *BCR::ABL1* RQ-PCR at the same timepoint. However, the outcome of patients achieving MRD negativity by either of the three MRD assays was not significantly different despite a slower MRD clearance by *BCR::ABL1*

RQ-PCR. For instance, the 5-year EFS of patients achieving MRD negativity at TP1, TP2, and TP3 on AALL1122 was 60·0% (95% CI: 40·5–75·0), 56·2% (95% CI: 42·1–68·2), and 53·3% (95% CI: 41·4–63·9) by Ig/TCR PCR; 63·0% (95% CI: 48·7–74·3), 58·4% (95% CI: 46·0–69·0), and 54·3% (95% CI: 43·3–64·1) by flow cytometry; and 66·7% (95% CI: 5·4–94·5), 57·1% (95% CI: 17·2–83·7), and 66·7% (95% CI: 37·5–84·6) by *BCR::ABL1* RQ-PCR, respectively [37]. Adult Ph$^+$ ALL studies utilized predominantly *BCR::ABL1* RQ-PCR as the primary MRD assay and complete molecular response at three months by *BCR::ABL1* RQ-PCR has been shown to be an independent predictor of outcome in several studies [32, 42–44]. Recently, the clonoSEQ next-generation sequencing (NGS) MRD assay also showed high concordance rate with the Ig/TCR PCR MRD assay. Interestingly, the more sensitive NGS MRD assay still detects microscopic residual leukemia in about 10% of patients who were deemed MRD negative by Ig/TCR PCR [45]. Whether the increased sensitivity of NGS MRD assay could further define prognostically relevant MRD levels in the TKI era warrants prospective assessment in future trials.

Discrepancies between MRD assays have revealed a distinct subgroup of Ph$^+$ ALL patients that phenocopy CML biology. Zuna et al. identified 20–25% of children with Ph$^+$ ALL have discordant MRD (negative by Ig/TCR but positive by DNA-based *BCR::ABL1* genomic breakpoint MRD) in which the *BCR::ABL1* fusion persists in the non-blastic compartment such as myeloid cells, non-ALL B cells, T cells, reminiscent of CML disease [46]. Children with CML-like phenotype had an outcome that was similar to other children with Ph$^+$ ALL (5-year EFS/OS 49%/73% vs. 60%/75%, respectively). Importantly, there was a trend toward superior prognosis among CML-like patients who underwent CR1 HSCT compared to those treated with chemotherapy plus TKI alone (5-year EFS 81% vs. 47%; $p = 0.06$), as demonstrated in previous reports [46, 47]. The development of a DNA-based *BCR::ABL1* MRD to rapidly identify these CML-like patients without requiring cell-sorting facilities could potentially be used in prospective trials for risk stratification and/or CR1 HSCT treatment allocation.

Additional genomic abnormalities have emerged as potential novel biomarkers which may help to inform Ph$^+$ ALL prognostication. *IKZF1* gene deletions, including deletions of the entire gene and deletions of specific exons, are present in approximately 70% cases of Ph$^+$ ALL (compared with about 15% of pediatric Ph-negative B-ALL), and appear to confer adverse prognostic significance. In the COG AALL0622 trial, the presence of *IKZF1* deletion was significantly associated with worse EFS/OS compared with wild-type *IKZF1* (5-year EFS/OS of 52% and 80% vs. 82% and 100%, respectively; $p = 0.04$). More importantly, even among patients who were classified SR based upon early favorable MRD response, *IKZF1* deletion remained prognostic, suggesting that *IKZF1* gene status could help to identify high-risk patients among those with favorable early MRD response [11]. In Ph-negative ALL, the AEIOP-BFM group has defined a subgroup of *IKZF1*-deleted patients they labeled as *IKZF1^{plus}*: these patients had co-occurrence of deletions of *CDKN2A*, *CDKN2B*, *PAX5* or *PAR1* (in the absence of *ERG* deletion) and appeared to have worse prognosis than other *IKZF1*-deleted patients [48]. The prognostic relevance of *IKZF1^{plus}* in pediatric Ph$^+$ ALL has not yet been reported, but adult Ph$^+$ ALL studies have confirmed the adverse prognostic impact of *IKZF1^{plus}*. Foa et al. reported that DFS was significantly worse among patients with *IKZF1^{plus}* compared to those with *IKZF1* deletion alone or no *IKZF1* deletion (64% vs. 92% vs. 100%; $p = 0.03$) [31]. In a large retrospective study of 100 adult Ph$^+$ ALL patients treated with hyper-CVAD and dasatinib or ponatinib, the presence of *IKZF1^{plus}* was independently associated with poor OS [32].

Other genomic aberrations have also been reported to have prognostic relevance, but this awaits further confirmation. In the first COG trial for Ph$^+$ ALL with imatinib (AALL0031), the 5-year EFS of patients with only the t(9;22) translocation was 86% compared to 51% for those with secondary chromosomal abnormalities ($p = 0.05$) [7]. Several adult studies have shown the adverse prognostic impact of the p210 fusion transcript when compared to the p190 fusion transcript [49, 50]. In contrast, the 5-year EFS/OS of children with the p190 transcript variant ($n = 71$) treated on the international AALL1122 trial was 49.1% (95% CI: 37.2–60.0)/75.3% (95% CI: 63.7–83.7) and 75.0% (95% CI: 46.3–89.8) and 100.0% (95% CI: 100.0–100.0) for patients with p210 transcript ($n = 15$), respectively [37]. Finally, *BCR::ABL1* kinase domain mutations constitute the primary mechanism of acquired resistance leading to relapse in adult Ph⁺ ALL [51, 52]. The presence of kinase domain mutations at relapse or even at diagnosis when using more sensitive technologies was associated with a high risk of relapse and consequently, inferior outcome in some studies [49, 50, 53]. In pediatric Ph⁺ ALL, the incidence of acquired ABL1 kinase domain mutations is rather low, possibly due to the concomitant administration of TKI along with a more intensive chemotherapy regimen compared to that used in adult Ph⁺ ALL [54]. Using the ultra-sensitive droplet digital polymerase chain reaction, 3 out of 23 patients with *EBF1::PDGFRB* Ph-like ALL were found to harbor subclonal gatekeeper T681I mutations at diagnosis and its presence was associated with a trend toward a higher likelihood of relapse [55]. In summary, advances in molecular diagnostics and our improved understanding of disease biology have led to the discovery of several potential novel prognostic factors that in the future could help refine risk stratification.

12.6 Future Directions and Conclusion

Despite survival improvement in pediatric Ph⁺ ALL with the introduction of TKI into treatment protocols, the cumulative incidence of relapse and the treatment-related mortality in Ph⁺ ALL remain higher than in Ph-negative ALL, highlighting the need for further treatment optimization in the TKI era. As treatment intensification using conventional cytotoxic chemotherapy has reached its limit, novel therapeutic avenues investigating the incorporation of immunotherapeutic agents, such as blinatumomab or the anti-CD22 antibody drug conjugate, inotuzumab ozogamicin, into a chemotherapy plus TKI backbone may help to reduce relapse rates while minimizing the treatment-related morbidity and mortality risks associated with intensive chemotherapy backbones. Chemotherapy-sparing approaches via the addition of immunotherapy plus TKI in adult Ph⁺ ALL illustrate the rapidly changing treatment landscape. As an example, the GIMEMA LAL2116 D-ALBA trial recently demonstrated promising early outcomes using consolidation with blinatumomab and dasatinib within a chemotherapy-free backbone. Among 61 evaluable patients, 60% achieved a molecular response after two cycles of blinatumomab and dasatinib which increased to 81% after four cycles. With a median follow-up of 18 months, the 1-year DFS and OS were 88% and 95%, respectively [31]. More recently, the results of the phase 2 single-institution trial testing the combination of blinatumomab with the third-generation multikinase inhibitor, ponatinib, yielded the best outcomes in newly diagnosed adults with Ph⁺ ALL with 1-year EFS and OS both reported to be 95% [56]. The combination of blinatumomab and ponatinib resulted in an earlier and deeper complete molecular response than blinatumomab and dasatinib. Importantly, only 1 out of 40 patients underwent CR1 HSCT in the blinatumomab and ponatinib cohort, whereas 23 out of 61 patients received HSCT consolidation in CR1 in the D-ALBA trial (blinatumomab with dasatinib). These results provide compelling rationale to test the incorporation of immunotherapeutic agents (such as blinatumomab) into current TKI-based pediatric regimens for pediatric Ph⁺ ALL and ABL-class fusion-positive ALL, either in addition or as a replacement for some of the more morbid cytotoxic chemotherapy phases of treatment. Finally, for rare, high-risk patient subsets such as Ph⁺ ALL and ABL-class fusion-positive ALL, international collaborative efforts are essential to conduct sufficiently powered precision medicine trials in order to advance the field and improve outcomes (Tables 12.2 and 12.3).

Table 12.2 Clinical and biological similarities between Ph+ ALL and ABL-class fusion-positive ALL

	Ph+ ALL	ABL-class fusion-positive ALL
Prevalence	3–5%	2–3%
Sex predominance	M > F	M > F
Presenting features	>10 years old Higher WBC > 100 x 10^9/L	>10 years old Higher WBC > 100 × 10^9/L
IKZF1 alteration	~70%	~70%
Early response	Poor prednisone response High rates of induction failure High end-induction/consolidation MRD positivity	Poor prednisone response High rates of induction failure High end-induction/consolidation MRD positivity
Outcomes (pre-TKI)	5-year DFS: 28%; OS:40%	5-year EFS: 59.1%; OS: 76.1%
Sensitivity	Imatinib/dasatinib	Imatinib/dasatinib

Table 12.3 Spectrum of ABL-class fusion-positive ALL

3′ kinase genes	Estimated frequency	5′ fusion partner genes
ABL1	33% of ABL-class fusions	*CENPC, CNTRL,* ***ETV6****, FOXP1, INPP5D, LSM14A, NUP153,* ***NUP214****, RANBP2,* ***RCSD1****, SFPQ, SHIP1, SNX1, SNX2, SPTNA1, ZMIZ1*
ABL2	7% of ABL-class fusions	*EZR, PAG1,* ***RCSD1****, ZC3HAV1*
CSF1R	8% of ABL-class fusions	*NUMA1, MEF2D,* ***SSBP2****, TBL1XR1*
PDGFRB	52% of ABL-class fusions	*ATF7IP,* ***EBF1****, ETV6, GOLGA4, PACSIN2, SNX29, SSBP2, TNIP1, ZEB2, ZMYND8, ZNF608*
KIT	Very rare	*G3BP2*
PDGFRA	Very rare	*FIP1L1*

The most common 5′ partner genes are highlighted in bold

References

1. Aricò M, et al. Outcome of treatment in children with Philadelphia chromosome-positive acute lymphoblastic leukemia. N Engl J Med. 2000;342(14):998–1006.
2. Aricò M, et al. Clinical outcome of children with newly diagnosed Philadelphia chromosome-positive acute lymphoblastic leukemia treated between 1995 and 2005. J Clin Oncol. 2010;28(31):4755–61.
3. Hunger SP, Mullighan CG. Redefining ALL classification: toward detecting high-risk ALL and implementing precision medicine. Blood. 2015;125(26):3977–87.
4. Bernt KM, Hunger SP. Current concepts in pediatric Philadelphia chromosome-positive acute lymphoblastic leukemia. Front Oncol. 2014;4:54.
5. Fielding AK. Treatment of Philadelphia chromosome-positive acute lymphoblastic leukemia in adults: a broader range of options, improved outcomes, and more therapeutic dilemmas. Am Soc Clin Oncol Educ Book. 2015:e352–9.
6. Schultz KR, et al. Improved early event-free survival with imatinib in Philadelphia chromosome-positive acute lymphoblastic leukemia: a children's oncology group study. J Clin Oncol. 2009;27(31):5175–81.
7. Schultz KR, et al. Long-term follow-up of imatinib in pediatric Philadelphia chromosome-positive acute lymphoblastic leukemia: Children's oncology group study AALL0031. Leukemia. 2014;28(7):1467–71.
8. Biondi A, et al. Imatinib after induction for treatment of children and adolescents with Philadelphia-chromosome-positive acute lymphoblastic leukaemia (EsPhALL): a randomised, open-label, intergroup study. Lancet Oncol. 2012;13(9):936–45.
9. Biondi A, et al. Imatinib treatment of paediatric Philadelphia chromosome-positive acute lymphoblastic leukaemia (EsPhALL2010): a prospective, intergroup, open-label, single-arm clinical trial. Lancet Haematol. 2018;5(12):e641–52.
10. Biondi A, et al. Long-term follow up of pediatric Philadelphia positive acute lymphoblastic leukemia treated with the EsPhALL2004 study: high white blood cell count at diagnosis is the strongest prognostic factor. Haematologica. 2019;104(1):e13–6.
11. Slayton WB, et al. Dasatinib plus intensive chemotherapy in children, adolescents, and young adults with Philadelphia chromosome-positive acute lymphoblastic leukemia: results of Children's oncology group trial AALL0622. J Clin Oncol. 2018;36(22):2306–14.
12. Cerchione C, Locatelli F, Martinelli G. Dasatinib in the management of pediatric patients with Philadelphia chromosome-positive acute lymphoblastic leukemia. Front Oncol. 2021;11:632231.
13. Aubert L, et al. Therapeutic approach and outcome of children with Philadelphia chromosome-positive

acute lymphoblastic leukemia at first relapse in the era of tyrosine kinase inhibitors: an SFCE retrospective study. Pediatr Blood Cancer. 2022;69(2):e29441.
14. Den Boer ML, et al. A subtype of childhood acute lymphoblastic leukaemia with poor treatment outcome: a genome-wide classification study. Lancet Oncol. 2009;10(2):125–34.
15. Mullighan CG, et al. Deletion of IKZF1 and prognosis in acute lymphoblastic leukemia. N Engl J Med. 2009;360(5):470–80.
16. Harvey RC, et al. Rearrangement of CRLF2 is associated with mutation of JAK kinases, alteration of IKZF1, Hispanic/Latino ethnicity, and a poor outcome in pediatric B-progenitor acute lymphoblastic leukemia. Blood. 2010;115(26):5312–21.
17. Roberts KG, et al. Targetable kinase-activating lesions in Ph-like acute lymphoblastic leukemia. N Engl J Med. 2014;371(11):1005–15.
18. Reshmi SC, et al. Targetable kinase gene fusions in high-risk B-ALL: a study from the Children's oncology group. Blood. 2017;129(25):3352–61.
19. Roberts KG, et al. High frequency and poor outcome of Philadelphia chromosome-like acute lymphoblastic leukemia in adults. J Clin Oncol. 2017;35(4): 394–401.
20. Leoni V, Biondi A. Tyrosine kinase inhibitors in BCR-ABL positive acute lymphoblastic leukemia. Haematologica. 2015;100(3):295–9.
21. den Boer ML, et al. Outcomes of paediatric patients with B-cell acute lymphocytic leukaemia with ABL-class fusion in the pre-tyrosine-kinase inhibitor era: a multicentre, retrospective, cohort study. Lancet Haematol. 2021;8(1):e55–66.
22. Slayton WB, et al. How we approach Philadelphia chromosome-positive acute lymphoblastic leukemia in children and young adults. Pediatr Blood Cancer. 2020;67(10):e28543.
23. Tran TH, Tasian SK. Has Ph-like ALL superseded Ph+ ALL as the least favorable subtype? Best Pract Res Clin Haematol. 2021;34(4):101331.
24. Vettenranta K, et al. What is the role of HSCT in Philadelphia-chromosome-positive and Philadelphia-chromosome-like ALL in the tyrosine kinase inhibitor era? Front Pediatr. 2021;9:807002.
25. Nowell PC, Hungerford DA. Chromosome studies on normal and leukemic human leukocytes. J Natl Cancer Inst. 1960;25:85–109.
26. Rowley JD. Letter: a new consistent chromosomal abnormality in chronic myelogenous leukaemia identified by quinacrine fluorescence and Giemsa staining. Nature. 1973;243(5405):290–3.
27. Quintás-Cardama A, Cortes J. Molecular biology of bcr-abl1-positive chronic myeloid leukemia. Blood. 2009;113(8):1619–30.
28. Vairy S, Tran TH. IKZF1 alterations in acute lymphoblastic leukemia: the good, the bad and the ugly. Blood Rev. 2020;44:100677.
29. Churchman ML, et al. Efficacy of Retinoids in IKZF1-mutated BCR-ABL1 acute lymphoblastic leukemia. Cancer Cell. 2015;28(3):343–56.
30. Churchman ML, Mullighan CG. Ikaros: exploiting and targeting the hematopoietic stem cell niche in B-progenitor acute lymphoblastic leukemia. Exp Hematol. 2017;46:1–8.
31. Foà R, et al. Dasatinib-Blinatumomab for Ph-positive acute lymphoblastic leukemia in adults. N Engl J Med. 2020;383(17):1613–23.
32. Sasaki Y, et al. Genetic correlates in patients with Philadelphia chromosome-positive acute lymphoblastic leukemia treated with hyper-CVAD plus dasatinib or ponatinib. Leukemia. 2022;36(5):1253–60.
33. Tran TH, Hunger SP. The genomic landscape of pediatric acute lymphoblastic leukemia and precision medicine opportunities. Semin Cancer Biol. 2022;84:144–52.
34. Iacobucci I, et al. G3BP2-KIT drives leukemia amenable to kinase inhibition in Ph-like ALL. Blood Adv. 2022;6(11):3255–9.
35. Tran TH, Tasian SK. Clinical screening for Ph-like ALL and the developing role of TKIs. Hematology Am Soc Hematol Educ Program. 2022;2022(1):594–602.
36. Cario G, et al. Relapses and treatment-related events contributed equally to poor prognosis in children with ABL-class fusion positive B-cell acute lymphoblastic leukemia treated according to AIEOP-BFM protocols. Haematologica. 2020;105(7):1887–94.
37. Hunger SP, et al. Dasatinib with intensive chemotherapy in de novo paediatric Philadelphia chromosome-positive acute lymphoblastic leukaemia (CA180-372/COG AALL1122): a single-arm, multicentre, phase 2 trial. Lancet Haematol. 2023;10(7):e510–20.
38. Shen S, et al. Effect of Dasatinib vs Imatinib in the treatment of pediatric Philadelphia chromosome-positive acute lymphoblastic leukemia: a randomized clinical trial. JAMA Oncol. 2020;6(3):358–66.
39. Hunger SP, et al. CA180-372: an international collaborative phase 2 trial of Dasatinib and chemotherapy in pediatric patients with newly diagnosed Philadelphia chromosome positive acute lymphoblastic leukemia. Blood. 2017;130(Suppl 1):98.
40. Thastrup M, et al. Central nervous system involvement in childhood acute lymphoblastic leukemia: challenges and solutions. Leukemia. 2022;36(12):2751–68.
41. Cazzaniga G, et al. Predictive value of minimal residual disease in Philadelphia-chromosome-positive acute lymphoblastic leukemia treated with imatinib in the European intergroup study of post-induction treatment of Philadelphia-chromosome-positive acute lymphoblastic leukemia, based on immunoglobulin/T-cell receptor and BCR/ABL1 methodologies. Haematologica. 2018;103(1):107–15.
42. Daver N, et al. Final report of a phase II study of imatinib mesylate with hyper-CVAD for the front-line treatment of adult patients with Philadelphia chromosome-positive acute lymphoblastic leukemia. Haematologica. 2015;100(5):653–61.
43. Chalandon Y, et al. Randomized study of reduced-intensity chemotherapy combined with imatinib in adults with Ph-positive acute lymphoblastic leukemia. Blood. 2015;125(24):3711–9.

44. Jabbour E, et al. Treatment of adults with Philadelphia chromosome-positive acute lymphoblastic leukemia-from intensive chemotherapy combinations to chemotherapy-free regimens: a review. JAMA Oncol. 2022;8(9):1340–8.
45. Tran TH, et al. Minimal residual disease comparison between Ig/TCR PCR versus NGS assays in children with Philadelphia chromosome-positive acute lymphoblastic leukemia: a report from the COG AALL1631 study. J Clin Oncol. 2022;40:10023.
46. Hovorkova L, et al. Monitoring of childhood ALL using BCR-ABL1 genomic breakpoints identifies a subgroup with CML-like biology. Blood. 2017;129(20):2771–81.
47. Zuna J, et al. Minimal residual disease in BCR::ABL1-positive acute lymphoblastic leukemia: different significance in typical ALL and in CML-like disease. Leukemia. 2022;36(12):2793–801.
48. Stanulla M, et al. IKZF1(plus) defines a new minimal residual disease-dependent very-poor prognostic profile in pediatric B-cell precursor acute lymphoblastic leukemia. J Clin Oncol. 2018;36(12):1240–9.
49. DeBoer R, et al. Clinical impact of ABL1 kinase domain mutations and IKZF1 deletion in adults under age 60 with Philadelphia chromosome-positive (Ph+) acute lymphoblastic leukemia (ALL): molecular analysis of CALGB (Alliance) 10001 and 9665. Leuk Lymphoma. 2016;57(10):2298–306.
50. Wieduwilt MJ, et al. Dasatinib and dexamethasone followed by hematopoietic cell transplantation for adults with Ph-positive ALL. Blood Adv. 2021;5(22):4691–700.
51. Soverini S, et al. Contribution of ABL kinase domain mutations to imatinib resistance in different subsets of Philadelphia-positive patients: by the GIMEMA working party on chronic myeloid leukemia. Clin Cancer Res. 2006;12(24):7374–9.
52. Soverini S, et al. Philadelphia-positive patients who already harbor imatinib-resistant Bcr-Abl kinase domain mutations have a higher likelihood of developing additional mutations associated with resistance to second- or third-line tyrosine kinase inhibitors. Blood. 2009;114(10):2168–71.
53. Pfeifer H, et al. Kinase domain mutations of BCR-ABL frequently precede imatinib-based therapy and give rise to relapse in patients with de novo Philadelphia-positive acute lymphoblastic leukemia (Ph+ ALL). Blood. 2007;110(2):727–34.
54. Chang BH, et al. Imatinib resistant BCR-ABL1 mutations at relapse in children with Ph+ ALL: a Children's Oncology Group (COG) study. Br J Haematol. 2012;157(4):507–10.
55. Tran TH, et al. The EBF1-PDGFRB T681I mutation is highly resistant to imatinib and dasatinib in vitro and detectable in clinical samples prior to treatment. Haematologica. 2021;106(8):2242–5.
56. Jabbour E, et al. Ponatinib and blinatumomab for Philadelphia chromosome-positive acute lymphoblastic leukaemia: a US, single-centre, single-arm, phase 2 trial. Lancet Haematol. 2023;10(1):e24–34.

Part IV

Immunotherapy in ALL

13 The Role for Immunotherapy in Childhood Acute Lymphoblastic Leukemia

Franco Locatelli, Martin Schrappe, and Francesca del Bufalo

Although the survival rate of pediatric patients with acute lymphoblastic leukemia (ALL) has considerably improved over the past few decades and nowadays it approaches 90%, disease recurrence remains the main cause of treatment failure in childhood ALL and the long-term outcome of relapsed patients is still unsatisfactory [1]. Indeed, relapsed/refractory ALL remains a leading cause of mortality in children with cancer. Prognostic factors for patients experiencing leukemia relapse are the duration of first remission, the immunophenotype of the malignant clone, site of relapse, and recurrent very high-risk genetic features, including KMT2A rearrangements, t(1;19), t (17;19); hypodiploidy, TP53 mutations [1]. Novel treatments based on the use of either monoclonal antibodies (mAbs) or even more innovative immunotherapies hold promise for these children and several breakthroughs in the treatment of ALL have been achieved with these strategies [2]. Novel immunotherapy approaches are under investigation also in newly diagnosed patients with the goal of not only decreasing the recurrence rate but also sparing the acute and chronic toxicities associated with intensive, multi-agent chemotherapy courses, which may have a particularly detrimental effect in subjects with a long expectancy of life.

The most relevant results in the use of immunotherapy strategies have been obtained in patients with B-ALL: by targeting CD19 and/or CD22, several different approaches have been tested so far (see Fig. 13.1). Blinatumomab, a bispecific antibody able to simultaneously bind the CD3 molecule expressed on the cell surface of T cells and the CD19 antigen on leukemia cells, is the first T-cell engager molecule approved for the treatment of both adult and pediatric patients with relapsed/refractory (r/r) B-ALL after the results obtained in prospective clinical studies [3, 4]. In particular, a phase I/II trial identified the recommended dose in children with full-blown r/r B-ALL (5 μg/m^2/day for 1 week and then 15 μg/m^2/day for 3 additional weeks) and demonstrated that the drug can induce complete remission (CR) in about 40% of patients [4]. In a large proportion of these patients, morphological CR was associated with negative measurable residual disease (MRD). A subsequent

F. Locatelli (✉)
Pediatric Haematology/Oncology and Cell and Gene Therapy Department – IRCCS, Bambino Gesù Children's Hospital, Rome, Italy

Department of Life Sciences, Catholic University of the Sacred Heart, Rome, Italy
e-mail: franco.locatelli@opbg.net

M. Schrappe
Department of Pediatrics I, Pediatric Hematology/Oncology, ALL-BFM Study Group, Christian Albrechts University Kiel and University Hospital Schleswig-Holstein, Campus Kiel, Kiel, Germany
e-mail: m.schrappe@pediatrics.uni-kiel.de

F. del Bufalo
Pediatric Haematology/Oncology and Cell and Gene Therapy Department – IRCCS, Bambino Gesù Children's Hospital, Rome, Italy
e-mail: francesca.delbufalo@opbg.net

G. Escherich, V. Conter (eds.), *Acute Lymphoblastic Leukemia in Children and Adolescents*, Pediatric Oncology, https://doi.org/10.1007/978-3-031-71180-0_13

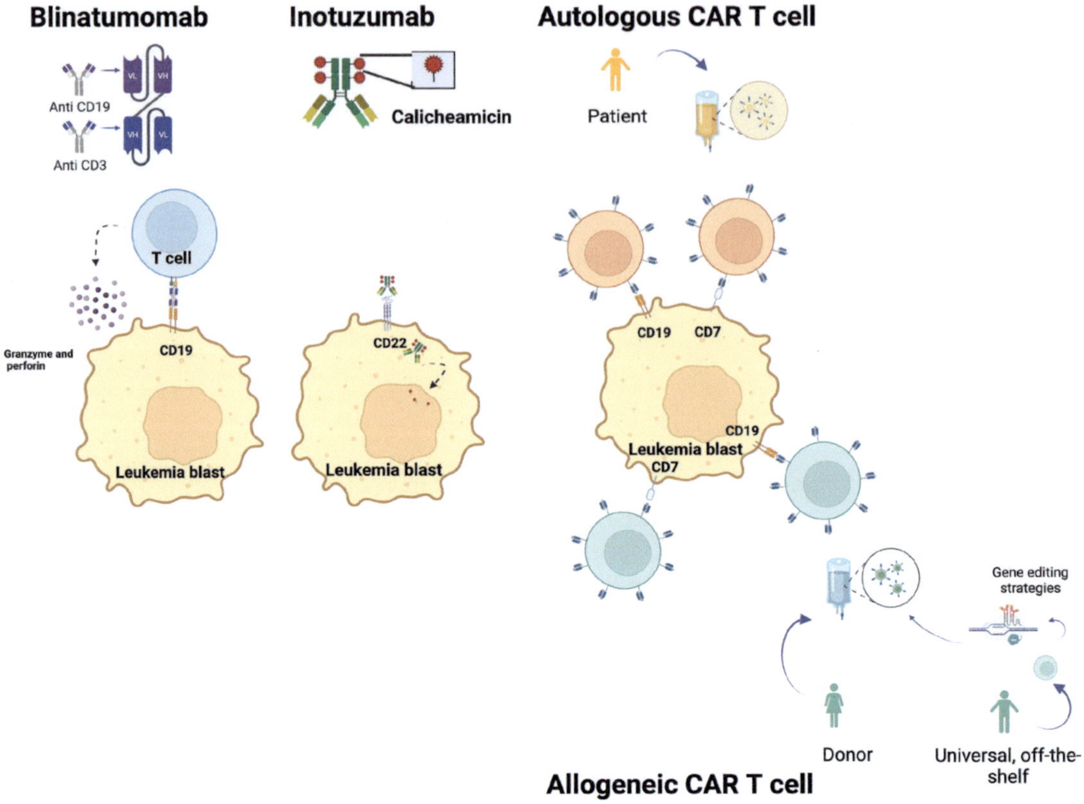

Fig. 13.1 Main immunotherapy approaches for acute lymphoblastic leukemia. Bispecific T-cell engager (BiTE) targeting CD19 (Blinatumomab) (left panel); antibody-drug conjugate targeting CD22 and delivering calicheamicin to blasts (Inotuzumab) (middle panel); CD19 or CD7 targeting CAR-T cells (right panel), either autologous (upper panel) or allogeneic (lower panel)

expanded access study showed that the probability of obtaining CR after treatment with blinatumomab inversely correlates with the BM blast percentage and that patients treated in morphological CR but with molecularly resistant disease may achieve MRD negativity in 90% of cases [5]. Two randomized clinical trials recently proved the superiority of blinatumomab over conventional chemotherapy as consolidation treatment before allogeneic HSCT in children with high-risk or intermediate-risk, first relapse of B-ALL, resulting in improved disease-free survival, lower incidence of posttransplantation disease recurrence, and significantly reduced toxicity [6, 7]. Even more recently, blinatumomab has been studied also in standard-risk first relapse B-ALL in a phase 3 trial, in which blinatumomab was intercalated to continuation chemotherapy before maintenance, and tested against standard chemotherapy courses [8]. The study demonstrated a benefit of the blinatumomab-containing arm in patients with a bone marrow relapse, with or without extramedullary involvement. By contrast, no advantage related to the use of blinatumomab was recorded in patients with isolated extramedullary relapse, likely due to the limited ability of the agent to cross the blood–brain barrier [8]. In newly diagnosed patients with high-risk B-ALL, the prospective clinical trial AIEOP-BFM ALL 2017 focused on the reduction of treatment-related complications in children stratified to the high-risk group by replacing parts of the highly intensive consolidation phase with two courses of blinatumomab. In this randomized trial, after the first consolidation block, high-risk patients were randomized to receive either two courses of conventional consolidation (blocks HR-2 and HR-3), or two 28-day courses of blinatumomab at 15 μg/m²/day administered by continuous IV infusion (with a 2-week treatment-free interval). Although the efficacy data are still to be reported, the safety analysis demonstrated that the toxicity profile of blinatumomab is much more favorable as compared to the intensive cytotoxic agent-based approach using chemotherapy blocks [9]. Van der Sluis and colleagues investigated in a phase II trial the safety and efficacy of one course of blinatumomab added to the Interfant-06 backbone in 30 infants with newly diagnosed KMT2A-rearranged B-ALL [10]. Blinatumomab was employed at the end of induction therapy, before the administration of consolidation therapy. No toxic effects meeting the definition of the primary endpoint occurred. Remarkably, the 2-year probability of disease-free survival (DFS) was 81.6% and that of overall survival (OS) was 93.3%; these results compare very favorably with the corresponding values of 49.4% and 62.1% recorded in the Interfant-06 study protocol, suggesting that blinatumomab may lower the high incidence of relapses which occur frequently and early during therapy in this peculiar type of B-ALL [11]. A prospective trial, Interfant 21, aimed at validating these promising results on the use of blinatumomab in intermediate or high-risk infants with newly diagnosed KMT2A-rearranged B-ALL has just started. Peculiar toxicities associated with the use of blinatumomab include cytokine release syndrome (CRS), whose frequency and severity correlate with the leukemia burden and usually occur during the first days of administration of the drug, and neurotoxicity, mainly represented by seizures. These toxicities are commonly manageable with the temporary discontinuation of the drug and with the use of steroids or interleukin-6 neutralizing antibodies, whenever needed. Children with constitutional trisomy 21, especially if older than 10 years, seem to be at particular risk of developing neurotoxicity and thus may be elective candidates to be prophylactically treated with anti-epileptic drugs.

Another extremely promising immunotherapy is represented by inotuzumab, a humanized anti-CD22 monoclonal antibody bound to calicheamicin, a potent cytotoxic agent, causing cell death by inducing double-strand DNA breaks. [12] Results from an adult phase III study showed the superiority of weekly inotuzumab over standard intensive chemotherapy, with significantly greater CR rates, MRD negativity, and duration of remission [13]. In the pediatric population, data on the safety and efficacy of Inotuzumab have recently been published: the recommended dose was established at 1.8 mg/m²/course, fractionated in three doses with an initial loading dose as in adults, and the overall response rate of the antibody–drug conjugate was 80% [14]. The phase 2 part of the same study confirmed the very high response rate in multiple relapse setting, as well as in patients relapsing after allogeneic stem cell transplantation [15]. The mechanism of resistance to inotuzumab still needs to be elucidated and deserves further investigation. The combination of inotuzumab with a modified R3 reinduction regimen of chemotherapy (5-day blocks of 20 mg/m² dexamethasone, weekly vincristine) did not show any advantage deriving from the addition of chemotherapy to the mAb, suggesting that the anti-leukemia effect displayed by inotuzumab could not be susceptible to a further increase with conventional cytotoxic agents [16]. Several pediatric cooperative groups are testing inotuzumab in children with newly diagnosed B-ALL. In particular, the ALLTogether group is investigating the use of inotuzumab in a prospective clinical trial (NCT04307576) during consolidation for newly diagnosed ALL patients with persistent high MRD level, while the Children Oncology Group (COG) is testing the agent in a phase 3 randomized trial in newly diagnosed high-risk CD22-positive BCP-ALL (NCT03959085). The international consortium on relapsed ALL (IntReALL group) is conducting two prospective randomized clinical trials in standard- and high-risk first-relapse B-ALL comparing one course of inotuzumab vs. the classical R3 reinduction scheme, with the goals of improving the MRD negativity in patients at the end of induction therapy and to improve the patient's final outcome. A particular concern related to the use of inotuzumab is the occurrence of sinusoidal obstruction syndrome (SOS), likely due to the calicheamicin component. This complication has been frequently recorded in patients subsequently treated with allogeneic hematopoietic stem cell transplantation, but it can be diagnosed also during subsequent chemotherapy administration, especially if thioguanine is employed [17]. Strategies to reduce the risk of SOS after allogeneic stem cell transplantation in patients treated with inotuzumab are based on the choice of not administering more than three courses of inotuzumab and trying to prolong the time elapsed between the last course of the drug and transplantation, by using some bridging therapy.

The most sophisticated form of immunotherapy is represented by engineering T cells to express a chimeric antigen receptor (CAR) resulting from the fusion of the heavy and light chain variable regions of a mAb to the cytotoxic ζ chain of a T-cell receptor (TCR) (first-generation CAR), with the inclusion of either one or two co-stimulatory molecules (second- and third-generation CAR). The most widely used co-stimulatory domains include CD28 and 4-1BB. Several studies have been conducted on B-ALL by using second-generation CAR constructs different in terms of costimulatory domains and viral platform, and all consistently showed an antitumor efficacy exceeding expectations, with CR rates ranging from 70% up to 90% [18, 19, 20]. An international, multicenter, global study (ELIANA) confirmed these unprecedented results, thus leading to the approval by both FDA and EMA of tisagenlecleucel for the treatment of children and young adults (up to the age of 25 years) with r/r B-ALL [21]. In particular, tisagenlecleucel (which includes 4-1BB as co-stimulatory domain) is approved for patients with ALL resistant to conventional therapy, for those relapsing after an allograft and for subjects who have experienced two previous relapses. Recently, the 3-year update of the ELIANA study was published confirming an overall remission rate of 82%, with a 3-year event-free survival (EFS) of 44% [22]. CD19-targeting CAR T cells are able to induce similar results across cytogenetic categories and are associated with promising outcomes also in infants [23]. In addition, some preliminary evidence of the efficacy of CD19-targeting CAR T cells in patients with central nervous system (CNS) involvement has been reported, especially if disease control is achieved before infusion of the cell product [24, 25].

Some drawbacks limit the success rate of CAR T-cell therapy, including failure to generate CAR T cells and non-target antigen toxicities, such as CRS and neurotoxicity, whose frequency and severity largely depend on leukemia burden at the time of CAR T-cell infusion. A duration of B-cell aplasia (BCA) shorter than 3–6 months [26] and a high-disease burden were reported to be independently associated with inferior EFS [27]. Thus, these findings are to be considered to decide if patients reaching CR after CD19-targeting CAR T cells should be offered a subsequent allograft to optimize the chance of eradicating the leukemia population. Importantly, a substantial proportion of patient relapses and CD19dim or negative recurrence is an important cause of treatment failure because of alternative exon splicing forms of the CD19 gene where exon 2 is lost [28]. In order to reduce the risk of immunological escape, bispecific CAR T cells simultaneously targeting different surface antigens are currently being tested. The report of six adults affected by r/r B-ALL treated with CD19/CD22 CAR T cells shows that all the treated patients obtained CR; however, 50% of them relapsed 3–10 months after treatment [29]. Several aspects of the treatment with CAR T cells still need to be fully elucidated and optimized. Among these, the choice of the best bridging treatment to control the disease during the manufacturing window is still largely unexplored. Concerning the impact of previously administered immunotherapies on the benefit deriving from CAR T-cell administration, Dourthe et al. recently reported that patients previously exposed to blinatumomab as bridging therapy had lower probability of benefiting from CAR T cells [30]. However, these results were not confirmed by a larger study published by Myers and colleagues who showed that only blinatumomab non-responders had lower complete remission rates to

CD19-targeting CAR T cells, while the CR rate and the EFS of blinatumomab-naive patients and blinatumomab non-responders was superimposable [31].

A recent German real-world experience showed another important obstacle to the efficacy of autologous CAR T cells. Interestingly, the authors showed that in patients relapsing after allogeneic transplantation, the use of tisagenlecleucel within 6 months from the allograft is associated with significantly worse long-term outcomes and shorter duration of B-cell aplasia (BCA) than those recorded in patients relapsing >6 months after transplantation [32]. These findings suggest a lower persistence of CAR T cells generated early after allogeneic stem cell transplantation and the authors speculate that they may be associated with an incomplete restoration of polyclonal and functional T cells early after transplantation. To overcome this obstacle, CAR T cells generated directly from the transplant donor have been employed. Two major strategies have made their way to the clinics showing promising results: the use of donor-derived allogeneic T cells and the use of off-the-shelf, gene-edited universal T cells. The former approach has been shown to be associated with no rejection by the patient, limited risk of graft-versus-host disease, promising long-term persistence, and promising antitumor efficacy but is limited by the availability of a cell donor [33]. Universal, off-the-shelf CAR T cells represent a fascinating approach, potentially readily available for every patient in need of treatment, and showed an acceptable toxicity profile and promising efficacy. The limited long-term persistence and the consistent risk of relapse after their infusion suggests, however, the need to further optimize the approach [34].

The results of immunotherapies for the treatment of T-ALL have been less encouraging, and several specific hurdles still need to be overcome, including the lack of tumor-specific surface antigen (with the subsequent risk of T-cell aplasia), and, for CAR T cells, the risk of transducing blasts and the occurrence of fratricide. CD38 represents an interesting target for immunotherapy, being expressed in a high proportion of T-ALL blasts. The use of the CD38-directed monoclonal antibody daratumumab (a monoclonal antibody approved as monotherapy and in combination with standard-of-care regimens for newly diagnosed and r/r multiple myeloma that induces lysis through cytotoxic mechanisms such as complement-dependent, cell-mediated lysis, and antibody-dependent cellular phagocytosis) has demonstrated efficacy against T-ALL in preclinical studies and few patients and was investigated in a phase II study in pediatric and young adult patients with relapsed/refractory T-cell ALL (NCT03384654) [35, 36]. In a non-randomized phase 1–2 trial, daratumumab was used in combination with standard four-drug re-induction (vincristine, prednisone, PEG-asparaginase, and doxorubicin). Among 24 T-ALL pediatric patients, 41.7% (n = 10) achieved CR at the end of induction therapy, while the overall response rate achieved at any time during treatment was 83.3% [37]. The use of CAR T cells has been explored only preliminarily in patients with T-ALL. To date, only the results of the use of CD7-edited, allogeneic T cells expressing a CD7-directed CAR T cell on two patients affected by T-ALL have been reported, both obtaining MRD-negative CR [38]. In order to overcome the risk of blast contamination in the drug product, third-party, off-the-shelf products have been exploited. In particular, Chiesa and colleagues recently reported their experience on the first three patients treated with CD7-directed, universal, off-the-shelf CAR T cells generated using base-editing technology and showed that the approach is feasible and was able to induce MRD-negative CR in two out of three patients, the third, unfortunately, developing a fatal fungal infection [39]. Besides the use of gene-edited allogeneic T cells with a knockout of the T-cell receptor (TCR) α-chain, another strategy to develop allogeneic CAR-cell products avoiding the risks of graft-versus-host disease is represented by the use of different cell platforms lacking allogeneic reactivity, such as natural killer (NK) cells. CAR NK cells targeting CD19 have shown extraordinary early results in both preclinical [40] and clinical studies [41], encouraging further clinical exploration. Allogeneic cytokine-induced killer cells also can represent another interesting off-the-shelf product, “with promising results reported in a phase I/II trial in B-ALL [42]. Besides allogeneic products, an interesting autologous approach was developed by the group of Campana by co-expressing in T cells the CAR construct and a protein-expression blocker (PEBL) able to retain the CD7 protein in the endoplasmic reticulum/Golgi apparatus, thus preventing fratricide and enabling the successful manufacturing of CAR T cells [43]. The clinical testing of the approach is undergoing and results are eagerly awaited.

In summary, it is easy to predict that, in the forthcoming years, the therapeutic scenario of childhood ALL will be characterized by the introduction of several immunotherapy approaches not only in patients with r/r ALL, but also in the whole treatment strategy of newly diagnosed patients. Indeed, despite the long-term OS of about 90% currently reached with the available standard-of-care poly-chemotherapy regimens, the need to replace toxic elements with newer, more selective anti-leukemia agents is clear and pediatric front-line regimens are also moving toward significant changes, with the introduction of antibodies and even CAR T-cell therapy, but also other targeted agents like menin inhibitors for specific subgroups, such as children with KMT2A-rearranged leukemia [44].

References

1. Locatelli F, Schrappe M, Bernardo ME, Rutella S. How I treat relapsed childhood acute lymphoblastic leukemia. Blood. 2012;120(14):2807–16.
2. Batlevi CL, Matsuki E, Brentjens RJ, Younes A. Novel immunotherapies in lymphoid malignancies. Nat Rev Clin Oncol. 2016;13(1):25–40.
3. Topp MS, Gokbuget N, Stein AS, et al. Safety and activity of blinatumomab for adult patients with relapsed or refractory B-precursor acute lymphoblastic leukaemia: a multicentre, single-arm, phase 2 study. Lancet Oncol. 2015;16(1):57–66.
4. von Stackelberg A, Locatelli F, Zugmaier G, et al. Phase I/phase II study of Blinatumomab in pediatric patients with relapsed/refractory acute lymphoblastic leukemia. J Clin Oncol. 2016;34(36):4381–9.
5. Locatelli F, Zugmaier G, Mergen N, et al. Blinatumomab in pediatric patients with relapsed/refractory acute lymphoblastic leukemia: results of the RIALTO trial, an expanded access study. Blood Cancer J. 2020;10:77.
6. Locatelli F, Zugmaier G, Rizzari C, et al. Effect of Blinatumomab vs chemotherapy on event-free survival among children with high-risk first-relapse B-cell acute lymphoblastic leukemia. A randomized clinical trial. JAMA. 2021;325(9):843–54. https://doi.org/10.1001/jama.2021.0987.
7. Brown PA, Ji L, Xu X, et al. Effect of Postreinduction therapy consolidation with Blinatumomab vs chemotherapy on disease-free survival in children, adolescents, and young adults with first relapse of B-cell acute lymphoblastic leukemia. A randomized clinical trial. JAMA. 2021;325(9):833–42. https://doi.org/10.1001/jama.2021.0669.
8. Hogan LE, Brown PA, Ji L, Xu X, Devidas M, Bhatla T, et al. Children's oncology group AALL1331: phase III trial of Blinatumomab in children, adolescents, and young adults with low-risk B-cell ALL in first relapse. J Clin Oncol. 2023;41(25):4118–29.
9. Schrappe M, Locatelli F, Valsecchi MG, Cario G, et al. Pediatric patients with high-risk B-cell ALL in first complete remission may benefit from less toxic immunotherapy with Blinatumomab – results from randomized controlled phase 3 trial AIEOP-BFM ALL 2017. Blood. 2023;142(Suppl 1):825.
10. van der Sluis IM, de Lorenzo P, Kotecha RS, Attarbaschi A, et al. Blinatumomab added to chemotherapy in infant lymphoblastic leukemia. N Engl J Med. 2023;388(17):1572–81.
11. Pieters R, De Lorenzo P, Ancliffe P, Aversa LA, et al. Outcome of infants younger than 1 year with acute lymphoblastic leukemia treated with the Interfant-06 protocol: results from an international phase III randomized study. J Clin Oncol. 2019;37(25):2246–56.
12. Jabbour E, O'Brien S, Ravandi F, Kantarjian H. Monoclonal antibodies in acute lymphoblastic leukemia. Blood. 2015;125(26):4010–6.
13. Kantarjian HM, DeAngelo DJ, Stelljes M, et al. Inotuzumab Ozogamicin versus standard therapy for acute lymphoblastic leukemia. N Engl J Med. 2016;375(8):740–53.
14. Brivio E, Locatelli F, Lopez-Yurda M, et al. A phase I study of inotuzumab ozogamicin in pediatric relapsed/refractory acute lymphoblastic leukemia (ITCC-059 study). Blood. 2020:blood.2020007848.
15. Pennesi E, Michels N, Brivio E, van der Velden VHJ, et al. Inotuzumab ozogamicin as single agent in pediatric patients with relapsed and refractory acute lymphoblastic leukemia: results from a phase II trial. Leukemia. 2022;36(6):1516–24.
16. Pennesi E, Brivio E, Ammerlaan ACJ, Jiang Y, et al. Inotuzumab ozogamicin combined with chemotherapy in pediatric B-cell precursor CD22+ acute lymphoblastic leukemia: results of the phase IB ITCC-059 trial. Haematologica. 2024;4 https://doi.org/10.3324/haematol.2023.284409.
17. O'Brien MM, Ji L, Shah NN, Rheingold SR, Bhojwani D, Yuan CM, et al. Phase II trial of Inotuzumab Ozogamicin in children and adolescents with relapsed or refractory B-cell acute lymphoblastic leukemia: Children's oncology group protocol AALL1621. J Clin Oncol. 2022;40(9):956–67.

18. Davila ML, Riviere I, Wang X, et al. Efficacy and toxicity management of 19-28z CAR T cell therapy in B cell acute lymphoblastic leukemia. Sci Transl Med. 2014;6(224):224ra25.
19. Maude SL, Frey N, Shaw PA, et al. Chimeric antigen receptor T cells for sustained remissions in leukemia. N Engl J Med. 2014;371(16):1507–17.
20. Lee DW, Kochenderfer JN, Stetler-Stevenson M, et al. T cells expressing CD19 chimeric antigen receptors for acute lymphoblastic leukaemia in children and young adults: a phase 1 dose-escalation trial. Lancet. 2015;385(9967):517–28.
21. Maude SL, Laetsch TW, Buechner J, et al. Tisagenlecleucel in children and young adults with B-cell lymphoblastic leukemia. N Engl J Med. 2018;378(5):439–48.
22. Laetsch TW, Maude SL, Rives S, et al. Three-year update of Tisagenlecleucel in pediatric and young adult patients with relapsed/refractory acute lymphoblastic leukemia in the ELIANA trial. J Clin Oncol. 2023;41(9):1664–9.
23. Ghorashian S, Jacoby E, De Moerloose B, et al. Tisagenlecleucel therapy for relapsed or refractory B-cell acute lymphoblastic leukaemia in infants and children younger than 3 years of age at screening: an international, multicentre, retrospective cohort study. Lancet Haematol. 2022;9(10):e766–75.
24. Leahy AB, Newman H, Li Y, et al. CD19-targeted chimeric antigen receptor T-cell therapy for CNS relapsed or refractory acute lymphocytic leukaemia: a post-hoc analysis of pooled data from five clinical trials. Lancet Haematol. 2021;8(10):e711–e22.
25. Jacoby E, Ghorashian S, Vormoor B, et al. CD19 CAR T-cells for pediatric relapsed acute lymphoblastic leukemia with active CNS involvement: a retrospective international study. Leukemia. 2022;36(6):1525–32.
26. Pulsipher MA, Han X, Maude SL, Laetsch TW, et al. Next-generation sequencing of minimal residual disease for predicting relapse after Tisagenlecleucel in children and young adults with acute lymphoblastic leukemia. Blood Cancer Discov. 2022;3(1):66–81.
27. Schultz LM, Baggott C, Prabhu S, Pacenta HL, et al. Disease burden affects outcomes in pediatric and young adult B-cell lymphoblastic leukemia after commercial Tisagenlecleucel: a pediatric real-world chimeric antigen receptor consortium report. J Clin Oncol. 2022;40(9):945–55.
28. Sotillo E, Barrett D, Black KL, et al. Convergence of acquired mutations and alternative splicing of CD19 enables resistance to CART-19 immunotherapy. Cancer Discov. 2015;5(12):1282–95.
29. Dai H, Wu Z, Jia H, et al. Bispecific CAR-T cells targeting both CD19 and CD22 for therapy of adults with relapsed or refractory B cell acute lymphoblastic leukemia. J Hematol Oncol. 2020;13(1):30.
30. Dourthe E, Rabian F, Yakouben K, et al. Determinants of CD19-positive vs CD19-negative relapse after tisagenlecleucel for B-cell acute lymphoblastic leukemia. Leukemia. 2021;35(12):3383–93.
31. Myers RM, Taraseviciute A, Steinberg SM, Lamble AJ, et al. Blinatumomab nonresponse and high-disease burden are associated with inferior outcomes after CD19-CAR for B-ALL. J Clin Oncol. 2022;40(9):932–44.
32. Bader P, Rossig C, Hutter M, et al. CD19 CAR T cells are an effective therapy for posttransplant relapse in patients with B-lineage ALL: real-world data from Germany. Blood Adv. 2023;7(11):2436–48.
33. Del Bufalo F, Becilli M, Rosignoli C, De Angelis B, et al. Allogeneic, donor-derived, second-generation, CD19-directed CAR-T cells for the treatment of pediatric relapsed/refractory BCP-ALL. Blood. 2023;142(2):146–57.
34. Benjamin R, Graham C, Yallop D, et al. Genome-edited, donor-derived allogeneic anti-CD19 chimeric antigen receptor T cells in paediatric and adult B-cell acute lymphoblastic leukaemia: results of two phase 1 studies. Lancet. 2020;396(10266):1885–94.
35. Bride KL, Vincent TL, Im SY, et al. Preclinical efficacy of daratumumab in T-cell acute lymphoblastic leukemia. Blood. 2018;131(9):995–9.
36. Ofran Y, Ringelstein-Harlev S, Slouzkey I, et al. Daratumumab for eradication of minimal residual disease in high-risk advanced relapse of T-cell/CD19/CD22-negative acute lymphoblastic leukemia. Leukemia. 2020;34(1):293–5.
37. Hogan LE, Bhatla T, Teachey DT, Sirvent FJB, Moppett J, Puyó PV, et al. Efficacy and safety of daratumumab (DARA) in pediatric and young adult patients (pts) with relapsed/refractory T-cell acute lymphoblastic leukemia (ALL) or lymphoblastic lymphoma (LL): results from the phase 2 DELPHINUS study. J Clin Oncol. 2022;40(16_suppl):10001.
38. Li S, Wang X, Yuan Z, et al. Eradication of T-ALL cells by CD7-targeted universal CAR-T cells and initial test of Ruxolitinib-based CRS management. Clin Cancer Res. 2021;27(5):1242–6.
39. Chiesa R, Georgiadis C, Syed F, et al. Base-edited CAR7 T cells for relapsed T-cell acute lymphoblastic leukemia. N Engl J Med. 2023;389(10):899–910.
40. Quintarelli C, Sivori S, Caruso S, et al. Efficacy of third-party chimeric-antigen receptor modified peripheral blood natural killer cells for adoptive cell therapy of B–cell precursor acute lymphoblastic leukemia. Leukemia. 2020;34:1102–15.
41. Liu E, Marin D, Banerjee P, et al. Use of CAR-transduced natural killer cells in CD19-positive lymphoid tumors. N Engl J Med. 2020;382:545–53.
42. Magnani CF, Gaipa G, Lussana F, et al. Sleeping beauty-engineered CAR T cells achieve antileukemic activity without severe toxicities. J Clin Invest. 2020;130(11):6021–33.
43. Png YT, Vinanica N, Kamiya T, et al. Blockade of CD7 expression in T cells for effective chimeric antigen receptor targeting of T-cell malignancies. Blood Adv. 2017;1(25):2348–60.
44. Issa GC, Aldoss I, DiPersio J, Cuglievan B, et al. The menin inhibitor revumenib in KMT2A-rearranged or NPM1-mutant leukaemia. Nature. 2023;615(7954):920–4.

CAR T in Childhood Acute Lymphoblastic Leukemia

14

Friso Calkoen and Jochen Buechner

14.1 Introduction

The improvements of chimeric antigen receptor (CAR) T cell therapy in the last decade has augmented the therapeutic options for children and young adults with relapsed refractory B-cell precursor ALL (BCP-ALL). The overall goal of this chapter is to provide insights into the concept of CAR T cell therapy for ALL. The clinical use and the future challenges of this novel therapy are discussed.

14.2 The Anatomy of CAR T Cell Therapy

The aim of CAR T cell therapy (CAR T) is to specifically redirect healthy T cells to malignant cells by gene transfer of a CAR construct. A CAR construct consists of an extracellular antigen recognition domain, a transmembrane domain, and an intracellular cytoplasmic signaling domain. The antigen recognition domain is typically a single-chain variable fragment (scFv), derived from a monoclonal antibody and is responsible for specifically recognizing a protein or antigen present on the surface of cancer cells (Fig. 14.1). The concept of directing T cells via an artificial receptor to target cells was first developed by Eshar and colleagues in Israel and concomitantly by the research group headed by Kurosowa [2, 3]. The first generation of CAR T cells, directed against HIV and solid tumors, had only one signaling domain, the CD3z chain [4, 5]. The addition of costimulatory domains, providing signal II in T-cell stimulation in second-generation CARs improved the proliferation, function and persistence of the effector cells [6, 7]. Directing T cells to CD19, a transmembrane protein of importance for intrinsic B cell signaling and widely expressed on normal and malignant B-cells, was shown to be very efficient to eliminate malignant CD19+ cells in vitro [8, 9]. Initial clinical trials in adults with treatment refractory CD19+ chronic lymphoblastic leukemia (CLL) achieved complete response rates from 30% to 50% [10]. The introduction of CD19 directed CAR T in BCP-ALL and B-NHL with complete response rates over 70% boosted the CAR T development [11–14].

F. Calkoen (✉)
Princess Maxima Center for Pediatric Oncology, Utrecht, The Netherlands
e-mail: f.g.j.calkoen-2@prinsesmaximacentrum.nl

J. Buechner
Department of Pediatric Hematology and Oncology, Oslo University Hospital, Oslo, Norway

G. Escherich, V. Conter (eds.), *Acute Lymphoblastic Leukemia in Children and Adolescents*, Pediatric Oncology, https://doi.org/10.1007/978-3-031-71180-0_14

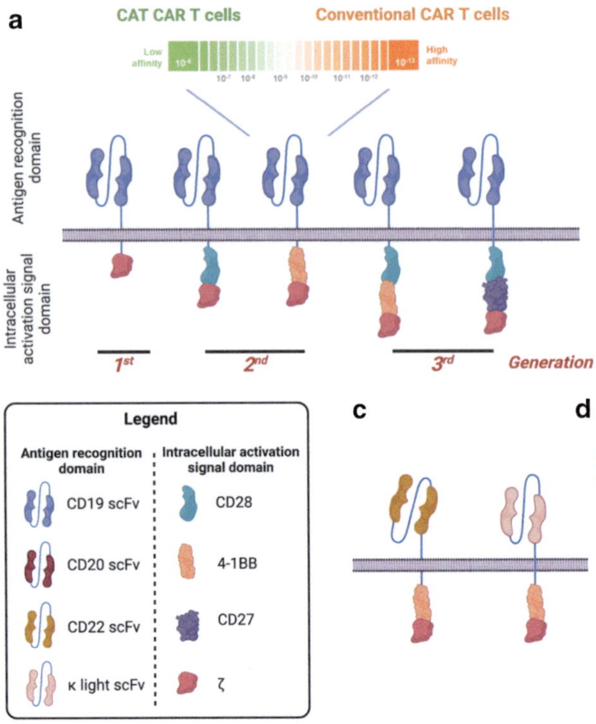

Fig. 14.1 Visual summary of different chimeric antigen receptor (CAR) designs to target B-cell malignancies. CD19 CAR has been tested in many clinical trials so far. Different generations of CD19 CAR have been developed including a second-generation CD19 CAR with low affinity for the CD19 antigen (CAT CAR) (**a**). Several groups proposed strategies to improve the long-term efficacy of the CD19 CAR by armored CAR constructs capable of expressing both CD19 CAR and other molecules such as CD40L, interleukin 18 (IL-18), or programmed death 1 (PD1) capable of improving cytotoxic activity, reducing the exhaustion profile, and sustaining the proliferation and persistence of CAR T cells (**b**). In addition to CD19, other B-cell antigens have been investigated and CARs have been generated and tested in preclinical and early-stage human clinical studies (e.g., CD22 and k light chain) (**c**). To avoid tumor escape, bispecific CARs have been developed targeting, for example, CD19 and CD20 or CD22 (**d**). To improve the safety profile and generate a tool to mitigate/abrogate side effects, a suicide gene based on an inducible caspase 9 (iC9) has been developed and validated (**e**). previously published in Buechner et al. Buechner et al. [1]

14.3 CAR T Cell Therapy in BCP-ALL

In 2013, the first two children, both with chemorefractory BCP-ALL, were treated with CD19 CAR T [15]. These children received CTL019 (later developed as tisagenlecleucel), an autologous, second-generation anti-CD19 CAR T cell product composed of a scFv from the recombinant monoclonal murine antibody clone FMC63 for CD19 antigen recognition, a CD8-α hinge region, a 4-1BB (CD137) costimulatory domain and CD3ζ as a signaling domain utilizing a lentiviral transduction [9]. The clinical course of these patients highlights the challenges in CAR T cell therapy with respect to toxicity and efficacy. Both patients experienced severe life-threatening systemic inflammation, an entity now well known as cytokine release syndrome (CRS). The use of a blocking antibody of the IL-6 receptor, tocilizumab, was initiated based on extensive cytokine profiling in the first child treated. As discussed later in this chapter, tocilizumab became a pivotal drug of CRS management. Both patients survived CRS and had a complete response at early evaluation.

The overall remission rate (ORR), including CR and CR with incomplete hematologic recovery in the first phase I/II CAR T cell trial with tisagenlecleucel (NCT01626495 and NCT01029366) at the Children's Hospital of Philadelphia was 90%, with 22 of 25 evaluable patients achieving a minimal residual disease (MRD)-negative CR [16]. This led to the subsequent phase II trial ENSIGN (NCT02228096) further investigating tisagenlecleucel in a multicenter setting with centralized manufacturing. The trial enrolled 73 patients of whom 58 were infused. The ORR within 6 months of infusion was 69%. Subsequently, the international pivotal ELIANA phase II trial (NCT02435849), investigated the safety and efficacy of tisagenlecleucel in pediatric patients with relapsed (either ≥ 2nd relapse or relapse after allogeneic hematopoietic stem cell transplantation, HSCT) or refractory BCP-ALL at 25 study sites in 11 countries across North America, Europe, Asia, and Australia [11]. In the primary publication, 75 infused patients (aged 3–23 years at enrolment) were reported, of whom 61% had relapsed after prior HSCT. Sixty-one patients (81%) were in CR/CRi within 3 months post infusion. The last update from this trial with 79 patients infused at a median follow-up of 38.8 months reported an estimated EFS of 44% and estimated OS of 63% among all infused patients at 3 years. The probability of CAR T cell persistence, measured by persistent B-cell aplasia at 12 and 24 months, was 71% and 59%, respectively [17].

No significant difference in RFS was seen when patients who underwent consolidating therapy including HSCT were censored in the analysis (3-year RFS 52% and 47.8% with or without censoring for allogeneic stem-cell transplant and/or further anticancer therapies, respectively). This supports the potential of CAR T cells to serve as a single agent treatment option with long-term efficacy in children and young adults with relapsed/refractory BCP-ALL. Tisagenlecleucel is currently (as of May 2023) the only FDA and EMA approved CAR T cell therapy for patients with BCP-ALL under 18 years of age. Labeled indications are a second or higher relapse, a relapse post HSCT (in Europe), or refractory disease. After receiving marketing authorization, numerous groups and consortia have published "real-world experience" with tisagenlecleucel outside of clinical trials, confirming and extending the results from the initial registration trials [18–22]. Various other company sponsored trials evaluate the safety and efficacy of CD19-directed CAR T therapy in children with B cell malignancies (e.g., NCT02625480, NCT04245839, and NCT03853616).

Although patients with active CNS disease or younger than 3 years were excluded from the registration trials, numerous consortia collecting data from "real-world use" of tisagenlecleucel have demonstrated comparable efficacy of CAR T cell therapy in extramedullary disease [23–25]. Infants with ALL, irrespective of KMT2A status benefit from CAR T cell therapy in a similar manner [22, 26]. CAR T cell therapy is well tolerated in ALL patients with Down syndrome, with a similar toxicity profile and outcomes as in non-DS patients [27].

Although the early complete response rates after infusion (most often evaluated on day 28) is 80-90%, roughly half of the patients relapse post CD19 CAR T therapy, either with CD19- or CD19+ disease [18, 28]. It is important to define risk factors that predict CAR T failure and tailor patients who optimally benefit from this treatment, or may need further interventions [1]. KMT2A rearrangements, Philadelphia-positive/-like or hypodiploid disease, and cytogenetic risk factors otherwise used for risk stratification of BCP-ALL treatment are not predictive for outcome after CAR T therapy [29, 30]. Potential new genetic risk factors, associated with intrinsic resistance to CAR T cell cytotoxicity, include tp53 mutations and increased death-receptor pathway activation [31, 32]. Despite these improvements, the best predictors of outcome remain leukemic burden at infusion [33, 34], minimal residual disease-negative complete response on day 28 and the duration of CAR T cell persistence [19, 35].

14.3.1 CAR T Cell Manufacturing

The production process of autologous CAR T cells consists of a non-mobilized leukapheresis to collect T cells, activation of T cells, insertion of the CAR construct, expansion of CAR T cells, and of utmost importance, quality controls based on release criteria [36]. T cell apheresis is well tolerated, even in children between 6 and 10 kg, but requires experience and in children often a central venous catheter rather than peripheral venous cannulas [37, 38]. Patients should undergo a pre-collection evaluation including the washout of prior antineoplastic therapy and other drugs compromising T cell fitness, and the presence of uncontrolled infections. In addition, serology testing is mandatory depending on local policies, for example for hepatitis B, hepatitis C, toxoplasmosis, *Treponema pallidum*, and HIV. Local or product-related manuals include the specific wash-out times of drugs prior leukapheresis, as comparative studies to determine the required washout time have not been performed [36, 39]. T cell lytic agents such as anti-CD52 or anti-thymocyte globulin, and clofarabine, require a washout of at least 8 weeks. Highly immunosuppressive drugs like fludarabine or high dose cytarabine can cause prolonged lymphopenia hampering T cell apheresis for 4–6 weeks. Short acting chemotherapy and small molecules like tyrosine kinase inhibitors need approximately 7 days wash-out. A short course of steroids or hydroxyurea can be used to control disease while scheduling the leukapheresis as a 3-day washout can be accepted [39]. The transduction and expansion procedure takes generally 10-14 days. However, numerous efforts are made to shorten this process to limit in vitro T cell exhaustion [40]. The use of allogeneic "third-party" CAR T cells could overcome the production time, reduce the cost of manufacturing a patient-specific product and difficulties with timing of the leukapheresis. Currently, the benefit in BCP-ALL of long-lasting autologous CAR T cells outweighs the potential advantages of allogeneic products. This approach should not be mistaken for CAR T cell production from an apheresis product of the allogeneic HSCT donor.

The optimization of genetically engineered viral vectors in the 1980s was a critical step in the process of CAR T development [41]. Currently, viral transfection with either lentivirus or retrovirus is the most used platform to introduce the CAR construct in immune effector cells. Different ongoing efforts explore the feasibility and efficacy of virus-free transfection platforms. Regarding lentiviral or retroviral transfection, no evidence of recombination-competent virus or tumor transformation post infusion has been registered so far.

Quality control of the final product includes assays to assess safety and efficacy of the product [42]. These are subject to changes in a rapidly developing field. The FDA and EMA provide regular updates of directions for advanced therapy medicinal products (ATMPs).

14.3.2 Bridging Treatment

The goal of the bridging phase is to achieve or keep control of the leukemic disease, rather than obtaining a CR or even an MRD-negative remission prior infusion. High disease burden at infusion is associated with an increased risk of CRS [34, 43] and a higher risk of CD19-negative relapses post CAR T cell infusion [19]. Selecting the optimal bridging strategy depends on the responses to prior antileukemic therapy, disease load and biology, patient's specific toxicity profile and wash-out times before infusion. The patient should be kept in a good clinical condition, avoiding severe bone marrow aplasia, infections or organ dysfunction that all may complicate or even exclude the patient from CAR T cell infusion. Although the toxicity of immunotherapy as a bridging agent is limited, the use of blinatumomab and inotuzumab ozogamicin (InO) is not generally recommended. The use of CD19-directed therapy before CAR T cell infusion can select for CD19-negative clones resulting in inferior outcome of CD19 directed therapy [19, 44]. On the other hand, response to blinatumomab during bridging may indicate efficacy of subsequent CAR T. Myers *et al.* demonstrated that patients not responding to or developing CD19 dim disease during blinatumomab had an inferior outcome after CAR T [45]. Notably, in their study, CR rates and 6-month EFS for blinatumomab-exposed responders and blinatumomab-naïve patients were comparable.

A potential pitfall, particularly with the use of inotuzumab ozogamicin, can be that achieving a MRD-negative response in combination with a deep B-cell aplasia will lead to insufficient CD19 antigen exposure during consecutive CAR T [46]. Similar the 1-year EFS of 53.3% and OS of 77.8% in children and young adults treated with inotuzumab ozogamicin prior to the CAR T was comparable to published cohorts in a retrospective study of 39 patients treated in Europe and the United States [47]. Due to the retrospective nature of this study, the presence and importance of CD19 antigen at the moment of infusion could not be addressed as CD19 load and CAR T cell expansion data were lacking. To enable CAR T cell activation and subsequent expansion, minimal B cell recovery after inotuzumab ozogamicin, e.g., reappearance of hematogones in the bone marrow or detectable B cells in peripheral blood should be awaited before CAR T cells are infused.

14.3.3 Lymphodepleting Regimen

Addition of a lymphodepleting regimen prior to CAR T cell infusion was the first factor demonstrated to improve efficacy [48]. It removes consumptive cytokine "sink" by endogenous lymphocytes, enabling the adoptively transferred T cells a less competitive environment and greater access to IL-7, IL-15, and IL-21, which enhances their homeostatic expansion. The most used agents are cyclophosphamide (Cy) and fludarabine (Flu). Various dosages of Cy have been used ranging from a cumulative dose of 900 mg/m^2 to 3000 mg/m^2. Improved clinical outcome was reported in patients with B-NHL and B-ALL in the cohorts receiving higher doses of Cy. The myelosuppressive acute toxicity and the gonadotoxic long term toxicity of this drug should be taken into account when increasing the doses of this drug [49, 50]. In addition, numerous groups reported a beneficial effect on clinical outcome and CAR T cell expansion if Flu was included in the conditioning regimen [51–53]. Various lymphodepleting regimens are currently used in clinical studies or for commercial use. However, strategies mainly rely on the combination of Flu and Cy. In 2022, Dekker *et al.* and Fabrizio *et al.* reported an association between the Flu exposure and relapse after CAR T cell therapy [54, 55]. Whereas the first group measured the Flu exposure in plasma samples, the latter predicted the exposure based on body weight and renal function. Both came to a comparable clinically relevant cut-offs (an area under the curve of >14 mg•h/L of F-ara-ATP) predictive for persistence of B-cell aplasia and for relapse.

14.3.4 Post-infusion Monitoring

14.3.4.1 Toxicity

Early recognition of cell therapy related side effects and toxicity management have contributed to the successful implementation of CAR T cell therapy in the standard of care treatment protocols for relapsed/refractory B-cell malignancies. The description of the clinical course of the first child treated with CTL019 clearly exemplifies the importance of teamwork in early phase clinical trials [56]. Different consortia have contributed to toxicity management by sharing consensus guidelines for immune cell related toxicity management [39, 57]. Multidisciplinary teams including pediatric neurologist, ICU doctors and dedicated pharmacologists need be involved while implementing these toxicity guidelines for CAR T cell therapy.

14.3.4.2 Cytokine-Release Syndrome (CRS)

CAR T for ALL is often accompanied by severe or life-threatening toxicities [58–60]. The most common adverse event reported in clinical trials and from "real-world experiences" is cytokine-release syndrome (CRS), which occurs in the majority of patients (in 55-77% for CD19-directed products [11, 18, 19, 61]. CRS is an inflammatory syndrome characterized by elevated levels of inflammatory mediators, leading to fever and other characteristic clinical manifestations of varying severity [62]. CRS is observed not just with CAR T and other immune effector cell therapies, but has also been described in many patients treated with bispecific T cell engagers (BiTE), e.g., blinatumomab [63].

The systemic release of inflammatory cytokines from CAR T cells and bystander immune cells, triggered by target cell recognition and killing, is the primary cause of CRS. CAR T cells rapidly activate and proliferate upon antigen recognition ("on-target effect"), particularly in B-cell antigen-directed therapies. This leads to CAR T cell-mediated cytolysis of target cells and the release of numerous inflammatory cytokines and chemokines from activated CAR T cells, bystander immune cells, and non-immune cells. This widespread immune activation amplifies and defines the systemic inflammatory state associated with CRS [62].

Key inflammatory cytokines, including IL-6, interferon γ (IFN-γ), and IL-1, play central roles in CRS, although other cytokines and chemokines are also up-regulated. The specific cell types and their contributions to the onset and exacerbation of CRS are still being investigated. An initial burst of IFN-γ and TNF-α from CAR T cells stimulates immune cells and endothelial cells, triggering the release of other inflammatory mediators such as IL-6 and IL-1. Activated non-CAR T cells and myeloid cells, including monocytes, macrophages, and dendritic cells, serve as specific cellular sources of these cytokines and chemokines, contributing to the cascade of inflammation. Endothelial activation, evidenced by elevated levels of angiopoietin-2 (ANG2) and von Willebrand factor (VWF), is another hallmark feature observed in severe CRS [62].

Evidence from animal models suggests that myeloid-derived monocytes and macrophages, along with their inflammatory products, play a critical role. In the SCID-beige mouse model of CRS [64], macrophages and monocytes exhibited increased expression of IL-6, granulocyte colony-stimulating factor, macrophage colony-stimulating factor, and IL-12, with macrophages being the major producers of iNOS (inducible nitric oxide) leading to abundant production of nitric oxide (NO) which promotes vasodilation and hypotension. In the humanized mouse model [65], CRS was primarily mediated by monocytes, as shown by monocyte-specific ablation preventing CRS development in mice receiving CD19 CAR T cells.

The clinical presentation of CRS in patients undergoing CAR T-cell treatment typically begins 1–2 weeks after cell administration but can occur as early as one day after infusion, depending on product- and patient-specific factors. It is characterized by fever, malaise, fatigue, anorexia, myalgias, nausea, vomiting, headache, and changes in mental status, often resembling infection. From there, the severity, duration, and range of symptoms can vary greatly between patients, with severe cases experiencing hypotension, capillary leak, hypoxia, pulmonary edema, multiorgan failure, and potential death.

The timing of CRS onset, peak, and duration is influenced by various factors. The magnitude of CAR T cell activation and expansion directly affects the development and severity of CRS. Accordingly, disease burden has been identified as most significant predictor of severe CRS after CAR T therapy [66, 67]. Higher doses of CAR T cells [53, 61, 68] and CARs containing CD28 costimulatory domains are also associated with an increased risk and faster onset of CRS [57]. Most CRS cases typically resolve within a span of 7 to 8 days after the initial onset of symptoms. However, there have been documented instances where CRS persists for more than 30 days [69].

In 2019, the American Society for Transplantation and Cellular Therapy (ASTCT) published consensus recommendations aiming to establish standardized definitions and grading systems for cytokine-release syndrome (CRS) [70]. The grading system focuses on easily identifiable criteria at the bedside, specifically the presence of fever, with a temperature ≥ 38°C at the onset as necessary requirement for the diagnosis of CRS, and the degree of hypotension and hypoxia (Table 14.1). The ASTCT consensus system is now recommended by regulatory authorities for grading CRS within investigational/experimental clinical trials, as well as for evaluating commercially available CAR T-cell products.

To mitigate the risk of severe CRS, it is essential to evaluate patient-specific risk factors for CRS (e.g., the proliferative state of the disease, remission status, organ function, especially car-

Table 14.1 CRS consensus grading as published by Lee *et al.* [67]

CRS parameter	Grade 1	Grade 2	Grade 3	Grade 4
Fever[a]	Temperature ≥ 38 °C	Temperature ≥ 38 °C	Temperature ≥ 38 °C	Temperature ≥38 °C
			with	
Hypotension	None	Not requiring vasopressors	Requiring a vasopressor with or without vasopressin	Requiring multiple vasopressors (excluding vasopressin)
			and/or[b]	
Hypoxia	None	Requiring low-flow nasal[c] cannula or blow-by	Requiring high-flow nasal cannula[c], facemask, nonrebreather mask or venturi mask	Requiring positive pressure (CPAP, BiPAP, intubation and mechanical ventilation)

Organ toxicities associated with CRS may be graded according to CTCAE v5.0, but they do not influence CRS grading

[a]Fever is defined as temperature ≥38°C not attributable to any other cause. In patients who have CRS then receive anti-pyretic or anti-cytokine therapy such as tocilizumab or steroids, fever is no longer required to grade subsequent CRS severity. In this case, CRS grading is driven by hypotension and/or hypoxia

[b]CRS grade is determined by the more severe event: hypotension or hypoxia not attributable to any other cause

[c]Low-flow nasal cannula is defined as oxygen delivered ≤6L/min. High flow is defined as oxygen delivered at >6 L/min

diac function and arrhythmias, clinical signs of infection/inflammation), and product-specific risk factors (e.g., the nature of the costimulatory domain) already before the infusion of CAR T cells. Recommended minimum set of tests that should be performed at screening in order to assess organ function and patient eligibility include C-reactive protein (CRP), ferritin, lactate dehydrogenase (LDH), complete blood counts, comprehensive metabolic panel (including magnesium/phosphorus levels), kidney and liver function tests, and transthoracic echocardiogram (TTE) or multigated acquisition (MUGA) scan as well as an electrocardiogram [57, 71]. Additionally, assessing the disease burden through bone marrow evaluation and/or lumbar puncture is recommended. In cases where a patient exhibits fever and positive bacterial blood cultures prior to CAR T cell infusion, it is important to administer appropriate antibacterial agents. CAR T cell infusion should be delayed until the patient becomes afebrile and cultures return negative. Patients with active influenza infections should be treated with antiviral therapy and infusion held until resolution of major symptoms [57].

Early and high-quality supportive care plays a critical role in effectively managing CRS. After CAR T cell infusion, close monitoring is crucial. If patients receive CAR T cell products in an outpatient setting, admission should be considered at the first signs of toxicity, including fever, hypotension, or altered mental status [57]. The duration of monitoring for CRS and other toxicities should align with the recommendations provided in the product package insert or study protocol, typically spanning several weeks.

Management of CRS primarily involves targeting elevated cytokines, particularly interleukin-6 (IL-6). Tocilizumab, an IL-6 receptor-blocking antibody, was approved by the FDA in 2017 for the treatment of severe or life-threatening CAR T-induced CRS [72]. For pediatric patients, administration of tocilizumab is recommended at ASTCT grade 3 CRS. In cases of prolonged grade 2 CRS or intolerance to fever, tocilizumab may also be considered [57].

If CRS does not improve after one dose of tocilizumab, the addition of steroids alongside a second dose is warranted. If CRS fails to improve even after two doses of tocilizumab (and steroids), the use of third-line agents such as anakinra (IL-1 receptor antagonist), siltuximab (IL-6 antagonist), and high-dose methylprednisolone should be considered [57, 73].

If CRS remains unresponsive to tocilizumab and steroids, the possibility of infections should be reconsidered, and appropriate management should be initiated [73]. When utilizing steroids for CRS management, it is recommended to employ a rapid taper once symptoms begin to improve [57].

14.3.4.3 Immune Effector Cell-Associated Neurotoxicity Syndrome (ICANS)

Transient neurological complications have been documented in almost every trial that aimed to target T cells to CD19 [74], including studies involving CAR T cells and BiTEs [75, 76]. The incidence of ICANS appears to be highest in CD19-targeting CAR T cell therapies, possibly due to the robust and often rapid expansion of T cells observed with these products. The likelihood of experiencing neurological toxicity may vary depending on the specific product used and the disease condition of the patient. The most consistently identified factors associated with the development of neurotoxicity across studies are the disease burden and the peak expansion of CAR T cells [77]. Accordingly, patients with a high blast count prior to infusion or those treated with CAR T cell products containing CD28 may be at a higher risk of developing neurotoxicity following therapy [57]. Moreover, patients who experience grade 3-4 CRS are also at an increased risk of developing ICANS [77]. Other risk factors include extramedullary disease, younger age, preexisting neurological comorbidities, higher total CAR T cell doses, and cytopenias [57].

The current hypotheses regarding the pathophysiology of ICANS suggest that systemic inflammation and cytokine production after CAR T cell infusion initiate a series of events, including activation of endothelial cells and disruption of the blood–brain barrier [58, 78]. This process leads to increased levels of cytokines in the cerebral spinal fluid (CSF), and in severe cases, hemorrhage and cerebral edema. Severe ICANS is often accompanied by a coagulopathy [79, 80] and elevated levels of von Willebrand factor (vWF) and angiopoietin 2 (ANG2), markers indicating endothelial dysregulation.

Elevated levels of cytokines, including IL-6, in the CSF of patients with severe ICANS are likely due to both increased permeability of the blood–brain barrier and local production by activated microglia, astrocytes, and macrophages. The infiltration of T cells into the central nervous system (CNS) may also contribute to the neuropathology, as both CAR T and non-CAR T cells have been detected in the CSF of patients experiencing neurotoxicity, without concurrent CNS disease [58, 78, 79].

Common clinical manifestations of ICANS include confusion, delirium, expressive aphasia, weakness, tremor, headache, seizures, and altered level of consciousness. Aphasia, particularly anomia and word-finding difficulties, may serve as important early warning signs. Changes in handwriting have also been reported as an early indication of high-grade ICANS [57]. However, patients may present with additional signs and symptoms, including cerebral edema that require specific management strategies [81].

ICANS can occur concurrently with CRS, shortly after CRS symptoms subside, or as a delayed-onset condition up to one month after CAR T cell infusion. Typically, neurological events occur around 4-5 days after infusion and tend to resolve within 3-8 weeks [57]. Most cases of ICANS are fully reversible; however, long-term neuropsychiatric sequelae have been described [58, 82]. Subtle neurological signs, e.g., persistent severe postural tremors lasting >2 months after CAR, new migraines and various peripheral neuropathies have been reported and need specific awareness [81].

For patients who develop ICANS, the diagnostic workup should include tests to rule out other causes, especially infections and bleedings, and a coagulation status (including fibrinogen, prothrombin time, and international normalized ratio). As clinically indicated, and in most cases, a head CT/brain MRI, lumbar puncture, and electroencephalogram (EEG) may also be considered.

The grading of ICANS follows the ASTCT ICANS consensus grading system [70] (Tables 14.2 and 14.3), with mental status changes marking the onset of ICANS after CAR T cell therapy.

Table 14.2 ICANS consensus grading for adults as published by Lee *et al.* [67]

Neurotoxicity domain	Grade 1	Grade 2	Grade 3	Grade 4
ICE score[a]	7–9	3–6	0–2	0
Depressed level of consciousness[b]	Awakens spontaneously	Wakens to voice	Awakens to tactile stimulus	Patient is unarousable or requires vigorous or repetitive tactile stimuli to arouse. Stupor or coma
Seizure	None	None	Any clinical seizure focal or generalized that resolves rapidly or nonconvulsive seizures on EEG that resolve with intervention	Life-threatening prolonged seizure (> 5 min); or repetitive clinical or electrical seizures without return to baseline in between
Motor finding[c]	None	None	None	Deep focal motor weakness such as hemiparesis or paraparesis
Elevated ICP or cerebral edema	None	None	Focal/local edema on neuroimaging[d]	Diffuse cerebral edema on neuroimaging: decerebrate or decorticate posturing; or cranial nerve VI palsy; or papilledema; or Cushing's triad

ICANS grade is determined by the most severe event not attributable to any other cause

[a]A patient with ICE score of 0 may be classified as grade 3 ICANS if awake with global aphasia, but a patient with an ICE score of 0 may be classified as grade 4 ICANS if unarousable

[b]Depressed level of consciousness should be attributable to no other cause

[c]Tremors and myoclonus associated with immune effector cell therapies may be graded according to CTCAE v5.0, but they do not influence ICANS grading

[d]Intracranial hemorrhage with or without associated edema is not considered a neurotoxicity feature and is excluded from ICANS grading. It may be graded according to CTCAE v5.0

The evaluation includes an easily performed bedside encephalopathy assessment based on the ICE score for patients aged 12 years or older (Table 14.4) or the CAPD score for patients under 12 years old as described in Traube *et al.* [83] Other domains evaluated include the level of consciousness, motor symptoms, seizures, and signs of elevated intracranial pressure.

The management of ICANS should be tailored to the specific risks associated with the product and the patient [57, 71, 73, 84]. Tocilizumab, despite alleviating severe CRS, has not been effective in resolving ICANS symptoms. Its inability to penetrate the CNS and its potential to increase CSF IL-6 levels (by blocking the IL-6 receptor outside the CNS) have raised concerns about exacerbating neurotoxicity. Siltuximab, an anti-IL-6 antibody, and the IL-1 antagonist anakinra have been suggested as potential alternatives, but data on their safety and efficacy are lacking. Corticosteroids have shown success in managing ICANS, and even longer courses of steroids do not appear to compromise the effectiveness of cancer treatment [57, 71, 73, 84].

The management of neurotoxicity should take precedence over low-grade CRS [57]. When using steroids, at least two doses should be administered, and a rapid tapering regimen should be implemented once improvement is observed [57]. For patients treated with 4-1BB CAR T cell products, steroids may be considered for grade 2 ICANS, while they are recommended for grade 3 or 4 ICANS. In the case of CD28-costimulated CAR T cell products, steroids should be used for grade 2 ICANS to mitigate its duration and severity [57].

14.3.4.4 HLH/MAS

There is a significant overlap in the clinical features and laboratory abnormalities observed in

Table 14.3 ICANS consensus grading for children as published by Lee *et al.* [67]

Neurotoxicity domain	Grade 1	Grade 2	Grade 3	Grade 4
ICE score for children ≥12 years[a]	7–9	3–6	0–2	0
CAPD score for children age <12 years	1-8	1-8	≥9	Unable to perform CAPD
Depressed level of consciousness[b]	Awakens spontaneously	Wakens to voice	Awakens to tactile stimulus	Patient is unarousable or requires vigorous or repetitive tactile stimuli to arouse. Stupor or coma
Seizure (any age)	None	None	Any clinical seizure focal or generalized that resolves rapidly or nonconvulsive seizures on EEG that resolve with intervention	Life-threatening prolonged seizure (>5 min); or repetitive clinical or electrical seizures without return to baseline in between
Motor weakness (any age)[c]	None	None	None	Deep focal motor weakness such as hemiparesis or paraparesis
Elevated ICP or cerebral edema (any age)	None	None	Focal/local edema on neuroimaging[d]	Diffuse cerebral edema on neuroimaging: decerebrate or decorticate posturing; or cranial nerve VI palsy; or papilledema; or Cushing's triad

ICANS grade is determined by the most severe event not attributable to any other cause

[a]A patient with ICE score of 0 may be classified as grade 3 ICANS if awake with global aphasia, but a patient with an ICE score of 0 may be classified as grade 4 ICANS if unarousable

[b]Depressed level of consciousness should be attributable to no other cause

[c]Tremors and myoclonus associated with immune effector cell therapies may be graded according to CTCAE v5.0, but they do not influence ICANS grading

[d]Intracranial hemorrhage with or without associated edema is not considered a neurotoxicity feature and is excluded from ICANS grading. It may be graded according to CTCAE v5.0

Table 14.4 Immune cell effector score as published by Lee *et al.* [67]

ICE score
Orientation: orientation in year, month, city, hospital: 4 points
Naming: ability to name three objects: 3 points
Following commands: ability to follow simple commands: 1 point
Writing: ability to write a standard sentence: 1 point
Attention: ability to count backward from 100 by 10: 1 point

cytokine release syndrome (CRS), hemophagocytic lymphohistiocytosis (HLH), and macrophage activation syndrome (MAS) [85]. Most patients with moderate to severe CRS exhibit laboratory findings that meet the established criteria for HLH/MAS, including elevated levels of certain cytokines such as IFNγ, IL-10, sIL-2Rα, IL-6, IL-8, and GM-CSF. Therefore, when there is suspicion of HLH/MAS, it is appropriate to follow the clinical management guidelines for CRS initially [57].

However, there are cases where patients present with symptoms resembling grade 3 or 4 CRS, high fevers, extremely elevated ferritin levels, and persistent cytopenia weeks after the infusion [86]. In such instances, MAS may be the predominant condition, and it is often unresponsive to treatment with tocilizumab. Delayed coagulopathy, particularly hypofibrinogenemia that is disproportionately worse than changes in PT/INR, may serve as a characteristic feature of delayed onset HLH/MAS-like toxicity [57]. Close monitoring is necessary, and replacement therapy with cryoprecipitate or fibrinogen concentrate, depending on local availability, may be required.

For the treatment of late-onset HLH/MAS-like pathology not responding to tocilizumab, third-line agents used for CRS, such as anakinra and steroids, may be considered. Etoposide should be reserved as a last resort for patients who do not respond to other treatments [57].

14.3.4.5 Infectious Complications

Different factors contribute to the increased risk for opportunistic infections in CAR T cell recipients [87]. A thorough assessment of any ongoing active infection is mandatory prior to CAR T cell infusion as an already activated immune system might increase the severity of CRS. After infusion systemic infections can mimic CRS and therefore all patients with fever need an extensive workup and initiation of empiric antibiotic therapy. Prior treatment regimens including allogeneic stem cell transplantation, bridging therapy and the lymphodepleting regimen including fludarabine may require prophylaxis for pneumocystis pneumonia and HSV reactivation [39, 57]. The lymphodepleting regimen can cause a transient neutropenia; however, approximately 30% of the patients have prolonged neutropenia after 28 [16, 88], probably due to the cumulative bone marrow toxicity of previous therapy, lymphodepletion, and CRS/HLH, in patients with a reduced bone marrow reserve, e.g., post HSCT. The recommendations from the European Society for Blood and Marrow Transplantation (EBMT) are to use antifungal prophylaxis according to local guidelines in persisting neutropenia, whereas gram-negative prophylaxis is not recommended [39, 71]. Shortening the duration of neutropenia with G-CSF can be considered; however, GM-CSF is associated with increased risk of severe CRS and should be omitted in the first 28 days after CAR T cell infusion [39, 57]. Whereas cytopenias resolve spontaneously in most patients within the first 3 months, some patients experience prolonged cytopenias and severe bone marrow hypoplasia, which can be accompanied by transfusions dependency and/or infections. Some centers have reported their experience with unconditioned CD34+ stem cell boosts to safely reconstitute the bone marrow as a salvage therapy for severe hematotoxicity post CAR T [89–92]. An on-target, but off-tumor effect of CAR T cell therapy, and more pronounced in patients with persisting CAR T cells is B-cell aplasia leading to hypogammaglobulinemia in 50% of patients. It is recommended, based on expert opinion, and distracted from the experience in the allogeneic stem cell transplantation setting and in children with hypo- or agammaglobulinemia, to supplement with intravenous immunoglobulins (ivIg) or subcutaneous immunoglobulins (scIg) during infections, or if IgG levels fall below 4 g/L. [93]

14.4 Strategies to Improve the Efficacy of CAR T

The major limitations of long-lasting CAR T cell efficacy are early loss of CAR T cells and antigen escape by loss of CD19.

14.4.1 CAR T Cell Persistence

Early loss of B-cell aplasia within 6 months after infusion is associated with an increased risk of CD19-positive relapse [19, 35, 94, 95]. The full mechanism of loss of CAR T cells has not been elucidated but is multifactorial as persistence of CAR T cells requires a delicate balance of activation while limiting exhaustion. Minimal changes in the CAR T construct have significant impact. Fine tuning of the construct, the culture procedure and the apheresis material are explored to alter the balance between exhaustion and expansion [96, 97]. This has been longer known for the two most often used costimulatory molecules 41BB and CD28 [98]. Further optimization of CAR T cell efficacy is proposed by combination of different costimulatory domains (third generation) or addition of pro-inflammatory cytokines in the CAR construct (fourth generation) or TRUCK T cells redirected for antigen-unrestricted cytokine-initiated killing [99].

The intrinsic properties of the apheresis product contribute to the expansion capacity and persistence of CAR T cells [100]. During chemotherapy treatment children lose the naive and stem cell memory T cells which is associated with inferior CAR T cell expansion during production [96]. Specific clonal expansion of stem cell memory T cells was associated with longer persistence of CAR T cells in ALL patients [101]. Optimization of culture conditions and selection procedures during production is an option to increase the percentage of naive/stem cell memory T cells in the apheresis product [102]. Children and young adults relapsing within 6 months after HSCT have an inferior outcome after CAR T cell therapy (18% in patients relapsing within 6 months versus 55% thereafter) [20]. It has been hypothesized that T cell fitness contributes to the inferior results. The use of donor-derived T cells as source for the CAR T cell manufacturing has shown promising results [103, 104].

For patients not achieving a complete remission after CAR T cell therapy or those experiencing CD19+ relapse, the development of recipient anti-CAR immune responses limiting CAR T cell survival is a potential mechanism underlying treatment failure [105]. Patients can develop T-cell and antibody mediated responses directed at the murine scFv antigen-binding domain of the CAR, which may lead to elimination of the CAR T cells [51, 106, 107]. CAR T cell therapy with a humanized CAR T cell, still containing 25% of the murine sequence showed promising response rates in patients with R/R BCP-ALL [75]. Humanized CAR T cells have also been demonstrated to be effective in achieving CR in patients after prior CAR T cell therapy. The CR rate was 64% in CAR exposed compared to 100% in CAR naïve patients [108]. Cao *et al.* reported on a similar association in 14 CAR naïve and 3 CAR exposed patients [109]. A recent update of this study demonstrates indeed a higher event-free survival in CAR naïve patients potentially explained by anti-CAR immunity despite humanization of the CAR T construct [110]. This is supported by a higher likelihood to lose circulating CAR T cells and recovery of B cells in CAR exposed patients. A CD28-based CAR T cell study targeting CD19 in non-Hodgkin lymphoma demonstrated that anti-CAR T cell responses result in lower, although not significant, CAR T cell levels in patients receiving a murine construct but not in those receiving a human CAR construct [111]. Various phase I studies have evaluated the use of fully human or humanized constructs [109, 112, 113]. The use of a human recognition domain might further reduce the immunogenicity of the CAR T cell product and overcome premature rejection, leading to improved outcome. Although anti-murine CAR responses increased after CAR T infusion, the presence of or a change in the immune response was not correlated to CAR efficacy or kinetics [114].

14.4.2 Antigen Escape

The first CAR T cell trials reported a high percentage of CD19-negative relapses [11]. In contrast to CD19-positive relapse, where CAR T cell loss leads to relapse, CD19-negative relapse occurs most often under CAR T cell pressure, as a consequence of several potential mechanisms [115]. Either preexisting CD19-negative clones expand or acquired mutations cause the loss or alteration of CD19 expression [116]. Sotillo *et al.* have reported various genetic alterations expressed in BCP-ALL in the CD19 domains recognized by the FMC63 scFv [117]. In addition, they describe BCP-ALL clones with mutations in the transmembrane part of the CD19 protein resulting in insufficient CD19 membrane expression.

Relapse due to lineage switch is rarer. A lineage switch is characterized by a genetically related clone with a different phenotype, most often resembling acute myeloid leukemia (AML). This phenomenon occurs more often in patients with underlying KMT2A fusion and is associated with an inferior outcome [29, 33].

Different clinical studies have addressed the potential of dual targeting the B-lineage marker CD22, a member of the immunoglobulin superfamily inhibiting the over activation of the B cell receptor complex. A fully humanized scFv targeting CD22 was developed at NCI [118]. Twenty-one children and young adults (age median 19; range 7-30 years) were infused in the phase I study. The complete response rate in the subgroup that received the recommended phase II dose was comparable to the CR rates seen in CD19 targeting studies (11 out of 15 patients). CAR T cells were detectable in 19 of 21 patients treated. Prior CD19 therapy or diminished expression of CD19 was not predictive for outcome in this study. However, relapse occurred in eight out of 12 responders, of whom seven had diminished CD22 expression. In the update of this trial it was shown that 30 out of 45 complete responders relapsed, with again the majority being CD22 negative or dim [119].

Dual targeting of two antigens simultaneously could decrease the antigen-negative relapse rate. Various strategies to target with multispecificity have been explored with different advantages and disadvantages. One vector encoding two CAR constructs, bicistronic, separated by a skipping sequence results in one T-cell expressing two independent CAR proteins with independent intracellular signaling domains. A single CAR targeting two different proteins, so called tandem CAR, may increase the binding and signaling. The manufacturing of two independent products that are infused simultaneously or sequentially is logistically and financially more challenging [120]. Alternatively, two vectors are used in the same manufacturing process resulting in a mixed product consisting of single-positive and dual-positive CAR T cells. Phase I studies in children and young adults with R/R B-ALL evaluated dual targeting. The AMELIA study assessed the safety and efficacy of a bicistronic CAR with the OX40 and 41BB costimulatory molecules in the CD19 and CD22 binding CAR, respectively [121]. The CAR showed a favorable safety profile and the response rate defined as morphological complete response with or without hematologic recovery on day 28 was 86% in 15 patients of whom 14 were CAR T naïve. The limitation of the product is the short persistence. Shalabi *et al.* report comparable findings in a bicistronic CAR T cell. Twenty patients were infused, the majority 14 out of 20 CAR naïve, and 12 out of 20 patients responded [122]. Because of short persistence of the CD19/CD22 CAR T, consolidation of a remission by HSCT was performed in responders if donor and financial situation allowed. Pan *et al.* are the first to report sequential infusion of CD19 and CD22 CAR T cells [123]. CD19 CAR T cells were administered to 20 pediatric patients. If CD19 CAR T cells were not detectable anymore in the peripheral blood CD22 CAR T cells were infused, with a median interval of 1.65 months. An MRD-negative CR was detected after CD19 CAR T cells in all patients. Seventeen out of 20 patients remain in complete remission at 18 months after infusion without HSCT consolidation reducing the rate of CD19-negative relapse compared to historical controls. Taken together, dual targeting has potential advantages over single targeting but currently does not show the same persistence as tisagenlecleucel.

14.4.3 Multiple CAR T Infusions

Longer persistence of CAR T cells measured by the presence of B-cell aplasia is associated with less CD19-positive relapses [35, 94]. In order to prolong persistence of B-cell aplasia, the administration of a second product has been hypothesized and small cohorts have been reported with limited efficacy [34, 124–126]. A second CAR T infusion for a relapse after the first CAR T infusion is associated with inferior complete response rates. Gauthier *et al.* reported a CR rate of 21% (three of 14 patients, and in only two an MRD-negative CR) in ALL [125]. However, factors improving CR rates after a second infusion were a higher cell dose compared to the first infusion, fludarabine–cyclophosphamide lymphodepletion prior second infusion, and NHL disease.

14.5 CAR T Cell Therapy for T-ALL

The rapid implementation of CAR T for B cell malignancies in children and adults, is not yet achieved in T-ALL. CAR T for T-ALL has several hurdles. The apheresis product often contains leukemic blasts. Persistence of the CAR T cells will result in long term T-cell aplasia, which would require a subsequent allogeneic stem cell transplantation. But most of all, fratricide occurs as the currently available antigens are not selective for

T-ALL blasts. For example, CD5 and CD7 are both expressed on healthy T-cells and T-ALL blasts. Genetic engineering is critical to remove the target antigen from the CAR T cells, e.g., by a protein expression blocker (PEBL) or base editing [127, 128]. The PEBL proteins, introduced in the T cells by the same retroviral vector as the CAR construct, block the surface expression of CD7 in T cells, preventing fratricide. Base editing uses CRISPR to inactivate the CD7 gene to prevent fratricide, the CD52 gene to escape from the lymphodepleting regimen used and the β-chain of the αβ-T cell receptor to prevent graft-versus-host disease as these cells were from an allogeneic donor. The first three patients treated with base-edited CAR T cells were recently reported [129]. Adapting the culture conditions, by adding ibrutinib and dasatinib during the ex vivo expansion step, to prevent fratricide during CAR T production or selecting naturally occurring CD7-negative T cells is an example for strategies that are currently explored to overcome these hurdles [130, 131]. Other targets for T-ALL currently under investigation are among others CD1a, the constant region of the TCR beta chain [132], and intracellular proteins like TdT [133]. The latter target requires T cell receptor-engineered T cells (TCR T) as TdT is an intracellular protein. Various phase I clinical trials have shown promising response rates in patients with T-ALL or T-LBL (lymphoblastic lymphoma) [134–137].

Recent preliminary data suggest that CD7-negative T cells evoke after administration of CD7-targeting CAR T cells. In addition, CD7-negative T cells showed ex vivo proliferation and cytokine production upon exposure to antigen stimulation [136]. However, in the majority of the clinical trials reported the CD7 targeting CAR T cells are a bridge to transplant [129, 135].

14.6 Conclusion

The development of CTL019 to an FDA and EMA approved licensed product (tisagenlecleucel) for relapsed/refractory BCP ALL has had major implications for the treatment of these resistant subtypes of ALL which historically have a poor prognosis. Where to position CAR T in the overall treatment landscape of ALL is still a matter of scientific debate [1] and this is addressed in ongoing studies (e.g., in primary ALL disease in the CASSIOPEIA study (NCT03876769). In recent years, steps have been made to implement adoptive cellular therapies for T-ALL; however, in this disease several hurdles need to be overcome.

References

1. Buechner J, Caruana I, Künkele A, et al. Chimeric antigen receptor T-cell therapy in paediatric B-cell precursor acute lymphoblastic leukaemia: curative treatment option or bridge to transplant? Front Pediatr. 2022:9. https://doi.org/10.3389/FPED.2021.784024.
2. Gross G, Waks T, Eshhar Z. Expression of immunoglobulin-T-cell receptor chimeric molecules as functional receptors with antibody-type specificity. Proc Natl Acad Sci U S A. 1989;86(24):10024–8. https://doi.org/10.1073/PNAS.86.24.10024.
3. Kuwana Y, Itoh S, Nagase F, Nakashima I, Kurosawa Y. Production of the constant domain of murine T-cell receptor beta-chain in Escherichia coli. FEBS Lett. 1987;219(2):360–4. https://doi.org/10.1016/0014-5793(87)80253-3.
4. Park JR, DiGiusto DL, Slovak M, et al. Adoptive transfer of chimeric antigen receptor re-directed cytolytic T lymphocyte clones in patients with neuroblastoma. Mol Ther. 2007;15(4):825–33. https://doi.org/10.1038/SJ.MT.6300104.
5. Walker RE, Bechtel CM, Natarajan V, et al. Long-term in vivo survival of receptor-modified syngeneic T cells in patients with human immunodeficiency virus infection. Blood. 2000;96(2):467–74.
6. Finney HM, Akbar AN, Lawson ADG. Activation of resting human primary T cells with chimeric receptors: costimulation from CD28, inducible costimulator, CD134, and CD137 in series with signals from the TCR zeta chain. J Immunol. 2004;172(1):104–13. https://doi.org/10.4049/JIMMUNOL.172.1.104.
7. Imai C, Mihara K, Andreansky M, et al. Chimeric receptors with 4-1BB signaling capacity provoke potent cytotoxicity against acute lymphoblastic leukemia. Leukemia. 2004;18(4):676–84. https://doi.org/10.1038/SJ.LEU.2403302.
8. Brentjens RJ, Santos E, Nikhamin Y, et al. Genetically targeted T cells eradicate systemic acute lymphoblastic leukemia xenografts. Clin Cancer Res. 2007;13(18 Pt 1):5426–35. https://doi.org/10.1158/1078-0432.CCR-07-0674.
9. Milone MC, Fish JD, Carpenito C, et al. Chimeric receptors containing CD137 signal transduction

domains mediate enhanced survival of T cells and increased antileukemic efficacy in vivo. Mol Ther. 2009;17(8):1453–64. https://doi.org/10.1038/MT.2009.83.
10. Porter D, Frey N, Melenhorst J, Blood WH. Randomized, phase ii dose optimization study of chimeric antigen receptor modified T cells directed against CD19 (CTL019) in patients with relapsed. Elsevier; 2014.
11. Maude SL, Laetsch TW, Buechner J, et al. Tisagenlecleucel in children and young adults with B-cell lymphoblastic leukemia. New Engl J Med. 2018;378(5):439–48. https://doi.org/10.1056/NEJMoa1709866.
12. Shah BD, Ghobadi A, Oluwole OO, et al. KTE-X19 for relapsed or refractory adult B-cell acute lymphoblastic leukaemia: phase 2 results of the single-arm, open-label, multicentre ZUMA-3 study. Lancet. 2021;398(10299):491–502. https://doi.org/10.1016/S0140-6736(21)01222-8.
13. Schuster SJ, Bishop MR, Tam CS, et al. Tisagenlecleucel in adult relapsed or refractory diffuse large B-cell lymphoma. N Engl J Med. 2019;380(1):45–56. https://doi.org/10.1056/NEJMOA1804980.
14. Neelapu SS, Locke FL, Bartlett NL, et al. Axicabtagene ciloleucel CAR T-cell therapy in refractory large B-cell lymphoma. N Engl J Med. 2017;377(26):2531–44. https://doi.org/10.1056/NEJMOA1707447.
15. Grupp SA, Kalos M, Barrett D, et al. Chimeric antigen receptor-modified T cells for acute lymphoid leukemia. N Engl J Med. 2013;368(16):1509–18. https://doi.org/10.1056/NEJMOA1215134.
16. Maude SL, Frey N, Shaw PA, et al. Chimeric antigen receptor T cells for sustained remissions in leukemia. N Engl J Med. 2014;371(16):1507–17. https://doi.org/10.1056/NEJMOA1407222.
17. Laetsch TW, Maude SL, Rives S, et al. Three-year update of tisagenlecleucel in pediatric and young adult patients with relapsed/refractory acute lymphoblastic leukemia in the ELIANA trial. J Clin Oncol. 2023;41(9):1664–9. https://doi.org/10.1200/JCO.22.00642.
18. Pasquini MC, Hu ZH, Curran K, et al. Real-world evidence of tisagenlecleucel for pediatric acute lymphoblastic leukemia and non-Hodgkin lymphoma. Blood Adv. 2020;4(21):5414–24. https://doi.org/10.1182/BLOODADVANCES.2020003092.
19. Dourthe ME, Rabian F, Yakouben K, et al. Determinants of CD19-positive vs CD19-negative relapse after tisagenlecleucel for B-cell acute lymphoblastic leukemia. Leukemia. 2021;35(12):3383–93. https://doi.org/10.1038/S41375-021-01281-7.
20. Bader P, Rossig C, Hutter M, et al. CD19 CAR T cells are an effective therapy for posttransplant relapse in patients with B-lineage ALL: real-world data from Germany. Blood Adv. 2023;7(11) https://doi.org/10.1182/BLOODADVANCES.2022008981.
21. Moskop A, Pommert L, Baggott C, et al. Real-world use of tisagenlecleucel in infant acute lymphoblastic leukemia. Blood Adv. 2022;6(14):4251–5. https://doi.org/10.1182/bloodadvances.2021006393.
22. Ghorashian S, Jacoby E, De Moerloose B, et al. Tisagenlecleucel therapy for relapsed or refractory B-cell acute lymphoblastic leukaemia in infants and children younger than 3 years of age at screening: an international, multicentre, retrospective cohort study. Lancet Haematol. 2022;9(10):e766–75. https://doi.org/10.1016/S2352-3026(22)00225-3.
23. Fabrizio VA, Phillips CL, Lane A, et al. Tisagenlecleucel outcomes in relapsed/refractory extramedullary ALL: A PEDIATRIC REAL WORLD CAR consortium report. Blood Adv. 2022;6(2):600–10. https://doi.org/10.1182/bloodadvances.2021005564.
24. Leahy AB, Newman H, Li Y, et al. CD19-targeted chimeric antigen receptor T-cell therapy for CNS relapsed or refractory acute lymphocytic leukaemia: a post-hoc analysis of pooled data from five clinical trials. Lancet Haematol. 2021;8(10) https://doi.org/10.1016/S2352-3026(21)00238-6.
25. Jacoby E, Ghorashian S, Vormoor B, et al. CD19 CAR T-cells for pediatric relapsed acute lymphoblastic leukemia with active CNS involvement: a retrospective international study. Leukemia. 2022;36(6):1525–32. https://doi.org/10.1038/S41375-022-01546-9.
26. Holland EM, Yates B, Ling A, et al. Characterization of extramedullary disease in B-ALL and response to CAR T-cell therapy. Blood Adv. 2022;6(7):2167–82. https://doi.org/10.1182/bloodadvances.2021006035.
27. Laetsch TW, Maude SL, Balduzzi A, et al. Tisagenlecleucel in pediatric and young adult patients with Down syndrome-associated relapsed/refractory acute lymphoblastic leukemia. Leukemia. 2022;36(6):1508–15. https://doi.org/10.1038/S41375-022-01550-Z.
28. Xu X, Sun Q, Liang X, et al. Mechanisms of relapse after CD19 CAR T-cell therapy for acute lymphoblastic leukemia and its prevention and treatment strategies. Front Immunol. 2019:10. https://doi.org/10.3389/FIMMU.2019.02664.
29. Leahy AB, Devine KJ, Li Y, et al. Impact of high-risk cytogenetics on outcomes for children and young adults receiving CD19-directed CAR T cell therapy. Blood. Published online December. 2021; https://doi.org/10.1182/BLOOD.2021012727.
30. Zwaan CM, Calkoen FGJ. Immunotherapy: genetically agnostic in BCP-ALL? Blood. 2022;139(14):2093–4. https://doi.org/10.1182/BLOOD.2022015618.
31. Pan J, Tan Y, Deng B, et al. Frequent occurrence of CD19-negative relapse after CD19 CAR T and consolidation therapy in 14 TP53-mutated r/r B-ALL children. Leukemia. 2020;34(12):3382–7. https://doi.org/10.1038/S41375-020-0831-Z.
32. Singh N, Lee YG, Shestova O, et al. Impaired death receptor signaling in leukemia causes antigen-

independent resistance by inducing CAR T-cell dysfunction. Cancer Discov. 2020;10(4):552–67. https://doi.org/10.1158/2159-8290.CD-19-0813.
33. Lamble AJ, Myers RM, Taraseviciute A, et al. Preinfusion factors impacting relapse immunophenotype following CD19 CAR T cells. Blood Adv. 2023;7(4):575–85. https://doi.org/10.1182/BLOODADVANCES.2022007423.
34. Schultz LM, Baggott C, Prabhu S, et al. Disease burden affects outcomes in pediatric and young adult B-cell lymphoblastic leukemia after commercial tisagenlecleucel: a pediatric real-world chimeric antigen receptor consortium report. J Clin Oncol. 2022;40(9):945–55. https://doi.org/10.1200/JCO.20.03585.
35. Pulsipher MA, Han X, Maude SL, et al. Next-generation sequencing of minimal residual disease for predicting relapse after tisagenlecleucel in children and young adults with acute lymphoblastic leukemia. Blood Cancer Discov. 2022;3(1):66–81. https://doi.org/10.1158/2643-3230.BCD-21-0095.
36. Laetsch TW, Yanik GA, Boyer MW, Rheingold SR. An owner's manual for CD19 "CAR"-T cell therapy in managing pediatric and young adult B-cell acute lymphoblastic leukemia. Blood Rev. 2021:50. https://doi.org/10.1016/J.BLRE.2021.100848.
37. Crocoli A, Martucci C, Persano G, et al. Vascular access in pediatric oncology and hematology: state of the art. Children. 2022;9(1) https://doi.org/10.3390/CHILDREN9010070.
38. Worel N, Holbro A, Vrielink H, et al. A guide to the collection of T-cells by apheresis for ATMP manufacturing—recommendations of the GoCART coalition apheresis working group. Bone Marrow Transpl. Published online. 2023; https://doi.org/10.1038/S41409-023-01957-X.
39. Hayden PJ, Roddie C, Bader P, et al. Management of adults and children receiving CAR T-cell therapy: 2021 best practice recommendations of the European Society for Blood and Marrow Transplantation (EBMT) and the Joint Accreditation Committee of ISCT and EBMT (JACIE) and the European Haematol. Ann Oncol. 2022;33(3):259–75. https://doi.org/10.1016/J.ANNONC.2021.12.003.
40. Dickinson MJ, Barba P, Jager U, et al. A novel autologous CAR-T therapy, YTB323, with preserved T-cell stemness shows enhanced CAR T-cell efficacy in preclinical and early clinical development. Cancer Discov. Published online May. 2023; https://doi.org/10.1158/2159-8290.CD-22-1276.
41. Van Overstraeten-Schlögel N, Beguin Y, Gothot A. Role of stromal-derived factor-1 in the hematopoietic-supporting activity of human mesenchymal stem cells. Eur J Haematol. 2006;76(6):488–93. https://doi.org/10.1111/j.1600-0609.2006.00633.x.
42. FDA. Considerations for the development of chimeric antigen receptor (CAR) T cell products; 2022.
43. Maude SL, Barrett D, Teachey DT, Grupp SA. Managing cytokine release syndrome associated with novel T cell-engaging therapies. Cancer J. 2014;20(2):119–22. https://doi.org/10.1097/PPO.0000000000000035.
44. Pillai V, Muralidharan K, Meng W, et al. CAR T-cell therapy is effective for CD19-dim B-lymphoblastic leukemia but is impacted by prior blinatumomab therapy. Blood Adv. 2019;3(22):3539–49. https://doi.org/10.1182/BLOODADVANCES.2019000692.
45. Myers RM, Taraseviciute A, Steinberg SM, et al. Blinatumomab nonresponse and high-disease burden are associated with inferior outcomes after CD19-CAR for B-ALL. J Clin Oncol. 2022;40(9):932–44. https://doi.org/10.1200/JCO.21.01405.
46. Krueger J, Bittencourt HNS, Rives S, et al. Tisagenlecleucel (Tisa) for relapsed/refractory (r/r) acute lymphoblastic leukemia (ALL): B2001X study focusing on prior exposure to blinatumomab (BLINA) and inotuzumab (INO). 2020;38(15_suppl):10518. https://doi.org/10.1200/JCO.2020.38.15_SUPPL.10518.
47. Ceolin V, Brivio E, van Tinteren H, et al. Outcome of chimeric antigen receptor T-cell therapy following treatment with inotuzumab ozogamicin in children with relapsed or refractory acute lymphoblastic leukemia. Leukemia. 2023;37(1):53–60. https://doi.org/10.1038/S41375-022-01740-9.
48. Zhang T, Cao L, Xie J, et al. Efficiency of CD19 chimeric antigen receptor-modified T cells for treatment of B cell malignancies in phase I clinical trials: a meta-analysis. Oncotarget. 2015;6(32):33961–71. https://doi.org/10.18632/ONCOTARGET.5582.
49. Curran KJ, Margossian SP, Kernan NA, et al. Toxicity and response after CD19-specific CAR T-cell therapy in pediatric/young adult relapsed/refractory B-ALL. Blood. 2019;134(26):2361–8. https://doi.org/10.1182/BLOOD.2019001641.
50. Hirayama AV, Gauthier J, Hay KA, et al. The response to lymphodepletion impacts PFS in patients with aggressive non-Hodgkin lymphoma treated with CD19 CAR T cells. Blood. 2019;133(17):1876–87. https://doi.org/10.1182/BLOOD-2018-11-887067.
51. Turtle CJ, Hanafi LA, Berger C, et al. CD19 CAR-T cells of defined CD4+:CD8+ composition in adult B cell ALL patients. J Clin Invest. 2016;126(6):2123–38. https://doi.org/10.1172/JCI85309.
52. Turtle CJ, Hanafi LA, Berger C, et al. Immunotherapy of non-Hodgkin's lymphoma with a defined ratio of CD8+ and CD4+ CD19-specific chimeric antigen receptor-modified T cells. Sci Transl Med. 2016;8(355) https://doi.org/10.1126/SCITRANSLMED.AAF8621.
53. Gardner RA, Finney O, Annesley C, et al. Intent-to-treat leukemia remission by CD19 CAR T cells of defined formulation and dose in children and young adults. Blood. 2017;129(25):3322–31. https://doi.org/10.1182/BLOOD-2017-02-769208.
54. Dekker L, Calkoen FG, Jiang Y, et al. Fludarabine exposure predicts outcome after CD19 CAR T-cell

therapy in children and young adults with acute leukemia. Blood Adv. 2022;6(7):1969–76. https://doi.org/10.1182/BLOODADVANCES.2021006700.

55. Fabrizio VA, Boelens JJ, Mauguen A, et al. Optimal fludarabine lymphodepletion is associated with improved outcomes after CAR T-cell therapy. 2022;6(7):1961–8.
56. Rosenbaum L. Tragedy, perseverance, and chance – the story of CAR-T therapy. N Engl J Med. 2017;377(14):1313–5. https://doi.org/10.1056/NEJMP1711886.
57. Maus MV, Alexander S, Bishop MR, et al. Society for Immunotherapy of Cancer (SITC) clinical practice guideline on immune effector cell-related adverse events. J Immunother Cancer. 2020;8(2) https://doi.org/10.1136/JITC-2020-001511.
58. Freyer CW, Porter DL. Cytokine release syndrome and neurotoxicity following CAR T-cell therapy for hematologic malignancies. J Allergy Clin Immunol. 2020;146(5):940–8. https://doi.org/10.1016/J.JACI.2020.07.025.
59. Levine JE, Grupp SA, Pulsipher MA, et al. Pooled safety analysis of tisagenlecleucel in children and young adults with B cell acute lymphoblastic leukemia. J Immunother Cancer. 2021;9(8) https://doi.org/10.1136/JITC-2020-002287.
60. Bedoya F, Frigault MJ, Maus MV. The flipside of the power of engineered T cells: observed and potential toxicities of genetically modified t cells as therapy. Mol Ther. 2017;25(2):314–20. https://doi.org/10.1016/J.YMTHE.2016.11.011.
61. Wayne AS, Huynh V, Hijiya N, et al. Three-year results from phase I of ZUMA-4: KTE-X19 in pediatric relapsed/refractory acute lymphoblastic leukemia. Haematologica. 2023;108(3):747–60. https://doi.org/10.3324/HAEMATOL.2022.280678.
62. Cobb DA, Lee DW. Cytokine release syndrome biology and management. Cancer J. 2021;27(2):119–25. https://doi.org/10.1097/PPO.0000000000000515.
63. Aldoss I, Khaled SK, Budde E, Stein AS. Cytokine release syndrome with the novel treatments of acute lymphoblastic leukemia: pathophysiology, prevention, and treatment. Curr Oncol Rep. 2019;21(1) https://doi.org/10.1007/S11912-019-0753-Y.
64. Giavridis T, Van Der Stegen SJC, Eyquem J, Hamieh M, Piersigilli A, Sadelain M. CAR T cell-induced cytokine release syndrome is mediated by macrophages and abated by IL-1 blockade. Nat Med. 2018;24(6):731–8. https://doi.org/10.1038/S41591-018-0041-7.
65. Norelli M, Camisa B, Barbiera G, et al. Monocyte-derived IL-1 and IL-6 are differentially required for cytokine-release syndrome and neurotoxicity due to CAR T cells. Nat Med. 2018;24(6):739–48. https://doi.org/10.1038/S41591-018-0036-4.
66. Tedesco VE, Mohan C. Biomarkers for Predicting Cytokine Release Syndrome following CD19-Targeted CAR T Cell Therapy. J Immunol. 2021;206(7):1561–8. https://doi.org/10.4049/JIMMUNOL.2001249.
67. Iglesias JR, Hernández F, de Iglesias RE. Histochemical study of ubiquinones in the central nuclei of the cerebellum of the mouse during its development. Histochemie. 1973;34(1):33–41. https://doi.org/10.1007/BF00304306.
68. Hay KA, Hanafi LA, Li D, et al. Kinetics and biomarkers of severe cytokine release syndrome after CD19 chimeric antigen receptor-modified T-cell therapy. Blood. 2017;130(21):2295–306. https://doi.org/10.1182/BLOOD-2017-06-793141.
69. Santomasso B, Bachier C, Westin J, Rezvani K, Shpall EJ. The other side of CAR T-cell therapy: cytokine release syndrome, neurologic toxicity, and financial burden. Am Soc Clin Oncol Educ Book. 2019;39(39):433–44. https://doi.org/10.1200/EDBK_238691.
70. Lee DW, Santomasso BD, Locke FL, et al. ASTCT consensus grading for cytokine release syndrome and neurologic toxicity associated with immune effector cells. Biol Blood Marrow Transplant. 2019;25(4):625–38. https://doi.org/10.1016/J.BBMT.2018.12.758.
71. Yakoub-Agha I, Chabannon C, Bader P, et al. Management of adults and children undergoing chimeric antigen receptor T-cell therapy: best practice recommendations of the European Society for Blood and Marrow Transplantation (EBMT) and the Joint Accreditation Committee of ISCT and EBMT (JACIE). Haematologica. 2020;105(2):297–316. https://doi.org/10.3324/HAEMATOL.2019.229781.
72. Le RQ, Li L, Yuan W, et al. FDA approval summary: tocilizumab for treatment of chimeric antigen receptor T cell-induced severe or life-threatening cytokine release syndrome. Oncologist. 2018;23(8):943–7. https://doi.org/10.1634/THEONCOLOGIST.2018-0028.
73. Jain MD, Smith M, Shah NN. How I treat refractory CRS and ICANS after CAR T-cell therapy. Blood. 2023;141(20) https://doi.org/10.1182/BLOOD.2022017414.
74. Grant SJ, Grimshaw AA, Silberstein J, et al. Clinical presentation, risk factors, and outcomes of immune effector cell-associated neurotoxicity syndrome following chimeric antigen receptor T cell therapy: a systematic review. Transplant Cell Ther. 2022;28(6):294–302. https://doi.org/10.1016/J.JTCT.2022.03.006.
75. Liu H, Xi R, Mao D, Zhao X, Wu T. Efficacy and safety of blinatumomab for the treatment of relapsed/refractory acute lymphoblastic leukemia: a systemic review and meta-analysis. Clin Lymphoma Myeloma Leuk. 2023;23(3):e139–49. https://doi.org/10.1016/J.CLML.2022.12.009.
76. Marrapodi MM, Mascolo A, di Mauro G, Mondillo G, Pota E, Rossi F. The safety of blinatumomab in pediatric patients with acute lymphoblastic leukemia: a systematic review and meta-analysis. Front Pediatr. 2022:10. https://doi.org/10.3389/FPED.2022.929122.

77. Santomasso BD, Park JH, Salloum D, et al. Clinical and biological correlates of neurotoxicity associated with CAR T-cell therapy in patients with B-cell acute lymphoblastic leukemia. Cancer Discov. 2018;8(8):958–71. https://doi.org/10.1158/2159-8290.CD-17-1319.
78. Pensato U, Muccioli L, Cani I, et al. Brain dysfunction in COVID-19 and CAR-T therapy: cytokine storm-associated encephalopathy. Ann Clin Transl Neurol. 2021;8(4):968–79. https://doi.org/10.1002/ACN3.51348.
79. Galli E, Sorà F, Hohaus S, et al. Endothelial activation predicts disseminated intravascular coagulopathy, cytokine release syndrome and prognosis in patients treated with anti-CD19 CAR-T cells. Br J Haematol. 2023;201(1) https://doi.org/10.1111/BJH.18596.
80. Buechner J, Grupp SA, Hiramatsu H, et al. Practical guidelines for monitoring and management of coagulopathy following tisagenlecleucel CAR T-cell therapy. Blood Adv. 2021;5(2):593–601. https://doi.org/10.1182/BLOODADVANCES.2020002757.
81. Santomasso BD, Gust J, Perna F. How I treat unique and difficult-to-manage cases of CAR T-cell therapy-associated neurotoxicity. Blood. 2023;141(20) https://doi.org/10.1182/BLOOD.2022017604.
82. Ruark J, Mullane E, Cleary N, et al. Patient-reported neuropsychiatric outcomes of long-term survivors after chimeric antigen receptor T cell therapy. Biol Blood Marrow Transplant. 2020;26(1):34–43. https://doi.org/10.1016/J.BBMT.2019.09.037.
83. Traube C, Silver G, Kearney J, et al. Cornell assessment of pediatric delirium: a valid, rapid, observational tool for screening delirium in the PICU*. Crit Care Med. 2014;42(3):656–63. https://doi.org/10.1097/CCM.0B013E3182A66B76.
84. Bhojwani D, Bansal R, Wayne AS. Managing therapy-associated neurotoxicity in children with ALL. Hematol Am Soc Hematol Educ Prog. 2021;2021(1):376–83. https://doi.org/10.1182/HEMATOLOGY.2021000269.
85. Teachey DT, Lacey SF, Shaw PA, et al. Identification of predictive biomarkers for cytokine release syndrome after chimeric antigen receptor T-cell therapy for acute lymphoblastic leukemia. Cancer Discov. 2016;6(6):664–79. https://doi.org/10.1158/2159-8290.CD-16-0040.
86. Hashmi H, Bachmeier C, Chavez JC, et al. Haemophagocytic lymphohistiocytosis has variable time to onset following CD19 chimeric antigen receptor T cell therapy. Br J Haematol. 2019;187(2):e35–8. https://doi.org/10.1111/BJH.16155.
87. Vora SB, Waghmare A, Englund JA, Qu P, Gardner RA, Hill JA. Infectious complications following CD19 chimeric antigen receptor T-cell therapy for children, adolescents, and young adults. Open Forum Infect Dis. 2020;7(5) https://doi.org/10.1093/OFID/OFAA121.
88. Wudhikarn K, Palomba ML, Pennisi M, et al. Infection during the first year in patients treated with CD19 CAR T cells for diffuse large B cell lymphoma. Blood Cancer J. 2020;10(8) https://doi.org/10.1038/S41408-020-00346-7.
89. Rejeski K, Burchert A, Iacoboni G, et al. Safety and feasibility of stem cell boost as a salvage therapy for severe hematotoxicity after CD19 CAR T-cell therapy. Blood Adv. 2022;6(16):4719–25. https://doi.org/10.1182/BLOODADVANCES.2022007776.
90. Gagelmann N, Wulf GG, Duell J, et al. Hematopoietic stem cell boost for persistent neutropenia after CAR T-cell therapy: a GLA/DRST study. Blood Adv. 2023;7(4):555–9. https://doi.org/10.1182/BLOODADVANCES.2022008042.
91. de Tena PS, Bailén R, Oarbeascoa G, et al. Allogeneic CD34-selected stem cell boost as salvage treatment of life-threatening infection and severe cytopenias after CAR-T cell therapy. Transfusion (Paris). 2022;62(10):2143–7. https://doi.org/10.1111/TRF.17071.
92. Mullanfiroze K, Lazareva A, Chu J, et al. CD34+-selected stem cell boost can safely improve cytopenias following CAR T-cell therapy. Blood Adv. 2022;6(16):4715–8. https://doi.org/10.1182/BLOODADVANCES.2022007572.
93. Kampouri E, Walti CS, Gauthier J, Hill JA. Managing hypogammaglobulinemia in patients treated with CAR-T-cell therapy: key points for clinicians. Expert Rev Hematol. 2022;15(4):305–20. https://doi.org/10.1080/17474086.2022.2063833.
94. Finney OC, Brakke H, Rawlings-Rhea S, et al. CD19 CAR T cell product and disease attributes predict leukemia remission durability. J Clin Invest. 2019;129(5):2123–32. https://doi.org/10.1172/JCI125423.
95. Ghorashian S, Furness C, Cummins M, et al. Intention to treat analysis of real-world outcomes following tisgenlecleucel therapy for pediatric and young adult ALL through a national access programme. Blood. 2020;136(Suppl 1):18–9. https://doi.org/10.1182/BLOOD-2020-138438.
96. Das RK, Vernau L, Grupp SA, Barrett DM. Naïve T-cell deficits at diagnosis and after chemotherapy impair cell therapy potential in pediatric cancers. Cancer Discov. 2019;9(4) https://doi.org/10.1158/2159-8290.CD-18-1314.
97. Feucht J, Sun J, Eyquem J, et al. Calibration of CAR activation potential directs alternative T cell fates and therapeutic potency. Nat Med. 2019;25(1):82–8. https://doi.org/10.1038/S41591-018-0290-5.
98. Long AH, Haso WM, Shern JF, et al. 4-1BB costimulation ameliorates T cell exhaustion induced by tonic signaling of chimeric antigen receptors. Nat Med. 2015;21(6):581–90. https://doi.org/10.1038/NM.3838.
99. Chmielewski M, Abken H. TRUCKs: the fourth generation of CARs. Expert Opin Biol Ther. 2015;15(8):1145–54. https://doi.org/10.1517/14712598.2015.1046430.

100. Singh N, Perazzelli J, Grupp SA, Barrett DM. Early memory phenotypes drive T cell proliferation in patients with pediatric malignancies. Sci Transl Med. 2016;8(320) https://doi.org/10.1126/SCITRANSLMED.AAD5222.
101. Biasco L, Izotova N, Rivat C, et al. Clonal expansion of T memory stem cells determines early anti-leukemic responses and long-term CAR T cell persistence in patients. Nat Cancer. 2021;2(6):629–42. https://doi.org/10.1038/S43018-021-00207-7.
102. Arcangeli S, Bove C, Mezzanotte C, et al. CAR T cell manufacturing from naive/stem memory T lymphocytes enhances antitumor responses while curtailing cytokine release syndrome. J Clin Invest. 2022;132(12) https://doi.org/10.1172/JCI150807.
103. Zhang C, Wang XQ, Zhang RL, et al. Donor-derived CD19 CAR-T cell therapy of relapse of CD19-positive B-ALL post allotransplant. Leukemia. 2021;35(6):1563–70. https://doi.org/10.1038/S41375-020-01056-6.
104. del Bufalo F, Becilli M, Rosignoli C, et al. Allogeneic, donor-derived, second-generation, CD19-CAR-T cell for the treatment of pediatric relapsed/refractory BCP-ALL. Blood. Published online May. 2023;12 https://doi.org/10.1182/BLOOD.2023020023.
105. Jensen MC, Popplewell L, Cooper LJ, et al. Antitransgene rejection responses contribute to attenuated persistence of adoptively transferred CD20/CD19-specific chimeric antigen receptor redirected T cells in humans. Biol Blood Marrow Transplant. 2010;16(9):1245–56. https://doi.org/10.1016/J.BBMT.2010.03.014.
106. Lamers CHJ, Willemsen R, Van Elzakker P, et al. Immune responses to transgene and retroviral vector in patients treated with ex vivo-engineered T cells. Blood. 2011;117(1):72–82. https://doi.org/10.1182/BLOOD-2010-07-294520.
107. Maus MV, Haas AR, Beatty GL, et al. T cells expressing chimeric antigen receptors can cause anaphylaxis in humans. Cancer Immunol Res. 2013;1(1):26–31. https://doi.org/10.1158/2326-6066.CIR-13-0006.
108. Maude SL, Pulsipher MA, Boyer MW, et al. Efficacy and safety of CTL019 in the first US phase II multicenter trial in pediatric relapsed/refractory acute lymphoblastic leukemia: results of an interim analysis. Blood. 2016;128(22):2801. https://doi.org/10.1182/BLOOD.V128.22.2801.2801.
109. Cao J, Wang G, Cheng H, et al. Potent anti-leukemia activities of humanized CD19-targeted Chimeric antigen receptor T (CAR-T) cells in patients with relapsed/refractory acute lymphoblastic leukemia. Am J Hematol. 2018;93(7):851–8. https://doi.org/10.1002/AJH.25108.
110. Myers RM, Li Y, Leahy AB, et al. Humanized CD19-targeted chimeric antigen receptor (CAR) T Cells in CAR-Naive and CAR-exposed children and young adults with relapsed or refractory acute lymphoblastic leukemia. J Clin Oncol. 2021;39(27):3044–55. https://doi.org/10.1200/JCO.20.03458.
111. Brudno JN, Lam N, Vanasse D, et al. Safety and feasibility of anti-CD19 CAR T cells with fully human binding domains in patients with B-cell lymphoma. Nat Med. 2020;26(2):270–80. https://doi.org/10.1038/S41591-019-0737-3.
112. Song F, Hu Y, Zhang Y, et al. Safety and efficacy of autologous and allogeneic humanized CD19-targeted CAR-T cell therapy for patients with relapsed/refractory B-ALL. J Immunother Cancer. 2023;11(2) https://doi.org/10.1136/JITC-2022-005701.
113. Wang S, Wang X, Ye C, et al. Humanized CD19-targeted chimeric antigen receptor T (CAR-T) cells for relapsed/refractory pediatric acute lymphoblastic leukemia. Am J Hematol. 2021;96(5):E162–5. https://doi.org/10.1002/AJH.26123.
114. Mueller KT, Grupp SA, Maude SL, et al. Tisagenlecleucel immunogenicity in relapsed/refractory acute lymphoblastic leukemia and diffuse large B-cell lymphoma. Blood Adv. 2021;5(23):4980–91. https://doi.org/10.1182/BLOODADVANCES.2020003844.
115. Aparicio-Pérez C, Carmona M, Benabdellah K, Herrera C. Failure of ALL recognition by CAR T cells: a review of CD 19-negative relapses after anti-CD 19 CAR-T treatment in B-ALL. Front Immunol. 2023;14:1165870. https://doi.org/10.3389/FIMMU.2023.1165870.
116. Fischer J, Paret C, El Malki K, et al. CD19 isoforms enabling resistance to CART-19 immunotherapy are expressed in B-ALL patients at initial diagnosis. J Immunother. 2017;40(5):187–95. https://doi.org/10.1097/CJI.0000000000000169.
117. Sotillo E, Barrett DM, Black KL, et al. Convergence of acquired mutations and alternative splicing of CD19 enables resistance to CART-19 immunotherapy. Cancer Discov. 2015;5(12):1282–95. https://doi.org/10.1158/2159-8290.CD-15-1020.
118. Fry TJ, Shah NN, Orentas RJ, et al. CD22-targeted CAR T cells induce remission in B-ALL that is naive or resistant to CD19-targeted CAR immunotherapy. Nat Med. 2018;24(1):20–8. https://doi.org/10.1038/NM.4441.
119. Shah NN, Highfill SL, Shalabi H, et al. CD4/CD8 T-cell selection affects chimeric antigen receptor (CAR) T-cell potency and toxicity: updated results from a phase I anti-CD22 CAR T-cell trial. J Clin Oncol. 2020;38(17):1938–50. https://doi.org/10.1200/JCO.19.03279.
120. Zhang Y, Li S, Wang Y, et al. A novel and efficient CD22 CAR-T therapy induced a robust antitumor effect in relapsed/refractory leukemia patients when combined with CD19 CAR-T treatment as a sequential therapy. Exp Hematol Oncol. 2022;11(1) https://doi.org/10.1186/S40164-022-00270-5.
121. Cordoba S, Onuoha S, Thomas S, et al. CAR T cells with dual targeting of CD19 and CD22 in pediatric and young adult patients with relapsed or refractory B cell acute lymphoblastic leukemia: a phase 1 trial. Nat Med. 2021;27(10):1797–805. https://doi.org/10.1038/S41591-021-01497-1.

122. Shalabi H, Qin H, Su A, et al. CD19/22 CAR T cells in children and young adults with B-ALL: phase 1 results and development of a novel bicistronic CAR. Blood. 2022;140(5):451–63. https://doi.org/10.1182/BLOOD.2022015795.
123. Pan J, Zuo S, Deng B, et al. Sequential CD19-22 CAR T therapy induces sustained remission in children with r/r B-ALL. Blood. 2020;135(5):387–91. https://doi.org/10.1182/BLOOD.2019003293.
124. Galletta TJ, Rubinstein JD, Krupski C, et al. Durable remissions achieved with reinfusion of CD19-directed CAR-T despite failure to induce or maintain B-cell aplasia and single-center experience with reinfusion of tisagenlecleucel. Pediatr Blood Cancer. 2023;70(5) https://doi.org/10.1002/PBC.30271.
125. Gauthier J, Bezerra ED, Hirayama AV, et al. Factors associated with outcomes after a second CD19-targeted CAR T-cell infusion for refractory B-cell malignancies. Blood. 2021;137(3):323–35. https://doi.org/10.1182/BLOOD.2020006770.
126. Holland EM, Molina JC, Dede K, et al. Efficacy of second CAR-T (CART2) infusion limited by poor CART expansion and antigen modulation. J Immunother Cancer. 2022;10(5) https://doi.org/10.1136/JITC-2021-004483.
127. Png YT, Vinanica N, Kamiya T, Shimasaki N, Coustan-Smith E, Campana D. Blockade of CD7 expression in T cells for effective chimeric antigen receptor targeting of T-cell malignancies. Blood Adv. 2017;1(25):2348–60. https://doi.org/10.1182/BLOODADVANCES.2017009928.
128. Georgiadis C, Rasaiyaah J, Gkazi SA, et al. Base-edited CAR T cells for combinational therapy against T cell malignancies. Leukemia. 2021;35(12):3466–81. https://doi.org/10.1038/S41375-021-01282-6.
129. Chiesa R, Georgiadis C, Syed F, et al. Base-edited CAR7 T cells for relapsed T-cell acute lymphoblastic leukemia. N Engl J Med. 2023;14 https://doi.org/10.1056/NEJMOA2300709. Published online June
130. Freiwan A, Zoine JT, Crawford JC, et al. Engineering naturally occurring CD7- T cells for the immunotherapy of hematological malignancies. Blood. 2022;140(25):2684–96. https://doi.org/10.1182/BLOOD.2021015020.
131. Watanabe N, Mo F, Zheng R, et al. Feasibility and preclinical efficacy of CD7-unedited CD7 CAR T cells for T cell malignancies. Mol Ther. 2023;31(1):24–34. https://doi.org/10.1016/J.YMTHE.2022.09.003.
132. Maciocia PM, Wawrzyniecka PA, Philip B, et al. Targeting the T cell receptor β-chain constant region for immunotherapy of T cell malignancies. Nat Med. 2017;23(12):1416–23. https://doi.org/10.1038/NM.4444.
133. Ali M, Giannakopoulou E, Li Y, et al. T cells targeted to TdT kill leukemic lymphoblasts while sparing normal lymphocytes. Nat Biotechnol. 2022;40(4):488–98. https://doi.org/10.1038/S41587-021-01089-X.
134. Lu P, Liu Y, Yang J, et al. Naturally selected CD7 CAR-T therapy without genetic manipulations for T-ALL/LBL: first-in-human phase 1 clinical trial. Blood. 2022;140(4):321–34. https://doi.org/10.1182/BLOOD.2021014498.
135. Li Z, An N, Yang K, et al. Donor CD7 Chimeric Antigen Receptor T Cell Bridging to Allogeneic Hematopoietic Stem Cell Transplantation for T Cell Hematologic Malignancy. Transplant Cell Ther. 2023;29(3):167–73. https://doi.org/10.1016/J.JTCT.2022.11.013.
136. Pan J, Tan Y, Wang G, et al. Donor-derived CD7 chimeric antigen receptor T cells for T-cell acute lymphoblastic leukemia: first-in-human, phase I trial. J Clin Oncol. 2021;39(30):3340–51. https://doi.org/10.1200/JCO.21.00389.
137. Hu Y, Zhou Y, Zhang M, et al. Genetically modified CD7-targeting allogeneic CAR-T cell therapy with enhanced efficacy for relapsed/refractory CD7-positive hematological malignancies: a phase I clinical study. Cell Res. 2022;32(11):995–1007. https://doi.org/10.1038/S41422-022-00721-Y.

Part V

Strategies for Patients with Lymphoblastic Lymphoma

Stratification and Treatment of Lymphoblastic Lymphoma

15

Andishe Attarbaschi

15.1 Introduction

Lymphoblastic disorders, including both acute lymphoblastic leukaemia (ALL) and lymphoblastic lymphoma (LBL), account for one-third of all malignancies diagnosed in childhood and adolescence [1, 2]. Among non-Hodgkin lymphomas (NHL) LBL is the second most common entity comprising 25–30% of all cases. Lymphoblastic lymphomas are histopathologically and cytomorphologically indistinguishable from ALL as both diseases are derived from precursor T and B cells [3]. The distinction of ALL and LBL is arbitrarily based on the amount of infiltration of blast cells in the bone marrow (BM) with patients having ≥25% blast cells being classified as ALL and patients having <25% blast cells being classified as LBL.

Although ALL and LBL appear grossly identical on a morphological level, share similar molecular aberrations and respond well to identical therapies, there is an ongoing debate on whether they are distinct disorders or lie on a spectrum of the same disease [4–6]. The development of multiagent chemotherapy regimens, regularly applied in multinational trials during the last 40 years, together with the standardisation of the diagnostic work-up at initial diagnosis and during treatment, have yielded excellent outcomes of LBL, with event-free survival (EFS) and overall survival (OS) rates exceeding 80% [1, 2, 7, 8].

15.2 Epidemiology

The incidence of LBL in Western countries is approximately 0.2–0.3 cases per year among 100,000 children <15 years of age. The median age at diagnosis is 9 years and not significantly different between B-lymphoblastic lymphoma (B-LBL; 8.0 years) and T-lymphoblastic lymphoma (T-LBL; 8.8. years) [9]. With a male-to-female ratio of 2.5:1, T-LBL shows a male predominance, while there are no differences in sex distribution for B-LBL (0.9:1) [9]. The majority of LBL cases is of T-cell precursor origin (75%) and the remaining 25% of cases of B-cell precursor origin [9–11]. Mixed phenotype

A. Attarbaschi (✉)
Department of Paediatric Haematology and Oncology, St. Anna Children's Hospital, Department of Paediatrics and Adolescent Medicine, Medical University of Vienna, Vienna, Austria
e-mail: andishe.attarbaschi@stanna.at

G. Escherich, V. Conter (eds.), *Acute Lymphoblastic Leukemia in Children and Adolescents*, Pediatric Oncology, https://doi.org/10.1007/978-3-031-71180-0_15

acute leukaemia (MPAL) phenotypes are rarely seen [12, 13].

15.3 Aetiology

The aetiology of LBL is not yet elucidated, but children with inborn errors of immunity such as ataxia telangiectasia, Nijmegen breakage syndrome, and constitutional mismatch repair diseases carry an increased risk for developing LBL [14–16]. Clinical management of LBL in patients with ataxia telangiectasia and Nijmegen breakage syndrome is challenging with regard to both the delivery of optimal lymphoma treatment and the excessive toxicities related to the intense chemotherapy usually needed [14, 15]. Consensus recommendations for the diagnostic and therapeutic management of haematological malignancies in children with DNA double-strand break disorders have been recently published, but are out of the scope of the present chapter [17].

15.4 Classification

15.4.1 Histology

The pathology of LBL, which is a small, blue round cell tumour, follows the World Health Organisation (WHO) classification of 2022 and is usually characterised by uniform infiltrates of small to medium-sized mononuclear cells consistent with blast cells (Fig. 15.1) [13]. The infiltrates can show increased mitoses and tingible body macrophages, thus imparting a starry-sky appearance. The morphological diagnosis of LBL can be usually performed on tumour touch imprints and BM as well as on malignant body fluid cytospins

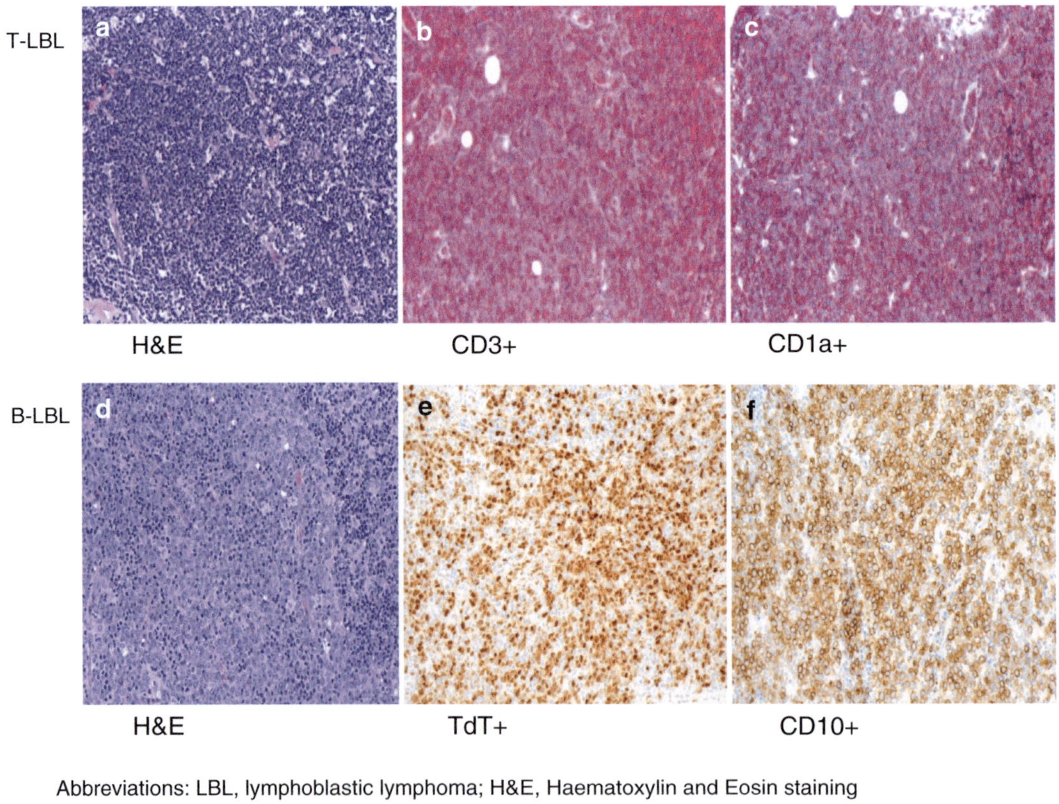

Fig. 15.1 Histopathology of T-LBL: (**a**) haematoxylin and eosin stain, (**b**) surface CD3 positivity, and (**c**) CD1a positivity. Histopathology of B-LBL: (**d**) haematoxylin and eosin stain, (**e**) TdT positivity, and (**f**) and CD10 positivity

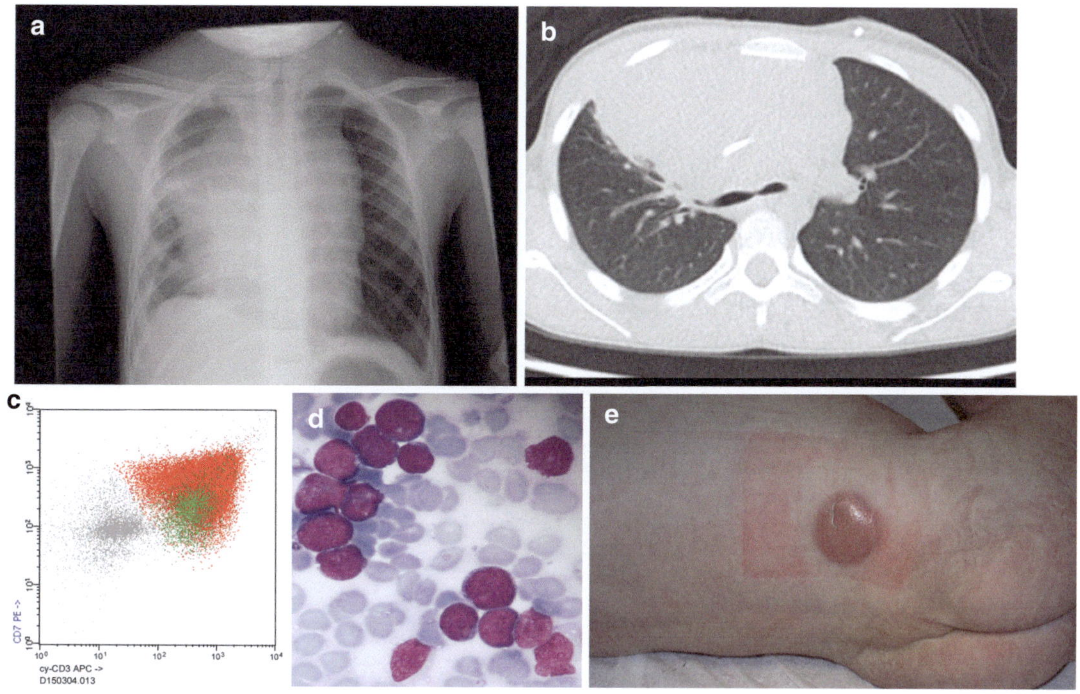

Fig. 15.2 Diagnostic work-up in patients with lymphoblastic lymphoma: (**a**, **b**) Chest X-ray and thoracic CT with a mediastinal mass in T-LBL, (**c**) Flow cytometric immunophenotyping of T-LBL, (**d**) cytomorphology of lymphoblastic lymphoma, and (**e**) skin involvement of B-LBL

and follows the French–American–British (FAB) classification, which differentiates between an L1 and L2 subtype (Fig. 15.2) [18, 19]. Due to the development of multicolour flow cytometry techniques, allowing an exact immunophenotyping of LBL, the cytomorphological distinction between the FAB L1 and L2 subtype has completely lost its significance. However, the basic cytomorphological assessment of May-Grünwald–Giemsa-stained BM smears, tumour touch imprints and body fluid cytospins is still the easiest, most rapid and cost-effective way of LBL diagnosis [18]. Cytochemical reactions, including acid phosphatase reaction, might help differentiate T from B lymphoblasts [20].

15.4.2 Immunophenotype

The WHO classification of 2022 and European Group for Immunological Classification of Leukemias (EGIL) have published exact guidelines for immunohistochemistry and immunophenotyping of LBL (Fig. 15.1, Table 15.1) [10, 13, 21]. The gold standard for the diagnosis of T-LBL is the expression of cytoplasmic or surface CD3. The presence of T-lymphoblasts is further established by the expression of immature markers such as TdT, CD99, or CD1a. Expression of other markers such as CD2, CD4, CD5, CD7, or CD8 is not as specific, but used to subclassify T-LBL according to the stage of differentiation of the T-lymphoblasts. A new T-LBL subtype of potential importance is the so-called early T-cell precursor (ETP) LBL, originally described for T-ALL [22–25]. The ETP immunophenotype is defined by 1) a negative expression of CD1a, CD8, and myeloperoxidase, 2) a positive expression of ≥1 myeloid marker (CD34, CD117, HLA-DR, CD13, CD33, CD11b, and CD65) and CD7, and (3) a negative or dim expression of CD5, defined by an expression in <75% of the blast cells and 1 log lower fluorescence intensity than of mature T cells. The B-LBL immunophenotype is defined by a variable combination of B-cell markers such as

Table 15.1 Immunological classification of LBL according to the EGIL criteria for acute lymphoblastic leukaemia (A) and biphenotypic acute leukaemia (BAL) (B)

A	
Lineage	Marker
All T-ALLs	sCD3 or cCD3+, TdT+, CD34-, HLA-DR-
Pro-T ALL	CD7+
Pre-T ALL	CD2+ and/or CD5+ and/or CD8+
Cortical T-ALL	CD1a+
Mature T-ALL	sCD3+, CD1a-
α/ß + T-ALL	Anti-TCRα/ß+
γ/δ + T-ALL	Anti-TCRγ/δ+
All B-ALLs	CD19+ and/or CD22+ and/or cCD79a+, TdT+, CD34+, HLA-DR+
Pro-B ALL	No further marker
Common ALL	CD10+
Pre-B ALL	Cytoplasmic μ chain+, (CD10+)
Mature B-AL	sIg + or cIg + (or sIg/κ chain+ or sIg/λ chain+)
Abbreviations:	*s* surface, *c* cytoplasmic, *TCR* T-cell receptor, *Ig* immunoglobulin
	ALL acute lymphoblastic leukaemia, *AL* acute leukaemia

B			
Myeloid lineage	T-lineage	B-lineage	Points
MPO	CD3	cCD79	2
Lysozyme	Anti-TCRα/ß+	IgM	
	Anti-TCRγ/δ+	CD22	
CD13	CD2	CD19	1
CD33	CD5	CD10	
CD65	CD8	CD20	
CD117	CD10		
CD14	TdT	TdT	0.5
CD15	CD7	CD24	
CD64	CD1a		
Abbreviations:	*MPO* myeloperoxidase, *c* cytoplasmic, *TCR* T-cell receptor		
BAL definition:	When scores are >2 points for both myeloid and T- or B-lymphoid lineages		

CD19, CD22, cCD79a, and PAX5. Other markers such as CD34, TdT, CD10, and cytoplasmic μ chain are used to subclassify B-LBL according to the stage of differentiation of the B lymphoblasts. An MPAL immunophenotype has also been reported for LBL and follows the respective criteria of the WHO classification of 2022 and EGIL (biphenotypic acute leukaemia score, Table 15.1) [10, 13, 21].

15.4.3 Genetic Alterations

Recurrent chromosomal alterations in number and structure can be identified in almost all cases of ALL in childhood and adolescence, being associated with prognosis, and regularly used for treatment stratification [26, 27]. Although genetic aberrations such as the *BCR::ABL1*, *ETV6::RUNX1* and *TCF3::PBX1* fusion genes, *KMT2A* rearrangements, alterations of chromosome 21, and high-hyperdiploidy have been reported in B-LBL patients, their respective incidence and prognostic relevance are unknown [1, 28–33]. Other recurrent B-ALL alterations such as deletions of key B-cell haematopoietic factors such as *IKZF1*, *CDKN2A/B*, *PAX5*, *ETV6*, and *EBF1* are recurrently found in B-LBL, but also with an unknown incidence, as compared with B-ALL [34, 35].

In T-LBL, most translocations involve the gene locus of the α/δ chain of the T-cell receptor (TCR) on chromosome 14q11 or the gene locus of the β chain of the TCR on chromosome 7q35

[28, 36]. The fusion gene partners are variable and their respective incidence and prognostic significance unclear. Recent sophisticated research, performed on a multinational level, has identified two candidate genes of strong prognostic relevance for T-LBL: *NOTCH1* and *FBXW7* [36–40]. Mutations of *NOTCH1* and/or *FBXW7* at recurrent hotspots are found in approximately 50% of T-LBL patients and associated with an improved response to therapy and final outcome [36–40]. In contrast, other markers of molecular research in T-LBL, such as the loss of heterozygosity at chromosomal region 6q14–24 (LOH6q), mutations of *PTEN or KMT2D,* and the absence of biallelic TCR γ gene locus deletion, have been shown to carry an adverse prognosis in T-LBL [36, 40–44]. Intriguingly, a recent analysis showed that the negative impact of *PTEN* mutations is completely abrogated by *NOTCH1* mutations (EFS: 91% ± 9%) [41, 45]. Another molecular marker of interest in pediatric T-LBL is *miR-223,* which directly targets SIK1, an anti-metastatic protein [46]. As over-expression of *miR-223* was shown to reduce SIK1 expression, thereby promoting tumour cell growth, migration, and invasion of T-LBL in vitro, its expression levels were measured in a cohort of 67 Italian T-LBL patients and correlated with outcome [46]. Multivariable analysis revealed that a high level of *miR-223* was the only independent risk factor for an inferior prognosis and thus might be useful for treatment stratification in childhood T-LBL. Nevertheless, mutations of *NOTCH1* and/or *FBXW7* proved as the most robust prognostic factors in a number of studies and thus were set to be used as the novel biologic stratification markers in T-LBL in the multinational LBL-2018 trial [36–40].

15.5 Clinical Presentation at Diagnosis

The clinical symptoms of a patient with LBL depend on the extent of disease spread. The patient's history is often very short as LBL is a highly proliferative disease. Patients with T-LBL usually present with a mass in the anterior mediastinum involving the thymus and lymph nodes (LN) (Fig. 15.2), although any LN region can be involved [1, 28, 47]. Patients can present with chronic cough, wheezing or hoarseness, dyspnoea, other respiratory distress such as nasal flaring and suprasternal and intercostal retractions, chest swelling and pain, pericardial tamponade with low-output cardiac failure, or a superior vena cava syndrome with facial and neck oedema, jugular venous distension, and headache. Reasons are local tumour effects such as the compression of the upper and lower respiratory tract and of the superior vena cava, and accompanying pericardial and pleural effusions. Involvement of the BM may impair normal haematopoiesis resulting in cytopenia(s) with corresponding symptoms, but, as T-LBL is only diagnosed in case of <25% blast cells in the BM, signs of BM failure are usually not as prominent as in ALL patients. Symptoms of central nervous system (CNS) disease are rarely observed, but may include headache, neck rigidity, impaired vision, seizures, and cranial nerve palsies. Clinical features of B-LBL patients may vary considerably with the peripheral LN, BM, skin (Fig. 15.2) and bone (multifocal) being the most common sites of involvement [5, 47–50].

15.6 Diagnosis

The diagnosis of LBL is based on the clinical evaluation of the patient, laboratory work-up, histopathological and cytomorphological analyses of paraffin-embedded and fresh tumour samples, and imaging studies (Table 15.2, Fig. 15.2). A primary goal at initial presentation is to establish the diagnosis as soon as possible, but to avoid life-threatening situations. As children and adolescents with T-LBL usually have a high initial tumour burden, serious complications due to spontaneous tumour lysis syndrome or local tumour effects may already be seen at diagnosis [51]. T-LBL patients with a mass in the anterior mediastinum, which often leads to respiratory distress and an upper inflow congestion, require rapid diagnosis and commencement of treatment. However, anaesthesia needed for the surgical diagnostic procedures carries a high anaesthesiologic risk, and, in particular, when trying to end

Table 15.2 Initial diagnostic work-up in patients with lymphoblastic lymphoma

List of parameters
Complete clinical status (esp. liver, spleen, testicles, CNS)
Signs of infection or bleeding); Karnofsky score; B-symptoms
Laboratory (Na, K, Cl, P, Ca, Mg, uric acid, LDH, creatinine, urea, liver transaminases, immunoglobulins, CRP, coagulation)
Blood group, optional: TPMT status, APCR
Serologies: Virology (CMV, HSV, VZV, EBV, HIV), toxoplasmosis, Lues
Surveillance cultures (gram-positive and gram-negative bacteria, Candida)
BM aspirate and biopsy for morphology, genetics and phenotyping (MDD)
PB for morphology and phenotyping (MDD)
CSF with cell count and cytospins for morphology, genetics, and phenotyping
Malignant effusions with cytospins for morphology, genetics, and phenotyping
ECG, echocardiography, EEG
Ophthalmological examination (fundus)
Pregnancy test for female adolescents
Imaging procedures:
Chest X-ray
Ultrasound of lymph nodes, mediastinum, abdomen, pelvis, and testes
MRI of the involved regions: Neurocranium, mediastinum, abdomen, pelvis, and spine/spinal cord
CT of the involved regions: Mediastinum, lungs
FDG-PET-CT/MRI: According to local standards and availability

CNS central nervous system, *LDH* lactate dehydrogenase, *CRP* C-reactive protein, *TPMT* thiopurine methyltransferase, *APCR* activated protein C resistance, *BM* bone marrow, *PB* peripheral blood, *MDD* minimal disseminated disease, *CSF* cerebrospinal fluid, ECG echocardiography, *EEG* electroencephalography, *MRI* magnetic resonance imaging, *CT* computed tomography, *FDG-PET* fluoro-desoxy glucose positron emission tomography

anaesthesia tracheal collapse could occur. Thus, a minimally invasive procedure, preferentially done under local anaesthesia, is usually pursued to establish a diagnosis. Such procedures include punctures of initially existing body cavity effusions or of the BM. Fine needle aspirations of peripheral LN may be occasionally acceptable. If, however, a primary diagnosis of the T-LBL is not possible because of the threatening clinical situation, early admission to an intensive care unit is crucial and beginning an empirical cytoreductive corticosteroid prephase is warranted. Tumour material should be obtained after a maximum of 48–72 h to confirm the diagnosis. Alternatively, patients may undergo endotracheal intubation under general anaesthesia, allowing mechanical ventilation, having the diagnostic surgical procedures performed while intubated, and be extubated only at a time when a reduction in tumour size has been achieved and when there is no more risk of an anaesthesiologic incident.

The complete standard diagnostic work-up always includes a thorough physical examination, especially of all peripheral LN regions on both sides of the diaphragm, the liver, spleen and testicles. The diagnosis is completed by the collection of laboratory parameters (blood counts, tumour lysis parameters such as potassium, calcium, phosphorus, lactate dehydrogenase, uric acid and creatinine as well as coagulation and liver parameters). Flow cytometry of the peripheral blood and BM may detect minimal disseminated disease (MDD) on a submicroscopical level, whereby the diagnosis of T- or B-LBL could be suspected, but the number of cells may not be sufficient for comprehensive and reliable molecular-genetic analyses [52–54].

Imaging studies include a chest X-ray and computed tomography as well as an ultrasound of the neck, axillae, supraclavicular and infraclavicular region, groin and abdomen (kidney infiltration, LN, liver and spleen size). Cranial computed or magnetic resonance imaging to rule out lymphomatous infiltrations is also recommended for LBL. For special sites of involvement, a local magnetic resonance (ear–nose–throat area, abdomen, skeleton, epidural tumour) or computed tomography (lung) is obligatory.

The definite BM and CNS status has to be assessed by punctures of both compartments [20]. As LBL is morphologically indistinguishable from ALL, their distinction is arbitrarily made by the number of blast cells in the BM taking into account the cut-off of 25% blast cells; patients with ≥5% and < 25% blast cells in the BM are defined as LBL with BM involvement (stage IV disease). With regard to the definition of CNS disease, the following criteria are used [20]: CNS1: no blast cells on cerebral spinal fluid cytospins (irrespective of the white blood cell number in the Fuchs–Rosenthal chamber), CNS2: <5 white blood cells/μl and unequivocally identifiable blast cells, and CNS3 (stage IV disease): ≥5 white blood cells/μl and unequivocally identifiable blast cells, and/or cerebral and/or medullary infiltrates on imaging and/or cranial nerve palsies that cannot be explained by extradural lesions.

Staging of LBL was originally based on the St. Jude's (Murphy) staging system, but due to an international effort, has been evolved to the International Paediatric NHL Staging System which includes, in particular, modifications with regard to specific sites of involvement such as the skin, bone, BM, and CNS (Table 15.3) [55, 56]. Notably, BM disease is found in 15–20% and 30–40% of T- and B-LBL patients, respectively, and CNS disease in approximately 5% of both

Table 15.3 International Paediatric Non-Hodgkin Lymphoma Staging System (A) including additional staging information (B)

A	
Stage	Definition
Stage I	Single tumour with exclusion of mediastinum and abdomen (N; EN; B or S: EN-B, EN-S)
Stage II	Single EN tumour with regional node involvement
	≥ two N areas on same side of diaphragm
	Primary GI tract tumour (usually in ileocecal area), ± involvement of associated mesenteric nodes, that is completely resectable
	(if malignant ascites or extension of tumour to adjacent organs, it should be regarded as stage III)
Stage III	≥ two EN tumourtumours (including EN-B or EN-S) above and/or below diaphragm
	≥ two N areas above and below diaphragm
	Any intrathoracic tumour (mediastinal, hilar, pulmonary, pleural, or thymic)
	Intra-abdominal and retroperitoneal disease, including liver, spleen, kidney, and/or ovary localizations
	Regardless of degree of resection (except primary GI tract tumour [usually in ileocecal region]
	± involvement of associated mesenteric nodes that is completely resectable)
	Any paraspinal or epidural tumour, regardless of whether other sites are involved
	Single B lesion with concomitant involvement of EN and/or nonregional N sites
Stage IV	Any of the above findings with initial involvement of CNS (stage IV CNS), BM (stage IV BM),
	Or both (stage IV combined) based on conventional methods
Abbreviations:	*B* bone, *BM* bone marrow, *EN* extranodal, *N* nodal, *S* skin

B	
Site	Additional staging information
BM involvement	Stage IV disease, resulting from BM involvement, is currently defined by morphologic evidence of ≥5% blasts or lymphoma cells by BM aspiration;
	This applies to any histologic subtype and will be maintained in IPNHLSS.
	For each stage, type and degree of BM involvement (by BM aspiration) should be specified, using abbreviations below to identify involvement:
	BMm: BM positivity by morphology (specify % lymphoma cells)
	BMi: BM positivity by immunophenotypic methods (immunohistochemical or flow cytometric analysis; specify % lymphoma cells)

(continued)

Table 15.3 (continued)

B	
Site	Additional staging information
	BMc: BM positivity by cytogenetic or FISH analysis (specify % lymphoma cells)
	BMmol: BM positivity by molecular techniques (PCR based; specify level of involvement)
	Same approach should be used for PB involvement (ie, PBm, PBi, PBc, PBmol).
	Definition of BM involvement should be obtained from analysis of bilateral BM aspirates and BM biopsy
CNS involvement	Stage IV disease, CNS is considered involved in case of:
	Any CNS tumour mass (identified by imaging techniques [i.e. CT, MRI])
	Cranial nerve palsy that cannot be explained by extradural lesions
	Blasts morphologically identified in CSF
	Condition that defines CNS positivity should be specified: CNS positive/mass, CNS positive/palsy, CNS positive/blasts
	CSF status: CSF positivity is based on morphologic evidence of lymphoma cells
	CSF should be considered positive when any no. of blasts is detected
	CSF unknown (not performed, technical difficulties)
	Similar to BM, type of CSF involvement should be described whenever possible:
	CSFm: CSF positivity by morphology (specify no. of blasts/μL)
	CSFi: CSF positivity by immunophenotype methods (immunohistochemical or flow cytometric analysis; specify % lymphoma cells)
	CSFc: CSF positive by cytogenetic or FISH analysis (specify % lymphoma cells)
	CSFmol: CSF positivity by molecular techniques (PCR based; specify level of involvement)

Based on data from Refs. [55, 56]
BM bone marrow, *CT* computed tomography, *FISH* fluorescent in situ hybridization, *IPNHLSS* international Paediatric non-Hodgkin lymphoma staging system, *MRI* magnetic resonance imaging, *PB* peripheral blood, *PBc* PB positivity by cytogenetic or FISH analysis, *PBi* PB positivity by immunophenotype methods, *PBm* PB positivity by morphology, *PBmol* PB positivity by molecular techniques, *PCR* polymerase chain reaction

entities [1, 2, 28]. Due to the very frequent involvement of the mediastinum, the majority of T-LBL patients present with at least stage III disease, whereas limited stage I/II disease is found ≥50% of the B-LBL patients [5, 9, 47, 48].

15.7 Prognostic Factors

Since the early 1980s, it has been well established that the choice of treatment in paediatric NHL is the most important prognostic factor and depends on whether the disease is localized or disseminated and whether the disease is lymphoblastic or non-lymphoblastic (i.e. mature B-cell neoplasms) [57, 58]. As a consequence, patients with LBL are usually treated with protocols designed for childhood ALL [59]. The delineation of further prognostic factors in LBL is needed to identify a subgroup with an excellent outcome, which can be achieved with a therapy of minimal acute and long-term toxicities, and a subgroup at risk, for whom augmentation of therapy and/or novel targeted approaches are needed. The latter aim is of utmost importance as, in particular, T-LBL relapses usually have a fatal outcome [60].

The inferior prognostic relevance of characteristics such as adolescent age, infant age, female sex, advanced disease stages and poor response of a mediastinal mass after a 7-day prednisone pre-phase or at the end of induction therapy has been shown for T-LBL in several trials, but not reproduced consistently by others [9, 30, 61–64]. Thus, to date, almost all study groups are still using stage of disease to stratify both T- and B-LBL patients into two risk groups. Outcomes of the EURO-LB 02 trial showed that stage of disease is still a prognostic marker, with stage I/II B-LBL patients doing significantly better than stage III/IV B-LBL patients, who even received a delayed intensification element [7]. However, using stage of disease in T-LBL to discriminate between a low- and high-risk group appears useless as the number of stage I/II disease in T-LBL is extremely low (i.e. EURO-LB 02 trial: 8 out of 233 T-LBL patients had stage I/II disease) [7]. While earlier trials found that stage IV T-LBL has a better outcome than stage III T-LBL, the EURO-LB 02 study showed superimposable EFS rates [7, 65].

Besides molecular genetics, response to therapy, as measured on a sub-microscopical level in the BM during the patient's early disease course (MRD, minimal residual disease), using either quantitative polymerase chain reaction-based patient-specific immunoglobulin and TCR gene rearrangements or flow cytometry, is the most important prognostic factor in childhood ALL [26, 66, 67]. Several trials have demonstrated that MDD at diagnosis as measured by flow cytometry in BM has the potential of being used as a stratification parameter in LBL [52, 54, 68, 69]. In a study performed by the St. Jude's Children's Research Hospital, 77 of 99 T-LBL patients had MDD in BM with a median of 0.22% blast cells. Two-year EFS was 68.1% ± 11.1% for patients with ≥1% blast cells in BM versus 90.7% ± 4.4% for those with lower levels of BM involvement ($P = 0.031$); EFS for patients with ≥5% blast cells was 51.9% ± 18.0% ($P = 0.009$) [52]. In an Italian study, MDD was detected in 32 of 65 T- and B-LBL patients [53]. Applying a cut-off level of 3%, 5-year EFS was 60% ± 22% for patients with >3% blast cells versus 83% ± 6% for patients with <3% blast cells in BM ($P = 0.04$). Nevertheless, to date, large-scale confirmation of these findings is lacking.

Currently, the dimensions of the mediastinal tumour appear to be the only disease marker to quantify treatment response in T-LBL. While the persistence of a large tumour mass after induction therapy (<70% regression on day 33 in the NHL-BFM (Berlin–Frankfurt–Münster) trials) is usually regarded as treatment failure and has been used to upgrade patients into high-risk therapy arms, the significance of a small residual mass is not yet completely clear [62, 70]. Trial NHL-BFM 90 revealed that local relapse in the mediastinum was indeed mostly responsible for treatment failure, but it did not show that patients with a persistent tumour at day 33 (incomplete regression, but ≥70%) or after completion of early intensification (day 63, any residual tumour) had a significantly worse prognosis compared with those whose tumour regressed completely [62]. Local relapses were diagnosed with a comparable frequency in patients with and without a residual tumour at both time points. However, a British study reported that children with a persistent mediastinal mass after 60 days of therapy had a dismal prognosis [63]. This discrepancy between the two studies might be due to differences in intensity or combinations of chemotherapy; the British protocols did not include high-dose methotrexate or cyclophosphamide.

In order to elucidate the prognostic relevance of treatment response by imaging, other methods than magnetic resonance imaging or computed tomography during the patient's early disease course, such as 18-fluorodeoxyglucose positron emission tomography, are currently under investigation [71–73]. Importantly, with the development of standardized definitions for response assessment in paediatric NHL by the International Paediatric Non-Hodgkin Lymphoma Response Criteria, data obtained from new and more sensitive technologies, that are now being widely used for disease evaluation, will be taken into account, providing a standardized means for reporting and comparing treatment response [74].

15.8 Treatment

15.8.1 Primary Disease

An increase in the cure rates for children and adolescents with LBL, from 10% in the 1950s to 80–85% nowadays, has been obtained with modern chemotherapeutic regimens [1, 28, 59]. A first major step was the introduction of a multiagent chemotherapy by Wollner et al. in the 1970s with the LSA_2-L_2 protocol, that was established in the United States (Memorial Sloan Kettering Cancer Center) and included elements known to be effective against ALL and LBL [57]. The ten-drug combination therapy, consisting of an induction, consolidation, and maintenance therapy, was given for a total treatment duration of 3 years. Intrathecal methotrexate was added in all therapy phases. Most patients underwent radiation therapy of the local tumour but no prophylactic cranial irradiation. The regimen was superior to pulse-like therapies as proven by randomized studies [58, 75]. Finally, it became the gold standard and was applied worldwide with several modifications [57].

At the same time, in Europe, the ALL-BFM protocol was developed and used in its unchanged form for LBL [76]. The main differences from the LSA_2-L_2 protocol were lower cumulative dosages of drugs with a risk of long-term adverse sequelae, i.e. the alkylating agents (which harbour the risk of secondary malignancies and infertility), and the potentially cardiotoxic anthracyclines. Additionally, no routine local irradiation was given to the mediastinum, thereby reducing the life-long increased risk of secondary malignancies in the radiation field. From the beginning, systemic methotrexate was part of the BFM regimen and was soon escalated to four cycles of 5 g/m^2/24 h given as consolidation therapy [77]. Prior to consolidation, the NHL-BFM regimen (Fig. 15.3 and Table 15.4) includes a 5-week induction and early 4-week intensification therapy (protocol I, phases a and b) [7, 62]. Patients with stage III/IV disease also undergo a delayed intensification phase (protocol II) [7, 62, 70]. For all patients, maintenance treatment with 6-mercaptopurine and methotrexate is scheduled for a total treatment duration of 2 years. Until trial NHL-BFM 90, all patients with stage III/IV disease received prophylactic cranial irradiation (12 Gy) [62]. Finally, trial NHL-BFM 90 for T-LBL resulted in an EFS rate of 90%. B-LBL patients included in trials NHL-BFM 86 and 90 had an EFS of 73% [48].

Current LBL protocols are mostly derived from either the LSA_2-L_2 protocol or the NHL-BFM protocol which both achieved the first durable remissions in paediatric patients with LBL [57, 59]. Using ALL-type treatment regimens, long-term EFS rates of 68–90% (Table 15.5) can be achieved in childhood LBL nowadays, with the EURO-LB 02 trial being the last multinational study accomplished in Europe (5-year EFS: 82 ± 2%) [7, 8, 59, 62, 64, 65, 70, 75, 77–92].

An interesting trial in LBL came from the international BFM Study Group and showed that escalating Capizzi-based methotrexate (C-MTX) in combination with the NHL-BFM backbone resulted in an EFS of 90.8% in 58 LBL patients [93]. CNS-directed treatment was based on frequent intrathecal injections. The Children's Oncology Group (COG) study AALL0434 evaluated the safety and efficacy of multiagent chemotherapy with C-MTX in paediatric T-LBL and reported preliminary data using nelarabine in high-risk patients [88, 94, 95]. The trial enrolled 299 patients, high-risk patients had ≥1% MDD in BM at diagnosis or received prior corticosteroid treatment. Induction failure was defined as failure to achieve a partial response at the end of the 4-week induction. All patients received the augmented BFM (ABFM) C-MTX regimen and high-risk patients were randomised to 0 or 6 5-day courses of nelarabine incorporated into the ABFM

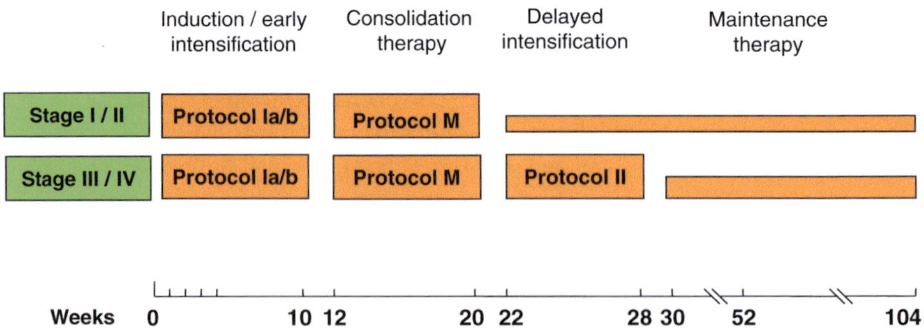

Fig. 15.3 Treatment strategy in lymphoblastic lymphoma according to the NHL-BFM Study Group

Table 15.4 Treatment protocols used in trial NHL-BFM 90 / trial EURO-LB 02

Protocol phase	Dosage	Days
Cytoreductive pre-phase		
Prednisone	60 mg/m²/d	1–7
Methotrexate (it)	12 mg[b]	1
Induction protocol Ia		
Prednisone (oral or iv)	60 mg/m²/d	8–28, then tapered over 3 × 3 days
Vincristine (iv)	1.5 mg/m² (max 2 mg)	8, 15, 22, 29
Daunorubicin (iv over 1 h)	30 mg/m²	8, 15, 22, 29
Native *E. Coli* L-asparaginase[a] (iv over 1 h)	10.000 IU/m²	12, 15, 18, 21, 24, 27, 30, 33
Methotrexate (it)	12 mg[b]	12, 19, 26, 33
Early intensification protocol Ib		
Cyclophosphamide (iv over 1 h)	1000 mg/m²	36, 64
Cytarabine (iv)	75 mg/m²	38–41, 45–48, 52–55, 59–62
6-Mercaptopurine (oral)	60 mg/m²	36–63
Methotrexate (it)	12 mg[b]	45, 59
Consolidation protocol M		
6-Mercaptopurine (oral)	25 mg/m²	1–56
Methotrexate (iv over 24 h)	5 g/m²	8, 22, 36, 50
Methotrexate (it)	12 mg[b]	8, 22, 36, 50
For stages III and IV only: delayed intensification		
Protocol IIa		
Dexamethasone (oral or iv)	10 mg/m²	1–21, then tapered over 3 × 3 days
Vincristine (iv)	1.5 mg/m² (max 2 mg)	8, 15, 22, 29
Doxorubicin (iv over 1 h)	30 mg/m²	8, 15, 22, 29
Native *E. coli* L-asparaginase[a] (iv over 1 h)	10.000 IU/m²	8, 11, 15, 18
Protocol IIb		
Cyclophosphamide (iv over 1 h)	1000 mg/m²	36
Cytarabine (iv)	75 mg/m²	38–41, 45–48
Methotrexate (it)	12 mg[b]	38, 45
6-Thioguanine (oral)	60 mg/m²	36–49
Maintenance		
6-Mercaptopurine (oral)	50 mg/m²	Daily until 24 month of total therapy
Methotrexate (oral)	20 mg/m²	Weekly until 24 month of total therapy

Based on data from references [7, 62]
iv, intravenously, *it* intrathecally, *h* hour(s), *mo* months
[a]In ongoing trial LBL-2018, native *E. Coli* L-asparaginase was replaced by PEG-L-asparaginase 2500 IU/m² in protocol Ia (days 12 and 26) and in protocol IIa (day 8)
[b]Dose of IT methotrexate was adjusted for children <3 years of age

protocol. Patients with induction failure were nonrandomly assigned to ABFM C-MTX + nelarabine. No patients received prophylactic cranial radiation. For the whole cohort, the 4-year EFS and OS were 84.7% ± 2.3% and 89.0% ± 2.0%. The 4-year disease-free survival (DFS) from end-induction was 85.9% ± 2.6%. There was no difference in DFS observed between the high-risk and standard-risk groups (P = 0.29) or by treatment regimen (P = 0.55). Nelarabine did not show an advantage for high-risk patients [88]. Importantly, CNS relapse occurred in only four patients. In summary, the COG AALL0434 protocol showed excellent outcomes in one of the largest trials ever conducted for patients with primary T-LBL [88]. The COG ABFM regimen with C-MTX provided

Table 15.5 Treatment results of selected trials in lymphoblastic lymphoma between 1977 and 2017

Authors	Publication year	Study Group	Period	Protocol	Protocol backbone	No. of patients	EFS
Anderson et al.	1993	CCG	1977–1982	CCG-551	LSA2-L2	124 (T- and B-LBL, III/IV)	64%
Patte et al.	1992	SFOP	1981–1989	LMT81	Modified LSA2-L2	84 (T- and B-LBL)	75%
Tubergen et al.	1995	CCG	1983–1990	CCG-502	LSA2-L2 vs. ADCOMP	143 vs. 138 (T- and B-LBL)	74 vs. 64%
Abromowitch	2008	COG	1994–1997	COG-5941	Modified LSA2-L2	85 (T- and B-LBL, III, IV)	78%
Reiter et al.	1995	BFM	1986–1990	NHL-BFM 86	ALL-BFM-derived	77 (T- and B-LBL)	78%
Reiter et al.	2000	BFM	1990–1995	NHL-BFM 90	ALL-BFM-derived	105 (T-LBL)	90%
Burkhardt et al.	2006	BFM	1995–2001	NHL-BFM 95	ALL-BFM-derived	156 (T-LBL III/IV)	82%
Uyttebroeck et al.	2008	EORTC	1989–1998	CLG 58881	NHL-BFM ALL-derived	119 (T-LBL)	77.5%
Uyttebroeck et al.	2012	EORTC	1998–2008	CLG 58951	NHL-BFM ALL-derived	74 (T-LBL)	85%
Asselin et al.	2011	POG	1996–2001	POG-9404	DFCI ALL-derived	137 (T-LBL, III/IV)	84.6%
Bergeron et al.	2015	SFOP	1997–2003	LMT96	Modified NHL-BFM ALL-derived	79 (T-LBL)	85%
Pillon et al.	2009	AIEOP	1992–1997	AIEOP LNH-92	Modified LSA2-L2	55 (T- and B-LBL)	69%
Pillon et al.	2015	AIEOP	1997–2007	AIEOP LNH-97	Modified LSA2-L2	114 (T- and B-LBL)	74%
Sandlund et al.	2009	St. Jude	1992–2002	St. Jude NHL13	T-ALL-derived	41 (T-LBL, III/V)	82.9%
Termuhlen et al.	2013	COG	2000–2005	COG-A5971	CCG ALL vs. NHL-BFM 95	254 (T- and B-LBL, III/IV)	80–84%
Landmann et al.	2017	EICNHL	2003–2008	EURO-LB 02	NHL-BFM 90-derived	319 (T- and B-LBL)	82%
Gao et al.	2015	SCMC	2007–?	Three protocols	NHL-BFM 90–/95-derived	96 (T- & B-LBL)	68%
Sekimizu et al.	2018	JPLL	2018–2024	LLB-NHL3	De-intensified ALL-BFM-derived	48 planned (T- and B-LBL, I/II)	NA
Sunami et al.	2016	JPLL	2004–2010	ALB-NHL3	ALL-BFM-derived	136 (T- and B-LBL, III/IV)	77.9%
Hayashi et al.	2020	COG	2010–2014	AALL0434	Augmented ALL-BFM-derived	299 (T-LBL)	84.7%
Teachey et al.	2022	COG	2014–2017	AALL1231	Augmented ALL-BFM-derived	209 (T-LBL)	81.2%

N number, *EFS* event-free survival, *CCG* Children's Cancer Group, *SFOP* Société Française d'Oncologie Pédiatrique, *COG* Children's Oncology Group, *BFM* Berlin-Frankfurt-Münster, *EORTC* European Organisation for Research and Treatment of Cancer, *POG* Paediatric Oncology Group, *AIEOP* Associazione Italiana di Ematologia e Oncologia Pediatrica, *EICNHL* European Intergroup for Childhood Non-Hodgkin Lymphoma, *SCMC* Shanghai Children's Medical Centre, *JPLL* Japanese Paediatric Leukaemia/Lymphoma Study Group, *NHL* non-Hodgkin lymphoma, *CLG* Children's Leukaemia Group, *ALL* acute lymphoblastic leukaemia, *DFCI* Dana Farber Cancer Institute, *NA* not applicable excellent EFS and OS without cranial irradiation. The COG study AALL1231, randomising patients to the addition of bortezomib, a proteasome inhibitor, on a COG BFM backbone showed that patients with T-LBL had improved EFS and OS with bortezomib: 4-year EFS (76.5% ± 5.1% versus 86.4% ± 4.0%; $P = 0.041$); and 4-year OS (78.3% ± 4.9% versus 89.5% ± 3.6%; $P = 0.009$) [96]. The COG A5971 study reported excellent results for 66 B-LBL cases with a 5-year EFS of 90% for 42 patients with localized disease and only one relapse among 24 patients with disseminated disease [8, 97]. Similar excellent results for localized B-LBL have been reported by the French LMT96 study and the EORTC 58881 and 58951 trials [64, 81, 98].

Although LBLs are radiosensitive malignancies, local irradiation as a routine measure has been abandoned since the introduction and use of highly effective chemotherapy. However, there is a lack of sufficient information to define the role of local radiation therapy in patients with an inadequate early response of the mediastinal tumour to chemotherapy. With respect to the high cure rates, omission of prophylactic and therapeutic cranial radiation therapy in children receiving highly active, CNS-directed systemic and intrathecal chemotherapy seems to be justified, although a slight increase of CNS-involving relapses has been observed since trial NHL-BFM 95 [7, 70]. In order to reduce the rate of CNS-involving recurrences, the multinational LBL-2018 trial is randomising the corticosteroid in induction therapy for all patients, with the more effective dexamethasone being tested against the standard substance prednisone. The role of surgery in the treatment of LBL is confined to diagnostic procedures, which should be restricted to the least invasive interventions to gain sufficient tumour material.

15.8.2 Progression and Relapse

Refractory and relapsed (r/r) LBL still has a dismal outcome, with survival rates of only 10–30% [60, 99]. The largest analysis reported to date by the international BFM Study Group showed survival rates of 27 ± 3% for 177 T-LBL patients and 52 ± 10% for 34 B-LBL patients [100]. There were almost no survivors in T-LBL patients without allogeneic haematopoietic stem cell transplantation (allo-HSCT). As a consequence, it is currently recommended that second-line treatment should comprise intense treatment courses derived from high-risk ALL or relapsed ALL protocols followed by allo-HSCT. These treatment recommendations also apply for r/r B-LBL patients, apart from the rare cases of late relapses which could be cured with intense chemotherapy alone [100].

15.9 Novel Therapies

Potential drugs of interest in treatment of T-lymphoblastic diseases are either targeting pathways like NOTCH-, PI3K-AKT-mTOR-, JAK-STAT-, and MAPK-pathways, the cell cycle regulation, the proteasome, epigenetic markers, or based on immunotherapeutic concepts [1, 28, 96, 101–103]. Only a limited number of drugs are, however, under investigation in r/r T-LBL. The armamentarium of novel drugs for treatment of B-LBL could be greater due to the fascinating developments in r/r B-ALL, but, as r/r B-LBL is an ultrarare disease, it is not an attractive standalone cohort of patients for drug developments [104, 105].

15.9.1 Chemotherapy-Based Approaches

The NECTAR study T2008–002 tested whether addition of etoposide and cyclophosphamide to the nucleoside analogue nelarabine could improve response rates over single-agent nelarabine for r/r T-ALL and T-LBL [106, 107]. The overall best response rate was 38% (8/21), with 33% (4/12) responses in the T-ALL and 44% (4/9) responses in the T-LBL group. These response rates were similar to those observed with single-agent nelarabine and suggest that the addition of cyclophosphamide and etoposide to nelarabine does not increase the response rate beyond that obtained with single-agent nelarabine in children with first relapse of T-ALL and T-LBL [106, 107].

15.9.2 Antibody-Based Therapies

Chimeric or purely genetically engineered monoclonal antibodies (mAB) attach themselves to a specific tumour surface antigen, which leads to the activation of natural killer cells and macrophages. After activation, they release cytotoxic granules to kill the tumour cells in a process called antibody-mediated cellular cytotoxicity. mABs have the advantage of being tumour-specific instead of patient-specific and can therefore be produced industrially, stored easily and used immediately without waiting times. Although most trials have focused on r/r ALL, recent trials have started enrolling both types of lymphoblastic disorders by including a separate treatment arm for r/r LBL [106].

Unconjugated mAB currently under investigation in the therapy of r/r paediatric T-ALL and T-LBL include daratumumab and isatuximab, which are directed against CD38 [108, 109]; study results are still pending. Conjugated mABs that are currently increasingly used in r/r B-lymphoblastic disorders include inotuzumab ozogamicin. Inotuzumab ozogamicin is an mAB directed against CD22 and to which the spindle poison calicheamicin is bound. The very high remission induction rates described to date in r/r B-ALL, in conjunction with a very high proportion of MRD responders, are so promising that inotuzumab ozogamicin will be randomly tested against conventional polychemotherapy in re-induction therapy of first standard- and high-risk B-ALL relapse [110, 111]. Bispecific T-cell engagers (BiTEs) consist of two single-chain variable fragments connected by a flexible linker. They activate T cells because one side binds to the CD3 receptor of the T lymphocytes and the other side to the tumour antigen, resulting in T-cell-mediated cytolysis of the tumour cells. Blinatumomab, a CD19/CD3 BiTE, is approved for the treatment of children with r/r B-ALL [112, 113]. Blinatumomab seems to be particularly effective in the MRD setting and therefore appears to have its place in the consolidation elements [104, 114, 115]. In a recent randomized study of first high-risk ALL relapse, survival rates, molecular remission rates, and the toxicity profile were significantly more advantageous in the blinatumomab group as compared to the standard chemotherapy group, so that blinatumomab as a bridge to allo-HSCT is considered the new standard of care for first high-risk B-ALL relapse right before allo-HSCT [116]. An analogous role in r/r B-LBL could be envisioned for both blinatumomab and inotuzumab ozogamicin.

15.9.3 Allogeneic Stem Cell Transplantation and Adoptive Cell Therapies

The immunotherapeutic efficacy of allo-HSCT in the treatment of ALL and r/r LBL has been demonstrated [100, 117, 118]. The prerequisite for this procedure, however, is the achievement of a complete remission before. It is international consensus that all r/r T-LBL cases and very early and early relapsed B-LBL cases should undergo allo-HSCT in second complete remission [100]. According to the results of the FORUM (For Omitting Radiation Under Majority Age) trial in childhood ALL the conditioning regimen should be based on total body irradiation and etoposide [117].

The concept of combining MHC-independent antigen recognition of mAB and effector function of T cells led to the development and clinical validation of chimeric antigen receptor (CAR) T cells. The advantages of CAR T cells over mAB are manifold and are mainly based on the ability of CAR T cells to eliminate tumour cells directly, on proliferation upon activation, and on a better penetration into, i.e. the CNS. In addition, CAR T cells may provide permanent protection against the recurrence of leukemia and lymphoma, i.e. they are curative and, unlike allo-HSCT, do not require prior complete remission. Results obtained in patients with lymphoproliferative B-cell diseases (i.e. ELIANA study) with CD19-

targeting CAR T cells led to approval of tisagenlecleucel by the Food and Drug Administration and, subsequently, by the European Medicines Agency [119]. Both approved therapy with tisagenlecleucel for children and young adults (up to 25 years of age) with B-ALL in ≥2. relapse, in refractory disease or in relapse after allo-HSCT.

Although the prognosis of primary T-LBL and B-LBL is very good, salvage rates of r/r diseases are particularly unfavourable, since in many cases the remission needed for the curative use of a consolidating allo-HSCT is not achieved [60, 100]. The major obstacle to the development of effective CAR T cells for T-lymphoblastic diseases is that the surface marker profile of malignant T cells overlaps with that of activated T lymphocytes. The promising "Anti-CD7 Protein Expression Blocker (PEBL) CAR T-Cell Therapy for Relapsed and Refractory T-Lineage Acute Lymphoblastic Leukaemia (CARTALL)" study (NCT05043571) in Singapore is testing the safety and efficacy of a CAR T-cell construct targeting the surface marker CD7, which is highly expressed in almost all cases of T-ALL (and T-LBL), including ETP-ALL. In order to prevent a "fratricide effect" of the T cells, the CD7 expression of the CAR T cells is effectively downregulated with the expression of an anti-CD7-PEBL (anti-CD7-PEBL-CAR T cells) The study allows for the inclusion of patients, 6 months to 65 years old, with r/r T-ALL and could be a major breakthrough in the highly anticipated CAR T-cell therapy of T-lymphoblastic diseases and used as bridge to allo-HSCT.

15.10 Conclusion

Despite the high cure rates of nearly 80–85% in children and adolescents with LBL, delineation of biology-driven stratification factors and further improvement in survival and reduction of the still considerable treatment-related toxicity, especially for patients with advanced stages of the disease, are important goals of future studies.

References

1. Burkhardt B, Hermiston ML. Lymphoblastic lymphoma in children and adolescents: review of current challenges and future opportunities. Br J Haematol. 2019;185(6):1158–70.
2. Schmidt E, Burkhardt B. Lymphoblastic lymphoma in childhood and adolescence. Pediatr Hematol Oncol. 2013;30(6):484–508.
3. Borowitz MJC, JK C, Downing JR, Le Beau MM, Arber DA. Precursor Lymphoid Neoplasms. In: Swerdlow SHC E, Harris NL, Jaffe ES, Plieri SA, Stein H, Thiele J, editors. WHO classification of tumours of haematopoietic and lymphoid tissue. Lyon: International Agency for Research on Cancer (IARC); 2017. p. 200–13.
4. Burkhardt B. Paediatric lymphoblastic T-cell leukaemia and lymphoma: one or two diseases? Br J Haematol. 2010;149(5):653–68.
5. Kroeze E, Arias Padilla L, Bakker M, Boer JM, Hagleitner MM, Burkhardt B, et al. Pediatric precursor B-cell lymphoblastic malignancies: from Extramedullary to medullary involvement. Cancers (Basel). 2022;14(16)
6. Uyttebroeck A, Vanhentenrijk V, Hagemeijer A, Boeckx N, Renard M, Wlodarska I, et al. Is there a difference in childhood T-cell acute lymphoblastic leukaemia and T-cell lymphoblastic lymphoma? LeukLymphoma. 2007;48(9):1745–54.
7. Landmann E, Burkhardt B, Zimmermann M, Meyer U, Woessmann W, Klapper W, et al. Results and conclusions of the European intergroup EURO-LB02 trial in children and adolescents with lymphoblastic lymphoma. Haematologica. 2017;102(12):2086–96.
8. Termuhlen AM, Smith LM, Perkins SL, Lones M, Finlay JL, Weinstein H, et al. Disseminated lymphoblastic lymphoma in children and adolescents: results of the COG A5971 trial: a report from the Children's oncology group. Br J Haematol. 2013;162(6):792–801.
9. Burkhardt B, Zimmermann M, Oschlies I, Niggli F, Mann G, Parwaresch R, et al. The impact of age and gender on biology, clinical features and treatment outcome of non-Hodgkin lymphoma in childhood and adolescence. Br J Haematol. 2005;131(1):39–49.
10. Béné MC, Nebe T, Bettelheim P, Buldini B, Bumbea H, Kern W, et al. Immunophenotyping of acute leukemia and lymphoproliferative disorders: a consensus proposal of the European LeukemiaNet work package 10. Leukemia. 2011;25(4):567–74.
11. Oschlies I, Burkhardt B, Chassagne-Clement C, d'Amore ES, Hansson U, Hebeda K, et al. Diagnosis and immunophenotype of 188 pediatric lymphoblastic lymphomas treated within a randomized prospective trial: experiences and preliminary recommendations from the European childhood lymphoma pathology panel. Am J Surg Pathol. 2011;35(6):836–44.

12. Matutes E, Pickl WF, Van't Veer M, Morilla R, Swansbury J, Strobl H, et al. Mixed-phenotype acute leukemia: clinical and laboratory features and outcome in 100 patients defined according to the WHO 2008 classification. Blood. 2011;117(11):3163–71.
13. Alaggio R, Amador C, Anagnostopoulos I, Attygalle AD, Araujo IBO, Berti E, et al. The 5th edition of the World Health Organization classification of Haematolymphoid Tumours: lymphoid neoplasms. Leukemia. 2022;36(7):1720–48.
14. Attarbaschi A, Carraro E, Abla O, Barzilai-Birenboim S, Bomken S, Brugieres L, et al. Non-Hodgkin lymphoma and pre-existing conditions: spectrum, clinical characteristics and outcome in 213 children and adolescents. Haematologica. 2016;101(12):1581–91.
15. Bienemann K, Burkhardt B, Modlich S, Meyer U, Moricke A, Bienemann K, et al. Promising therapy results for lymphoid malignancies in children with chromosomal breakage syndromes (ataxia teleangiectasia or Nijmegen-breakage syndrome): a retrospective survey. Br J Haematol. 2011;155(4): 468–76.
16. Bomken S, van der Werff Ten Bosch J, Attarbaschi A, Bacon CM, Borkhardt A, Boztug K, et al. Current understanding and future research priorities in malignancy associated with inborn errors of immunity and DNA repair disorders: the perspective of an interdisciplinary working group. Front Immunol. 2018;9:2912.
17. Pastorczak A, Attarbaschi A, Bomken S, Borkhardt A, van der Werff Ten Bosch J, Elitzur S, et al. Consensus recommendations for the clinical Management of Hematological Malignancies in patients with DNA double stranded break disorders. Cancers (Basel). 2022;14(8)
18. Bennett JM, Catovsky D, Daniel MT, Flandrin G, Galton DA, Gralnick HR, et al. Proposals for the classification of the acute leukaemias. French-American-British (FAB) co-operative group. Br J Haematol. 1976;33(4):451–8.
19. Mann G, Attarbaschi A, Steiner M, Simonitsch I, Strobl H, Urban C, et al. Early and reliable diagnosis of non-Hodgkin lymphoma in childhood and adolescence: contribution of cytomorphology and flow cytometric immunophenotyping. Pediatr Hematol Oncol. 2006;23(3):167–76.
20. van der Does-van den Berg A, Bartram CR, Basso G, Benoit YC, Biondi A, Debatin KM, et al. Minimal requirements for the diagnosis, classification, and evaluation of the treatment of childhood acute lymphoblastic leukemia (ALL) in the "BFM family" cooperative group. Med Pediatr Oncol. 1992;20(6):497–505.
21. Bene MC, Castoldi G, Knapp W, Ludwig WD, Matutes E, Orfao A, et al. Proposals for the immunological classification of acute leukemias. European Group for the Immunological Characterization of Leukemias (EGIL). Leukemia. 1995;9(10):1783–6.
22. Coustan-Smith E, Mullighan CG, Onciu M, Behm FG, Raimondi SC, Pei D, et al. Early T-cell precursor leukaemia: a subtype of very high-risk acute lymphoblastic leukaemia. Lancet Oncol. 2009;10(2):147–56.
23. Dworzak MN, Buldini B, Gaipa G, Ratei R, Hrusak O, Luria D, et al. AIEOP-BFM consensus guidelines 2016 for flow cytometric immunophenotyping of pediatric acute lymphoblastic leukemia. Cytometry B Clin Cytom. 2018;94(1):82–93.
24. Zhang J, Ding L, Holmfeldt L, Wu G, Heatley SL, Payne-Turner D, et al. The genetic basis of early T-cell precursor acute lymphoblastic leukaemia. Nature. 2012;481(7380):157–63.
25. Haydu JE, Ferrando AA. Early T-cell precursor acute lymphoblastic leukaemia. Curr Opin Hematol. 2013;20(4):369–73.
26. Pui CH, Carroll WL, Meshinchi S, Arceci RJ. Biology, risk stratification, and therapy of pediatric acute leukemias: an update. J Clin Oncol. 2011;29(5):551–65.
27. Brady SW, Roberts KG, Gu Z, Shi L, Pounds S, Pei D, et al. The genomic landscape of pediatric acute lymphoblastic leukemia. Nat Genet. 2022;54(9):1376–89.
28. Burkhardt B, Mueller S, Khanam T, Perkins SL. Current status and future directions of T-lymphoblastic lymphoma in children and adolescents. Br J Haematol. 2016;173(4):545–59.
29. Boddu P, Yin CC, Kanagal-Shamanna R, Tang G, Thakral B, Kadia T, et al. An unsuspected finding of t(9;22): a rare case of Philadelphia chromosome-positive B-lymphoblastic lymphoma. Case Rep Hematol. 2017;2017:2413587.
30. Mann G, Attarbaschi A, Burkhardt B, Niggli F, Klapper W, Ludwig WD, et al. Clinical characteristics and treatment outcome of infants with non-Hodgkin lymphoma. Br J Haematol. 2007;139(3):443–9.
31. Shirai R, Osumi T, Sato-Otsubo A, Nakabayashi K, Mori T, Yoshida M, et al. Genetic features of B-cell lymphoblastic lymphoma with TCF3-PBX1. Cancer Rep (Hoboken). 2022;5(9):e1559.
32. Ahlmann M, Meyer C, Marschalek R, Burkhardt B, Koehler G, Klapper W, et al. Complex MLL rearrangement in non-infiltrated bone marrow in an infant with stage II precursor B-lymphoblastic lymphoma. Eur J Haematol. 2014;93(4):349–53.
33. Insuasti-Beltran G, Butros L, Foucar K. Concurrent t(4;11) and t(1:19) in a pediatric patient with B-lymphoblastic leukemia/lymphoma (B-ALL): a case report and review of the literature. J Assoc Genet Technol. 2013;39(4):195–7.
34. Lones MA, Heerema NA, Le Beau MM, Sposto R, Perkins SL, Kadin ME, et al. Chromosome abnormalities in advanced stage lymphoblastic lymphoma of children and adolescents: a report from CCG-E08. Cancer GenetCytogenet. 2007;172(1):1–11.
35. Meyer JA, Zhou D, Mason CC, Downie JM, Rodic V, Abromowitch M, et al. Genomic characterization of pediatric B-lymphoblastic lymphoma and

B-lymphoblastic leukemia using formalin-fixed tissues. Pediatr Blood Cancer. 2017;64(7):e26363.
36. Bonn BR, Rohde M, Zimmermann M, Krieger D, Oschlies I, Niggli F, et al. Incidence and prognostic relevance of genetic variations in T-cell lymphoblastic lymphoma in childhood and adolescence. Blood. 2013;121(16):3153–60.
37. Basso K, Mussolin L, Lettieri A, Brahmachary M, Lim WK, Califano A, et al. T-cell lymphoblastic lymphoma shows differences and similarities with T-cell acute lymphoblastic leukemia by genomic and gene expression analyses. Genes Chromosomes Cancer. 2011;50(12):1063–75.
38. Park MJ, Taki T, Oda M, Watanabe T, Yumura-Yagi K, Kobayashi R, et al. FBXW7 and NOTCH1 mutations in childhood T cell acute lymphoblastic leukaemia and T cell non-Hodgkin lymphoma. Br J Haematol. 2009;145(2):198–206.
39. Baleydier F, Decouvelaere AV, Bergeron J, Gaulard P, Canioni D, Bertrand Y, et al. T cell receptor genotyping and HOXA/TLX1 expression define three T lymphoblastic lymphoma subsets which might affect clinical outcome. ClinCancer Res. 2008;14(3):692–700.
40. Callens C, Baleydier F, Lengline E, Ben Abdelali R, Petit A, Villarese P, et al. Clinical impact of NOTCH1 and/or FBXW7 mutations, FLASH deletion, and TCR status in pediatric T-cell lymphoblastic lymphoma. J Clin Oncol. 2012;30(16): 1966–73.
41. Balbach ST, Makarova O, Bonn BR, Zimmermann M, Rohde M, Oschlies I, et al. Proposal of a genetic classifier for risk group stratification in pediatric T-cell lymphoblastic lymphoma reveals differences from adult T-cell lymphoblastic leukemia. Leukemia. 2016;30(4):970–3.
42. Burkhardt B, Bruch J, Zimmermann M, Strauch K, Parwaresch R, Ludwig WD, et al. Loss of heterozygosity on chromosome 6q14-q24 is associated with poor outcome in children and adolescents with T-cell lymphoblastic lymphoma. Leukemia. 2006;20(8):1422–9.
43. Khanam T, Sandmann S, Seggewiss J, Ruether C, Zimmermann M, Norvil AB, et al. Integrative genomic analysis of pediatric T-cell lymphoblastic lymphoma reveals candidates of clinical significance. Blood. 2021;137(17):2347–59.
44. Gutierrez A, Dahlberg SE, Neuberg DS, Zhang J, Grebliunaite R, Sanda T, et al. Absence of biallelic TCRgamma deletion predicts early treatment failure in pediatric T-cell acute lymphoblastic leukemia. J Clin Oncol. 2010;28(24):3816–23.
45. Bandapalli OR, Zimmermann M, Kox C, Stanulla M, Schrappe M, Ludwig WD, et al. NOTCH1 activation clinically antagonizes the unfavorable effect of PTEN inactivation in BFM-treated children with precursor T-cell acute lymphoblastic leukemia. Haematologica. 2013;98(6):928–36.
46. Pomari E, Lovisa F, Carraro E, Primerano S, D'Amore ESG, Bonvini P, et al. Clinical impact of miR-223 expression in pediatric T-cell lymphoblastic lymphoma. Oncotarget. 2017;8(64):107886–98.
47. Minard-Colin V, Brugières L, Reiter A, Cairo MS, Gross TG, Woessmann W, et al. Non-Hodgkin lymphoma in children and adolescents: Progress through effective collaboration, current knowledge, and challenges ahead. J Clin Oncol. 2015;33(27):2963–74.
48. Neth O, Seidemann K, Jansen P, Mann G, Tiemann M, Ludwig WD, et al. Precursor B-cell lymphoblastic lymphoma in childhood and adolescence: clinical features, treatment, and results in trials NHL-BFM 86 and 90. MedPediatrOncol. 2000;35(1):20–7.
49. Geethakumari PR, Hoffmann MS, Pemmaraju N, Hu S, Jorgensen JL, O'Brien S, et al. Extramedullary B lymphoblastic leukemia/lymphoma (B-ALL/B-LBL): a diagnostic challenge. Clin Lymphoma Myeloma Leuk. 2014;14(4):e115–8.
50. Maitra A, McKenna RW, Weinberg AG, Schneider NR, Kroft SH. Precursor B-cell lymphoblastic lymphoma. A study of nine cases lacking blood and bone marrow involvement and review of the literature. Am J Clin Pathol. 2001;115(6):868–75.
51. Coiffier B, Altman A, Pui CH, Younes A, Cairo MS. Guidelines for the management of pediatric and adult tumor lysis syndrome: an evidence-based review. J Clin Oncol. 2008;26(16):2767–78.
52. Coustan-Smith E, Sandlund JT, Perkins SL, Chen H, Chang M, Abromowitch M, et al. Minimal disseminated disease in childhood T-cell lymphoblastic lymphoma: a report from the children's oncology group. J Clin Oncol. 2009;27(21):3533–9.
53. Mussolin L, Buldini B, Lovisa F, Carraro E, Disaro S, Nigro LL, et al. Detection and role of minimal disseminated disease in children with lymphoblastic lymphoma: the AIEOP experience. Pediatr Blood Cancer. 2015;62(11):1906–13.
54. Trinquand A, Plesa A, Abdo C, Subtil F, Aladjidi N, Rigaud C, et al. Toward pediatric T lymphoblastic lymphoma stratification based on minimal disseminated disease and. Hema. 2021;5(10):e641.
55. Murphy SB. Classification, staging and end results of treatment of childhood non-Hodgkin's lymphomas: dissimilarities from lymphomas in adults. SeminOncol. 1980;7(3):332–9.
56. Rosolen A, Perkins SL, Pinkerton CR, Guillerman RP, Sandlund JT, Patte C, et al. Revised international pediatric non-Hodgkin lymphoma staging system. J Clin Oncol. 2015;33(18):2112–8.
57. Wollner N, Burchenal JH, Lieberman PH, Exelby P, D'Angio G, Murphy ML. Non-Hodgkin's lymphoma in children. A comparative study of two modalities of therapy. Cancer. 1976;37(1):123–34.
58. Anderson JR, Wilson JF, Jenkin DT, Meadows AT, Kersey J, Chilcote RR, et al. Childhood non-Hodgkin's lymphoma. The results of a randomized therapeutic trial comparing a 4-drug regimen (COMP) with a 10-drug regimen (LSA2-L2). N Engl J Med. 1983;308(10):559–65.
59. Teachey DT, O'Connor D. How I treat newly diagnosed T-cell acute lymphoblastic leukemia and

T-cell lymphoblastic lymphoma in children. Blood. 2020;135(3):159–66.
60. Burkhardt B, Reiter A, Landmann E, Lang P, Lassay L, Dickerhoff R, et al. Poor outcome for children and adolescents with progressive disease or relapse of lymphoblastic lymphoma: a report from the berlin-Frankfurt-muenster group. J Clin Oncol. 2009;27(20):3363–9.
61. Burkhardt B, Oschlies I, Klapper W, Zimmermann M, Woessmann W, Meinhardt A, et al. Non-Hodgkin's lymphoma in adolescents: experiences in 378 adolescent NHL patients treated according to pediatric NHL-BFM protocols. Leukemia. 2011;25(1):153–60.
62. Reiter A, Schrappe M, Ludwig WD, Tiemann M, Parwaresch R, Zimmermann M, et al. Intensive ALL-type therapy without local radiotherapy provides a 90% event-free survival for children with T-cell lymphoblastic lymphoma: a BFM group report. Blood. 2000;95(2):416–21.
63. Shepherd SF, A'Hern RP, Pinkerton CR. Childhood T-cell lymphoblastic lymphoma--does early resolution of mediastinal mass predict for final outcome? The United Kingdom Children's Cancer Study Group (UKCCSG). Br J Cancer 1995;72(3):752–756.
64. Uyttebroeck A, Suciu S, Laureys G, Robert A, Pacquement H, Ferster A, et al. Treatment of childhood T-cell lymphoblastic lymphoma according to the strategy for acute lymphoblastic leukaemia, without radiotherapy: long term results of the EORTC CLG 58881 trial. EurJCancer. 2008;44(6):840–6.
65. Kobayashi R, Takimoto T, Nakazawa A, Fujita N, Akazai A, Yamato K, et al. Inferior outcomes of stage III T lymphoblastic lymphoma relative to stage IV lymphoma and T-acute lymphoblastic leukemia: long-term comparison of outcomes in the JACLS NHL T-98 and ALL T-97 protocols. Int J Hematol. 2014;99(6):743–9.
66. Maurer-Granofszky M, Schumich A, Buldini B, Gaipa G, Kappelmayer J, Mejstrikova E, et al. An extensive quality control and quality assurance (QC/QA) Program significantly improves inter-laboratory concordance rates of flow-Cytometric minimal residual disease assessment in acute lymphoblastic leukemia: an I-BFM-FLOW-network report. Cancers (Basel). 2021;13(23).
67. van der Velden VH, Panzer-Grumayer ER, Cazzaniga G, Flohr T, Sutton R, Schrauder A, et al. Optimization of PCR-based minimal residual disease diagnostics for childhood acute lymphoblastic leukemia in a multi-center setting. Leukemia. 2007;21(4):706–13.
68. Mussolin L, Damm-Welk C, Pillon M, Woessmann W. Minimal disease monitoring in pediatric non-Hodgkin's lymphoma: current clinical application and future challenges. Cancers (Basel). 2021;13(8)
69. Stark B, Avigad S, Luria D, Manor S, Reshef-Ronen T, Avrahami G, et al. Bone marrow minimal disseminated disease (MDD) and minimal residual disease (MRD) in childhood T-cell lymphoblastic lymphoma stage III, detected by flow cytometry (FC) and real-time quantitative polymerase chain reaction (RQ-PCR). Pediatr Blood Cancer. 2009;52(1):20–5.
70. Burkhardt B, Woessmann W, Zimmermann M, Kontny U, Vormoor J, Doerffel W, et al. Impact of cranial radiotherapy on central nervous system prophylaxis in children and adolescents with central nervous system-negative stage III or IV lymphoblastic lymphoma. J ClinOncol. 2006;24(3):491–9.
71. Nakatani K, Nakamoto Y, Watanabe K, Saga T, Higashi T, Togashi K. Roles and limitations of FDG PET in pediatric non-Hodgkin lymphoma. Clin Nucl Med. 2012;37(7):656–62.
72. Sioka C. The utility of FDG PET in diagnosis and follow-up of lymphoma in childhood. Eur J Pediatr. 2013;172(6):733–8.
73. Bardi E, Csoka M, Garai I, Szegedi I, Muller J, Gyorke T, et al. Value of FDG-PET/CT examinations in different cancers of children, focusing on lymphomas. Pathol Oncol Res POR. 2014;20(1):139–43.
74. Sandlund JT, Guillerman RP, Perkins SL, Pinkerton CR, Rosolen A, Patte C, et al. International pediatric non-Hodgkin lymphoma response criteria. J Clin Oncol. 2015;33(18):2106–11.
75. Anderson JR, Jenkin RD, Wilson JF, Kjeldsberg CR, Sposto R, Chilcote RR, et al. Long-term follow-up of patients treated with COMP or LSA2L2 therapy for childhood non-Hodgkin's lymphoma: a report of CCG-551 from the Childrens cancer group. J Clin Oncol. 1993;11(6):1024–32.
76. Muller-Weihrich S, Beck J, Henze G, Jobke A, Kornhuber B, Lampert F, et al. BFM study 1981/83 of the treatment of highly malignant non-Hodgkin's lymphoma in children: results of therapy stratified according to histologic immunological type and clinical stage. Klin Padiatr. 1984;196(3):135–42.
77. Reiter A, Schrappe M, Parwaresch R, Henze G, Muller-Weihrich S, Sauter S, et al. Non-Hodgkin's lymphomas of childhood and adolescence: results of a treatment stratified for biologic subtypes and stage--a report of the Berlin-Frankfurt-Munster Group. JClinOncol. 1995;13(2):359–72.
78. Patte C, Kalifa C, Flamant F, Hartmann O, Brugieres L, Valteau-Couanet D, et al. Results of the LMT81 protocol, a modified LSA2L2 protocol with high dose methotrexate, on 84 children with non-B-cell (lymphoblastic) lymphoma. MedPediatrOncol. 1992;20(2):105–13.
79. Pillon M, Arico M, Mussolin L, Carraro E, Conter V, Sala A, et al. Long-term results of the AIEOP LNH-97 protocol for childhood lymphoblastic lymphoma. Pediatr Blood Cancer. 2015;62(8):1388–94.
80. Pillon M, Piglione M, Garaventa A, Conter V, Giuliano M, Arcamone G, et al. Long-term results of AIEOP LNH-92 protocol for the treatment of pediatric lymphoblastic lymphoma: a report of the Italian Association of Pediatric Hematology and Oncology. Pediatr Blood Cancer. 2009;53(6):953–9.
81. Uyttebroeck A, Suciu S, Plat G, Laureys G, Costa V, Rohrlich P, et al. Dexamethasone (DEX) versus

prednisone (PRED) in T-cell non Hodgkin lymphoma (T-NHL): results of the randomized phase III trial 58951 of the EORTC children leukemia group. Br J Haematol. 2012;159(Suppl. 1):37.
82. Asselin BL, Devidas M, Wang C, Pullen J, Borowitz MJ, Hutchison R, et al. Effectiveness of high-dose methotrexate in T-cell lymphoblastic leukemia and advanced-stage lymphoblastic lymphoma: a randomized study by the Children's oncology group (POG 9404). Blood. 2011;118(4):874–83.
83. Bergeron C, Coze C, Segura C, Pacquement H, Gandemer V, Ducassou S, et al. Treatment of childhood T-cell lymphoblastic lymphoma-long-term results of the SFOP LMT96 trial. Pediatr Blood Cancer. 2015;62(12):2150–6.
84. Sandlund JT, Pui CH, Zhou Y, Behm FG, Onciu M, Razzouk BI, et al. Effective treatment of advanced-stage childhood lymphoblastic lymphoma without prophylactic cranial irradiation: results of St Jude NHL13 study. Leukemia. 2009;23(6):1127–30.
85. Abromowitch M, Sposto R, Perkins S, Zwick D, Siegel S, Finlay J, et al. Shortened intensified multi-agent chemotherapy and non-cross resistant maintenance therapy for advanced lymphoblastic lymphoma in children and adolescents: report from the Children's oncology group. Br J Haematol. 2008;143(2):261–7.
86. Sekimizu M, Fujimoto J, Takimoto T, Tsurusawa M, Horibe K, Sunami S. Phase II Clinical Trial for Newly Diagnosed Children and Adolescents with Localized Lymphoblastic Lymphoma (Japanese Leukemia/Lymphoma Study Group Trial LLB-NHL03) : Study Protocol for Nationwide Multicenter Trial. Acta Med Okayama. 2018;72(4):427–30.
87. Sunami S, Sekimizu M, Takimoto T, Mori T, Mitsui T, Fukano R, et al. Prognostic impact of intensified maintenance therapy on children with advanced lymphoblastic lymphoma: a report from the Japanese pediatric leukemia/lymphoma study group ALB-NHL03 study. Pediatr Blood Cancer. 2015;63:451.
88. Hayashi RJ, Winter SS, Dunsmore KP, Devidas M, Chen Z, Wood BL, et al. Successful outcomes of newly diagnosed T lymphoblastic lymphoma: results from Children's oncology group AALL0434. J Clin Oncol. 2020;38(26):3062–70.
89. Tubergen DG, Krailo MD, Meadows AT, Rosenstock J, Kadin M, Morse M, et al. Comparison of treatment regimens for pediatric lymphoblastic non-Hodgkin's lymphoma: a Childrens cancer group study. J Clin Oncol. 1995;13(6):1368–76.
90. Lymphoma Study Group SGoHtSoPCMA. Lymphoma study Group Committee of Pediatrics Chinese Anti-Cancer A [A collaborative study of children with lymphoblastic non-Hodgkin's lymphoma in China]. Zhonghua Er Ke Za Zhi. 2015;53(12):931–7.
91. Gao YJ, Pan C, Tang JY, Lu FJ, Chen J, Xue HL, et al. Clinical outcome of childhood lymphoblastic lymphoma in Shanghai China 2001-2010. Pediatr Blood Cancer. 2014;61(4):659–63.
92. Sun XF, Xia ZJ, Zhen ZJ, Xiang XJ, Xia Y, Ling JY, et al. Intensive chemotherapy improved treatment outcome for Chinese children and adolescents with lymphoblastic lymphoma. Int J Clin Oncol. 2008;13(5):436–41.
93. Sterba J, Kovacs G, Matus M, Bubanska E, Kyr M, Krenova Z, et al. Capizzi methotrexate with BFM backbone without craniospinal irradiation is effective treatment for pediatric lymphoblastic lymphoma: results from 5 countries with I-BFM LL 09 protocol. Br J Haematol. 2015;171(Suppl.1):33.
94. Cohen MH, Johnson JR, Justice R, Pazdur R. FDA drug approval summary: nelarabine (Arranon) for the treatment of T-cell lymphoblastic leukemia/lymphoma. Oncologist. 2008;13(6):709–14.
95. Dunsmore KP, Winter SS, Devidas M, Wood BL, Esiashvili N, Eisenberg N, Briegel N, Hayashi RJ, Gastier-Foster JM, Carroll AJ, Heerema N, Asselin B, Rabin KR, Zweidler-McKay P, Raetz RA, Loh ML, Winick NJ, Carroll WL, Hunger S. COG AALL0434: a randomized trial testing nelarabine in newly diagnosed t-cell malignancy. J Clin Oncol. 2018:10500.
96. Teachey DT, Devidas M, Wood BL, Chen Z, Hayashi RJ, Hermiston ML, et al. Children's oncology group trial AALL1231: a phase III clinical trial testing Bortezomib in newly diagnosed T-cell acute lymphoblastic leukemia and lymphoma. J Clin Oncol. 2022;40(19):2106–18.
97. Termuhlen AM, Smith LM, Perkins SL, Lones M, Finlay JL, Weinstein H, et al. Outcome of newly diagnosed children and adolescents with localized lymphoblastic lymphoma treated on Children's oncology group trial A5971: a report from the Children's oncology group. Pediatr Blood Cancer. 2012;59(7):1229–33.
98. Ducassou S, Ferlay C, Bergeron C, Girard S, Laureys G, Pacquement H, et al. Clinical presentation, evolution, and prognosis of precursor B-cell lymphoblastic lymphoma in trials LMT96, EORTC 58881, and EORTC 58951. Br J Haematol. 2011;152(4):441–51.
99. Mitsui T, Mori T, Fujita N, Inada H, Horibe K, Tsurusawa M. Retrospective analysis of relapsed or primary refractory childhood lymphoblastic lymphoma in Japan. Pediatr Blood Cancer. 2009;52:591.
100. Burkhardt B, Taj M, Garnier N, Minard-Colin V, Hazar V, Mellgren K, et al. Treatment and outcome analysis of 639 relapsed non-Hodgkin lymphomas in children and adolescents and resulting treatment recommendations. Cancers (Basel). 2021;13(9)
101. De Smedt R, Peirs S, Morscio J, Matthijssens F, Roels J, Reunes L, et al. Preclinical evaluation of second generation PIM inhibitors for the treatment of T-cell acute lymphoblastic leukemia and lymphoma. Haematologica. 2018;104:e17.
102. Delgado-Martin C, Meyer LK, Huang BJ, Shimano KA, Zinter MS, Nguyen JV, et al. JAK/STAT pathway inhibition overcomes IL7-induced glucocorticoid resistance in a subset of human T-cell acute lymphoblastic leukemias. Leukemia. 2017;31(12):2568–76.

103. Raetz EA, Teachey DT. T-cell acute lymphoblastic leukemia. Hematology Am Soc Hematol Educ Program. 2016;2016(1):580–8.
104. Brivio E, Baruchel A, Beishuizen A, Bourquin JP, Brown PA, Cooper T, et al. Targeted inhibitors and antibody immunotherapies: novel therapies for paediatric leukaemia and lymphoma. Eur J Cancer. 2022;164:1–17.
105. Bogaerts J, Sydes MR, Keat N, McConnell A, Benson A, Ho A, et al. Clinical trial designs for rare diseases: studies developed and discussed by the international rare cancers initiative. Eur J Cancer. 2015;51(3):271–81.
106. Whitlock JA, Malvar J, Dalla-Pozza L, Goldberg JM, Silverman LB, Ziegler DS, et al. Nelarabine, etoposide, and cyclophosphamide in relapsed pediatric T-acute lymphoblastic leukemia and T-lymphoblastic lymphoma (study T2008-002 NECTAR). Pediatr Blood Cancer. 2022;69(11):e29901.
107. Zwaan CM, Kowalczyk J, Schmitt C, Bielorai B, Russo MW, Woessner M, et al. Safety and efficacy of nelarabine in children and young adults with relapsed or refractory T-lineage acute lymphoblastic leukaemia or T-lineage lymphoblastic lymphoma: results of a phase 4 study. Br J Haematol. 2017;179(2):284–93.
108. Bride KL, Vincent TL, Im SY, Aplenc R, Barrett DM, Carroll WL, et al. Preclinical efficacy of daratumumab in T-cell acute lymphoblastic leukemia. Blood 2018;131(9):995–9.
109. Boissel N, Chevallier P, Doronin V, Griskevicius L, Maschan A, McCloskey J, et al. Isatuximab monotherapy in patients with refractory T-acute lymphoblastic leukemia or T-lymphoblastic lymphoma: phase 2 study. Cancer Med. 2022;11(5):1292–8.
110. Brivio E, Locatelli F, Lopez-Yurda M, Malone A, Diaz-de-Heredia C, Bielorai B, et al. A phase 1 study of inotuzumab ozogamicin in pediatric relapsed/refractory acute lymphoblastic leukemia (ITCC-059 study). Blood. 2021;137(12):1582–90.
111. Pennesi E, Michels N, Brivio E, van der Velden VHJ, Jiang Y, Thano A, et al. Inotuzumab ozogamicin as single agent in pediatric patients with relapsed and refractory acute lymphoblastic leukemia: results from a phase II trial. Leukemia. 2022;36(6):1516–24.
112. von Stackelberg A, Locatelli F, Zugmaier G, Handgretinger R, Trippett TM, Rizzari C, et al. Phase I/phase II study of Blinatumomab in pediatric patients with relapsed/refractory acute lymphoblastic leukemia. J Clin Oncol. 2016;34(36):4381–9.
113. Gore L, Locatelli F, Zugmaier G, Handgretinger R, O'Brien MM, Bader P, et al. Survival after blinatumomab treatment in pediatric patients with relapsed/refractory B-cell precursor acute lymphoblastic leukemia. Blood Cancer J. 2018;8(9):80.
114. Locatelli F, Eckert C, Hrusak O, Buldini B, Sartor M, Zugmaier G, et al. Blinatumomab overcomes poor prognostic impact of measurable residual disease in pediatric high-risk first relapse B-cell precursor acute lymphoblastic leukemia. Pediatr Blood Cancer. 2022;69(8):e29715.
115. Locatelli F, Maschan A, Boissel N, Strocchio L, Alam N, Pezzani I, et al. Pediatric patients with acute lymphoblastic leukemia treated with blinatumomab in a real-world setting: results from the NEUF study. Pediatr Blood Cancer. 2022;69(4):e29562.
116. Locatelli F, Zugmaier G, Rizzari C, Morris JD, Gruhn B, Klingebiel T, et al. Effect of Blinatumomab vs chemotherapy on event-free survival among children with high-risk first-relapse B-cell acute lymphoblastic leukemia: a randomized clinical trial. JAMA. 2021;325(9):843–54.
117. Peters C, Dalle JH, Locatelli F, Poetschger U, Sedlacek P, Buechner J, et al. Total body irradiation or chemotherapy conditioning in childhood ALL: a multinational, randomized, noninferiority phase III study. J Clin Oncol. 2021;39(4):295–307.
118. Gross TG, Hale GA, He W, Camitta BM, Sanders JE, Cairo MS, et al. Hematopoietic stem cell transplantation for refractory or recurrent non-hodgkin lymphoma in children and adolescents. Biol Blood Marrow Transplant. 2009;16(2):223–30.
119. Maude SL, Laetsch TW, Buechner J, Rives S, Boyer M, Bittencourt H, et al. Tisagenlecleucel in children and young adults with B-cell lymphoblastic leukemia. N Engl J Med. 2018;378(5):439–48.

Part VI

Strategies for Patients with Relapse of ALL

16 Biology and Treatment of Relapsed Acute Lymphoblastic Leukemia

Peter M. Hoogerbrugge, Melanie M. Hagleitner, and Arend von Stackelberg

16.1 Introduction

Major progress has been made in the management of relapsed acute lymphoblastic leukemia (ALL) in the last decades. Improved knowledge of the molecular biology of relapsed disease, better stratification based on risk-factors for poor outcome, the implementation of new drugs in relapsed-ALL protocols and the use of novel immunotherapy and cellular therapy provide chances of survival in previously incurable patients as illustrated in Fig. 16.1.

With current contemporary upfront-treatment regimens, approximately 85–90% of children diagnosed with ALL can be cured. The relapse rate of children with ALL on current treatment protocols ranges from 8% to 15% [3, 4]. As survival after relapsed ALL is approximately 50%, children dying from relapsed ALL is still a large proportion of the mortality in childhood cancer. In addition, cure in relapsed ALL so far could only be achieved at high costs in terms of toxicity due to intensive chemotherapy courses, often in combination with irradiation and stem cell transplantation. Newer, potentially more effective and less toxic treatment regimens including cellular immunotherapy with chimeric antigen receptor T-cells (CARTs), immunotherapy using bispecific T-cell engagers and drugs targeted to lymphoblastic cells (inotuzumab, daratumumab) may improve the therapy of children with relapsed ALL in the near future. In the current chapter, we will review the biology of relapsed ALL, current treatment modalities and future prospects of relapsed ALL in children.

P. M. Hoogerbrugge (✉)
Princess Maxima Center for Pediatric Oncology, Utrecht, The Netherlands

Dutch Childhood Oncology Group, Utrecht, The Netherlands
e-mail: p.m.hoogerbrugge@prinsesmaximacentrum.nl

M. M. Hagleitner
Princess Maxima Center for Pediatric Oncology, Utrecht, The Netherlands
e-mail: m.m.hagleitner-2@prinsesmaximacentrum.nl

A. von Stackelberg
Charité Universitätsmedizin, Berlin, Germany
e-mail: arend.stackelberg@charite.de

G. Escherich, V. Conter (eds.), *Acute Lymphoblastic Leukemia in Children and Adolescents*, Pediatric Oncology, https://doi.org/10.1007/978-3-031-71180-0_16

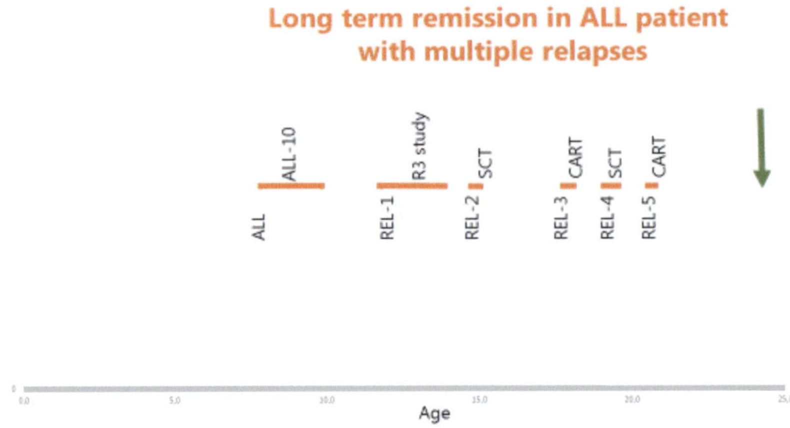

Fig. 16.1 The history of a 25-year-old patient in sixth remission of ALL after five relapses since initial diagnosis at the age of 7 till latest follow-up (green arrow) at age 25. After initial therapy according to the Dutch DCOG-ALL10 protocol [1], she suffered from a late relapse treated according to the international R3-relapse ALL study [2]. For subsequent relapses, she was treated with stem cell transplantation (SCT) preceded by chemotherapy reinduction, experimental CART therapy, second SCT preceded by chemotherapy and commercial CART therapy preceded by inotuzumab (orange lines). At latest follow-up, she was in complete remission with persisting circulating CARTs and B-cell aplasia

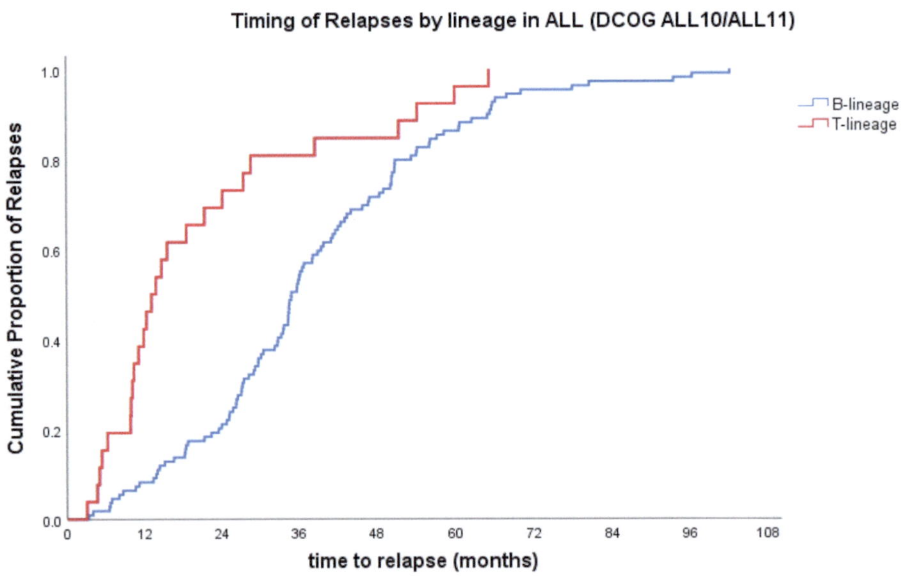

Fig. 16.2 Time of relapse after start of initial therapy in relapsed ALL-patients

16.2 Biology of Relapsed ALL

The far majority of ALL relapses occur during treatment or within the first 2 years after cessation of treatment (Fig. 16.2), although relapses have been reported to occur even after 10 years from diagnosis. In these very late relapses, detailed molecular analysis is needed to discriminate relapsed ALL from a second de novo ALL [5, 6]. The majority of relapses occur in the bone marrow (BM), either in an isolated form or combined with involvement of another site, mainly central nervous system (CNS) or the testes. Isolated CNS or testicular relapse or, much less frequently, relapse involving other extramedullary sites, e.g., bone or uterus, may also occur [7].

It is known for long time, that relapsed ALL is more drug-resistant than ALL at initial diagnosis. For example, Klumper at al [8]. reported that cells from children with relapsed ALL were significantly more resistant to glucocorticoids, L-asparaginase, anthracyclines, and thiopurines, but not to vinca alkaloids, cytarabine, ifosfamide, and epipodophyllotoxins. Particularly, a large difference was observed in glucocorticoid resistance between ALL cells at initial diagnosis and at relapse in this and other [9, 10] studies. In clinical studies, the increased drug resistance of relapsed ALL is reflected by poorer response rates on remission induction treatment as compared to response rate in upfront treatment (Table 16.1).

Although much has been learned, the biology of relapsed ALL and the molecular mechanisms behind the increased drug resistance remain to be elucidated. In their hallmark paper comparing the genomes at initial diagnosis with relapse samples in 61 matched-paired samples using analysis of copy number abnormalities (CNAs), Mullighan et al. [17] reported that in approximately half of the patients clonal evolution occurred from ancestral clones. In approximately one third, clonal evolution was seen from clones that were already present at lower frequency in the leukemic cells at initial diagnosis. In 8% of the patients, no differences were seen in the CNAs between samples at initial diagnosis and relapse. In few patients, the initial and relapse samples were fully discordant, suggesting the presence of a second ALL instead of a relapse. Szczepanski et al. [5] confirmed this latter finding in their study in which 36% of late (more than 30 months after diagnosis) occurring T-ALL "relapses" were actually a second T-ALL rather than a relapse of the original clone.

Table 16.1 Response (morphology and MRD level) of initial ALL, LR/IR, and HR relapsed ALL after modern (re)induction therapy

	Morphology CR	MRD <0.01%	References
Initial ALL	98–99	60–82	[3, 4, 11]
LR/IR relapsed ALL	96–97	40–50	[2, 12]
HR relapsed ALL	55–70	20–30	[2, 12–16]

Genomic studies on relapsed ALL additionally showed that the (minor) clones contributing to the relapse contain genetic alterations that made them more resistant to chemotherapy, including alterations in *NR3C1, NR3C2, TP53, NT5C2, FPGS, CREBBP, MSH2, MSH6, PMS2, WHSC1, PRPS1,* and *PRPS2* [18]. These alterations may already have been present in these clones at diagnosis of the initial leukemia, or may have been acquired during initial treatment [10, 19].

16.3 Historical Perspective of Relapsed ALL

Improvement of treatment for newly diagnosed ALL in the last decades resulted in much better outcome for children with ALL in recent years as compared to decades ago. This means that it is likely that features of relapsed ALL cells after earlier, less intensive, treatment differ from those of patients recently treated with novel treatment regimens. Gaynon et al. reported in 1998 [20] that "patients with late relapses after inferior treatment had a somewhat superior survival," but more recent data are lacking.

Early observations in the 1970s already showed that a second complete remission (CR) could be achieved in 50–80% of children with various remission reinduction strategies consisting of two to four drugs [21–24]. This led to a more systematic approach of four-drug reinduction strategies for relapsed ALL, consisting of prednisone, vincristine, asparaginase, and daunorubicin (or high-dose Cytarabine [24]) and intrathecal therapy. In protocol 8303 of the Pediatric Oncology Group [22], four-drug induction resulted a 82% second remission of high-risk patients relapsing early (within 6 months) after cessation of upfront therapy. This percentage could be increased to 87% by additional therapy with teniposide and cytarabine. Remarkably, also in 83% of very early relapses occurring within 18 months after first complete remission (CR1), a second complete remission (CR2) could be achieved. Similarly, Henze et al. [24] reported 88% CR2 rate in high risk, early relapses occurring within 6 months of cessation of therapy using four-drug induction with cytarabine instead of daunorubicin. Remission induction rate with similar four-drug induction therapy in high-risk relapses in the current era is much lower ranging from 50% to 65% [12, 25]. This confirms that early relapsing patients on modern upfront treatment regimens differ from patients relapsing early on older, less intensive treatment regimens. In contrast, remission-induction rates in low or standard risk relapses, was and is generally above 90–95% [2, 12–14, 16, 25].

Although a second remission could be achieved in a majority of relapsed patients also in the 1980s and 1990s of the previous century, the outcome of relapsed ALL was still dismal. For example, Woods et al. [26] reported more than four decades ago that the outcome of relapsed ALL was less than 3%. They and others [26–30] also reported that survival was better when the patients were treated with allogeneic stem cell transplantation (SCT), which was disputed by others [31–33].

Analysis of the role of SCT in treatment of children with relapsed ALL was difficult as prospective randomized trials on consolidation with or without SCT were lacking. A major problem in comparing the effect of intensive consolidation therapy versus SCT in these days was the selection process for children receiving SCT. For example, children relapsing shortly after reinduction or suffering from major toxicities were excluded for SCT. However, in case control analyses, a tendency toward better survival in children treated with SCT as compared to chemotherapy was reported [34]. With improving the safety of SCT, and the knowledge that the outcome of SCT in children with low or absent minimal residual disease at time of transplant was superior to the outcome in patients with higher disease load at SCT, resulted in better insight in the role of SCT in relapsed ALL, leading in the last decades to the policy to offer transplant to high-risk patients and patients with standard risk relapses that poorly respond to induction (see below).

16.4 Diagnosis of Relapsed ALL

Most current relapsed ALL trials use the site of relapse as one of the stratifying characteristics, with isolated marrow relapse, isolated extramedullary relapse and combined relapse as options. For decades, isolated marrow relapse has been defined as M3 marrow after initial complete remission with no other sites involved. Isolated extramedullary relapse (IEM) has been defined as extramedullary involvement with M1 marrow. Extramedullary mostly is central nervous system (CNS) or testicles. CNS relapse is defined as CNS3 (>5WBC/μL cerebrospinal fluid with identifiable blasts), cranial nerve palsies or cerebral mass. Testicular relapse is defined as testicular enlargement with ALL infiltration confirmed either by biopsy or imaging. Less frequently, biopsy-proven extramedullary relapses occur at other sites, e.g., lymph nodes, skin, bone or female genital organs [7]. Combined relapses historically have been defined as extramedullary relapse with ≥5% blasts in the bone marrow. Recently, a so-called Ponte di Legno consortium consisting of representatives of the larger ALL study groups worldwide, suggested to reformulate the definition of bone marrow relapse to more than 5% if confirmed by one additional sensitive test, e.g., immunophenotyping or PCR-based techniques [35]. If these sensitive tests are not available in case of M2 marrow, a confirmative marrow puncture at least 1 week later confirming the presence of M2 marrow is needed to diagnose a marrow relapse. The consortium suggested to define isolated CNS relapse as CNS 3, or CNS2 confirmed by other positive test ≥1 week later for isolated CNS relapses. Combined relapses are defined as any BM relapse combined with any extramedullary relapse [35]. In clinical studies, the "classical definitions" may still be used, e.g., if comparison with historical controls is one of the study questions.

16.5 Risk Stratification of Relapsed ALL

The duration of first remission, site of relapse and immunophenotype of the disease have been identified as the most important clinical risk factors for outcome in relapsed ALL.

In their pivotal studies, the international Berlin–Frankfurt–Münster (I-BFM) study group [36], UK [37] and the Children's Cancer Group [20] described the relevance of duration of first remission and site of relapse. For example, Tallen et al. [36] reported 17% event-free survival (EFS) in early marrow relapses versus 43% and 53% in late marrow or isolated CNS relapses, respectively. Accordingly, Gaynon et al. [20] reported EFS ranging from 6% in very early marrow relapses to 80% in late isolated CNS relapses.

T-lineage ALL appeared to be a high-risk factor for treatment failure in relapsed ALL. For example, Reismüller et al. [38] reported that survival of relapsed T-ALL was poorer than the survival of relapsed B-lineage ALL (21 vs. 37%). Most relapses of T-ALL occur early (Fig. 16.2) and remission-reinduction rate is historically low between 30 and 40% [39].

Using the risk-factors (duration of first remission, site of relapse, immunophenotype), the ALL-REZ BFM study group defined three (SR–IR–HR [40]) or four (S1–S4 [41]) strategy groups (Table 16.2).

Most study groups use risk group stratification similar to the criteria shown in Table 16.2, sometimes with minor modifications. For example, in trials of the Children's Oncology Group (COG) the cutoff point for early versus very early is 24 months after diagnosis, instead of 18 months CR1 as used in I-BFM-based protocols. In the IntReALL-2010 study, the IR and SR groups are combined to one SR arm.

In most clinical trials reported so far, genetic alterations of the relapse are not used as factors for risk-group stratification. However, the presence of *IKZF1* deletions, *TP53* alterations, *KMT2A::AFF1* t(4;11) translocation are related to poorer outcome [42, 43]. Eckert et al. [25] described in patients with high-risk (HR) relapses that recurrence was seen more frequently in those with a *TCF3* rearrangement, *TP53* deletions or mutations or hypodiploidy. In the R3-UK trial, deletions targeting *TP53, NR3C1, BTG1,* and *NRAS* were associated with inferior outcome in standard risk relapsed ALL patients, but in high-risk relapsed patients, the genetic risk group did not significantly influence outcome [44]. Also, in the recent COG AALL1331 trial, patients with unfavorable cytogenetics (hypodiploidy, *KMT2A*-rearrangement and iAMP21) tended toward poorer response to remission reinduction and survival [45].

16.6 Treatment of Patients with Relapsed ALL

During the last decades, many trials on relapsed ALL have been performed (for recent reviews: see [46–48]. In most studies, the strategy included induction of second complete remission with intensive conventional chemotherapy, followed by consolidation and reintensification. Subsequently, either maintenance treatment or allogeneic SCT was applied as consolidation therapy. Based on national frontline strategies, two approaches have been applied for post-induction treatment. The AIEOP, BFM, and

Table 16.2 Risk group stratification

	Immunophenotype: B-lineage			Immunophenotype: T-lineage		
Time point	IEM	Combined BM	Isolated BM	IEM	Combined BM	Isolated BM
Very early[a]	IR/S2	HR/S4	HR/S4	IR/S2	HR/S4	HR/S4
Early[b]	IR/S2	HR/S2	HR/S3	IR/S2	HR/S4	HR/S4
Late[c]	SR/S1	IR/S2	IR/S2	SR/S1	HR/S4	HR/S4

[a]Within 18 months after initial diagnosis
[b]After 18 months from initial diagnosis and within 6 months after cessation of frontline therapy
[c]After 6 months of cessation of frontline treatment

COPRALL groups have successfully applied relatively intensive, short multi-drug so-called R1-R2/F1-F2 courses [24, 38], followed by treatment-free intervals to allow hematopoietic regeneration, whereas the COG and UK-ALL-relapse groups applied a more continuous approach with repetitive application of relatively less intensive chemotherapy.

After standard four-drug reinduction treatment (vincristine, asparaginase, anthracycline, prednisone), or after reinduction using intermediate dose MTX (1 g/m^2) and high-dose cytarabine instead of anthracyclines [24], a second morphological remission can be achieved in most patients. Parker et al. [49] reported improved survival in patients treated with Mitoxantrone instead of Idarubicin, and therefore, many modern reinduction regimens in relapsed ALL studies include mitoxantrone. In patients with late relapses, CR2 rates of >95% can be achieved [2, 12, 15, 22, 50], whereas in early relapses, remission reinduction rate is only between 60 and 70% [12, 25, 51, 52] in most studies, without much improvement in the last decades, necessitating the use of new drugs to reinduce remission in high-risk, early relapses.

Due to better results in up-front ALL treatment, the number of relapses decreased. This was one of the reasons for many European study-groups (AIEOP, UKALL, ALL-REZ BFM, COPRALL, DCOG [50, 52–56]) and study groups from outside Europe (Australia) to join forces in collaborative relapse trials, the so-called IntReALL studies. These collaborative groups provide opportunities to study targeted compounds in rare subgroups of relapsed-ALL patients. In the next paragraphs, we will briefly review the results of recent relapsed-ALL trials.

16.7 Treatment of Patients with Late Bone Marrow Relapse of BCP-ALL

The last decades, survival of patients with late B-cell precursor (BCP) ALL relapses ranges from 50 to 80% [2, 15, 57–59]. Table 16.3 summarizes these studies. Like in frontline protocols, the end-of-reinduction minimal residual disease (MRD) appeared to be a major risk factor for outcome in relapsed ALL [54, 63]. For example, Eckert et al. reported that standard-risk patients treated according to the ALL-REZ-BFM95/96 study showed EFS of 76% (n = 46) in patients that had MRD of $<10^{-3}$, whereas patients with MRD $\geq 10^{-3}$ (n = 34) had only 18% EFS. Similar data were reported by others [2, 12]. In their pivotal paper, the ALL-REZ group showed that event-free survival of non-high-risk relapsed ALL patients with high MRD at end of reinduction increased from 18% in historical controls treated with chemotherapy only, to 64% in similar patients treated with allogeneic SCT [60]. Based on these and other studies [2, 15], most current trials apply SCT in patients with late bone-marrow relapses only in patients with high MRD at end of reinduction, whereas patients with low or negative MRD at end of reinduction have good outcomes without allogeneic SCT. Following standard four-drug reinduction regimen, 40–50% of the patients suffering from late marrow relapses have poor MRD responses after reinduction therapy, and therefore are generally treated with SCT.

Recently, the results of two large studies including late bone marrow relapses have been reported in patients with BCP-ALL. In the IntReALL-SR 2010 study, a randomization comparing the ALL-REZ BFM 2002 arm (arm A) with the UKALL-R3 arm (arm B) was performed. Patients with late relapse and good MRD response at end of reinduction had comparable EFS in both arms with EFS of 68% in arm A and 69% in arm B, both arms without SCT. Patients with late bone marrow relapses and poor MRD response, and therefore treated with alloSCT, also had comparable EFS in both arms with 66% and 69% in arms A and B respectively. This study confirmed that the outcome in patients with poor MRD response could be improved to levels similar to patients with good MRD response, if allogeneic SCT was applied in the poor-MRD group [59].

In the COG AALL1331 study [14], patients with low risk relapsed BCP-ALL and a good MRD response after reinduction were random-

Table 16.3 Recent clinical trials for ALL in the first relapse: bone marrow relapse of BCP-ALL

Study	Population	Patients	EFS (%)	OS (%)	Allo SCT	Remark/conclusion
AALL01P2, Raetz [12]	BCP, CR1 < 36 months BCP, CR1 18–36 months BCP, CR1 ≥ 36 months	16 39 45	13 45 84		No data on post induction regimen with or without SCT.	
UKALL-R3, Parker [2]	BCP and T, late (>6 months after stop frontline therapy)	228	60	72	120/228	
REZ-BFM 90 von Stackelberg [56]	Early BCP (BM, IEM and combined) Late BCP (BM, IEM and combined)	112 147	21 48		Recommended Not recomm.	No benefit increased MTX in induction
IntReALL-2010 von Stackelberg [59]	BCP, late isolated BM, late and early combined	299	48		If poor MRD response EOI	No difference ALL-REZ BFM 2002 and UKALL-R3
BFM 2002 Eckert [60]	BCP, late BM (92/109), good MRD response EOI BCP, late BM (92/109), poor MRD response EOI	109 99	70 64	73 68	22/107 81/98	SCT not needed in late relapses with good EOI MRD response SCT improved survival in late relapses with poor EOI MRD response
AALL1331 Brown [61]	BCP intermediate/high risk (see text), Blina. In consolidation BCP intermediate/high risk (see text), no Blina. In consolidation.	105 103	54 39	71 58	74/105 44/103	Blinatumomab in consolidation more effective and less toxic than chemotherapy
NCT 02393859 Locatelli [62]	BCP high-risk relapse, consolidation with two chemo courses + Blina BCP high-risk relapse, consolidation with three chemo courses (no Blina.)	54 54	58 28	81 56	48/54 38/54	Blinatumomab in consolidation more effective and less toxic than chemotherapy
AALL1331 Hogan [14]	BCP low-risk relapse, consolidation with two chemo courses + three Blina. Blocks BCP low-risk relapse, consolidation with four chemo courses (no Blina.)	87 87	72 54	97 85	No	Blina. Improved survival in low-risk BM relapses
Eckert, R3 and ALL-REZ 2002 [25].	BCP-HR relapse	278	26	32	>90%	CR2 rate 54%

ized to treatment according to chemotherapy similar to the UKALL-R3 trial versus treatment in which the R3 block 3 was replaced by three cycles of blinatumomab. Patients did not receive allogeneic SCT. The 4-year EFS (72%) and OS (97%) in patients with late marrow relapses and good MRD response treated with Blinatumomab were significantly better than in patients treated according to the control arm (see Table 16.3). In the Blinatumomab-treated arm, EFS was in the same range, and OS slightly higher than reported in the IntReALL-2010-SR study (69% EFS and 87% OS), in which no Blinatumomab was given [59]. However, in the IntReALL-2010-SR study, also patients with poor MRD-response were included, which makes the groups less comparable. In the COG AALL1331 study, the toxicity in the blinatumomab arm was very well tolerable and significantly lower than in the control arm.

Both in earlier trials [55] and more recent trials [14, 64], similar results were presented in patients with late isolated bone marrow relapse and late combined bone marrow relapse.

In summary, in patients with late bone marrow relapses of BCP-ALL, survival rates around 60–70% can be achieved. Approximately half of the patients with late bone marrow relapses have poor MRD responses after induction and therefore are currently stratified to SCT. Peters et al. [65] clearly showed that in childhood ALL, conditioning regimens containing total body irradiation (TBI) were superior to chemotherapy-only conditioning regimens. Therefore, in current trials the patients with late bone marrow relapse and poor MRD-response are treated with TBI, at the cost of late toxicities. Studies to further improve the survival at lower costs of toxicity are currently being developed, including the use of Blinatumomab and Inotuzumab to both improve survival and reduce the number of patients that stratify for SCT. Additionally, studies to the role of CART-cells in patients with first relapse of ALL may reveal whether CART treatment can be curative in this group of patients, thereby further reducing the number of patients needing SCT.

16.8 Treatment of Patients with Early Bone Marrow Relapse of BCP-ALL

For more than two decades, it is known that survival after early bone marrow relapses of ALL is dismal with chemotherapy only, whereas EFS of 30–40% can be achieved in children treated with SCT [40, 66]. Eckert et al. [25] clearly showed that children that suffer from early marrow relapse are hard to cure, with only 64% successful reinduction due to 5% induction deaths and 31% induction failures. EFS and OS were 26% and 33%, respectively. Similar data have been reported by Raetz et al. [12]. In the study of Eckert et al., a minority of 18 of 207 patients achieving CR2 received chemotherapy but were not transplanted, of whom 15 relapsed, stressing that with chemotherapy only, these children have a very poor chance of survival.

In the group of patients relapsing early, those relapsing very early (within 18 months of achieving first remission on upfront therapy) are at even higher risk of poor outcome with only 13% 1-year EFS as compared to 45% in patients relapsing between 18 and 36 after CR1 [12] . Eckert et al. reported that induction failure was higher in patients with very early relapse as compared to early relapse, but if CR2 could be achieved, EFS was similar in both groups [25]. As survival in patients relapsing very early, as well as in patients with high-risk genetics at relapse, is still poor, this group of patients is candidate for investigating novel agents early in treatment, e.g., inotuzumab and/or CART.

A major improvement in the outcome of children with early marrow relapse has recently been reported in two studies [61, 62] on the effect of blinatumomab, a CD3/CD19-directed bispecific T-cell engaging molecule. In the randomized clinical trial reported by Locatelli et al. [62], one cycle of blinatumomab was compared to a third consolidation chemotherapy block, followed, in both arms, by SCT. In the study reported by Brown et al. [61], patients received a 4-week reinduction chemotherapy course, followed by randomized assignment to receive two cycles of Blinatumomab or two cycles of multiagent chemotherapy, subsequently followed by SCT. In both trials, independent trial monitoring committees recommended premature termination of the study because patients in the Blinatumomab arms of both studies had better DFS and OS (see Table 16.3), less serious toxicity and higher rates of MRD-negativity prior to SCT. Both these studies [61, 62] show that in high-risk patient with aggressive forms of ALL that relapsed on, or shortly after, modern intensive upfront-treatment, immunotherapy can markedly improve outcome.

In the study of Brown et al., blinatumomab treatment was started directly after reinduction therapy, whereas in the study of Locatelli et al. two consolidation courses with intensive chemotherapy were given prior to blinatumomab. OS in these studies was in the blinatumomab arms 73 and 80%. Of note, these OS rates are calculated after induction (Brown) or after two consolidation courses (Locatelli), implicating, that OS of high-risk relapsed ALL is still lower, as induction failure (up to 30%) and death in induction (5%) occur commonly in these patients [25]. Both studies urge to further investigate the replacement of chemotherapy by immunotherapy. Promising agents that may be further studied in this patient population include CART and Inotuzumab (see chapters on Immunotherapy and CART therapy).

16.9 Treatment of Patients with Isolated Extramedullary Relapses of BCP-ALL

The incidence of isolated extramedullary relapses, like the incidence of bone marrow relapses, has decreased in the last decades due to improved frontline protocols. Of relapses, the percentage of IEM relapses is approximately 20%, relatively independent on the frontline protocol [67]. In IEM, leukemic cells have been protected from chemotherapy by biologic blood–tissue barriers in sanctuary sites such as the central nervous system and testes. To completely eradicate the relapsed disease from these sanctuary sites, local therapy in addition to systemic chemotherapy is indicated. In the vast majority of "isolated" extramedullary relapses, bone marrow involvement at the submicroscopic level is present [68], stressing the necessity of systemic chemotherapy in addition to local therapy.

In CNS relapses, cranial irradiation and enhanced intrathecal therapy is indicated. The most recommended dosage is 18 Gy, although 24 Gy has been used effectively as well [69]. In their COG AALL02P2 study, Hastings et al. [58] investigated whether the dosage of cranial irradiation could be reduced to 12 Gy in patients with late isolated CNS relapse. Their study showed inferior EFS (albeit, similar OS) after 12 Gy as compared to 18 Gy cranial irradiation. Limitations in this study were the small sample size and protocol non-adherence. In a recent study, Stackelberg et al. [59] showed in a randomized IntReALL-SR-2010 trial that the outcome of patients with IEM relapses was better if treated according to the ALL-REZ BFM 2002 strategy than in patients treated according to the UK-ALLR3 arm of the study. Most likely, this was due to the more intensive systemic high-dose methotrexate and cytarabine treatment, as well as to the more intensive intrathecal triple-therapy regimen in the ALL-REZ BFM 2002 strategy.

In testicular relapses, local therapy may differ between study groups. Most study groups recommend local irradiation of both testes at 24 Gy independent on whether one or both testes are involved. Unfortunately, this causes a complete loss of hormonal function. Therefore, ALL REZ BFM relapse strategies have recommended to remove a clinically involved testis and to irradiate a contralateral clinically and biopsy-proven not involved testis with 15 Gy, or with 18 Gy if the biopsy of the contralateral testis showed leukemic infiltration, aiming to preserve hormonal functions. The incidence of isolated testicular relapse decreased with high-dose methotrexate and intensive corticosteroid use in upfront-ALL protocols (recently reviewed by Nguyen et al. [70]).

Like in medullary relapses, the duration of CR1 is also in IEM relapses a major determinant of EFS and OS (Table 16.4). In their analysis of recent UK trials, Krishnan et al. [67] reported that the vast majority of isolated CNS relapses was either very early (37–43%) or early (38–46%), with less than 20% of patients suffering from late relapses. Similar data are published by others [36, 71, 72]. In most modern treatment protocols, patients with early and very early IEM relapses, as well as patients with late relapses but poor bone marrow MRD response after reinduction, are treated with allo-SCT, combined with cranial irradiation. For late relapses with good MRD response, chemotherapy plus local therapy, generally after completion of intensive treatment, is recommended [15, 36, 59, 69].

Table 16.4 Recent clinical trials for ALL in the first relapse: isolated extramedullary relapse

Study	Population	Patients	EFS (%)	OS (%)	SCT	Remark/conclusion
POG 9412 (56)	CR1 < 18 months CR1 ≥ 18 months 71 BCP, 5 T-lineage; CNS	24 52	51 77	57 86	No No	Outcome after late relapse better than after early
POG AALL02P2 [58]	BCP, CR1 > 18 months; CNS	118	64	79	No	12 Gy cranial irr. Inferior to 18 Gy
UKALL-R3 [69]	T and B-lineage, early and late; CNS	80	38	51	39/80 patients	24 Gy cranial irr.
COG AALL0433 [15]	Very early CNS	29	41	52	7/29 patients	–
BFM-90 (35)	Very early Early and late CNS and testis	12 19 and 4	33 47 and 50	– –	– –	
IntReALL-2010 [59]	ALL-REZ BFM 2002 UKALL-R3 Late and early, CNS and testis	40 45	82 43	– –	– –	In IEM, ALL-REZ BFM 2002 more effective than UKALL-R3
COPRALL-97 (52)	BCP CR1 < 24 months BCP CR1 ≥ 24 months CNS and testis	35 33	31 61	40 76	13/35 patients 1/33 patients	
AALL1331 [14]	BCP low-risk relapse, consolidation with two chemo courses + three Blina. Blocks BCP low-risk relapse, consolidation with four chemo courses (no Blina.) CNS and testis	40 41	37 39	76 69	No	Blina. Did not improve outcome in low-risk IEM relapses

Hogan et al. [14] showed that in isolated CNS relapses, in contrast to marrow relapses, blinatumomab did not improve survival most likely due to the impermeability of the blood–brain barrier for blinatumomab. As Inotuzumab does not cross the blood–brain barrier either, beneficial effects of inotuzumab on isolated CNS relapses are not expected, but data are lacking so far. Similarly, data on efficacy of blinatumomab and inotuzumab on isolated testicular relapses are lacking.

In contrast to the immunotherapeutic drugs blinatumomab and inotuzumab, which hardly cross the blood–brain barrier, the long-lasting presence of immunotherapeutic CARTs has been reported in the central nervous tissue [73, 74]. In 15 patients with isolated CNS relapses, approximately 45% EFS with more than 90% OS was reported [73]. These data indicate that the role of CART treatment in relapsed IEM deserves further study.

16.10 Relapsed T-Cell ALL

Relapsed T-ALL mostly occurs early or very early after first remission (Fig. 16.2). If a patient seems to have a relapse more than 3 years after initial diagnosis, the "relapse" possibly will be a second T-ALL as can be diagnosed by comparing results of detailed genetic analysis of diagnosis and relapse samples [5].

In relapsed ALL, T-ALL phenotype has since long been recognized as an adverse prognostic sign also in multivariate analyses [36, 46, 51, 75] and regarded as an indication for treatment according to high-risk strategies including SCT. This holds both for medullary relapses and isolated extramedullary relapses. The chance of achieving a second CR is only in the order of 30% after "classical four-drug induction" [12, 25]. By adding Nelarabine in their pivotal phase 2 study, Berg et al. reported CR2 rates around 50% in patients in first and early relapse [76].

Whitlock et al. showed that adding cyclophosphamide/etoposide to the nelarabine therapy did not increase remission reinduction rate as compared to Nelarabine single agent therapy [77].

Recently, Horton et al. [78] investigated the addition of the proteasome inhibitor Bortezomib on the reinduction rate in relapsed ALL. They reported an encouraging CR2 rate of 68% in relapsed T-ALL patients. However, MRD lower than 0.01% was reported in only four evaluable of 22 patients, of whom 3 (75%) were still alive at 3-years follow-up. In contrast 16 evaluable of 22 patients had poor MRD-response (>0.01%), of which only 7 (43%) were alive at 3-year follow-up. Based on these promising results, Teachey et al. randomized the addition of Bortezomib to a modified augmented Berlin-Frankfurt-Münster chemotherapy backbone [79] in the COG trial AALL1231 in upfront patients with T-ALL. The 4-year EFS and OS for arm A (no bortezomib) versus arm B (bortezomib) were 80.1% vs. 83.8% (EFS, p = 0.131) and 85.7% versus 88.3% (OS, p = 0.085). In the recent IntReALL-2010 trial for high-risk relapses, the addition of bortezomib is investigated in high-risk relapsed patients, including T-ALL relapses, in a randomized study [80].

Based on promising antitumor activity of BCL-2/BCL-X_L protein family inhibitors venetoclax and navitoclax, Pullarkat et al. [81] performed a phase I study combining venetoclax with low-dose navitoclax in relapsed/refractory ALL. They observed a promising CR rate of 53% in heavily pretreated patients with relapsed/refractory T-ALL, indicating that further studies to implementing this combination of drugs is indicated.

Despite the implementation of Nelarabine and Bortezomib in clinical studies, treatment of patients with relapsed T-ALL still uniformly rely on inducing deep CR2 followed by allo-SCT. Although this treatment is very intense and comes at the cost of major toxicities, less than 50% of children with relapsed T-ALL reaching SCT can be cured [82], leading to overall cure rate of 20–30%. Richter-Pechańska et al. [83] reported a so-called ultra-high-risk group of relapsed T-ALL patients carrying mutations in *TP53*, *MSH6*, *USP7*, *NRAS*, *KRAS*, *CNOT3*, and *IL7R* genes with fatal outcome.

With current poor prognosis of relapsed T-ALL despite aggressive therapy, individualized precision medicine approaches for patients with T-ALL in first relapse are urgently needed [84]. First candidates for these precision medicine approaches are patients with aberrant JAK-STAT signaling, who might benefit from JAK-STAT inhibitors. Patients with *ABL*-class fusions may benefit from tyrosine kinase inhibitors added to conventional chemotherapy. As preclinical efficacy of the anti-CD38 monoclonal antibodies daratumumab [85] and isatuximab [86] for T-ALL has been reported, these drugs are also being investigated in children with relapsed/refractory T-ALL expressing the CD38 protein.

Obviously, based on the promising results of CARTs in relapsed/refractory BCP-ALL, major effort has been put in generating anti-T-ALL CARTs. Possible targetable antigens include CD1a, CD5, and CD7, of which anti-CD7 CARTs are most advanced in clinical studies. Potential complications in anti-T-cell CART are "fratricide" (e.g., anti-CD7 CARTs killing other, CD7-carrying CARTs) and killing of T-cells in the patient, thereby introducing the status of severe combined immunodeficiency. Despite these caveats, initial studies reporting clinical efficacy have been reported using autologous [87] and allogeneic anti-CD7 CART-cells [88–90].

16.11 Miscellaneous Groups of Patients with Relapsed ALL

Both the COG and IntReALL consortia recognized that patients with high-risk cytogenetics and very early relapses had a poor outcome [25, 43]. High-risk genetics included hypodiploidy; *TP53* alterations; and *TCF3-HLF*, *TCF3-PBX1*, *MLL-AF4* translocations. In these patients, and in patients with very early relapses, the effect of inotuzumab on induction rate as compared to classical induction with UKALL-R3 induction, is explored in a phase 2 study [91]. In contrast, an excellent outcome has been reported by

Gandemer et al. [92] in patients with relapsed *ETV6/RUNX1*-positive ALL, reaching 80% in children with *ETV6/RUNX1* positive, late relapses. The role of CART therapy in patients with high-risk genetics looks promising. Although Gu et al. reported that patients carrying *TP53* mutations showed also after CART a worse outcome [93], they and Leahy et al. [94] reported that in patients with other high-risk cytogenetics, outcome after CART therapy was comparable to outcome in patients without high-risk cytogenetics. Therefore, clinical trials including CART therapy are urgently needed for patients with high-risk cytogenetics and very early relapses.

Patients with Down syndrome are known to be more prone to severe toxicities upon the intensive treatment regimens, with or without SCT, that are needed in relapsed ALL [95, 96]. Therefore, these children should be candidates to replace toxic components of relapse-ALL treatment with novel, immunotherapeutic agents like blinatumomab, inotuzumab, and CARTs [97, 98]. So far, however, children with Down syndrome have been excluded for many clinical trials [98], a policy that urgently needs reconsideration.

Until recently, the outcome of patients with second or subsequent relapse, or patients with relapse after allogeneic SCT, was considered dismal [99]. As shown in Fig. 16.1, nowadays with blinatumomab, inotuzumab, and CARTs [100, 101], a new effective immune-therapeutic repertoire is available for successful treatment of patients with second or greater relapses of BCP-ALL. In addition, these patients are candidates to study novel therapeutic approaches with targeted drugs [102].

16.12 Conclusion

Major improvements have been made in the therapy of childhood relapsed BCP-ALL. Challenges for the next years will be to implement newer, less toxic and more targeted treatment as the improved survival comes at great costs in terms of toxicity, especially if allogeneic SCT with TBI-based conditioning is needed to achieve improved survival. Prospective studies to evaluate the role of CART therapy in preventing the need for allogeneic SCT could help reducing the numbers of SCTs needed.

In contrast, children with relapsed T-ALL still suffer a poor outcome, and novel, effective agents are urgently needed. To study the possible role of agents, international collaboration in large trials is urgently warranted.

References

1. Pieters R, de Groot-Kruseman H, Van der Velden V, Fiocco M, van den Berg H, de Bont E, et al. Successful therapy reduction and intensification for childhood acute lymphoblastic leukemia based on minimal residual disease monitoring: study ALL10 from the Dutch childhood oncology group. J Clin Oncol. 2016;34(22):2591–601.
2. Parker C, Krishnan S, Hamadeh L, Irving JAE, Kuiper RP, Révész T, et al. Outcomes of patients with childhood B-cell precursor acute lymphoblastic leukaemia with late bone marrow relapses: long-term follow-up of the ALLR3 open-label randomised trial. Lancet Haematol. 2019;6(4):e204–e16.
3. Pieters R, de Groot-Kruseman H, Fiocco M, Verwer F, Van Overveld M, Sonneveld E, et al. Improved outcome for ALL by prolonging therapy for IKZF1 deletion and decreasing therapy for other risk groups. J Clin Oncol. 2023;41(25):4130–42.
4. Maloney KW, Devidas M, Wang C, Mattano LA, Friedmann AM, Buckley P, et al. Outcome in children with standard-risk B-cell acute lymphoblastic leukemia: results of Children's oncology group trial AALL0331. J Clin Oncol. 2020;38(6):602–12.
5. Szczepanski T, van der Velden VH, Waanders E, Kuiper RP, Van Vlierberghe P, Gruhn B, et al. Late recurrence of childhood T-cell acute lymphoblastic leukemia frequently represents a second leukemia rather than a relapse: first evidence for genetic predisposition. J Clin Oncol. 2011;29(12):1643–9.
6. Waanders E, Scheijen B, Jongmans MC, Venselaar H, van Reijmersdal SV, van Dijk AH, et al. Germline activating TYK2 mutations in pediatric patients with two primary acute lymphoblastic leukemia occurrences. Leukemia. 2017;31(4):821–8.
7. Lissat A, van Schewick C, Steffen IG, Arakawa A, Bourquin JP, Burkhardt B, et al. Other (non-CNS/testicular) extramedullary localizations of childhood relapsed acute lymphoblastic leukemia and lymphoblastic lymphoma-a report from the ALL-REZ study group. J Clin Med. 2021;10(22)
8. Klumper E, Pieters R, Veerman AJ, Huismans DR, Loonen AH, Hählen K, et al. In vitro cellular drug resistance in children with relapsed/refractory acute lymphoblastic leukemia. Blood. 1995;86(10):3861–8.

9. Hongo T, Fujii Y. In vitro chemosensitivity of lymphoblasts at relapse in childhood leukemia using the MTT assay. Int J Hematol. 1991;54(3):219–30.
10. Irving JA. Towards an understanding of the biology and targeted treatment of paediatric relapsed acute lymphoblastic leukaemia. Br J Haematol. 2016;172(5):655–66.
11. O'Connor D, Moorman AV, Wade R, Hancock J, Tan RM, Bartram J, et al. Use of minimal residual disease assessment to redefine induction failure in pediatric acute lymphoblastic leukemia. J Clin Oncol. 2017;35(6):660–7.
12. Raetz EA, Borowitz MJ, Devidas M, Linda SB, Hunger SP, Winick NJ, et al. Reinduction platform for children with first marrow relapse of acute lymphoblastic leukemia: a children's oncology group study [corrected]. J Clin Oncol. 2008;26(24):3971–8.
13. Eckert C, Groeneveld-Krentz S, Kirschner-Schwabe R, Hagedorn N, Chen-Santel C, Bader P, et al. Improving stratification for children with late bone marrow B-cell acute lymphoblastic leukemia relapses with refined response classification and integration of genetics. J Clin Oncol. 2019;37(36):3493–506.
14. Hogan LE, Brown PA, Ji L, Xu X, Devidas M, Bhatla T, et al. Children's oncology group AALL1331: phase III trial of Blinatumomab in children, adolescents, and young adults with low-risk B-cell ALL in first relapse. J Clin Oncol. 2023;41(25):4118–29.
15. Lew G, Chen Y, Lu X, Rheingold SR, Whitlock JA, Devidas M, et al. Outcomes after late bone marrow and very early central nervous system relapse of childhood B-acute lymphoblastic leukemia: a report from the children's oncology group phase III study AALL0433. Haematologica. 2021;106(1):46–55.
16. Raetz EA, Cairo MS, Borowitz MJ, Lu X, Devidas M, Reid JM, et al. Re-induction chemoimmunotherapy with epratuzumab in relapsed acute lymphoblastic leukemia (ALL): phase II results from Children's oncology group (COG) study ADVL04P2. Pediatr Blood Cancer. 2015;62(7):1171–5.
17. Mullighan CG, Phillips LA, Su X, Ma J, Miller CB, Shurtleff SA, et al. Genomic analysis of the clonal origins of relapsed acute lymphoblastic leukemia. Science. 2008;322(5906):1377–80.
18. Li B, Brady SW, Ma X, Shen S, Zhang Y, Li Y, et al. Therapy-induced mutations drive the genomic landscape of relapsed acute lymphoblastic leukemia. Blood. 2020;135(1):41–55.
19. Roberts KG, Mullighan CG. The biology of B-progenitor acute lymphoblastic leukemia. Cold Spring Harb Perspect Med. 2020;10(7).
20. Gaynon PS, Qu RP, Chappell RJ, Willoughby ML, Tubergen DG, Steinherz PG, et al. Survival after relapse in childhood acute lymphoblastic leukemia: impact of site and time to first relapse – the children's cancer group experience. Cancer. 1998;82(7):1387–95.
21. Amadori S, Spiriti MA, Meloni G, Pacilli L, Papa G, Mandelli F. Combination chemotherapy for marrow relapse in children and adolescents with acute lymphocytic leukaemia. Scand J Haematol. 1981;26(4):292–6.
22. Buchanan GR, Rivera GK, Boyett JM, Chauvenet AR, Crist WM, Vietti TJ. Reinduction therapy in 297 children with acute lymphoblastic leukemia in first bone marrow relapse: a pediatric oncology group study. Blood. 1988;72(4):1286–92.
23. Cornbleet MA, Chessells JM. Bone-marrow relapse in acute lymphoblastic leukaemia in childhood. Br Med J. 1978;2(6130):104–6.
24. Henze G, Fengler R, Hartmann R, Kornhuber B, Janka-Schaub G, Niethammer D, et al. Six-year experience with a comprehensive approach to the treatment of recurrent childhood acute lymphoblastic leukemia (ALL-REZ BFM 85). A relapse study of the BFM group. Blood. 1991;78(5):1166–72.
25. Eckert C, Parker C, Moorman AV, Irving JA, Kirschner-Schwabe R, Groeneveld-Krentz S, et al. Risk factors and outcomes in children with high-risk B-cell precursor and T-cell relapsed acute lymphoblastic leukaemia: combined analysis of ALLR3 and ALL-REZ BFM 2002 clinical trials. Eur J Cancer. 2021;151:175–89.
26. Woods WG, Nesbit ME, Ramsay NK, Krivit W, Kim TH, Goldman A, et al. Intensive therapy followed by bone marrow transplantation for patients with acute lymphocytic leukemia in second or subsequent remission: determination of prognostic factors (a report from the University of Minnesota Bone Marrow Transplantation Team). Blood. 1983;61(6):1182–9.
27. Bacigalupo A, Van Lint MT, Frassoni F, Occhini D, Pittaluga PA, Comelli A, et al. Allogeneic bone marrow transplantation versus chemotherapy for childhood acute lymphoblastic leukaemia in second remission. Bone Marrow Transplant. 1986;1(1):75–80.
28. Johnson FL, Thomas ED, Clark BS, Chard RL, Hartmann JR, Storb R. A comparison of marrow transplantation with chemotherapy for children with acute lymphoblastic leukemia in second or subsequent remission. N Engl J Med. 1981;305(15):846–51.
29. Niethammer D, Dopfer R, Klingebiel T, Riehm H, Schellong G, Henze G, et al. Actual role and perspectives of BMT in children. Bone Marrow Transplant. 1989;4(Suppl 4):7–11.
30. Sanders JE, Thomas ED, Buckner CD, Doney K. Marrow transplantation for children with acute lymphoblastic leukemia in second remission. Blood. 1987;70(1):324–6.
31. Chessells JM, Rogers DW, Leiper AD, Blacklock H, Plowman PN, Richards S, et al. Bone-marrow transplantation has a limited role in prolonging second marrow remission in childhood lymphoblastic leukaemia. Lancet. 1986;1(8492):1239–41.
32. Harrison G, Richards S, Lawson S, Darbyshire P, Pinkerton R, Stevens R, et al. Comparison of allogeneic transplant versus chemotherapy for relapsed childhood acute lymphoblastic leukaemia in the

MRC UKALL R1 trial. MRC childhood leukaemia working party. Ann Oncol. 2000;11(8):999–1006.
33. Pinkel D. Allogeneic bone marrow transplantation in children with acute leukemia: a practice whose time has gone. Leukemia. 1989;3(3):242–4.
34. Hoogerbrugge PM, Gerritsen EJ, vd Does-van den Berg A, vd Berg H, Zwinderman AH, Hermans J, et al. Case-control analysis of allogeneic bone marrow transplantation versus maintenance chemotherapy for relapsed ALL in children. Bone Marrow Transplant. 1995;15(2):255–9.
35. Buchmann S, Schrappe M, Baruchel A, Biondi A, Borowitz M, Campbell M, et al. Remission, treatment failure, and relapse in pediatric ALL: an international consensus of the Ponte-di-Legno consortium. Blood. 2022;139(12):1785–93.
36. Tallen G, Ratei R, Mann G, Kaspers G, Niggli F, Karachunsky A, et al. Long-term outcome in children with relapsed acute lymphoblastic leukemia after time-point and site-of-relapse stratification and intensified short-course multidrug chemotherapy: results of trial ALL-REZ BFM 90. J Clin Oncol. 2010;28(14):2339–47.
37. Lawson SE, Harrison G, Richards S, Oakhill A, Stevens R, Eden OB, et al. The UK experience in treating relapsed childhood acute lymphoblastic leukaemia: a report on the medical research council UKALLR1 study. Br J Haematol. 2000;108(3):531–43.
38. Reismüller B, Attarbaschi A, Peters C, Dworzak MN, Pötschger U, Urban C, et al. Long-term outcome of initially homogenously treated and relapsed childhood acute lymphoblastic leukaemia in Austria – a population-based report of the Austrian Berlin-Frankfurt-Münster (BFM) Study Group. Br J Haematol. 2009;144(4):559–70.
39. Raetz EA, Teachey DT. T-cell acute lymphoblastic leukemia. Hematology Am Soc Hematol Educ Program. 2016;2016(1):580–8.
40. Borgmann A, von Stackelberg A, Hartmann R, Ebell W, Klingebiel T, Peters C, et al. Unrelated donor stem cell transplantation compared with chemotherapy for children with acute lymphoblastic leukemia in a second remission: a matched-pair analysis. Blood. 2003;101(10):3835–9.
41. von Stackelberg A, Völzke E, Kühl JS, Seeger K, Schrauder A, Escherich G, et al. Outcome of children and adolescents with relapsed acute lymphoblastic leukaemia and non-response to salvage protocol therapy: a retrospective analysis of the ALL-REZ BFM study group. Eur J Cancer. 2011;47(1):90–7.
42. Hof J, Kox C, Groeneveld-Krentz S, Bandapalli OR, Karawajew L, Schedel K, et al. NOTCH1 mutation, TP53 alteration and myeloid antigen expression predict outcome heterogeneity in children with first relapse of T-cell acute lymphoblastic leukemia. Haematologica. 2017;102(7):e249–e52.
43. Krentz S, Hof J, Mendioroz A, Vaggopoulou R, Dörge P, Lottaz C, et al. Prognostic value of genetic alterations in children with first bone marrow relapse of childhood B-cell precursor acute lymphoblastic leukemia. Leukemia. 2013;27(2):295–304.
44. Irving JA, Enshaei A, Parker CA, Sutton R, Kuiper RP, Erhorn A, et al. Integration of genetic and clinical risk factors improves prognostication in relapsed childhood B-cell precursor acute lymphoblastic leukemia. Blood. 2016;128(7):911–22.
45. Bhatla THL, Xu X, et al. Prognostic importance of cytogenetic subgroups in relapse risk stratification in children and young adults with first relapsed B-ALL: a children's oncology group. Study AALL1331. Blood. 2022;140:3476–7.
46. Bhojwani D, Pui CH. Relapsed childhood acute lymphoblastic leukaemia. Lancet Oncol. 2013;14(6):e205–17.
47. Locatelli F, Schrappe M, Bernardo ME, Rutella S. How I treat relapsed childhood acute lymphoblastic leukemia. Blood. 2012;120(14):2807–16.
48. Hunger SP, Raetz EA. How I treat relapsed acute lymphoblastic leukemia in the pediatric population. Blood. 2020;136(16):1803–12.
49. Parker C, Waters R, Leighton C, Hancock J, Sutton R, Moorman AV, et al. Effect of mitoxantrone on outcome of children with first relapse of acute lymphoblastic leukaemia (ALL R3): an open-label randomised trial. Lancet. 2010;376(9757):2009–17.
50. Rizzari C, Valsecchi MG, Aricò M, Miniero R, Messina C, De Rossi G, et al. Outcome of very late relapse in children with acute lymphoblastic leukemia. Haematologica. 2004;89(4):427–34.
51. Einsiedel HG, von Stackelberg A, Hartmann R, Fengler R, Schrappe M, Janka-Schaub G, et al. Long-term outcome in children with relapsed ALL by risk-stratified salvage therapy: results of trial acute lymphoblastic leukemia-relapse study of the Berlin-Frankfurt-Münster group 87. J Clin Oncol. 2005;23(31):7942–50.
52. van den Berg H, de Groot-Kruseman HA, Damen-Korbijn CM, de Bont ES, Schouten-van Meeteren AY, Hoogerbrugge PM. Outcome after first relapse in children with acute lymphoblastic leukemia: a report based on the Dutch childhood oncology group (DCOG) relapse all 98 protocol. Pediatr Blood Cancer. 2011;57(2):210–6.
53. Domenech C, Mercier M, Plouvier E, Puraveau M, Bordigoni P, Michel G, et al. First isolated extramedullary relapse in children with B-cell precursor acute lymphoblastic leukaemia: results of the Cooprall-97 study. Eur J Cancer. 2008;44(16):2461–9.
54. Paganin M, Zecca M, Fabbri G, Polato K, Biondi A, Rizzari C, et al. Minimal residual disease is an important predictive factor of outcome in children with relapsed 'high-risk' acute lymphoblastic leukemia. Leukemia. 2008;22(12):2193–200.
55. Roy A, Cargill A, Love S, Moorman AV, Stoneham S, Lim A, et al. Outcome after first relapse in childhood acute lymphoblastic leukaemia – lessons from the United Kingdom R2 trial. Br J Haematol. 2005;130(1):67–75.

56. von Stackelberg A, Hartmann R, Bührer C, Fengler R, Janka-Schaub G, Reiter A, et al. High-dose compared with intermediate-dose methotrexate in children with a first relapse of acute lymphoblastic leukemia. Blood. 2008;111(5):2573–80.
57. Barredo JC, Devidas M, Lauer SJ, Billett A, Marymont M, Pullen J, et al. Isolated CNS relapse of acute lymphoblastic leukemia treated with intensive systemic chemotherapy and delayed CNS radiation: a pediatric oncology group study. J Clin Oncol. 2006;24(19):3142–9.
58. Hastings C, Chen Y, Devidas M, Ritchey AK, Winick NJ, Carroll WL, et al. Late isolated central nervous system relapse in childhood B-cell acute lymphoblastic leukemia treated with intensified systemic therapy and delayed reduced dose cranial radiation: a report from the Children's oncology group study AALL02P2. Pediatr Blood Cancer. 2021;68(12):e29256.
59. von Stackelberg A, et al. ALL-REZ BFM 2002 is associated with improved outcome as compared to ALL-R3 in children with standard risk isolated CNS relapse of acute lymphoblastic leukemia, while maintaining comparable results in patients with bone marrow relapse. Results of the multi-national, multi-center trial IntReALL SR 2010. Blood. 2022;140:3247–9.
60. Eckert C, Henze G, Seeger K, Hagedorn N, Mann G, Panzer-Grümayer R, et al. Use of allogeneic hematopoietic stem-cell transplantation based on minimal residual disease response improves outcomes for children with relapsed acute lymphoblastic leukemia in the intermediate-risk group. J Clin Oncol. 2013;31(21):2736–42.
61. Brown PA, Ji L, Xu X, Devidas M, Hogan LE, Borowitz MJ, et al. Effect of Postreinduction therapy consolidation with Blinatumomab vs chemotherapy on disease-free survival in children, adolescents, and young adults with first relapse of B-cell acute lymphoblastic leukemia: a randomized clinical trial. JAMA. 2021;325(9):833–42.
62. Locatelli F, Zugmaier G, Rizzari C, Morris JD, Gruhn B, Klingebiel T, et al. Effect of Blinatumomab vs chemotherapy on event-free survival among children with high-risk first-relapse B-cell acute lymphoblastic leukemia: a randomized clinical trial. JAMA. 2021;325(9):843–54.
63. Eckert C, Biondi A, Seeger K, Cazzaniga G, Hartmann R, Beyermann B, et al. Prognostic value of minimal residual disease in relapsed childhood acute lymphoblastic leukaemia. Lancet. 2001;358(9289):1239–41.
64. von Stackelberg A. Personal Communication. 2022.
65. Peters C, Dalle JH, Locatelli F, Poetschger U, Sedlacek P, Buechner J, et al. Total body irradiation or chemotherapy conditioning in childhood ALL: a multinational, randomized, noninferiority phase III study. J Clin Oncol. 2021;39(4):295–307.
66. Boulad F, Steinherz P, Reyes B, Heller G, Gillio AP, Small TN, et al. Allogeneic bone marrow transplantation versus chemotherapy for the treatment of childhood acute lymphoblastic leukemia in second remission: a single-institution study. J Clin Oncol. 1999;17(1):197–207.
67. Krishnan S, Wade R, Moorman AV, Mitchell C, Kinsey SE, Eden TO, et al. Temporal changes in the incidence and pattern of central nervous system relapses in children with acute lymphoblastic leukaemia treated on four consecutive Medical Research Council trials, 1985–2001. Leukemia. 2010;24(2):450–9.
68. Hagedorn N, Acquaviva C, Fronkova E, von Stackelberg A, Barth A, zur Stadt U, et al. Submicroscopic bone marrow involvement in isolated extramedullary relapses in childhood acute lymphoblastic leukemia: a more precise definition of "isolated" and its possible clinical implications, a collaborative study of the resistant disease Committee of the International BFM study group. Blood. 2007;110(12):4022–9.
69. Masurekar AN, Parker CA, Shanyinde M, Moorman AV, Hancock JP, Sutton R, et al. Outcome of central nervous system relapses in childhood acute lymphoblastic leukaemia--prospective open cohort analyses of the ALLR3 trial. PLoS One. 2014;9(10):e108107.
70. Nguyen HTK, Terao MA, Green DM, Pui CH, Inaba H. Testicular involvement of acute lymphoblastic leukemia in children and adolescents: diagnosis, biology, and management. Cancer. 2021;127(17):3067–81.
71. Barredo JC, Hastings C, Lu X, Devidas M, Chen Y, Armstrong D, et al. Isolated late testicular relapse of B-cell acute lymphoblastic leukemia treated with intensive systemic chemotherapy and response-based testicular radiation: a children's oncology group study. Pediatr Blood Cancer. 2018;65(5):e26928.
72. Oskarsson T, Söderhäll S, Arvidson J, Forestier E, Montgomery S, Bottai M, et al. Relapsed childhood acute lymphoblastic leukemia in the Nordic countries: prognostic factors, treatment and outcome. Haematologica. 2016;101(1):68–76.
73. Jacoby E, Ghorashian S, Vormoor B, De Moerloose B, Bodmer N, Molostova O, et al. CD19 CAR T-cells for pediatric relapsed acute lymphoblastic leukemia with active CNS involvement: a retrospective international study. Leukemia. 2022;36(6):1525–32.
74. Leahy AB, Newman H, Li Y, Liu H, Myers R, DiNofia A, et al. CD19-targeted chimeric antigen receptor T-cell therapy for CNS relapsed or refractory acute lymphocytic leukaemia: a post-hoc analysis of pooled data from five clinical trials. Lancet Haematol. 2021;8(10):e711–e22.
75. Nguyen K, Devidas M, Cheng SC, La M, Raetz EA, Carroll WL, et al. Factors influencing survival after relapse from acute lymphoblastic leukemia: a Children's oncology group study. Leukemia. 2008;22(12):2142–50.
76. Berg SL, Blaney SM, Devidas M, Lampkin TA, Murgo A, Bernstein M, et al. Phase II study of nelarabine (compound 506U78) in children and young

adults with refractory T-cell malignancies: a report from the Children's oncology group. J Clin Oncol. 2005;23(15):3376–82.
77. Whitlock JA, Malvar J, Dalla-Pozza L, Goldberg JM, Silverman LB, Ziegler DS, et al. Nelarabine, etoposide, and cyclophosphamide in relapsed pediatric T-acute lymphoblastic leukemia and T-lymphoblastic lymphoma (study T2008-002 NECTAR). Pediatr Blood Cancer. 2022;69(11):e29901.
78. Horton TM, Whitlock JA, Lu X, O'Brien MM, Borowitz MJ, Devidas M, et al. Bortezomib reinduction chemotherapy in high-risk ALL in first relapse: a report from the Children's oncology group. Br J Haematol. 2019;186(2):274–85.
79. Teachey DT, Devidas M, Wood BL, Chen Z, Hayashi RJ, Hermiston ML, et al. Children's oncology group trial AALL1231: a phase III clinical trial testing Bortezomib in newly diagnosed T-cell acute lymphoblastic leukemia and lymphoma. J Clin Oncol. 2022;40(19):2106–18.
80. von Stackelberg A, IntReALL HR. International Study for Treatment of High Risk Childhood Relapsed ALL 2010. 2010. https://www.ClinicalTrialsgov/show/NCT03590171.
81. Pullarkat VA, Lacayo NJ, Jabbour E, Rubnitz JE, Bajel A, Laetsch TW, et al. Venetoclax and Navitoclax in combination with chemotherapy in patients with relapsed or refractory acute lymphoblastic leukemia and lymphoblastic lymphoma. Cancer Discov. 2021;11(6):1440–53.
82. Burke MJ, Verneris MR, Le Rademacher J, He W, Abdel-Azim H, Abraham AA, et al. Transplant outcomes for children with T cell acute lymphoblastic leukemia in second remission: a report from the Center for International Blood and Marrow Transplant Research. Biol Blood Marrow Transplant. 2015;21(12):2154–9.
83. Richter-Pechańska P, Kunz JB, Hof J, Zimmermann M, Rausch T, Bandapalli OR, et al. Identification of a genetically defined ultra-high-risk group in relapsed pediatric T-lymphoblastic leukemia. Blood Cancer J. 2017;7(2):e523.
84. Network GCP. International proof of concept therapeutic stratification trial of molecular anomalies in relapsed or refractory HEMatological malignancies in children. 2023. https://www.ichgcpnet/clinical-trials-registry/NCT05740449.
85. Bride KL, Vincent TL, Im SY, Aplenc R, Barrett DM, Carroll WL, et al. Preclinical efficacy of daratumumab in T-cell acute lymphoblastic leukemia. Blood 2018;131(9):995–9.
86. Wang A, Song Z, Zheng G, Nicolazzi C, Fromm JR, Shehu E, et al. Evaluation of preclinical activity of Isatuximab in patients with acute lymphoblastic leukemia. Mol Cancer Ther. 2021;20(10):1916–25.
87. Lu P, Liu Y, Yang J, Zhang X, Yang X, Wang H, et al. Naturally selected CD7 CAR-T therapy without genetic manipulations for T-ALL/LBL: first-in-human phase 1 clinical trial. Blood. 2022;140(4):321–34.
88. Pan J, Tan Y, Wang G, Deng B, Ling Z, Song W, et al. Donor-derived CD7 chimeric antigen receptor T cells for T-cell acute lymphoblastic leukemia: first-in-human. Phase I Trial J Clin Oncol. 2021;39(30):3340–51.
89. Li S, Wang X, Yuan Z, Liu L, Luo L, Li Y, et al. Eradication of T-ALL cells by CD7-targeted universal CAR-T cells and initial test of Ruxolitinib-based CRS management. Clin Cancer Res. 2021;27(5):1242–6.
90. Chiesa R, Georgiadis C, Syed F, Zhan H, Etuk A, Gkazi SA, et al. Base-edited CAR7 T cells for relapsed T-cell acute lymphoblastic leukemia. N Engl J Med. 2023;389(10):899–910.
91. 2022-000186-40 EN. https://www.clinicaltrialsregister.eu/ctr-search/trial/2022-000186-40/BE#F. 2022.
92. Gandemer V, Chevret S, Petit A, Vermylen C, Leblanc T, Michel G, et al. Excellent prognosis of late relapses of ETV6/RUNX1-positive childhood acute lymphoblastic leukemia: lessons from the FRALLE 93 protocol. Haematologica. 2012;97(11):1743–50.
93. Gu J, Liu S, Cui W, Dai H, Cui Q, Yin J, et al. Identification of the predictive models for the treatment response of refractory/relapsed B-cell ALL patients receiving CAR-T therapy. Front Immunol. 2022;13:858590.
94. Leahy AB, Devine KJ, Li Y, Liu H, Myers R, DiNofia A, et al. Impact of high-risk cytogenetics on outcomes for children and young adults receiving CD19-directed CAR T-cell therapy. Blood. 2022;139(14):2173–85.
95. Gupta S, Sutradhar R, Pequeno P, Hitzler JK, Liu N, Nathan PC. Risks of late mortality and morbidity among survivors of childhood acute leukemia with down syndrome: a population-based cohort study. Cancer. 2022;128(6):1294–301.
96. Meyr F, Escherich G, Mann G, Klingebiel T, Kulozik A, Rossig C, et al. Outcomes of treatment for relapsed acute lymphoblastic leukaemia in children with down syndrome. Br J Haematol. 2013;162(1):98–106.
97. Laetsch TW, Maude SL, Balduzzi A, Rives S, Bittencourt H, Boyer MW, et al. Tisagenlecleucel in pediatric and young adult patients with down syndrome-associated relapsed/refractory acute lymphoblastic leukemia. Leukemia. 2022;36(6):1508–15.
98. Rabin K, Izraeli S, Hijiya N, Hitzler J. Need for new thinking: treatment of relapsed leukemia in children with down syndrome. Pediatr Blood Cancer. 2019;66(6):e27644.
99. Reismüller B, Peters C, Dworzak MN, Pötschger U, Urban C, Meister B, et al. Outcome of children and adolescents with a second or third relapse of acute lymphoblastic leukemia (ALL): a population-based analysis of the Austrian ALL-BFM (Berlin-Frankfurt-Münster) study group. J Pediatr Hematol Oncol. 2013;35(5):e200–4.

100. Stackelberg AV, Jäschke K, Jousseaume E, Templin C, Jeratsch U, Kosmides D, et al. Tisagenlecleucel vs. historical standard of care in children and young adult patients with relapsed/refractory B-cell precursor acute lymphoblastic leukemia. Leukemia. 2023;37(12):2346–55.
101. Laetsch TW, Maude SL, Rives S, Hiramatsu H, Bittencourt H, Bader P, et al. Three-year update of Tisagenlecleucel in pediatric and young adult patients with relapsed/refractory acute lymphoblastic leukemia in the ELIANA trial. J Clin Oncol. 2023;41(9):1664–9.
102. Teachey DT, Pui CH. Comparative features and outcomes between paediatric T-cell and B-cell acute lymphoblastic leukaemia. Lancet Oncol. 2019;20(3):e142–e54.

HSCT in the First CR and in the Subsequent CRs: Indications and Conditioning Regimens

17

Silvia Nucera, Francesca Limido, and Adriana Balduzzi

17.1 Hematopoietic Stem Cell Transplantation: Historical Perspective

Hematopoietic stem cell transplantation (HSCT) is the first cellular immunotherapy established in humans in 1955, by the group of the Nobel laureate E. Donnall Thomas. Despite an initial enthusiasm, all 200 patients transplanted between 1957 and 1967 eventually died [1]. This led to a temporary stop of the procedure and prompted intensive research studies, which allowed the discovery of HLA system, tissue compatibility and graft-versus-host disease (GvHD) in animal models. In 1968 HSCT was resumed and the first successful attempts were performed in patients with immune deficiencies. Only in the subsequent years, HSCT was applied to patients affected with hematological malignancies and aplastic anemia. Despite most HSCT were performed from HLA-identical siblings and despite prophylaxis with methotrexate, around 50% of the patients presented with GvHD. A first grading system for GvHD was proposed in 1974. In the same year the treatment with anti-thymoglobulin (ATG) for acute GvHD was also proposed [1, 2]. As the first attempts of HSCT for patients affected with acute leukemia were performed in patients with refractory disease, most patients subsequently died of relapse. The use of unrelated donors and of G-CSF-mobilized peripheral blood cells was implemented in the late 1980s. Progresses in supportive therapy, in particular for the management of infections, and the introduction of less toxic conditioning regimens (reduced intensity or reduced toxicity), were achieved in the 1990s and led to the tremendous expansion of the field [1]. Due to the significant improvements in patients' outcome, the number of total HSCT performed worldwide steadily increased in the last decades. In 2019 the number of HSCT performed worldwide reached 1.5 million, as reported by the Worldwide Network for Blood & Marrow Transplantation (WBMT). As will be discussed further in the chapter, the next challenge for HSCT will be to improve the outcome, particularly for malignant diseases, and reduce toxicity, both in terms of short-term morbidity as well as long-term sequelae.

17.1.1 Hematopoietic Stem Cell Transplantation for Acute Lymphoblastic Leukemia

HSCT may be indicated for a small proportion of patients with newly diagnosed ALL (in the first complete remission, CR1) and for the majority of

S. Nucera · F. Limido · A. Balduzzi (✉)
Tettamanti Center and Pediatrics, Fondazione IRCCS San Gerardo dei Tintori, Monza, Italy

School of Medicine and Surgery, University of Milano Bicocca, Milan, Italy
e-mail: silvia.nucera@unimib.it; f.limido@campus.unimib.it; adriana.balduzzi@unimib.it

G. Escherich, V. Conter (eds.), *Acute Lymphoblastic Leukemia in Children and Adolescents*, Pediatric Oncology, https://doi.org/10.1007/978-3-031-71180-0_17

those who achieve a CR after disease recurrence (the second complete remission or the third, CR2, CR3). The potential curative role of allogeneic HSCT is based both on the use of high dose chemo/radiotherapy and on the immunological activity of infused donor cells (graft vs. leukemia effect, GvL) [2].

As a general concept, the choice of the preparative regimen, which precedes the infusion of donor cells, is of pivotal importance for the outcome of HSCT [2]. It includes the conditioning regimen and the prophylaxis for graft-versus-host disease (GvHD), which mostly depends on type and compatibility of donor, and stem cell source. Together, these treatments are aimed to:

1. Eradicate residual malignant cells.
2. Provide sufficient immune suppression of the host, to ensure engraftment and prevent rejection of donor cells.
3. Create "room" in the stem cell niches of the recipient's bone marrow for the homing and the engraftment of donor stem cells.

17.2 Indications for HSCT in ALL

The indications for allogeneic HSCT in childhood ALL have evolved over time, driven both by improvements in treatment outcome by chemotherapy regimens and a better understanding of risk factors. This includes innovative methods for detecting minimal residual disease (MRD), allowing to tailor the intensity of therapy based on the risk status of each patient and incorporate novel agents in the upfront treatment.

When a matched donor, either an HLA-identical sibling (MSD) or a matched unrelated donor (MUD) is not available, alternative donor sources, like cord blood (CB), mismatched unrelated donors (MMUD), or haploidentical family donors (MMD) become valuable clinical options, nowadays with promising results [3–7].

17.2.1 Indications for HSCT in ALL-CR1

Patients who are eligible for HSCT in CR1 are only those with high-risk cytogenetic features and/or inadequate response to chemotherapy, which can be defined by levels of MRD at the end of induction or consolidation phase. Leukemia features associated with high-risk (HR) include *KMT2A-AFF1* [t(4;11), *MLL-AF4*], low hypodiploidy, gene fusion *TCF3-HLF* [t(17;19)], and the combination of *IKZF1* deletion co-occurring with any of *CDKN2A* or *CDKN2B* (only homozygous deletions), *PAX5*, and/or *PAR1* (*CRLF2*) in the absence of *ERG* deletions (*IKZF1*plus).

Most study groups define these patients based on an estimated event-free survival (EFS) probability lower than 50%, considering specific biological features and response to treatment. The main study groups present some differences in HSCT indications, which will be discussed in this paragraph. However, the different protocols agree on some aspects that have been established by previous trials.

Of note, a cooperative prospective study from Balduzzi et al. assessed the advantages in terms of survival on a cohort of 357 children diagnosed between 1995 and 2000 with very high risk (VHR) ALL (including T-cell immunophenotype with poor prednisone response (PPR) or PPR with WBC $\geq 100 \times 10^9$/L at diagnosis; positivity for t(9;22) or t(4;11)). The patients were assigned to the HSCT arm based on the availability of an HLA-matched related donor or chemotherapy (genetic randomization). The study showed a benefit from transplantation, with a significant improvement of 5-year disease-free survival (DFS) after transplant compared to chemotherapy alone (57% vs. 41%, hazard ratio 0·67). Among patients with T-ALL, HSCT was associated with a 5-year DFS of 62%, versus 54% in the chemotherapy arm [8].

In the AIEOP-BFM (Associazione Italiana Ematologia Oncologia Pediatrica—Berlin–Frankfurt–Münster) ALL 2017 trial, the eligibility to HSCT depends on a combination of genetic background of the disease and MRD response. Patients with translocation t(17;19), resulting in the *TCF3-HLF* fusion transcript, represent a rare subset with low sensitivity to conventional chemotherapy and a dismal prognosis with 100% mortality in previous patients' cohorts but a good response to blinatumomab [9, 10]. In these cases,

Table 17.1 Current indications for hematopoietic stem cell transplant (HSCT) in the AIEOP-BFM ALL 2017 study

	PCR-MRD TP1 negative	PCR-MRD TP1 or TP2 positive and TP2 < 5×10^{-4}	PCR-MRD TP2 ≥ 5×10^{-4} and < 5×10^{-3}	PCR-MRD TP2 ≥ 5×10^{-3}	No PCR-MRD result
TCF3-HLF	MMD	MMD	MMD	MMD	MMD
No CR d33	No	MD	MMD	MMD	MMD
KMT2A-AFF1	No	MD	MD	MMD	MD
Hypodiploidy <44 chr or DNA index <0.8	No	MD	MD	MMD	MD
*IKZF*plus and FCM-MRD d15 ≥ 10%	No	MD	MD	MMD	MD
*IKZF*plus and FCM-MRD d15 < 10%	No	No	MD	MMD	MD
T-ALL + PPR and/or FCM-MRD d15 ≥ 10%	No	No	MD	MMD	MD
None of above features	No	No	MD	MMD	No

AIEOP-BFM Associazione Italiana Ematologia Oncologia Pediatrica—Berlin–Frankfurt–Münster, *MRD* minimal residual disease, *PCR* polymerase chain reaction, *FCM* flow cytometry, *MD* matched donor, *MMD* mismatched donor, *TP1* time point 1, *TP2* time point 2, *CR* complete remission, *d33* day 33, *d15* day 15, *PPR* prednisone poor response, *FCM-MRD d15* flow cytometry MRD on day 15

Table 17.2 Current indications for hematopoietic stem cell transplant (HSCT) by cooperative study group COG (Children's Oncology Group)

B-ALL	
	Hypodiploidy + EOC MRD positive
	IF + EOC MRD detectable
	HR + EOC MRD detectable
	SR + EOC MRD ≥1%
T-ALL	
	EOC MRD ≥ 0,1%
	IF

ALL acute lymphoblastic leukemia, EOC, end of consolidation, *MRD* minimal residual disease, *HR* high-risk, *SR* standard-risk, *IF* induction failure

early consideration of HSCT from a matched donor (MD) or MMD is warranted as soon as CR is achieved, regardless of MRD response.

For the other categories (i.e. *KMT2A-AFF1* gene fusion, hypodiploidy, *IKFZ*plus, T-ALL with poor prednisone response or primary induction failure -PIF), the indications to HSCT and the type of donor vary according to MRD with MD preferred over MMD as shown in Table 17.1.

As shown in Table 17.2, according to the Children's Oncology Group (COG), MRD positivity at end of consolidation (EOC) is the most prominent prognostic factor in combination with genetic features or immune-phenotype. This is because patients exhibiting EOC MRD <0.01% have a superior 5-year survival rate of 79%, as opposed to those with ≥0.01%, who have a survival rate of 39% [11, 12]. Besides HSCT, a subset of patients with B-lineage ALL may qualify for participation in a currently ongoing phase II study evaluating the use of commercial anti-CD19 CAR T cells (tisagenlecleucel) for patients with high MRD (flow-MRD >10^{-4}) at the EOC (CASSIOPEIA study, NCT03876769).

For the COG, T-ALL with EOC MRD > 0.1% constitutes an indication for HSCT. This differs from the approach of the AIEOP-BFM group which designates patients with T-cell ALL as high risk if they present additional features such as PPR, FCM-MRD d15 ≥ 10% blasts, non-remission on day 33 (d33) in adjunction to PCR-MRD on day 78 (d78) ≥5×10^{-4}.

The ALLTogether1 protocol (ATP) marks the inaugural clinical investigation (NCT03911128) formulated by the collaborative ALLTogether consortium, working collaboratively to establish a standardized European treatment protocol. This consortium comprises the study groups from the Nordic countries NOPHO (Sweden, Denmark, Norway, Finland, Iceland, Lithuania, and Estonia), UKALL (the UK), DCOG (the Netherlands), COALL (Germany), BSPHO (Belgium), PHOAI (Ireland), SHOP (Portugal), and SFCE (France) [13]. According to this proto-

Table 17.3 Current indications for hematopoietic stem cell transplant (HSCT) by cooperative study group ALLTogether1 protocol

All patients	
	MRD ≥0.05% at TP2
B-ALL	
	MRD ≥5% at TP1 and ≥ 0.5% at TP1.5 (d50)
	Patients with t(17;19)/*TCF3-HLF*, irrespective of MRD levels
	Age ≥ 16 years at diagnosis and *KMT2A* rearrangement
	Age ≥ 16 years at diagnosis with any high-risk criterion: MRD ≥5% at TP1 MRD ≥0.01% at TP2
	Patients with increasing MRD following CAR-T treatment in CASSIOPEIA
T-ALL	
	MRD ≥5% at TP1 and ≥ 0.5% at TP1.5
	Age < 16 years, MRD ≥5% at TP1, <0.5% TP1.5 but detectable at TP2
	Patients with extramedullary disease that has not responded adequately by TP2
	Age ≥ 16 years at diagnosis with MRD ≥5% at TP1

MRD minimal residual disease, *TP2* time point 2, *TP1* time point 1, *TP1.5* time point 1.5, *d50* day 50, *CAR* chimeric antigen receptor

col, all patients with MRD ≥0.05% at TP2 (day 71/78) have indications for HSCT, independently from other characteristics. The same applies for patients with *TCF3-HLF* rearrangement, as for the AIEOP-BFM protocol. In this protocol, differently from COG and AIEOP-BFM age > 16 is also accounted for *KMT2A*-rearranged patients and for HR patients, both for B-ALL and T-ALL. Specific characteristics are shown in Table 17.3.

17.2.2 Indications for HSCT in ALL-CR2

The management of relapsed ALL continues to pose significant challenges, with survival rates significantly lower than those of first-line treatment [14]. Despite some progress in outcomes over the past few decades, approximately half of the children experiencing the first relapse of ALL achieve long-term survival, and the prognosis becomes dismal with second or subsequent relapses [14].

Risk stratification for relapsed ALL considers factors such as the time elapsed from diagnosis to relapse (very early, early or late relapse), the presence of bone marrow and/or extramedullary involvement (BM isolated, combined or extramedullary isolated), and immunophenotype (B or T) [15–17]. The treatment strategy for the population at poor prognosis aims to achieve a second CR through intensive chemotherapy and consolidate it by HSCT to improve DFS. As for frontline treatment, MRD has a crucial prognostic impact also on relapsed ALL as patients who undergo HSCT with high levels of MRD experience poor outcome [18]. Therefore, novel approaches to reduce disease burden (MRD negativity or < 0.01%), such as immunotherapy, are warranted [14, 19].

Immunophenotype impacts on prognosis, as relapsed T-ALL carries a significantly worse outcome compared to B-ALL, with relapsed T-ALL being associated with 25% survival [14, 20, 21]. Due to the unsatisfactory outcome of patients with T-cell ALL relapse treated solely with chemotherapy, HSCT has become the standard approach in most collaborative groups. However, the success of HSCT relies on achieving remission through reinduction therapy.

The IntReALL (International study for treatment of childhood relapsed ALL 2010 with standard therapy, systematic integration of new agents, and establishment of standardized diagnostic and research) 2010 study, identifies two categories: standard (SR) and high-risk (HR) relapse. According to this protocol, HSCT should be considered for any child displaying HR features. In this category, MRD impacts on the choice of donor. For SR patients, the indication to HSCT depends on timing and MRD response, as shown in Table 17.4.

The indications from the COG are consistent with those from IntReALL protocol, matching the site of relapse and MRD response but do not take into account the timing of relapse as shown in Table 17.5.

Table 17.4 Current indications for hematopoietic stem cell transplant (HSCT) by IntReALL 2010 protocol in CR2 (second complete remission)

SR		EOI MRD neg	EOI MRD positive	No EOI MRD result
	Late isolated or combined BM relapse B-ALL	No	MMD	MD
	Early combined BM relapse	MD	MMD	MMD
		Time of relapse		
		Early	Late	
	Isolated extramedullary	MD	No	
HR				
	Very early isolated extramedullary relapse of B-ALL or T-ALL	MD or MMD		
	Early isolated or any very early BM relapse of B-ALL	MD or MMD		
	Any BM relapse of T-ALL	MD or MMD		
	Time point of relapse:			
	Very early: < 18 months after primary diagnosis and < 6 months after completion of primary therapy			
	Early: ≥ 18 months after primary diagnosis and < 6 months after completion of primary therapy			
	Late: ≥ 6 months after completion of primary therapy			

MRD minimal residual disease, *ALL* acute lymphoblastic leukemia, *HR* high risk, *SR* standard risk, *MD* matched donor, *MMD* mismatched donor, *EOI* end of induction, *BM* bone marrow

Table 17.5 Current indications for hematopoietic stem cell transplant (HSCT) by cooperative study group COG (Children's Oncology Group) in CR2 (second complete remission)

B-ALL	
	Extramedullary relapse: Early or late with EOI MRD > 0,1%
	Marrow relapse: Early or late with EOI MRD > 0,1%
T-ALL	
	Any relapse

MRD minimal residual disease, *ALL* acute lymphoblastic leukemia

17.2.3 CR3 or More

All working groups agree on the eligibility for HSCT of all patients with ALL in third complete remission (CR3) or higher, despite the significantly increased risk of subsequent relapse, irrespective of the type of available donor [22].

Given the unfavorable outcome associated with a second relapse, alternative potentially curative therapies, such as CAR T-cell therapy or innovative immunotherapies, have emerged. However, the decision for subsequent HSCT as a consolidation therapy depends on factors such as the longevity of CAR T-cells post-infusion.

17.2.4 Philadelphia Chromosome-Positive (Ph+) ALL

The introduction of tyrosine kinase inhibitors (TKIs) together with intensive chemotherapy significantly improved Philadelphia chromosome-positive (Ph+) ALL outcome, allowing to achieve complete remission. This has reduced the role of HSCT in Ph + ALL and Philadelphia chromosome-like (Ph-like) ALL [23–25]. The indications for HSCT in the main pediatric protocols are based on MRD response and are summarized in Table 17.6.

In the EsPhALL 2017/ COGAALL1631 (NCT00287105) study, HSCT for consolidating remission in patients with Ph + or ABL-class fusion ALL patients is currently reserved for patients with MRD $\geq 5 \times 10^{-4}$ at EOC. In the ALLTogether 1 protocol, in patients with ABL-class fusions HSCT is instead indicated in cases with: 1) MRD ≥5% at TP1 (day 29) and rising at mid-consolidation (day 50); 2) MRD ≥0.05% at TP2 (day 71/78) [23, 26].

17.2.5 Infants

The Interfant-06 Study indicates HSCT for patients <6 months at diagnosis with WBC >300 × 10 [9]/L or exhibiting poor prednisone response. For these categories, MRD impacts on the choice of donor, while for patients who do not

Table 17.6 Current indications for hematopoietic stem cell transplant (HSCT) indications in Philadelphia-chromosome–positive (Ph+) ALL according to ALLTogether1 protocol and EsPhALL protocol

EsPhALL	ALLTogether1
EOC MRD $\geq 5 \times 10^{-4}$	MRD ≥5% at TP1 and rising at TP1.5
EOC MRD $< 5 \times 10^{-4}$ and positive at any level at end of HR3	MRD ≥0.05% at TP2

EsPhALL European study for pediatric Ph + ALL, *EOC* end of consolidation, *MRD* minimal residual disease, *TP1* time point 1, *TP1.5* time point 1.5 (day 50), *TP2* time point 2, *HR3* high-risk block 3

Table 17.7 Current indications for hematopoietic stem cell transplant (HSCT) for infants <1 year of age by Interfant 06 and COG (Children's Oncology Group)

Interfant-06	COG
KMT2A-AFF1 rearrangement	*KMT2A-AFF1* rearrangement
Age < 6 months and WBC ≥300.000/μl	EOC MRD positive
Age < 6 months and PPR	

WBC white blood cells, *EOC* end of consolidation, *MRD* minimal residual disease, *PPR* prednisone poor response

display the aforementioned features, the indication to HSCT depends on MRD response at EOC. While there is no definitive indication for HSCT in infant ALL COG Protocol, the HR group, characterized by *KMT2A* rearrangement and age less than 3 months at diagnosis, exhibits a survival rate as low as 20% [27]. Consequently, HSCT is frequently recommended in CR1 for individuals in this group who have positive MRD [27]. The indications to HSCT for infants are summarized in Tables 17.7 and 17.8.

A recent report from the FORUM trial compared treosulfan-based conditioning with busulfan-based conditioning for children below 4 years of age showing basically no difference between the two regimens except for a slight reduction in low-grade GvHD and survival for the treosulfan group which has to be further investigated [28].

In conclusion, among patients with ALL, infants remain the group with the worst prognosis. However, the advent of novel approaches will increase the probability for these patients to undergo HSCT with MRD negativity and this may in the end improve their outcome.

Table 17.8 Elements influencing immune reconstitution following hematopoietic stem cell transplantation (HSCT) and their impact on the process of immune recovery

Factor	Comment
Patient's age at HSCT	Younger patients have improved IR
Donor age	Younger donor cells show better engraftment and reduced NRM
Conditioning regimen	MAC regimens impair IR TBI directly damages thymus
Stem cell source	PBSCs are associated with faster T-cell recovery compared to BM and UCB UCB contains mostly antigen inexperienced naïve T cells
GvHD prophylaxis	ATLG severely impairs IR and damages thymic cells PTCy selectively spares Treg vs T conv. With ex vivo αβ T/CD19 cell depletion γδ T cells and NKs are the dominating subsets after HSCT
Acute or chronic GvHD	Steroids jeopardize lymphocyte, especially CD4, recovery

HSCT hematopoietic stem cell transplantation, *IR* immune reconstitution, *NRM* non-relapse mortality, *MAC* myeloablative conditioning, *TBI* total body irradiation, *PBSC* peripheral blood stem cell, *BM* bone marrow, *UCB* umbilical cord blood, *GvHD* graft-versus-host disease, *ATLG* anti-T lymphocyte globulin, *PTCy* post-transplantation cyclophosphamide

17.2.6 HSCT in Down Syndrome Patients

HSCT for Down syndrome (DS) patients with ALL is still a controversial matter. Data in literature show a post-HSCT survival rate of 19–48% [29, 30]. Death is mostly related to ALL relapse (often secondary to scarce pre-HSCT disease control) or treatment related mortality (TRM). Reducing intensity of conditioning regimen may reduce TRM but would increase relapse rate which is already high. Interestingly, one retrospective study where patients received methotrexate-based GvHD prophylaxis observed an incidence of GvHD of 90% [29]. On the other hand, when GvHD prophylaxis is based on other drugs the incidence of acute GvHD is around 30% as well as the chronic GvHD [30]. This may in part be linked to the reduced effectiveness of dose-adjusted prophylaxis with methotrexate but may also be in part related to the defective immune reconstitution due to preexisting thymic dysfunction intrinsic to DS. Furthermore, DS patients often display congenital heart defects or preexisting thyroid dysfunction, which may contribute to additional morbidity. Therefore, HSCT cannot be a standard option for DS-ALL patients. In particular, some front-line protocols such as the ALLTogether-1 do not stratify DS patients to HSCT in CR1 [26]. Alternative treatments such as CAR-T cells seem to be more promising than HSCT in this patients' category. A recent report showed that DS-ALL patients treated with tisagenlecleucel achieved comparable efficacy and safety outcomes as a cohort of patients without DS from the ELIANA trial [31].

17.2.7 HSCT in Li–Fraumeni Syndrome and Cancer Predisposition

Among cancer predisposition syndromes (CPS), Li–Fraumeni syndrome (LFS, MIM#151623) is the most common. LFS is a dominantly inherited condition caused by pathogenic germline variants in the *TP53* tumor suppressor gene. Children with LFS are predisposed to different neoplasms such as osteosarcoma, adrenocortical carcinoma, medulloblastoma, choroid plexus carcinoma, anaplastic rhabdomyosarcoma, and acute lymphoblastic leukemia [32].

Most frequently, in LFS ALL is characterized by hypodiploidy which is a high-risk feature and may pose the indication for HSCT, according to MRD response, in most treatment protocols.

In the past, hypodiploidy *per se* was a criterion for HSCT in CR1, due to the dismal prognosis [33, 34]. St. Jude Total Therapy studies (NCT00137111 and NCT00549848), however, showed that hypodiploid ALL patients achieving negative MRD at the end of induction (EOI) had a 5-year EFS of 85%, compared to 44% in patients with detectable MRD, suggesting that chemotherapy alone can effectively cure patients with hypodiploid ALL and that MRD is the most crucial prognostic indicator for childhood hypodiploid ALL [35]. Therefore nowadays, HSCT is no longer automatically recommended for patients with hypodiploidy in CR1.

In low-hypodiploid ALL, *TP53* mutations are present in the leukemic blasts of more than 90% of patients and nearly half of them are germline, which makes hypodiploid ALL a manifestation of Li–Fraumeni syndrome (LFS) [36]. Children with ALL and LFS have a dismal prognosis compared to the other children, with inferior event-free survival, disease- free survival and higher incidence of secondary neoplasms [32].

As studies on LFS patients are not available comparing HSCT outcome and conditioning regimens, these data can be inferred from hypodiploid ALL. A recent study on 131 pediatric patients with hypodiploid ALL from the COG showed that HSCT (with TBI-based conditioning regimen) did not improve the outcome of the patients in CR1 compared to those who did not undergo HSCT (with similar features and response to therapy) [36]. Besides, 12/61 patients undergoing HSCT developed secondary malignancies, compared to 3/52 who did not undergo HSCT. Comparable results derive from a parallel study on 272 patients from the Ponte di Legno Study Group [37]. Therefore, in hypodiploid patients, HSCT in CR1 may be substituted by immunotherapy with CAR-T cells [38]. It has to be established if CAR-T can offer an advantage in terms of survival and reduced toxicity.

The indication for HSCT in relapsed hypodiploid ALL poses an additional question as hypodiploid patients who relapse are more likely to undergo genetic screening for TP53 mutations (also due to an increased alertness toward the LFS), which rises the concern about secondary malignancies. Indeed, the choice of the best conditioning regimen for this patients' category is still a matter of debate. Ad hoc studies are needed to establish the correct indications and conditioning regimens for HSCT in LFS patients.

17.3 Considerations on the Choice of Donor in the Era of MMD

The prospective multicentric ALL SCT 2003 BFM trial (alongside with subsequent ALL SCT 2007 I-BFM trial, which is the international extension of the former to multiple Countries) was conducted to establish which type of donor would be the best for pediatric ALL patients [39, 40]. In particular, the study compared the outcome of 411 patients undergoing HSCT from a MSD or a highly compatible (9/10 or 10/10) MUD. Importantly, this trial established that, despite differences in engraftment kinetics and chronic GvHD incidence, patients undergoing HSCT from MSD or MUD had a similar overall survival, event-free survival and relapse incidence regardless of primary disease relapse risk [39].

A subsequent work from the BFM group compared the outcome of 148 patients undergoing HSCT from a MMD for high-risk and very high-risk patients. This study established that for high-risk patients undergoing HSCT from MMD the outcome is similar to high-risk patients undergoing HSCT from highly compatible MUD or MSD [41].

The use of MMD has increased in recent years due to the advent of improved supportive therapy and GvHD management. MMD HSCT donor availability for virtually all recipients is particularly important for ethnic groups scarcely represented in the worldwide donor registries. Furthermore, an easier availability of second donations for stem cell boosts, donor lymphocyte infusions or other cell products is almost invariably granted, as donors are most often parents, sometimes siblings or, more rarely, other close relatives to the patients.

However, the use of MMD has been historically hampered by the high incidence of severe GvHD. In order to overcome the alloreactivity of mismatched donor T cells, two different approaches aimed at eliminating donor alloreactive T cells have been developed: *in vivo* or *ex vivo* T-cell depletion. *Ex vivo* depletion is mainly based on selective elimination of TCR αβ T cell and CD19 B cells from the graft before infusion; as for *in vivo* T-cell depletion there are two major protocols: one is based on the administration of cyclophosphamide after transplant (PTCy), while the other is based on the administration of anti-thymocyte globulin (ATG; Beijing protocol) [42]. The use of αβ T/CD19-cell depletion in pediatric patients with ALL was shown for the first time by Locatelli and coworkers [43] in a single center phase I-II clinical trial (NCT01810120) on 80 patients whose outcome was comparable to an historical cohort of MUD and MSD from the same Center as well as from multiple Italian centers [44]. A follow-up study with additional 133 patients affected by ALL or acute myeloid leukemia (AML) recently confirmed similar findings as the previous study [45]. Consistently, a multicentric trial on pediatric and adult patients confirmed the feasibility of in vitro αβ T cell/CD19 depletion [46].

A different approach is based on *in vivo* T-cell depletion with administration of PTCy, in particular cyclophosphamide 50 mg/kg on days 3 and 4 (or days 3 and 5) after graft infusion. Initially applied in adult patients after reduced intensity conditioning [47], PTCy has recently been applied also in pediatric patients with acute leukemia. A multicentric retrospective trial showed the results of PTCy MMD transplant in 180 pediatric patients with ALL [48]. The reported incidence of GvHD is similar with the two T cell depletion approaches, ranging from 14 to 50% in the different studies, being mostly grade I–II [43, 46, 48]. One study even observed that the incidence of cGvHD is inferior with PTCy compared to matched donor HSCT in adult patients [49]. In terms of disease relapse, no differences are observed among the different studies, as it emerges that disease status prior to HSCT is the main predictor of subsequent relapse.

A third approach for *in vivo* T-cell depletion is the Beijing protocol, which is based on high-dose ATG and intense immune suppression with cyclosporin, mycophenolate, and methotrexate for G-CSF mobilized grafts. This protocol is mostly applied to MMD but can also be applied to other types of donors, such as MSD or MUD. Furthermore, MMD HSCT within the Beijing protocol was directly compared to standard MSD HSCT in ALL patients resulting in a superior outcome in terms of disease control.

As no direct comparison in a prospective randomized trial comparing the different MMD approaches is available, Kleinschmidt and coworkers recently reviewed the characteristics of the three platforms which result comparable in terms of outcome in ALL patients [42]. Despite this, the *in vivo* T-cell depletion is associated with a slightly shorter time to neutrophil and platelet engraftment compared to *ex vivo* T-cell depletion. On the other hand, the immune reconstitution pattern is significantly different between the two platforms. In the first 2–3 months after *ex vivo* αβ T/CD19-cell depletion lymphocytes are mainly constituted by natural killer cells (NKs) and γδ T cells which show a reduced GvHD potential but retain an anti-leukemic effect [42, 50, 51]. This is not the case for PTCy where CD3+ T-cell counts are significantly higher. PTCy selectively depletes proliferating T cells (which are mostly autoreactive T cells), while donor-derived naive T cells are not affected [42]. Furthermore, several studies suggest that among T cells that are spared by PTCy, there are T regulatory cells (Tregs) and an increased percentage of Tregs on the total T cells may help inducing tolerance.

Interestingly, the PTCy platform has been extended to other donors, in particular to MUD in adult patients receiving reduced intensity conditioning where PTCy proved superior to previously used GvHD prophylaxes [52]. However, a large study on 2320 adult patients showed that when using a myeloablative conditioning for malignant diseases (not only ALL) the outcome of PTCy MUD is slightly superior to PTCy MMD particularly in terms of GvHD, while no difference is observed in the incidence of relapse [53]. The authors therefore conclude that, if possible, MUD is still preferable to MMD. A similar prospective study should be performed in pediatric patients to establish which GvHD prophylaxis is the best for MUD and to compare the outcomes of MUD vs MMD with the same GvHD prophylaxis.

In the end, the choice of donor for ALL patients depends primarily on the indication for HSCT. If a matched donor (MSD or 9–10/10 MUD) is available, this is usually the first choice, particularly for patients in CR1, for whom most front-line protocols limit the application of MMD to very high-risk patients. For patients in CR2 or CR3, the indication for donor usually includes also MMD. In the next few years, however, it is very likely that the indications for MMD will increase also to high-risk patients in CR1, whenever a MUD was not available or when timing and date flexibility were an issue for a successful HSCT.

17.4 Choice of the Conditioning Regimen

The choice of the conditioning regimen depends on the primary indication for HSCT and patients' characteristics, mainly age and comorbidities. For children and adolescents with ALL, fully myeloablative conditionings are historically based on fractionated TBI (12 Gy in six fractions over 3 days, with or without lung shielding at 10 Gy) associated with chemotherapeutic drugs [39] for children above 2 years of age. On the other hand, for children below 2 years of age conditioning regimen was TBI-free, mainly based on busulfan, in combination with cyclophosphamide (120 mg/kg total dose) and etoposide (40 mg/kg total dose). The TBI-based conditioning regimen, associated with intravenous etoposide 60 mg/kg (upper total dose: 3600 mg), has been extensively evaluated in the ALL SCT 2003 BFM and ALL SCT 2007 I-BFM trials [39, 41, 54]. However, due to the impact of TBI on children, in particular in terms of long-term toxicities, a prospective randomized trial (Eudract no. 2012–003032-22, ClinicalTrials.gov: NCT01949129) was designed to evaluate the outcome after TBI-based versus chemotherapy-based conditioning regimens in patients over 4 years of age with ALL. The For Omitting Radiation Under Majority age (FORUM) trial indeed showed in the 413 patients randomized to TBI vs chemo-based conditioning regimens (busulfan- or treosulfan-based) a 2-year overall survival of 91% vs 75% (P 0.0001), cumulative incidence of relapse of 12% versus 33% (P 0.0001), treatment-related mortality of 2% vs 9% (P 0.0269) event free survival of 86% versus 58%, respectively [55]. These data led to the early discontinuation of random assignment for the study in 2019. Currently, TBI is the gold standard for children at least >4 years of age with high-risk ALL undergoing HSCT.

As for the youngest patients, the FORUM trial recommended chemotherapy-based conditioning regimens (either busulfan based or treosulfan according to the country of origin) under 4 years of age. The choice to avoid TBI for this category of patients relies mostly on the expected long-term toxicity associated with TBI.

17.4.1 Pharmacokinetics to Guide Conditioning Regimens

The application in the last two decades of real-time therapeutic drug monitoring (TDM) and dose adjustment for certain drugs, in particular busulfan, is currently routinely performed in most centers as it minimizes the risk of transplant-related complications, as well as of rejection. Busulfan has a narrow therapeutic window and high pharmacokinetic variability. Furthermore, initially, busulfan was administered orally, which increased the variability in the bioavailability for the patients, in particular for pediatric patients [56]. This had a significant impact on the incidence of complications and toxicities. To control busulfan exposure, the therapeutic window for busulfan recommended by the European Medicines Agency (EMA) is AUC6h 900–1500 μM·min. Doses >1500 μM·min are associated with a high incidence of sinusoidal obstruction syndrome (SOS) and acute GvHD, while doses <900 μM·min are associated with a higher incidence of relapse [56, 57]. As busulfan is mainly metabolized by glutathione-S-transferases (*GST*s), several studies have addressed the influence of genetic polymorphisms of *GST* on busulfan pharmacokinetics.

The association of these haplotypes with busulfan pharmacokinetics (PK) are still under investigation, but it appears clear that some haplotypes are associated with lower expression and others are associated with increased busulfan clearance.

In the last decade, treosulfan, an analogue of busulfan with an improved toxicity profile, has replaced busulfan in most conditioning regimens. Treosulfan is a prodrug that is metabolized into its monoepoxybutane (S,S-EBDM) and diepoxybutane (S,S-DEB) derivatives through nonenzymatic and pH-sensitive nucleophilic substitution. The toxicity profile for treosulfan is reportedly favorable compared to busulfan since the nonenzymatic transformation to biologically active metabolites occurs spontaneously under physiological conditions, bypassing hepatic metabolism and reducing the incidence of SOS [58, 59]. EMA authorized the use of treosulfan in conditioning regimens in adults and children >1 month of age in 2019.

The FORUM trial constituted the first large-scale study on the use of treosulfan in pediatric patients with ALL. Despite its favorable profile, in clinical practice, treosulfan administration is not routinely guided by pharmacokinetics in most centers. However, several studies associate Treosulfan exposure with early toxicity [58–61]. The recommended AUC for treosulfan is 3863 and 6037 mg·h/L [62]. A prospective study on a pediatric cohort of patients undergoing HSCT for nonmalignant and malignant conditions showed that, in patients receiving similar conditioning regimens, an AUC > 6000 mg·h/L is associated with a significantly higher transplant-related mortality. We expect that in the next few years, data from PK studies on treosulfan from the FORUM trial will shed light on the correct dosing for treosulfan and will define whether pharmakokinetics-based dosing of treosulfan, in a chemo-based conditioning regimen, may improve HSCT outcome. Whether such an outcome might equal the outcome achieved with a TBI-based conditioning will need to be addressed.

Clofarabine, a purine nucleoside analogue with anti-tumor activity, is approved for the treatment of children (<21 years) with relapsed or refractory ALL and was recently added to busulfan and fludarabine in the conditioning regimen for HSCT in pediatric hematological malignancies. Like treosulfan, also clofarabine is a prodrug that is metabolized intracellularly by phosphorylation. Optimal PK for clofarabine is meant to prevent graft rejection and excessive toxicity [63].

Overall, the development of personalized dosing in conditioning regimens will improve the outcomes of patients by sparing toxicity and graft failure compared to non-PK guided regimens. These data will need direct comparison with TBI to evaluate whether it was possible to spare children irradiation without increasing ALL relapse risk.

17.4.2 Impact of Conditioning Regimens on Post-HSCT Immune Reconstitution

A rapid and effective post-HSCT immune reconstitution (IR) significantly impacts on patient outcome as a poor or slow IR increases the risk of infections and disease relapse. IR occurs in different stages. The first subsets that recover after HSCT are myeloid cells (including monocytes and dendritic cells) and natural killer cells (NKs). Adaptive immunity recovers more slowly, with B cell and CD8 T cell numbers normalizing between 3 and 6 months after HSCT. The expansion of T and B cells in the first months after HSCT occurs mostly by peripheral expansion, which means that donor-derived lymphocytes proliferate to compensate the profound lymphopenia of the patient. This gives rise to oligoclonal T-cell receptor (TCR) and B-cell receptor (BCR) repertoire but allows a first line of protection from infections. Finally, thymic-dependent T cell reconstitution, particularly for the CD4 T cell compartment, may occur between 6 and 9 months after HSCT or later, depending on when tapering and discontinuation of immunosuppressants might take place [64].

There are several variables that impact on post-HSCT IR, some are intrinsic to the transplant, others depend on the specific development of complications. Table 17.8 summarizes the most widely known factors impacting on post-HSCT IR and how they influence immune recovery.

17.4.2.1 Patient Age and Donor Age

Both donor and recipient (patient) ages are important for immunological recovery and outcome post-HSCT. As thymic function physiologically declines with age, it is not surprising that a younger recipient age is correlated to improved thymus-dependent immune recovery after HSCT. However, also donor's age is an important risk factor for non-relapse mortality. Pediatric patients receiving grafts from younger donors have faster T-cell reconstitution (particularly for the CD4 T-cell subset), reduced risk of fungal infections, and higher disease-free survival. Older donor age is associated with lower naive CD4 T-cell counts on days +30 and + 80 after HSCT [65].

17.4.2.2 Conditioning Regimen

The process of IR is also influenced by conditioning regimen, including intensity of chemotherapy, use of radiation, and use of serotherapy. Overall, IR after myeloablative conditioning (MAC) is impaired compared to reduced intensity conditionings (RIC). As aforementioned, after the results of the FORUM trials, most ALL patients receive TBI-based conditioning, which is known to damage the thymus and impair its function, which is essential for full T cell reconstitution. In murine models, sublethal irradiation induces direct damage to thymic epithelium, including medullary epithelial cells (mTECs), which are important in negative selection. Thus, damage to mTEC may result in profound defects in central tolerance [65–67]. Besides direct damage to the epithelium, lymphoid progenitors contained in the thymus are also directly affected by radiation and undergo massive apoptosis [68].

17.4.2.3 Stem Cell Source

For HSCT, the stem cell graft can be derived from bone marrow (BM), peripheral blood (PB) or umbilical cord blood (UCB). Stem cell source impacts on the kinetics of engraftment and immune reconstitution. In particular, unmanipulated PB grafts contain a significantly higher number of lymphocytes (T and B cells) compared to BM and UCB grafts. On the other hand, UCB contains the lowest number of T cells, mostly immature. Besides intrinsic differences among the source, the GvHD prophylaxis used also differs according to the graft source, with PB grafts requiring a more intensive immune suppression to control donor-derived T cell activity. HSCT with UCB is associated with higher naive and memory B cell counts at 6 months after HCT compared to BM and PB grafts. In contrast, T cell reconstitution is delayed after UCB HCT, due to the lower initial T cell content and to the fact that UCB contains antigen-inexperienced naive T cells; therefore, T cell recovery is entirely thymic-dependent and consequently delayed. Furthermore, patients who receive UCB grafts have a slower recovery of thymopoiesis than patients receiving BM stem cells reflecting a lower thymic-derived naïve CD4 T cells at 6 months post HSCT. T cell reconstitution also differs between BM and PB recipients, with PB grafts being associated with faster lymphocyte recovery, in particular for CD4 T cells [64].

17.4.2.4 GvHD Prophylaxis

Preventing GvHD is of pivotal importance for the success of HSCT. Nevertheless, drugs used for GvHD prophylaxis significantly impact also on immune reconstitution. Drugs that have been historically used for GvHD prophylaxis include methotrexate, calcineurin inhibitors (including cyclosporin, tacrolimus, or sirolimus) and mycophenolate (MMF). These drugs are used for MUD, MSD, or MMD, with schedules varying according to institutional choice [69, 70]. All these drugs, however, affect lymphocyte function and proliferation, thus impacting on immune reconstitution.

The thymus, which is crucial for reconstitution of an adaptive immune system, undergoes direct damage by conditioning regimen. Besides, anti-thymoglobulin (ATLG/ATG) or alemtuzumab, also used for GvHD prophylaxis, can cause damage to lymphoid progenitors. ATG is produced in the laboratory by immunizing rabbits with human thymocytes. Another drug that is used for serotherapy is anti-T lymphoglobulin (ATLG) which are obtained by immunizing rabbits with Jurkat cell line. Although ATG and ATLG are commonly considered equivalent, their composition, as a consequence of the production methods, is slightly different as ATLG contains fewer antibodies to CD3, CD4, and HLA-DR and more antibodies to CD107. Therefore, ATLG is less effective in depleting peripheral blood mononuclear cells and dendritic cells and needs to be used at a much higher dose in vivo [2]. ATLG contains polyclonal antibodies which are directed against lymphoid progenitors but also thymic stroma, resulting in profound abatement of the thymic function [71]. Furthermore, for ATG, it has been shown that PK-driven dosing avoids over-exposure and significantly improves immune reconstitution [72].

Among chemotherapy agents, cyclophosphamide is associated with thymus toxicity and constitutes the basis for the PTCy platform, especially in the MMD approach. As aforementioned, PTCy selectively depletes proliferating alloreactive T cells, with a relative sparing of naïve and T regulatory cells. Recent data also show improved B cell reconstitution after PTCy, compared to other GvHD prophylaxis regimens [73].

On the other hand, as aforementioned, in the context of T-cell-depleted MMD, in particular in *ex vivo* αβ T/CD19-cell depletion, the main subsets that first appear after HSCT are NK cells and γδ T cells, while the number of total T cells are significantly reduced compared to MUD or MSD. Prompt NK recovery has been associated with improved outcome in different studies in MMD with PTCy, while delayed recovery is associated with viral reactivations [49]. On the other hand, in *ex vivo* αβ T/CD19 cell depletion, the number of NK cells at 1 month after HSCT is associated with lower incidence of relapse, in particular if the ratio between CD56 bright and CD56 dim favors the latter, which have been associated with a stronger GvL effect [74].

17.4.2.5 GvHD Therapy

Steroids constitute the first line of therapy for acute and chronic GvHD. However, double positive thymocytes are particularly sensitive to steroids and undergo apoptosis. Furthermore, studies from murine models show that GvHD per se can cause damage to thymic epithelium, thus impairing immune reconstitution and increasing the risk for alloreactivity, which, in turn, increases the risk for GvHD [67]. Besides steroids, all the drugs that are used to treat GvHD, by impairing T- or B-cell function, directly interfere with immune reconstitution. Overall, the presence of acute or chronic GvHD and the specific drugs to treat GVHD may deeply impair post-HSCT IR.

17.5 Concluding Remarks

As discussed in this chapter, the use of HSCT for ALL offers many advantages but also poses several questions which still remain unanswered. The important improvements in HSCT techniques, donor choice, conditioning regimens and complication management have significantly impacted on the survival of HSCT patients. In parallel, improvements in management of ALL patients, from front-line therapy to relapse, have increased the overall outcome and reduced the number of patients who need HSCT. On the other hand, in recent years and, most likely, in the near future, pediatric ALL patients who undergo HSCT present increasingly resistant/refractory ALL which has not responded to sophisticated therapies, such as CAR-T cells. We may even expect that ongoing and future HSCT studies might show outcomes which are inferior to what previously reported due to the selection of the patients who are refractory also to innovative therapies.

Finally, current results from HSCT trials, particularly from the FORUM trial, pose several questions. The first and most urgent deals with the toxicity of TBI-based conditioning regimen: while it significantly improves the patient cure rate, what will become of long-term toxicities? [75] Reducing the burden of long-term complications without jeopardizing the outcome is and will remain the future challenge in the field. The goal may be achieved through a change in the TBI administration (novel technique? lower dosing?) or the optimization of chemotherapy-based regimens, in case they could offer results comparable to TBI. The limitations of HSCT include the high burden of post-HSCT complications, caused by the direct toxicity of the conditioning regimen or by GvHD or GvHD-directed treatment, often associated with poor post-HSCT IR. To this aim, a better understanding of the mechanisms of IR and the development of strategies to enhance IR might further improve the outcome of HSCT patients.

In conclusion, despite the significant improvements in ALL cure rates and the availability of novel drugs and immunotherapeutic approaches, a proportion of ALL patients, with increasingly resistant diseases, still needs HSCT to pursue potential cure. The inclusion of haploidentical relatives substantially extended donor availability to virtually all patients. The efforts in the field in the next few years should aim at improving the long-term outcome in growing and most fragile patients.

Acknowledgments We are grateful to Dr. V. Conter and G. Escherich for their extensive support. We thank the principal investigators of multiple ongoing frontline ALL protocols, in particular Prof. M. Schrappe, Prof. M. M. Heyman, Prof. S. P. Hunger, Prof. L. L. Mignon, and Dr. T. T. Teachy, for giving the permission to share HSCT eligibility criteria.

References

1. Granot N, Storb R. History of hematopoietic cell transplantation: challenges and progress. Haematologica. 2020;105:2716–29.
2. Carreras E, Dufour C, Mohty M, Kröger N. The EBMT handbook: hematopoietic stem cell transplantation and cellular therapies. EBMT Handb Hematop Stem Cell Transplant Cell Ther. 2018:1–702.
3. Rocha V, Kabbara N, Ionescu I, Ruggeri A, Purtill D, Gluckman E. Pediatric related and unrelated cord blood transplantation for malignant diseases. Bone Marrow Transplant. 2009;44:653–9.
4. Berger M, Lanino E, Cesaro S, et al. Feasibility and outcome of Haploidentical hematopoietic stem cell transplantation with post-transplant high-dose cyclophosphamide for children and adolescents with hematologic malignancies: an AIEOP-GITMO retrospective multicenter study. Biol Blood Marrow Transplant. 2016;22:902–9.
5. Bader P, Kreyenberg H, Hoelle W, et al. Increasing mixed Chimerism is an important prognostic factor for unfavorable outcome in children with acute lymphoblastic leukemia after allogeneic stem-cell transplantation: possible role for pre-Emptive immunotherapy? J Clin Oncol. 2004;22:1696–705.
6. Beck JC, Cao Q, Trotz B, et al. Allogeneic hematopoietic cell transplantation outcomes for children with B-precursor acute lymphoblastic leukemia and early or late BM relapse. Bone Marrow Transplant. 2011;46:950–5.
7. Klein OR, Buddenbaum J, Tucker N, et al. Nonmyeloablative Haploidentical bone marrow transplantation with post-transplantation cyclophosphamide for pediatric and young adult patients with high-risk hematologic malignancies. Biol Blood Marrow Transplant. 2017;23:325–32.
8. Balduzzi A, Valsecchi MG, Uderzo C, et al. Chemotherapy versus allogeneic transplantation for

very-high-risk childhood acute lymphoblastic leukaemia in first complete remission: comparison by genetic randomisation in an international prospective study. Lancet. 2005;366:635–42.
9. Huang Y, Mouttet B, Warnatz HJ, et al. The leukemogenic TCF3-HLF complex rewires enhancers driving cellular identity and self-renewal conferring EP300 vulnerability. Cancer Cell. 2019;36:630–44.
10. Mouttet B, Vinti L, Ancliff P, et al. Durable remissions in TCF3-HLF positive acute lymphoblastic leukemia with blinatumomab and stem cell transplantation. Haematologica. 2019;104:e244–7.
11. Borowitz MJ, Wood BL, Devidas M, et al. Prognostic significance of minimal residual disease in high risk B-ALL: a report from Children's oncology group study AALL0232. Blood. 2015;126:964–71.
12. Teachey DT, O'Connor D. How i treat newly diagnosed T-cell acute lymphoblastic leukemia and T-cell lymphoblastic lymphoma in children. Blood. 2020;135:159–66.
13. Bartram J, Veys P, Vora A. Improvements in outcome of childhood acute lymphoblastic leukaemia (ALL) in the UK—a success story of modern medicine through successive UKALL trials and international collaboration. Br J Haematol. 2020;191:562–7.
14. Hunger SP, Raetz EA. How I treat relapsed acute lymphoblastic leukemia in the pediatric population. Blood. 2020;136:1803–12.
15. Nguyen K, Devidas M, Cheng SC, et al. Factors influencing survival after relapse from acute lymphoblastic leukemia: a Children's oncology group study. Leukemia. 2008;22:2142–50.
16. Einsiedel HG, Von Stackelberg A, Hartmann R, et al. Long-term outcome in children with relapsed ALL by risk-stratified salvage therapy: results of trial acute lymphoblastic leukemia-relapse study of the Berlin-Frankfurt-Münster group 87. J Clin Oncol. 2005;23:7942–50.
17. Gaynon PS, Qu RP, Chappell RJ, et al. Survival after relapse in childhood acute lymphoblastic leukemia: impact of site and time to first relapse--the children's cancer group experience. Cancer. 1998;82:1387–95.
18. Algeri M, Merli P, Locatelli F, Pagliara D. The role of allogeneic hematopoietic stem cell transplantation in pediatric leukemia. J Clin Med. 2021;10:10. https://doi.org/10.3390/jcm10173790.
19. Locatelli F, Zugmaier G, Rizzari C, et al. Effect of Blinatumomab vs chemotherapy on event-free survival among children with high-risk first-relapse B-cell acute lymphoblastic leukemia: a randomized clinical trial. JAMA J Am Med Assoc. 2021;325:843–54.
20. Borgmann A, Von Stackelberg A, Hartmann R, et al. Unrelated donor stem cell transplantation compared with chemotherapy for children with acute lymphoblastic leukemia in a second remission: a matched-pair analysis. Blood. 2003;101:3835–9.
21. Barrett AJ, Horowitz MM, Pollock BH, et al. Bone marrow transplants from HLA-identical siblings as compared with chemotherapy for children with acute lymphoblastic leukemia in a second remission. N Engl J Med. 1994;331:1253–8.
22. Merli P, Algeri M, Del Bufalo F, Locatelli F. Hematopoietic stem cell transplantation in pediatric acute lymphoblastic leukemia. Curr Hematol Malig Rep. 2019;14:94–105.
23. Vettenranta K, Dobšinská V, Kertész G, Svec P, Buechner J, Schultz KR. What is the role of HSCT in Philadelphia-chromosome–positive and Philadelphia-chromosome–like ALL in the tyrosine kinase inhibitor era? Front Pediatr. 2022;9:1–10.
24. Pui CH, Yang JJ, Hunger SP, et al. Childhood acute lymphoblastic leukemia: Progress through collaboration. J Clin Oncol. 2015;33:2938–48.
25. Aricò M, Schrappe M, Hunger SP, et al. Clinical outcome of children with newly diagnosed Philadelphia chromosome-positive acute lymphoblastic leukemia treated between 1995 and 2005. J Clin Oncol. 2010;28:4755–61.
26. Truong TH, Jinca C, Mann G, et al. Allogeneic hematopoietic stem cell transplantation for children with acute lymphoblastic leukemia: shifting indications in the era of immunotherapy. Front Pediatr. 2021;9:1–15.
27. Brown P, Pieters R, Biondi A. How I treat infant leukemia. Blood. 2019;133:205–14.
28. Bader P, Poetschger U, Dalle J-H, et al. Low rate of nonrelapse mortality in under 4-year-olds with ALL given chemo-conditioning for HSCT: phase III FORUM study. Blood Adv. 2023;8:416–28.
29. Goto H, Kaneko T, Shioda Y, et al. Hematopoietic stem cell transplantation for patients with acute lymphoblastic leukemia and down syndrome. Pediatr Blood Cancer. 2015;62:148–52.
30. Hitzler JK, He W, Doyle J, et al. Outcome of transplantation for acute lymphoblastic leukemia in children with down syndrome. Pediatr Blood Cancer. 2014;61:1126–8.
31. Laetsch TW, Maude SL, Balduzzi A, et al. Tisagenlecleucel in pediatric and young adult patients with down syndrome-associated relapsed/refractory acute lymphoblastic leukemia. Leukemia. 2022;36:1508–15.
32. Winter G, Kirschner-Schwabe R, Groeneveld-Krentz S, et al. Clinical and genetic characteristics of children with acute lymphoblastic leukemia and li-Fraumeni syndrome. Leukemia. 2021;35:1475–9.
33. Pui CH, Williams DL, Raimondi SC, et al. Hypodiploidy is associated with a poor prognosis in childhood acute lymphoblastic leukemia. Blood. 1987;70:247–53.
34. Raimondi SC, Zhou Y, Mathew S, et al. Reassessment of the prognostic significance of Hypodiploidy in pediatric patients with acute lymphoblastic leukemia. Cancer. 2003;98:2715–22.
35. Mullighan CG, Jeha S, Pei D, et al. Outcome of children with hypodiploid ALL treated with risk-directed therapy based on MRD levels. Blood. 2015;126:2896–9.
36. McNeer JL, Devidas M, Dai Y, et al. Hematopoietic stem-cell transplantation does not improve the poor

outcome of children with hypodiploid acute lymphoblastic leukemia: a report from children's oncology group. J Clin Oncol. 2019;37:780–9.
37. Pui CH, Rebora P, Schrappe M, et al. Outcome of children with hypodiploid acute lymphoblastic leukemia: a retrospective multinational study. J Clin Oncol. 2019;37:770–9.
38. Talleur AC, Maude SL. What is the role for HSCT or immunotherapy in pediatric hypodiploid B-cell acute lymphoblastic leukemia? Hematology (United States). 2020;20:508–11.
39. Peters C, Matthes-Martin S, Poetschger U, et al. Stem-cell transplantation in children with acute lymphoblastic leukemia: a prospective international multicenter trial comparing sibling donors with matched unrelated donors-The ALL-SCT-BFM-2003 trial. J Clin Oncol. 2015;33:1265–74.
40. Balduzzi A, Dalle JH, Wachowiak J, et al. Transplantation in children and adolescents with acute lymphoblastic leukemia from a matched donor versus an HLA-identical sibling: is the outcome comparable? Results from the international BFM ALL SCT 2007 study. Biol Blood Marrow Transplant. 2019;25:2197–210.
41. Dalle JH, Balduzzi A, Bader P, et al. Allogeneic stem cell transplantation from HLA-mismatched donors for pediatric patients with acute lymphoblastic leukemia treated according to the 2003 BFM and 2007 international BFM studies: impact of disease risk on outcomes. Biol Blood Marrow Transplant. 2018;24:1848–55.
42. Kleinschmidt K, Lv M, Yanir A, Palma J, Lang P, Eyrich M. T-cell-replete versus ex vivo T-cell-depleted Haploidentical Haematopoietic stem cell transplantation in children with acute lymphoblastic Leukaemia and other Haematological malignancies. Front Pediatr. 2021;9:9. https://doi.org/10.3389/fped.2021.794541.
43. Locatelli F, Merli P, Pagliara D, et al. Outcome of children with acute leukemia given HLA-haploidentical HSCT after ab T-cell and B-cell depletion. Blood. 2017;130:677–85.
44. Bertaina A, Zecca M, Buldini B, et al. Unrelated donor vs HLA-haploidentical a/b T-cell– and B-cell–depleted HSCT in children with acute leukemia. Blood. 2018;132:2594–607.
45. Merli P, Algeri M, Galaverna F, et al. TCRαβ/CD19 cell–depleted HLA-haploidentical transplantation to treat pediatric acute leukemia: updated final analysis. Blood. 2023;143:279. https://doi.org/10.1182/blood.2023021336.
46. Bethge WA, Eyrich M, Mielke S, et al. Results of a multicenter phase I/II trial of TCRαβ and CD19-depleted haploidentical hematopoietic stem cell transplantation for adult and pediatric patients. Bone Marrow Transplant. 2022;57:423–30.
47. Fuchs EJ. Human leukocyte antigen-haploidentical stem cell transplantation using T-cell-replete bone marrow grafts. Curr Opin Hematol. 2012;19: 440–7.
48. Ruggeri A, Galimard JE, Paina O, et al. Outcomes of unmanipulated haploidentical transplantation using post-transplant cyclophosphamide (PT-Cy) in pediatric patients with acute lymphoblastic leukemia. Transplant Cell Ther. 2021;27(424):e1–424.e9.
49. Rambaldi B, Kim HT, Reynolds C, et al. Impaired T- and NK-cell reconstitution after haploidentical HCT with posttransplant cyclophosphamide. Blood Adv. 2021;5:352–64.
50. Sperl D, Lang P, Benesch M, et al. Immunological recovery following HLA-matched CD3+ TCR αß+/CD19+ depleted hematopoietic stem cell transplantation in children. Pediatr Transplant. 2022;26:1–8.
51. Arnold DE, MacMath D, Seif AE, et al. Immune reconstitution following TCRαβ/CD19-depleted hematopoietic cell transplantation for hematologic malignancy in pediatric patients. Transplant Cell Ther. 2021;27(169):e1–169.e9.
52. Rimando J, McCurdy SR, Luznik L. How I prevent GVHD in high-risk patients: posttransplant cyclophosphamide and beyond. Blood. 2023;141:49–59.
53. Gooptu M, Romee R, St. Martin A, et al. HLA-haploidentical vs matched unrelated donor transplants with posttransplant cyclophosphamide-based prophylaxis. Blood. 2021;138:273–82.
54. Kuhlen M, Willasch AM, Dalle J-H, et al. Outcome of relapse after allogeneic HSCT in children with ALL enrolled in the ALL-SCT 2003/2007 trial. Br J Haematol. 2018;180:82–9.
55. Peters C, Dalle JH, Locatelli F, et al. Total body irradiation or chemotherapy conditioning in childhood all: a multinational, randomized, noninferiority phase III study. J Clin Oncol. 2021;39:295–307.
56. Ansari M, Théoret Y, Rezgui MA, et al. Association between busulfan exposure and outcome in children receiving intravenous busulfan before hematopoietic stem cell transplantation. Ther Drug Monit. 2014;36:93–9.
57. Ben Hassine K, Powys M, Svec P, et al. Total body irradiation forever? Optimising chemotherapeutic options for irradiation-free conditioning for paediatric acute lymphoblastic leukaemia. Front Pediatr. 2021;9:9. https://doi.org/10.3389/fped.2021.775485.
58. Rosser SPA, Lee S, Kohli S, et al. Evaluation of treosulfan cumulative exposure in paediatric patients through population pharmacokinetics and dosing simulations. Br J Clin Pharmacol. 2023;89:1413–24.
59. van der Stoep MYEC, Bertaina A, Moes DJAR, et al. Impact of Treosulfan exposure on early and long-term clinical outcomes in pediatric allogeneic hematopoietic stem cell transplantation recipients: a prospective multicenter study. Transplant Cell Ther. 2022;28(99):e1–99.e7.
60. van der Stoep MYEC, Bertaina A, ten Brink MH, et al. High interpatient variability of treosulfan exposure is associated with early toxicity in paediatric HSCT: a prospective multicentre study. Br J Haematol. 2017;179:772–80.
61. van der Stoep MYEC, Zwaveling J, Bertaina A, et al. Population pharmacokinetics of treosulfan in paediat-

ric patients undergoing hematopoietic stem cell transplantation. Br J Clin Pharmacol. 2019;85:2033–44.
62. Chiesa R, Standing JF, Winter R, et al. Proposed therapeutic range of Treosulfan in reduced toxicity pediatric allogeneic hematopoietic stem cell transplant conditioning: results from a prospective trial. Clin Pharmacol Ther. 2020;108:264–73.
63. Nijstad AL, Nierkens S, Lindemans CA, et al. Population pharmacokinetics of clofarabine for allogeneic hematopoietic cell transplantation in paediatric patients. Br J Clin Pharmacol. 2021;87:3218–26.
64. Bhatt ST, Bednarski JJ. Immune reconstitution in pediatric patients following hematopoietic cell transplant for non-malignant disorders. Front Immunol. 2020;11:1–7.
65. Velardi E, Clave E, Arruda LCM, Benini F, Locatelli F, Toubert A. The role of the thymus in allogeneic bone marrow transplantation and the recovery of the peripheral T-cell compartment. Semin Immunopathol. 2021;43:101–17.
66. Xiao S, Shterev ID, Zhang W, et al. Sublethal Total body irradiation causes long-term deficits in thymus function by reducing lymphoid progenitors. J Immunol. 2017;199:2701–12.
67. Chaudhry MS, Velardi E, Malard F, van den Brink MRM. Immune reconstitution after allogeneic hematopoietic stem cell transplantation: time to T up the thymus. J Immunol. 2017;198:40–6.
68. Calvo-Asensio I, Sugrue T, Bosco N, Rolink A, Ceredig R. DN2 thymocytes activate a specific robust DNA damage response to ionizing radiation-induced DNA double-strand breaks. Front Immunol. 2018;9:1–13.
69. Jamy O, Zeiser R, Bin CY. Novel developments in the prophylaxis and treatment of acute GVHD. Blood. 2023;142:1037–46.
70. Gooptu M, Antin JH. GVHD prophylaxis 2020. Front Immunol. 2021;12:1–13.
71. Mohty M. Mechanisms of action of antithymocyte globulin: T-cell depletion and beyond. Leukemia. 2007;21:1387–94.
72. Meesters-Ensing JI, Admiraal R, Ebskamp L, et al. Therapeutic drug monitoring of anti-thymocyte globulin in allogeneic stem cell transplantation: proof of concept. Front Pharmacol. 2022;13:1–8.
73. Teshima T, Boelens JJ, Matsuoka K. Novel insights into GVHD and immune reconstitution after allogeneic hematopoietic cell transplantation. Blood Cell Ther. 2023;6:6. https://doi.org/10.31547/bct-2022-023.
74. Diaz MA, Zubicaray J, Molina B, et al. Haploidentical stem cell transplantation in children with hematological malignancies using αβ+ t-cell receptor and cd19+ cell depleted grafts: high cd56dim /cd56bright nk cell ratio early following transplantation is associated with lower relapse incidenc. Front Immunol. 2019;10:1–10.
75. Diesch-Furlanetto T, Gabriel M, Zajac-Spychala O, Cattoni A, Hoeben BAW, Balduzzi A. Late effects after Haematopoietic stem cell transplantation in ALL, long-term follow-up and transition: a step into adult life. Front Pediatr. 2021;9:1–18.

Part VII

Toxicity and Late Effects Following ALL Treatment

18 Acute Toxicity and Late Effects Related to Acute Lymphoblastic Leukemia Treatment

Liv Andrés-Jensen, Camilla Grud Nielsen, Marry M. van den Heuvel-Eibrink, and Kjeld Schmiegelow

18.1 Introduction

The current high cure rate with the best contemporary chemotherapy for childhood ALL has come at a price [1, 2]. All patients encounter severe acute toxicities during therapy, including organ dysfunctions, and the majority of survivors are burdened by significant late effects [3], the vast majority of which are poorly understood, including their impact on post-treatment quality of life (QoL). Several late effects are long-term consequences of acute toxicities that occurred during chemotherapy (e.g., insulin-dependent diabetes after pancreatitis) [4], whereas others may emerge after discontinuation of therapy (e.g., osteonecrosis or second malignant neoplasm (SMN)) [5, 6]. Thus, the pattern of late effects after treatment of ALL will be affected by the duration of follow-up as well as the toxicity burden added for patients needing several lines of therapy due to up-front resistant disease, relapse, or second cancers.

As antileukemic therapy changes, so does the pattern of late effects [3]. Hematopoietic stem cell transplantation (hSCT), prophylactic cranial irradiation [7], and anthracyclines are used less frequently, while the use of glucocorticosteroids (including dexamethasone), asparaginase and vincristine have been intensified in first line therapy. Consequently, SMN, cognitive disturbances, reduced growth, hypothalamic/pituitary dysfunction, and heart failure become rarer, while osteonecrosis, musculoskeletal dysfunction, endocrine disturbances, and chemotherapy-induced peripheral neuropathy are more frequent. The long-term impact of recently introduced immunotherapies, including chimeric antigen receptor-modified T cells, is yet to be determined but is hoped to yield fewer late effects than traditional chemotherapies [8, 9].

Late effect studies often address subsets of patients, one or a few specific late effects, or have limited study power with few exceptions (Table 18.1).

There is an unmet need for international standardization for capturing and reporting late effects as a critical measure of treatment outcome. Such

L. Andrés-Jensen · C. G. Nielsen
Department of Pediatrics and Adolescent Medicine, Rigshospitalet, Copenhagen University Hospital, Copenhagen, Denmark
e-mail: liv.andres-jensen.02@regionh.dk; camilla.grud.nielsen@regionh.dk

M. M. van den Heuvel-Eibrink
Princess Máxima Center for Pediatric Oncology, Utrecht, The Netherlands
e-mail: m.m.vandenheuvel-eibrink@prinsesmaximacentrum.nl

K. Schmiegelow (✉)
Department of Pediatrics and Adolescent Medicine, Rigshospitalet, Copenhagen University Hospital, Copenhagen, Denmark

Faculty of Medicine, Institute of Clinical Medicine, University of Copenhagen, Copenhagen, Denmark
e-mail: Kjeld.Schmiegelow@regionh.dk

G. Escherich, V. Conter (eds.), *Acute Lymphoblastic Leukemia in Children and Adolescents*, Pediatric Oncology, https://doi.org/10.1007/978-3-031-71180-0_18

Table 18.1 Childhood cancer survivor cohorts

Cohort	Geographic	Established	Period of diagnosis	Cohort size	Survival at entry (years)	Age at diagnosis (years)	Diagnoses	Study design	Data collection
North American cohorts									
CCSS [10]	United States, Canada	1994	1970–1999	37,593	≥5	0–20	Leukemia, CNS, Hodgkin lymphoma, non-Hodgkin lymphoma, neuroblastoma, soft tissue sarcoma, Wilms, bone tumors	Retrospective, hospital-based cohort with prospective follow-up	Medical records, surveys
SJLIFE [11]	United States	2007	1962–2012	8245	≥5	0–24	All types	Retrospective, hospital-based cohort with prospective follow-up	Medical records, surveys, clinical visits
CAYACS [12]	British Columbia, Canada	2005	1970–2010	8735	0	0–24	All types	Retrospective population-based cohort with prospective follow-up	Registries, administrative databases, medical records
European cohorts									
BCCSS [13]	England, Wales, Scotland	1998	1940–2006	34,490	≥5	0–14	All types	Retrospective population-based cohort	Registries, surveys, medical records
ALiCCS [14]	Denmark, Finland, Iceland, Norway, Sweden	2010	1943–2012	33,160	≥1	0–19	All types	Retrospective population-based cohort	Nordic registries, medical records
SCCSS [15]	Switzerland	2007	1976–2018 (ongoing)	5737	≥5	0–20	All types	Retrospective population-based cohort with prospective follow-up	Registries, medical records, surveys

FCCSS [16]	Selected regions in France	2015	1946–1999	7670	≥5	0–19	All except leukemia	Retrospective hospital-based cohort with prospective follow-up	Hospital and insurance databases, surveys, clinical visits
LEA [17]	Selected regions in France (>75% of leukemia patients)	2004	1980–2019 (ongoing)	14,201	≥2	0–18	Leukemia	Retrospective hospital- and local registry-based cohort with prospective follow-up	Registries, medical records, surveys, clinical visits
LATER study [18]	Netherlands	2006	1963–2002	6165	≥5	0–18	All types	Retrospective hospital-based cohort with prospective follow-up	Registries, medical records, surveys, clinical visits
OTR [19]	Italy	1980	1960–2004	14,201	End of treatment	0–19	All types	Retrospective and prospective national hospital-based from AIEOP clinics with prospective follow-up	Regional registries, hospital data
European consortia									
PanCareSurFup [20]	European network established in 2008. Focus of cardiac disease, SMN and late mortality as well as establishing guidelines for optimal follow-up								
PanCareLIFE [21]	Focus on female infertility, cisplatin-induced ototoxicity and QoL								
PanCareFollowUp	Aiming to establish state-of-the-art late effects clinics based on international guidelines for surveillance								
Global ALL consortia									
PdL [22, 23]	International ALL consortia consisting of all major ALL groups across Europe, North America, Australia, Taiwan, and Japan. Established in 1995. Research focused on ALL outcome and toxicity								

Table inspired by Tables 1 and 2 in Norsker FN et al., *Pediatr. Clin. North Am.* 2020;67 (6):1033–1049 (PMID 33131533)

AIEOP Associazione Italiana di Ematologia e Oncologia Pediatrica, *ALiCCS* Adult Life after Childhood Cancer in Scandinavia, *BCCSS* British Childhood Cancer Survivor Study, *FCCSS* French Childhood Cancer Survivor Study, *LATER Study* Dutch Childhood Cancer Survivorship LATER Cohort Study, *LEA* The French Childhood Cancer Survivor Study for Leukaemia, *NA* not available, *OTR* The Italian Study on off-therapy Childhood Cancer Survivors, *PdL* Ponte di Legno consortium, *SCCSS* Swiss Childhood Cancer Survivor Study reporting should initially address the most severe and objective late effects [24], while subsequent and more comprehensive targets should include more subjective late conditions such as chronic fatigue, pain, self-reported QoL, and ability to comply with routine activities of daily living (ADL).

18.2 Organ-Specific Toxicities

18.2.1 Cardiovascular

Cardiovascular toxicities contribute substantially to the long-term burden of childhood antileukemic therapy [3, 25–30], and although a reduction in cumulative anthracycline dosing has resulted in decreased cardiac mortality among ALL survivors [31], a clear decline in the risk of nonfatal cardiac events has yet to be detected [29, 30], potentially due to limited follow-up in newer cohorts. Newer agents, such as chimeric antigen receptors, carry the risk of cytokine release syndrome, during which the release of pro-inflammatory cytokines and activated prostaglandins has been associated with cardiac failure, arrhythmias, vascular dysfunction, and coagulopathy [32, 33]. Potential long-term cardiac sequelae remain to be seen.

18.2.1.1 Heart Failure

Heart failure is primarily associated with chest irradiation as part of total body irradiation prior to stem cell transplantation, cumulative anthracycline doses $\geq$300 mg/m^2, and to a much lesser degree, cyclophosphamide and cytosine arabinoside [26, 34, 35]. Additional risk factors include young age at diagnosis, female sex, and cardiometabolic comorbidities such as hypertension, obesity, and diabetes [29, 35]. The mechanisms through which anthracyclines exert their acute cardiotoxic effects are not fully understood, but involve intracellular complex-forming with iron, leading to the production of free radicals and reactive oxygen species; depletion of glutathione peroxidase; and alterations of gene expression patterns, collectively resulting in apoptosis [26]. Furthermore, since cardiomyocytes are often terminally differentiated, they have limited capacity to regenerate, causing myocardial wall thinning after a certain threshold. Prospective studies find deterioration of cardiac function in most patients during anthracycline therapy [36]. Still, only a subset of patients have clinical symptoms during therapy, although these can arise years after therapy cessation due to progression of the underlying cardiomyopathy. The prevalence of self-reported (all grades) heart failure among long-term survivors is 2.4% [30], whereas the cumulative incidence of severe heart failure (grade 3–5 according to the Common Terminology Criteria for Adverse Events [CTCAE] grading system) [37] is 0.31–0.40% at 20 years after ALL diagnosis, depending on the decade of treatment [29]. Of note, subclinical cardiac abnormalities are seen in up to 30% of survivors, depending on follow-up time, even following low dose anthracycline exposure (e.g., 180 or 240 mg/m^2) [38], with no certain timepoint of a plateau being reached.

18.2.1.2 Arrhythmia

Cardiac arrhythmias arising during anticancer therapy can result from direct drug affection of molecular pathways involved in the electrical conduction system or, more commonly, secondary to endocardial or myocardial damage caused by infection, inflammation, ischemia, or radiation therapy [39, 40]. Risk is associated with alkylators and anthracyclines, but also newer agents, particularly tyrosine kinase inhibitors (TKIs) [40]. A recent Childhood Cancer Survivor Study (CCSS) performed among >6000 ALL survivors found a 20-year cumulative incidence of severe arrhythmias (requiring pacemakers or cardioversion) of 0.12, 0.08, and 0.05 corresponding to treatment decades 1970–1979, 1980–1989, and 1990–1999, respectively [29]. The hazard ratio decreased for each increasing decade, although the trend did not reach statistical significance [29]. A Swiss CCSS study compared 511 5-year survivors diagnosed with ALL between 1975 and 2005 with siblings and found no difference in the rate of (all grades) arrhythmias [30].

18.2.1.3 Heart Valve Disease

Heart valve dysfunction in the frame of ALL therapy is mainly associated with irradiation toward the cardiac field, infectious endocarditis, and (casuistically) Loeffler endocarditis [41–49], with valve replacement required in a small subset of cases [44, 47]. Most infectious cases are likely to resolve with aggressive antibacterial and antifungal therapy; however, some require surgical resection of the infectious vegetations [41, 46], and few require valvuloplasty [44, 47]. The proportion of patients developing valve dysfunction during ALL treatment is uncertain, and there are no follow-up studies of patients with endocarditis. However, the prevalence of severe heart valve disease at 20 years after ALL diagnosis is only 0.02–0.10% and comparable to that of siblings [29].

18.2.1.4 Coronary Artery Disease

Cardiac irradiation dose ≥15 Gy is the most consistently reported risk factor for coronary artery disease among ALL survivors [50]. Additional risk factors include alkylating drugs, antimetabolites, vinca alkaloids, and newer agents such as TKIs and vascular endothelial growth factor inhibitors [40, 50]. Cardiometabolic risk factors, themselves associated with antileukemic therapy, add to this risk [29, 50]. The cumulative incidence of severe coronary artery disease resulting in myocardial infarction, requiring angioplasty or resulting in death, was recently found to be 0.19–0.27% at 20 years after ALL diagnosis, and furthermore decreasing with increasing treatment era [29].

18.2.1.5 Thromboembolism (TE)

TE, primarily of venous origin, is among the most frequent and severe acute toxicities, occurring in 5% of children aged below 10 years at ALL diagnosis and 15–20% of children and adolescents aged 10–17.9 years, indicating that adolescent age is a significant risk factor [51]. Other risk factors include the leukemic state itself, central venous catheters, and being bedridden, while the main therapeutic risk factor is asparaginase, which causes a procoagulant state by reducing the hepatic synthesis of natural anticoagulants (antithrombin, heparin cofactor II, protein C, and protein S) [52–56]. Corticosteroids add to this state by increasing levels of coagulation factors VIII–IX and von Willebrand factor (vWF), and by limiting fibrinolysis through increased levels of plasminogen activator inhibitor 1 (PAI-1) [57, 58]. In addition, endothelial dysfunction, arising from mechanical (circulating blasts and central venous catheters) and biochemical (antileukemic drugs and inflammation) interactions, is thought to play a crucial role in thrombogenesis, although only few studies have investigated this is an ALL setting [59–61]. The individual risk profile is accentuated by leukemic factors (tumor lysis, mediastinal mass, inflammation, coinciding infections, and immobilization) [62–65], in addition to host factors (genotype, age, obesity, and possibly sex and non-O blood group) [51, 66–71]. Most cases resolve without sequelae; however, a subset experience long-term effects in the form of post-pulmonary embolism syndrome [72], post-thrombotic syndrome (after deep venous thrombosis) [73, 74], and cognitive impairments (following cerebral sinovenous thrombosis) [66, 75]. Evidence regarding the potential role of specific thromboprophylactic therapies is scarce due to few and insufficiently powered trials. Low-molecular-weight heparins might offer a prophylactic benefit during high-risk treatment phases such as induction [76]; however, trials are needed to validate this finding, and to investigate the potential role of other agents such as synthetic pentasaccharides, parenteral direct thrombin inhibitors, direct oral anticoagulants, and intravascular antithrombin-containing blood-derived products. Thromboembolism is primarily an acute toxicity. A study among 511 ALL survivors found no increased risk of venous thromboembolism or stroke after cessation of ALL therapy compared with siblings, and rates were very low in both groups [30].

18.2.2 Pulmonary

Pulmonary toxicities occurring during treatment are mainly of infectious origin or related to vascular events. Long-term pulmonary sequelae, including obstructive and restrictive ventilatory defects and impaired diffusion capacity, are rare except following TBI and high-dose alkylating agents in the setting of hSCT [77–79]. Patients treated with chemotherapy only may have a slightly increased risk of restrictive ventilatory patterns, particularly if exposed to high cumulative doses of anthracyclines, cytarabine, and cyclophosphamide at a young age [80]; however, lung function is generally within normal range [81]. A recent CCSS study reported a pulmonary cause standardized mortality ratio of 8.1 (95% CI: 3.8–17.0) among survivors of adolescent ALL and of 4.2 (95% CI: 1.0–16.7) among childhood ALL survivors treated between 1970 and 1999 [82]. Likewise, a British CCSS has reported increased respiratory mortality among non-AML childhood leukemia survivors with a pneumonia mortality standardized mortality ratio (SMR) of 8.9 (95% CI: 4.3–16.4), and an all cause respiratory mortality SMR of 4.8 (95% CI: 3.1–7.1) [81]. Importantly, the absolute excess risk is very low, and furthermore declining with more recent treatment eras, likely reflecting decreased use of hSCT [82, 83].

18.2.3 Renal

Acute nephrotoxicity is mainly associated with tumor lysis syndrome, the use of aminoglycosides, and high-dose MTX, the latter likely being caused by the precipitation of 7-OH-MTX crystals in the kidney [84, 85]. Glucarpidase rescue may be indicated in approximately 1% of patients despite vigorous hydration and alkalinization [86], with ethnicity, older age, and inherited genetic variations as potential risk factors [87]. Newer agents, such as TKIs, may aggravate the nephrotoxic effects of MTX [88]. Renal function normalizes within days to weeks in most cases, and several studies have failed to demonstrate an association with long-term renal dysfunction [89]. Other possible causes of acute renal impairment include tumor lysis syndrome, infections (including nephrotoxic antibiotics such as aminoglycosides and antifungal agents), and hSCT due to TBI, graft versus host disease (GvHD), and associated treatments [89–93]. Long-term outcomes related to individual acute renal effects are uncertain, but a Nordic registry study including 6843 childhood leukemia survivors treated since the 1940s found that 288 (4%) had a first hospital contact for any renal or urinary tract disease, corresponding to a standardized hospitalization rate ratio of 3.4 (95% CI: 3.0–3.8) and an absolute excess risk of 289 per 100,000 person-years (95% CI: 241–336), respectively [94]. The risk of long-term renal toxicities related to contemporary treatment regimens seems very low and is likely dominated by cases of urolithiasis [3].

18.2.4 Hepatic

Acute hepatotoxicity is mainly associated with 6-thioguanine, 6-mercaptopurine, MTX, irradiation, and hSTC, in addition to transfusion-acquired iron overload and cholestasis from prolonged parenteral nutrition [22, 95–97]. Sinusoidal-obstruction syndrome (SOS) is a vascular disease, characterized by hepatomegaly, hyperbilirubinemia, ascites, weight gain, and thrombocytopenia [98], and was once a rare complication outside the setting of hSCT; however, it has been reported in up to 10% of non-transplanted patients after the extension of asparaginase into maintenance phases, increasing the cytotoxic effects of 6-mercaptopurine in combination with MTX [99], and in up to 25% of patients treated with standard dose 6-thioguanine during maintenance therapy [95]. This risk is significantly increased among patients with low-activity *TPMT* variants as compared to *TPMT* wild-type patients [100]. The underlying pathophysiology leading to SOS is presumed to include drug-mediated injury to the sinusoidal endothelial cells, which are dissected from the underlying lining and form embolisms obstructing the hepatic microcirculation, which results in hepatocellular necrosis [95]. SOS and 6-thioguanine exposure is associated with long-term risk of adverse hepatic conditions, including splenomegaly, chronic thrombocytopenia, portal hypertension, esophageal varices, and fibrosis [96, 101–104]; however, evidence regarding late hepatic outcomes is generally sparse [105]. A Nordic register study including >6000 leukemia survivors found a hazard ratio of 1.7 (1.4–2.2) for hospitalization related to any liver disease when compared with CNS tumor survivors (the study did not include a cancer-naïve comparison group) [106].

18.2.5 Gastrointestinal

Gastrointestinal toxicity is common during ALL treatment and include constipation, nausea, vomiting, diarrhea, mucositis, and changes in the gastrointestinal microbiome which increases the risk of opportunistic infections, including *Clostridium difficile* [107, 108]. Treatment-related risk factors include anthracyclines, vinca alkaloids, alkylating agents, and abdominal radiation, and indirect factors include myelosuppression and altered microbiome [107, 109, 110]. Mucositis occurs in approximately half of the patients [107, 111] and spans from mild forms with erythematous lesions with intact mucosa to severe, painful forms with ulcerations penetrating fully into the submucosa [112]. The development of mucositis depends on both treatment and patient-related factors including neutropenia, low body weight, and elevated serum creatinine [113], and intestinal mucositis is associated with hypocitrullinemia reflecting a reduced number of functional enterocytes [110]. Affected patients are at increased risk for malnutrition as well as for systemic infections due to disrupted intestinal immunological barriers [110]. Most gastrointestinal toxicities are transient, but 7% of patients with ALL develops enteritis, typhlitis, or colitis, which are accompanied by risk of acute complications such as sepsis and intestinal obstruction as well as risk of long-term gastrointestinal complications (although rare) [114]. Management is conservative in most cases and includes broad-spectrum antibiotics and supportive care [115, 116]. A CCSS study evaluated self-reported gastrointestinal complications in >14,000 long-term childhood cancer survivors and found survivors to be at increased risk for developing gastrointestinal complications later in life compared to siblings. Complications included everything from nausea and heartburn to ileostomy/colostomy [109]. However, numbers were not reported specifically for ALL survivors and the risk for long-term gastrointestinal late effects are expected to be rare unless treated with hematopoietic stem cell transplantation.

18.2.6 Endocrine Conditions

Endocrine disorders represent the most common toxicities observed in children with ALL [117]. These side effects include mainly pituitary and gonadal dysfunctions, thyroid dysfunction, and metabolic syndrome (which includes overweight, dyslipidemia, hypertension, and insulin resistance). Patients suffering from asparaginase-associated pancreatitis during treatment are likely at higher risk of developing persistent insulin-dependent diabetes [4, 118, 119].

Treatment components are the most important determinants of these side effects, and since the omission of CNS irradiation and testicular irradiation in the majority of currently treated pediatric ALL patients, it is expected that in the future, these long-term side effects will occur less often than in historically treated ALL cohorts [2, 120]. This advancement is also due to enhancement of (molecular driven) treatment stratification which has decreased the proportion of patients that require high-dose stem cell transplantation as well as the adjustment of conditioning regimens. On the other hand, the impact of novel strategies, which includes immunotherapies, await prospective toxicity monitoring over the decades to come.

18.2.6.1 Growth Hormone Deficiency (GHD)

GHD has been reported as one of the first long-term side effects in several childhood ALL survivor cohorts (50% of the CNS-irradiated ALL survivors, 5% in children non-CNS irradiated), especially occurring when radiation dosages exceeded 20–24 Gy. GHD leads to impaired height, altered body composition, metabolic syndrome, resulting in enhanced risk of cardiovascular disease, neurocognitive impairment, as well as impaired quality of life [121–126].

Early studies revealed that the most prominent drop in height was observed in the first year of ALL treatment, and in the very young children (<4 years) [127, 128]. Growth velocity impairment during chemotherapy only is frequently observed in ALL patients, but typically not due to GHD. Hence, subsequent catch-up growth and achievement of adult height within the normal range is generally achieved [40, 124, 129, 130]. Still, female gender and younger age at diagnosis have remained risk factors associated with reduced final height in both irradiated and nonirradiated survivors [129, 131]. Importantly, most final adult height studies reflect protocols used during the 1970s–1990s, and follow-up of more recently treated patients are pending. Preliminary results indicate that also TKIs may induce impairment of final height, but larger cohort studies in CCS are lacking [132]

18.2.6.2 Gonadal Damage

Although precocious puberty, and hypothyroidism have been described, the gonadal axis seems less affected after CNS radiotherapy [130, 133]. Nevertheless, gonadal impairment can be seen in patients treated with high dosages of alkylating agents, HSCT and exposure of radiotherapy, as these strategies deprive the gonadal reserve as reflected by lower antral follicle counts (AFCs), and hampering of adequate hormone production [134–137]. This can lead to a delay of puberty, menstrual cycle problems, premature menarche, and infertility, as well as adverse effects on bone composition, muscle mass, and psychological well-being. The most significant treatment components associated with risk of gonadal insufficiency are alkylating agents and radiotherapy (local, TBI, and CNS) [138–140]. In males, azoospermia, and need for testosterone replacement have mainly been reported following testicular irradiation in cases of testicular relapse, spinal irradiation in girls, or as part of TBI, and not by CNS irradiation [141–144]. Following contemporary pediatric treatment strategies, it seems that gonadal function and pregnancy rates are hardly ever compromised in the majority of ALL patients, as the use of CNS irradiation, TBI, testicular irradiation and the use of (high dose of) alkylating agents are limited to a very restricted number of very high-risk ALL patients [138, 145–148].

International guidelines recommend systematic evaluations for signs indicating risk of premature menopause in post-pubertal survivors treated with potentially gonadotoxic chemotherapy and/or irradiation potentially exposing risk organs [140, 149–151].

Nevertheless, in current ALL therapy settings, it is important to inform all children with ALL and their families about their (even relatively low) risk. In general, extensive counselling and ovarian tissue preservation in girls is not necessary as fertility is not dramatically impaired [134, 148, 151–153]. In teenage boys, it is safe and of value to at least offer sperm preservation in all cases, as soon as CR is reached [149, 152]. More attention and counseling become relevant in high-risk ALL settings, and especially as soon as relapses occur, which require higher doses of alkylating agents and/or HSCT, with or without TBI settings [134, 149].

Currently, options for fertility preservation have become more accepted as standard of care, and successful puberty induction, as well as live birth after ovarian tissue cryopreservation (OTC) and transplantation of ovarian tissue, even from young children [148], has been reported now, indicating the importance to offer gonadal tissue preservation to the small subgroup of high-risk/relapse patients that benefit from HSCT, preferable at the status of complete remission to avoid harvest of residual leukemic cells.

18.2.6.3 Thyroid Dysfunction

TBI and craniospinal irradiation with scatter to the thyroid gland can cause hypo- and, more rarely, hyper-thyroidism. Although the risk of hypothyroidism 15 years after ALL diagnosis is reported at only 1.6% (CI: 1.1–2.1), the rate is significantly increased compared with siblings [154]. Importantly, survivors treated with cranial irradiation or chemotherapy only, do not seem to be at increased risk of thyroid dysfunction [124, 154, 155].

18.2.6.4 Metabolic Syndrome (MetS)

Several studies have reported (with various used definitions) increased risk of disproportional alterations in body composition (sarcopenic/obesity), hypertension, dyslipidemia, and insulin resistance/diabetes mellitus among childhood ALL survivors, altogether referred to as MetS [124, 131, 156–162]. The prevalence of MetS (and components) has been reported already at a young adult age in one third of all ALL survivors [123], which is far higher than in the normal population. Risk factors include female gender, cranial irradiation, and older age at evaluation [123, 162].

The dysmetabolic effects of cranial irradiation are likely mediated by hypothalamic–pituitary dysregulation of leptin sensitivity and growth hormone deficiency [124, 156, 162]. Although radiotherapy has gradually been omitted from frontline childhood ALL protocols, it has been replaced by intensified glucocorticosteroid therapy and extended asparaginase exposure, thereby potentially replacing one risk factor for MetS by others [156, 163] Corticosteroids can alter substrate oxidation and energy expenditure by suppressing growth hormone and inducing leptin resistance [156, 164, 165]. L-Asparaginase reduces insulin secretion and plasma insulin levels, while increasing insulin resistance, thereby acting synergistically with corticosteroids. In addition, AAP, or alternatively (partial) exposure of the pancreas to radiotherapy, ultimately can contribute to insulin-dependent diabetes (type 3c) in small subsets of ALL patients [1, 4, 158]. Clinical trials testing dietary and physical interventions to prevent or reduce MetS in childhood cancer survivors, are necessary to determine the efficacy for long-term survivors [166].

18.2.7 Osteogenic Side Effects in Children with ALL

Children treated for ALL are at risk for osteogenic side effects. These include impairment of bone mineral density and consequently increased risk of fractures, as well as the occurrence of symptomatic osteonecrosis (sON).

18.2.7.1 Osteoporosis

Nearly all studies show that ALL treatment leads to a substantial decline in bone mineral density (BMD) [167–171]. Risk factors include leukemia-related low BMD at diagnosis [164, 172], inadequate diet (low intake of D-vitamin and calcium), low level of weight-bearing physical activities, intensive glucocorticosteroids and high-dose methotrexate exposure, genetic susceptibility, and/or high dose of cranial irradiation [170, 173–175].

However, most ALL survivors reach their peak bone mass in adult life, and may even have the potential to retain peak bone mass longer than usual [172, 176–178]. If survivors fail to achieve expected normal peak bone mass during and following cessation of therapy, reduced BMD substantially increases the risk of osteoporotic fractures [168, 170, 179, 180]. The role of the cumulative dose of glucocorticoids as a risk factor has not been strongly confirmed so far, and studies that systematically include vertebral (asymptomatic) fractures in the research program are scarce [181]. The magnitude of BMD impairment due to applied TKIs and immunotherapy in subsets of ALL patients over the last decades, has not been investigated in large ALL survivor cohorts so far [182, 183].

Clinical risk prediction models for identifying ALL patients at risk for low BMD during and after treatment, as well as guidelines for surveillance and vitamin D supplementation, have now become available [170, 184–186].

18.2.7.2 Osteonecrosis (ON)

Osteonecrosis (ON) is a direct effect of ALL treatment and one of the most common and debilitating toxicities with a potentially long-term impact on daily function and QoL. A marked rise in the incidence of ON coincided with the introduction of dexamethasone in de novo ALL treatment, and with the ability to pursue magnetic resonance imaging (MRI) scanning, which is the golden standard to detect osteonecrosis [187]. Several clinical and radiological staging methods to determine the severity of osteonecrosis have been developed over the years. The most recent clinical classification was proposed by the Ponte di Legno

Toxicity Working Group which is based on osteonecrosis site and severity of symptoms in ALL patients [98]. A recently developed radiological grading system by Niinimäki and colleagues provides the first non-joint-specific radiological classification, which facilitates universal application [188]. It uses osteonecrosis site, as well as the amount of articular surface that is involved (<30% vs. ≥30%). The prognostic value of both classifications remains to be determined.

Osteonecrosis may be symptomatic or asymptomatic. Symptomatic osteonecrosis (sON) is most relevant, revealing (severe) pain, immobility, limitations in ADL, and sometimes even articular collapse, and systematic ON screening of asymptomatic ALL patients is not recommended. Symptoms present mainly in the weight-bearing joints [189, 190].

The prevalence of sON ranges between 10% and 20% [190]. The older patients reveal a longer interval between diagnosis of ALL and of ON [31]. ON is considered to occur through a combination of hypoperfusion caused by a combination of microthrombi, increased marrow pressure, and direct damage to the endothelial and smooth muscle cells in the nurturing arteries, accelerated by prothrombotic state, chemotherapy agents and systemic inflammation. The strongest risk factors for ON in children with ALL are female sex, higher age and hyperlipidemia, glucocorticoid (combined with asparaginase) exposure (cumulative dose and exposure time), cranial and gonadal irradiation, and race [188, 190, 191]. A trial implementing reduction of continuous exposure to dexamethasone found a reduction of ON occurrence, [192] but the benefit of implementing such "dexamethasone pulses" strategies in recent pediatric ALL trials seems to be neutralized by the intensified Asparaginase introduction over recent decades [193]. The occurrence of sON is independent of BMD; however, immobilization at time of sON occurrence increases the risk of BMD decline and subsequent fractures substantially [194]. Immobilization is the currently most used intervention strategy. Unfortunately, evidence-based efficient preventive or intervening (including surgical) strategies are currently not available. Use of bone modeling agents including bisphosphonates is reported to be of value to relieve pain only; however, recently, concerns regarding oncological safety have been raised [190, 195, 196]. sON seems to be reversible in 40% of the children in the first years after treatment; however, long-term follow-up studies after ALL treatment in children are currently lacking [189].

18.3 Dental

Both radiation and chemotherapy are associated with increased risk of dental developmental abnormalities such as tooth agenesis, microdontia, abnormal root development and enamel defects. The reported prevalence among childhood ALL survivors vary widely from 39% to 94% [197–199]; however, the studies with the highest frequency of dental abnormalities mirror treatment regimens used decades ago where radiotherapy was used more frequently. In 111 patients treated with chemotherapy only, microdontia and enamel hypoplasia were found in 28% and 46%, respectively [200]. The same study found strong association between cumulative doses of anthracycline >120 mg/m^2 and more severe dental aberrations. Chemotherapy-related abnormalities arising during dental development are irreversible and the effects of chemotherapy are amplified when administered at a young age where dental cells are highly proliferative, reflected in studies demonstrating that younger age at diagnosis is associated with more severe dental abnormalities [198–200]. Furthermore, high-intensity therapy is associated with the severity of dental abnormalities [199]. Conversely, the risk of caries has been demonstrated to be increased in patients diagnosed after or at the age of 5–6 years [200, 201], however, a population-based study found the increased risk of caries in childhood cancer survivors to be short-term [201]. Cranial irradiation is associated with dose-dependent increased risk for dental abnormalities and as little as 1–3 Gy is reported to damage ameloblasts and halt tooth development. Furthermore, cranial irradiation may also affect mandibular development resulting in craniofacial abnormalities [197, 198, 202].

18.4 Central Neurotoxicity

Childhood ALL patients receive multiple chemotherapeutic agents of which several may cause neurotoxicity. Around 7–13% of patients develop acute central nervous system (CNS) symptoms with seizures being the most common symptom [203–205]. CNS symptoms typically occur early in treatment and may be caused by defined CNS complications such as posterior reversible encephalopathy syndrome (PRES), sinovenous thrombosis (SVT), methotrexate (MTX)-related stroke-like syndrome, CNS bleeding, and encephalitis, or by systemic conditions such as infections or metabolic disturbances [203, 205].

PRES occurs in 1.6–4.5% of patients [206, 207] and presents typically with seizures, headaches, altered mental status, and visual impairment combined with transient but characteristic MRI findings. The pathogenesis of PRES is thought to include endothelial damage in the blood–brain barrier causing capillary hyperperfusion and consequent vasogenic edema [203]. The treatment of PRES is symptomatic and includes managing blood pressure.

MTX neurotoxicity occurs in 3–7% of patients who clinically presents with transient stroke-like symptoms, encephalopathy, speech disturbances, and seizures, [204, 208–210] and may result from disrupted CNS folate homeostasis and direct neuronal damage [211]. Stroke-like syndrome (SLS) occurs within 3 weeks after high-dose MTX (HDM)or intrathecal (IT) MTX with typical symptoms being focal weakness or hemiparesis, movement disorder, aphasia, or dysarthria, altered mental status or seizures [205, 212]. Most patients recover completely but severe cases may require months of intensive rehabilitation [208, 212]. Only a smaller group of patients (7–12, 9%) experience recurrent neurotoxicity when re-exposed to MTX, and the risk of recurrent MTX neurotoxicity should be balanced against the increased risk of relapse associated with omission of MTX. Recent studies support the continuation of MTX [204, 209]. MTX is also associated with leukoencephalopathy which may persist and is seen in both symptomatic and asymptomatic patients [209, 213]. Corticosteroids also affect cognitive functioning, sleep, and mood, and may induce acute psychosis [214].

Neurotoxicity is reported more frequently with newer immunotherapies, such as chimeric antigen receptor (CAR) T-cell therapy, with severe cases requiring intensive care for life-threatening seizures and cerebral edema [208, 215]. The long-term effects of these newer agents remain unknown.

Acute CNS symptoms often resolve, but some turn into permanent neurological sequelae, such as recurrent seizures, paralysis and movement disorders, and others may occur even years after treatment cessation. Persistent neurocognitive impairment has been reported in approximately 30–60% of childhood ALL survivors [216], but the decreased use of cranial radiotherapy in contemporary treatment protocols has improved neurocognitive outcomes. However, survivors treated with chemotherapy-only protocols remain at risk for long-term neurocognitive deficits with several domains affected such as processing speed, attention, intelligence, executive function, and working memory [217–224], which in turn affects academic achievement, educational attainment, and quality of life [225–227].

Risk factors for developing neurocognitive deficits are younger age at diagnosis, probably reflecting greater vulnerability of the developing brain, and higher treatment-intensity [216, 217, 225, 228]. Several other factors contribute to neurocognitive functioning, i.e., both individual factors such as patient age, sex, and genetic polymorphism, and environmental factors, such as socioeconomic status, education, and health-care access [227, 229]. Screening for neurocognitive late effects will allow for identification of those who might benefit from early interventions and is recommended in long-term follow-up care guidelines, e.g., in the United States [227, 229].

18.5 Peripheral Neurotoxicity

Chemotherapy-induced peripheral neuropathy (CIPN) is a common adverse effect mainly caused by vincristine (VCR) and is seen in approximately 80% of patients already after two months of treatment [230]. In severe cases CIPN may lead to dose reduction or treatment delay potentially compromising treatment efficacy. CIPN may persist even after treatment cessation, however, the reported prevalence varies widely reflecting varying assessment tools, diverse classifications of CIPN, and difficulties in accurately capturing PN in children [230].

Vincristine is a vinca alkaloid that inhibits the polymerization of microtubules and disrupts mitotic spindle formation leading to disruption of axonal transport. Combined with inflammatory processes these mechanisms result in neuropathy, affecting both sensory, motor, and autonomic nerves [231, 232].

Peripheral sensory neuropathy typically presents with a "stocking and glove" distribution reflecting the longest neurons being affected the most and classic symptoms include paresthesia, dysesthesia, numbness, and pain, leading to difficulties with fine motor tasks and walking. Peripheral motor neuropathy presents with distal muscle weakness and decreased deep tendon reflexes, whereas autonomic neuropathy may present with orthostatic hypotension and constipation [232, 233].

In a prospective study of 150 patients, 67.6% had persisting motor and/or sensory impairments 12 months post therapy [230], and another study found CIPN in 16% of 990 ALL survivors who were at least 5 year post diagnosis, suggesting that PN persists in a at least a group of survivors [234]. Some studies have also demonstrated worsening in CIPN after therapy cessation, the so-called coasting effect [232, 235]. Persistent CIPN may affect physical functioning contributing to an already increased risk of obesity in ALL survivors, in addition to reduced quality of life [236, 237].

Risk factors are not reported consistently, but a higher cumulative dose of vincristine is associated with increased risk for developing CIPN in several studies [233, 236]. However, in a recent study patients were randomized to receive vincristine and dexamethasone every 12 weeks vs. every 4 weeks, and most motor, sensory, functional and proxy-reported outcomes did not differ between treatment groups post therapy, possibly reflecting that CIPN develops early and persists, hence not benefitting from dose-reduction during maintenance [230]. Genetic factors is associated with prevalence and severity of CIPN [233], and a recent study found a risk variant in the CEP72 promoter region that associated with persistent motor neuropathy but also with chemosensitivity in a preclinical model, which indicate that vincristine drug doses could be personalized [234]. Also, drug interactions may interfere with the development of CIPN, e.g., antifungal azoles which inhibit cytochrome CYP3A4 involved in vinca alkaloid metabolism leading to excess vincristine exposure and severe neurotoxicity [233, 238].

Nerve-conduction studies have revealed mixed motor and sensory abnormalities in 15–68% ALL survivors [236, 239–241]. Interestingly, only 16% had both electrophysiological and clinical CIPN [236]. In general, there is poor agreement between self-reported symptoms, electrophysiological findings and clinically ascertained PN [242]. Furthermore, electrophysiological testing is painful and not suitable for routine evaluation of CIPN in children.

The identification of signs and symptoms of PN is crucial for interventions such as physical therapy to remediate symptoms [242]. However, clinical evaluation of PN is time-consuming and simple screening methods are warranted to identify those in need for specialized evaluation and treatment.

18.6 Common Underlying Toxic Effects

Despite diverse pathogenetic trajectories leading to distinct toxicities in individual patients, some general mechanisms exist. Leukemia, antileukemic drugs, radiation, supportive drugs, and the transformation of health-related behaviors collectively impact on all tissues, organ functions, and homeostasis in the individual organism. Overt adverse health conditions can result and present as local injury (e.g., bone fracture), loss of organ function (e.g., heart failure), or altered/gain of function (e.g., seizures), which resolve or progress over time. Alongside these rather well-defined disease entities are the more widespread, systemic reactions that involve inflammation, oxidative stress, and cellular aging, contributing to the overall shift in homeostasis for a limited or unlimited period. Such systemic reactions can sustain or exacerbate focal effects and act as independent risk factors that accelerate the development of typical age-related diseases such as diabetes, cardiovascular disease and neurocognitive impairment, which present decades earlier in childhood cancer survivors than in their peers [243]. Several studies have found signs of chronic inflammation in ALL survivors, defined by proinflammatory cytokines (e.g., tumor necrosis factor-α, IL-2, IL-10, IL-17a, and IL-1β), high-sensitivity C-reactive protein, intermediate monocytes, pro-inflammatory T-cell subsets, and advanced glycation of end products [105, 244–246]. The inflammatory state has furthermore been associated with endothelial cell activation [105], as well as accelerated cellular aging (inflammaging) [244, 247], both contributing to the aging phenotype. Reduced microbial diversity caused by antileukemic and antibacterial therapy in addition to mucosal damage [248], is seen to persist for years into survivorship and is thought to be a pivotal contributor to the risk of inflammation [248].

The vascular endothelial cells throughout the organism constitute a finite organ, however as they line the vessels supporting all organ functions and furthermore act as a metabolically active interface between multiple components of circulation and the underlying tissues, they could potentially play a central role for the development of acute toxicities (e.g., thrombosis, ON, SOS, and PRES) [60] as well as persistent systemic imbalances, such as chronic inflammation [249] and phenotypic frailty [250]. Nevertheless, only a very limited number of studies have investigated an association between endothelial dysfunction (ED) and toxicities in children with ALL.

Biological aging is characterized by loss of tissue or organ function or by hyperplastic pathologies, whereas the underlying cellular hallmarks of aging involve telomere attrition, genomic instability, epigenetic changes, mitochondrial dysfunction, cellular senescence (including an inflammatory phenotype), stem cell exhaustion, deregulated nutrient-sensing, and altered intercellular pathways of communication [251]. Several of these hallmarks have been linked to antileukemic exposures, such as anthracyclines, MTX, and radiation therapy, and some have been associated with frailty, impaired organ function, and risk of SMN among childhood cancer survivors, thus suggesting a functional link between antileukemic treatment and long-term morbidity [252, 253].

18.7 SMN

Although the development of a second malignant neoplasm (SMN) after diagnosis of childhood acute lymphoblastic leukemia (ALL) is a relatively rare event occurring in only a few percent of patients, several developments within the last decade call for attention to this adverse outcome [6].

First, as overall survival of childhood ALL has now reached 90% or more, the absolute proportion of deaths accounted for by SMN has grown.

Second, treatment-related myeloid neoplasia (t-MN) and lymphomas dominate with 80% having been diagnosed at 5–6 years from diagnosis of ALL. In contrast, 80% of central nervous system (CNS) tumors occur within 12–13 years from diagnosis of ALL, while 30 years of follow-up is needed before 80% of carcinomas have been diagnosed. Thus, the long-term risk of SMN will be underestimated, if follow-up is truncated after 8–10 years [6].

Third, as the use of both therapeutic and prophylactic CNS irradiation has been eliminated from many contemporary ALL protocols, the pattern of SMN will change accordingly [7]. Thus, CNS tumors will become rarer, and t-MN will dominate in publications from more recent decades.

Fourth, host genome sequencing of large cohorts has shown that a large proportion of patients have an underlying cancer prone syndrome (CPS; e.g., Li–Fraumeni syndrome) [10,

254], which emphasize that all patients with SMN should be explored for an underlying CPS, since this may guide treatment as well as surveillance of the patient and other carriers in the family for cancer development [11]. Although an underlying mechanism is yet to be detected, patients who harbor translocations in their ALL clone seem more likely to develop t-MN with *KMT2A* translocations, while those that have ALL with hyperdiploidy tend to develop t-MN with monosomy 7 [6].

Fifth, more common host genome variants, such as low activity *TPMT* and *NUDT15* variants, have also been linked to the risk of SMN in some [12, 13], although not all studies of patients being heterozygous for such variants, whereas he risk of SMN among the much rarer homozygous low variant patients remains to be determined [14]. Although their impact on the risk of SMN seem less profound than that of CPSs, they could also guide the intensity and duration of treatment with the drugs they associate to [12].

Sixth, large case studies such as that generated by the Ponte di Legno consortium with 642 SMN cases [6], have shown that most of the SMN subtypes do relatively well, although still inferior, compared with their primary counterparts with 5-year survival rates above 90% for patients with meningioma, Hodgkin lymphoma, thyroid carcinoma, basal cell carcinoma, and parotid gland tumor, and almost 70% for those with non-Hodgkin lymphoma. However, as patients with SMN are generally excluded from frontline protocols, the best therapeutic approach to these patients remains unclear. The two SMN subsets that stand out are CNS tumors, where overall survival was only 25% 10 years from diagnosis, and t-AML that had 5-year survival estimates for patients diagnosed before 2000 of 34.1% ± 6.3% [6].

There is a clear need for large collaborative efforts to (1) more systematically map the underlying biology behind SMN, and (when feasible) change the frontline ALL treatment accordingly to prevent their occurrence, and (2) establish more systematic and evidence-based treatment approaches to the SMN subsets, not least AML, as has been so in the frontline setting.

18.8 Integration of Toxicity in Outcome Evaluation

Traditional cancer outcome measures consist of overall survival and event-free survival, but for cancers with high survival rates, as for childhood ALL, these traditional outcome measures become insufficient, since they bypass the burden of therapy, of relevance for a growing population of survivors. Long-term toxicities are highly relevant to include in treatment outcome evaluation, but the lack of internationally standardized capturing and reporting of late effects has been a barrier.

Recently, ALL consortia across Europe, the United States, Asia, and Australia initiated a project aiming to prioritize and define the objectively most severe toxicities following the ALL treatment which are considered unacceptable. This work resulted in consensus definitions of 21 severe health conditions designated Severe Toxicities with examples being persistent organ failure and brain damage. The 21 severe toxicities are proposed to be integrated globally in treatment outcome evaluation as severe toxicity free survival (STFS) representing the proportion of patients cured without severe toxicities [24].

Systematic, consensus-based capturing of late effects will allow for comparison of severe toxicities across different treatment protocols and potentially reveal modifiable treatment-related factors associated with these conditions. Of note, the overall quality of life for the individual survivor reflects a complex combination of physiological, psychosocial, and socioeconomic factors, not encompassed by the STFS concept, which should rather be considered a first step toward integration of treatment sequelae with cancer outcome evaluation. Future reporting should also include lower-grade and subjective late-effects, which may be equally burdensome for the individual survivor. More comprehensive knowledge regarding the total health-related burden following cancer treatment will allow for subsequent evaluation of quality of life related to the most severe toxicities, which could reveal which conditions are the most burdensome for the survivors in questions, thus being the ones deserving most attention.

18.9 Future Directions

When the cure rate of ALL was dismal, late effects seemed a reasonable price to pay for cure. This is clearly not the case today. Although some subsets of ALL still have a poor prognosis (e.g., T-ALL resistant to induction therapy or t(17;19)/TCF3::HLF) the vast proportion of childhood ALL cases currently have cure rates well above 90%, and treatment reductions to avoid both acute and long-term toxicities are highly needed, either in a randomized setting or by comparisons with historical cohorts.

References

1. Wolthers BO, Frandsen TL, Abrahamsson J, Albertsen BK, Helt LR, Heyman M, et al. Asparaginase-associated pancreatitis: a study on phenotype and genotype in the NOPHO ALL2008 protocol. Leukemia. 2017;31(2):325–32.
2. Pui C-H, Yang JJ, Hunger SP, Pieters R, Schrappe M, Biondi A, et al. Childhood acute lymphoblastic leukemia: progress through collaboration. J Clin Oncol. 2015;33(27):2938–48.
3. Mulrooney DA, Hyun G, Ness KK, Bhakta N, Pui CH, Ehrhardt MJ, et al. The changing burden of long-term health outcomes in survivors of childhood acute lymphoblastic leukaemia: a retrospective analysis of the St Jude Lifetime Cohort Study. Lancet Haematol. 2019;6(6):e306–16.
4. Wolthers BO, Mogensen PR, Frandsen TL, Abrahamsson J, Behrendtz M, Heyman M, et al. Insulin-dependent diabetes: a chronic complication to acute pancreatitis in childhood acute lymphoblastic leukemia. Pediatr Blood Cancer. 2019;66(1):e27437.
5. Mogensen SS, Harila-Saari A, Mäkitie O, Myrberg IH, Niinimäki R, Vestli A, et al. Comparing osteonecrosis clinical phenotype, timing, and risk factors in children and young adults treated for acute lymphoblastic leukemia. Pediatr Blood Cancer. 2018;65(10):1–10.
6. Schmiegelow K, Levinsen MF, Attarbaschi A, Baruchel A, Devidas M, Escherich G, et al. Second malignant neoplasms after treatment of childhood acute lymphoblastic leukemia. J Clin Oncol. 2013;31(19):2469–76.
7. Vora A, Andreano A, Pui CH, Hunger SP, Schrappe M, Moericke A, et al. Influence of cranial radiotherapy on outcome in children with acute lymphoblastic leukemia treated with contemporary therapy. J Clin Oncol. 2016;34(9):919–26.
8. Fried S, Avigdor A, Bielorai B, Meir A, Besser MJ, Schachter J, et al. Early and late hematologic toxicity following CD19 CAR-T cells. Bone Marrow Transplant. 2019;54(10):1643–50.
9. Hansen DK, Dam M, Faramand RG. Toxicities associated with adoptive cellular therapies. Best Pract Res Clin Haematol. 2021;34(3):101287.
10. Robison LL, Mertens AC, Boice JD, Breslow NE, Donaldson SS, Green DM, et al. Study design and cohort characteristics of the Childhood Cancer Survivor Study: a multi-institutional collaborative project. Med Pediatr Oncol. 2002;38(4):229–39.
11. Hudson MM, Ehrhardt MJ, Bhakta N, Baassiri M, Eissa H, Chemaitilly W, et al. Approach for classification and severity grading of long-term and late-onset health events among Childhood Cancer Survivors in the St. Jude Lifetime Cohort. Cancer Epidemiol Biomarkers Prev. 2017;26(5):666–74.
12. McBride ML, Rogers PC, Sheps SB, Glickman V, Broemeling AM, Goddard K, et al. Childhood, adolescent, and young adult cancer survivors research program of British Columbia: objectives, study design, and cohort characteristics. Pediatr Blood Cancer. 2010;55(2):324–30.
13. Stevens M, Frobisher C, Hawkins M, Jenney M, Lancashire E, Reulen R, et al. The British Childhood Cancer Survivor Study: objectives, methods, population structure, response rates and initial descriptive information. Pediatr Blood Cancer. 2008;50(5):1018–25.
14. Asdahl PH, Winther JF, Bonnesen TG, De Fine LS, Gudmundsdottir T, Anderson H, et al. The Adult Life After Childhood Cancer in Scandinavia (ALiCCS) study: design and characteristics. Pediatr Blood Cancer. 2015;62(12):2204–10.
15. Kuehni CE, Rueegg CS, Michel G, Rebholz CE, Strippoli MPF, Niggli FK, et al. Cohort profile: the Swiss Childhood Cancer Survivor study. Int J Epidemiol. 2012;41(6):1553–64.
16. Demoor-Goldschmidt C, Allodji RS, Journy N, Rubino C, Zrafi WS, Debiche G, et al. Risk factors for small adult height in childhood cancer survivors. J Clin Oncol. 2020;38(16):1785–96.
17. Berbis J, Michel G, Baruchel A, Bertrand Y, Chastagner P, Demeocq F, et al. Cohort profile: the French Childhood Cancer Survivor Study for Leukaemia (LEA Cohort). Int J Epidemiol. 2015;44(1):49–57.
18. Teepen JC, Kremer LC, van der Heiden-van der Loo M, Tissing WJ, van der Pal HJ, van den Heuvel-Eibrink MM, et al. Clinical characteristics and survival patterns of subsequent sarcoma, breast cancer, and melanoma after childhood cancer in the DCOG-LATER cohort. Cancer Causes Control. 2019;30(9):909–22.
19. Bagnasco F, Caruso S, Andreano A, Valsecchi MG, Jankovic M, Biondi A, et al. Late mortality and causes of death among 5-year survivors of child-

hood cancer diagnosed in the period 1960–1999 and registered in the Italian Off-Therapy Registry. Eur J Cancer. 2019;2019(110):86–97.
20. Byrne J, Alessi D, Allodji RS, Bagnasco F, Bárdi E, Bautz A, et al. The PanCareSurFup consortium: research and guidelines to improve lives for survivors of childhood cancer. Eur J Cancer. 2018;2018(103):238–48.
21. Langer T, Clemens E, Broer L, Maier L, Uitterlinden AG, de Vries ACH, et al. Association of candidate pharmacogenetic markers with platinum-induced ototoxicity: PanCareLIFE dataset. Data Brief. 2020;32:106227.
22. Schmiegelow K, Attarbaschi A, Barzilai S, Escherich G, Leth Frandsen T, Halsey C, et al. Consensus definitions of 14 severe acute toxic eff ects for childhood lymphoblastic leukaemia treatment: a Delphi consensus. Lancet Oncol. 2016;17(17):231–9.
23. Pui CH, Schrappe M, Masera G, Nachman J, Gadner H, Eden OB, et al. Ponte di LEGNO WORKING GROUP: statement on the right of children with leukemia to have full access to essential treatment and report on the Sixth International Chilhood Acute Lymphoblastic Leukemia Workshop. Leukemia. 2004;18(6):1043–53.
24. Andrés-Jensen L, Attarbaschi A, Bardi E, Barzilai-Birenboim S, Bhojwani D, Hagleitner MM, et al. Severe toxicity free survival: physician-derived definitions of unacceptable long-term toxicities following acute lymphocytic leukaemia. Lancet Haematol. 2021;8(7):e513–23.
25. Lipshultz SE, Lipsitz SR, Mone SM, Goorin AM, Sallan SE, Sanders SP, et al. Female sex and higher drug dose as risk factors for late cardiotoxic effects of doxorubicin therapy for childhood cancer. N Engl J Med. 1995;332(26):1738–44.
26. Bansal N, Amdani S, Lipshultz ER, Lipshultz SE. Chemotherapy-induced cardiotoxicity in children. Expert Opin Drug Metab Toxicol. 2017;13(8):817–32.
27. Lipshultz SE, Colan SD, Gelber RD, Perez-Atayde AR, Sallan SE, Sanders SP. Late cardiac effects of doxorubicin therapy for acute lymphoblastic leukemia in childhood. N Engl J Med. 1991;324(12):808–15.
28. Kremer LCM, van der Pal HJH, Offringa M, van Dalen EC, Voute PA. Frequency and risk factors of subclinical cardiotoxicity after anthracycline therapy in children: a systematic review. Ann Oncol. 2002;13:819–29.
29. Mulrooney DA, Hyun G, Ness KK, Ehrhardt MJ, Yasui Y, Duprez D, et al. Major cardiac events for adult survivors of childhood cancer diagnosed between 1970 and 1999: report from the Childhood Cancer Survivor Study cohort. BMJ. 2020;368:l6794.
30. Hau EM, Caccia JN, Kasteler R, Spycher B, Suter T, Ammann RA, et al. Cardiovascular disease after childhood acute lymphoblastic leukaemia: a cohort study. Swiss Med Wkly. 2019;149(9–10):w20012.
31. Dixon SB, Chen Y, Yasui Y, Pui C-H, Hunger SP, Silverman LB, et al. Reduced morbidity and mortality in survivors of childhood acute lymphoblastic leukemia: a report from the Childhood Cancer Survivor study. J Clin Oncol. 2020;38(29):3418–29.
32. Burns EA, Gentille C, Trachtenberg B, Pingali SR, Anand K. Cardiotoxicity associated with anti-CD19 chimeric antigen receptor T-cell (CAR-T) therapy: recognition, risk factors, and management. Diseases. 2021;9(1):20.
33. Buechner J, Grupp SA, Hiramatsu H, Teachey DT, Rives S, Laetsch TW, et al. Practical guidelines for monitoring and management of coagulopathy following tisagenlecleucel CAR T-cell therapy. Blood Adv. 2021;5(2):593–601.
34. Silverman LB. Balancing cure and long-term risks in acute lymphoblastic leukemia. Hematology. 2014;2014(1):191–7.
35. Hutchins KK, Siddeek H, Franco VI, Lipshultz SE. Prevention of cardiotoxicity among survivors of childhood cancer. Br J Clin Pharmacol. 2017;83(3):455–65.
36. Mavinkurve-Groothuis AMC, Marcus KA, Pourier M, Loonen J, Feuth T, Hoogerbrugge PM, et al. Myocardial 2D strain echocardiography and cardiac biomarkers in children during and shortly after anthracycline therapy for acute lymphoblastic leukaemia (ALL): a prospective study. Eur Heart J Cardiovasc Imaging. 2013;14(6):562–9.
37. U.S. Department of Health and Human Services, National Institutes of Health, National Cancer Institute. Common Terminology Criteria for Adverse Events (CTCAE) Version 5.0; 2017.
38. Buza V, Rajagopalan B, Curtis AB. Cancer treatment-induced arrhythmias: focus on chemotherapy and targeted therapies. Circ Arrhythm Electrophysiol. 2017;10(8):e005443.
39. Chow EJ, Leger KJ, Bhatt NS, Mulrooney DA, Ross CJ, Aggarwal S, et al. Paediatric cardio-oncology: epidemiology, screening, prevention, and treatment. Cardiovasc Res. 2019;115:922–34.
40. Nikolousis E, Velangi M. Two cases of aspergillus endocarditis in non neutropenic children on chemotherapy for acute lymphoblastic leukaemia. Hematol Rep. 2011;3(1):20–1.
41. Chaudhary N, Vishwanath M, Pahuja M, Borker A. Candida albicans endocarditis in a child with acute lymphoblastic leukemia: a dreaded complication of intensive chemotherapy. Indian J Med Paediatr Oncol. 2013;34(1):28–30.
42. Keino D, Tsuzuki Y, Mori T, Kakuage S, Nakano M, Asoh K, et al. Infective endocarditis associated with acute leukemia: report of two cases. Pediatr Int. 2015;57(5):1017–20.
43. Son MH, Park ES, Seo J-H, Lim J-Y, Park C-H, Woo H-O, et al. Staphylococcal endocarditis presenting with a renal infarct in a patient with acute lymphoblastic leukemia. Cancer Res Treat. 2008;40(3):151.
44. Cone LA, Dreisbach L, Potts BE, Comess BE, Burleigh WA. Fatal Bacillus cereus endocardi-

tis masquerading as an anthrax-like infection in a patient with acute lymphoblastic leukemia: case report. J Heart Valve Dis. 2005;14(1):37–9.
45. Kowatari R, Suzuki Y, Daitoku K, Fukuda I. Cryptococcal infective endocarditis in a child with acute lymphocytic leukaemia. Interact Cardiovasc Thorac Surg. 2019;28(4):642–4.
46. Demaria RG, Durrleman N, Rispail P, Margueritte G, Macia JC, Aymard T, et al. Aspergillus flavus mitral valve endocarditis after lung abscess. J Heart Valve Dis. 2000;9(6):786–90.
47. Donahue TP. Loeffler's endocarditis resulting from acute lymphoblastic leukemia. Clin Cardiol. 2002;25(7):345.
48. Files MD, Zenel JA, Armsby LB, Langley SM. A child with eosinophilia, Loeffler endocarditis, and acute lymphoblastic leukemia. Pediatr Cardiol. 2009;30(4):530–2.
49. Armenian SH, Armstrong GT, Aune G, Chow EJ, Ehrhardt MJ, Ky B, et al. Cardiovascular disease in survivors of childhood cancer: insights into epidemiology, pathophysiology, and prevention. J Clin Oncol. 2018;36(21):2135–44.
50. Rank CU, Toft N, Tuckuviene R, Grell K, Nielsen OJ, Frandsen TL, et al. Thromboembolism in acute lymphoblastic leukemia: results of NOPHO ALL2008 protocol treatment in patients aged 1 to 45 years. Blood. 2018;131(22):2475–84.
51. Truelove E, Fielding AK, Hunt BJ. The coagulopathy and thrombotic risk associated with L-Asparaginase treatment in adults with acute lymphoblastic leukaemia. Leukemia. 2013;27(3):553–9.
52. Ramsay NKC, Coccia PF, Krivit W, Nesbit ME, Edson JR. The effect of L-asparaginase on plasma coagulation factors in acute lymphoblastic leukemia. Cancer. 1977;40(4):1398–401.
53. Zakarija A, Kwaan HC. Adverse effects on hemostatic function of drugs used in hematologic malignancies. Semin Thromb Hemost. 2007;33(4):355–64.
54. Appel IM, Hop WCJ, Van Kessel-Bakvis C, Stigter R, Pieters R. L-Asparaginase and the effect of age on coagulation and fibrinolysis in childhood acute lymphoblastic leukemia. Thromb Haemost. 2008;100(2):330–7.
55. Staddon JH, Smock KJ, Schiffman JD, Fluchel MN, Engel ME, Weyrich AS, et al. Pegasparaginase treatment alters thrombin generation by modulating the protein C and S system in acute lymphoblastic leukaemia/lymphoma. Blood Coagul Fibrinolysis. 2015;26(7):840–3.
56. van Zaane B, Nur E, Squizzato A, Gerdes VEA, Büller HR, Dekkers OM, et al. Systematic review on the effect of glucocorticoid use on procoagulant, anti-coagulant and fibrinolytic factors. J Thromb Haemost. 2010;8(11):2483–93.
57. Ozsoylu S. Effect of corticosteroids on coagulation tests. Acta Haematol. 1983;70(1):70.
58. Mukai M, Oka T. Mechanism and management of cancer-associated thrombosis. J Cardiol. 2018;72(2):89–93.
59. Levy-Mendelovich S, Barg AA, Kenet G. Thrombosis in pediatric patients with leukemia. Thromb Res. 2018;164:S94–7.
60. Andrés-Jensen L, Grell K, Rank CU, Albertsen BK, Tuckuviene R, Linnemann Nielsen R, et al. Endothelial dysfunction and thromboembolism in children, adolescents, and young adults with acute lymphoblastic leukemia. Leukemia. 2022;36(2):361–9.
61. Hijiya N, van der Sluis IM. Asparaginase-associated toxicity in children with acute lymphoblastic leukemia. Leuk Lymphoma. 2016;57(4):748–57.
62. Hernández-Espinosa D, Miñano A, Martínez C, Pérez-Ceballos E, Heras I, Fuster JL, et al. L-asparaginase-induced antithrombin type I deficiency: implications for conformational diseases. Am J Pathol. 2006;169(1):142–53.
63. Hongo T, Okada S, Ohzeki T, Ohta H, Nishimura S-I, Hamamoto K, et al. Low plasma levels of hemostatic proteins during the induction phase in children with acute lymphoblastic leukemia: a retrospective study by the JACLS. Pediatr Int. 2002;44(3):293–9.
64. Mitchell L, Hoogendoorn H, Giles AR, Vegh P, Andrew M. Increased endogenous thrombin generation in children with acute lymphoblastic leukemia: risk of thrombotic complications in L'Asparaginase-induced antithrombin III deficiency. Blood. 1994 Jan;83(2):386–91.
65. Klaassen ILM, Lauw MN, Fiocco M, van der Sluis IM, Pieters R, Middeldorp S, et al. Venous thromboembolism in a large cohort of children with acute lymphoblastic leukemia: risk factors and effect on prognosis. Res Pract Thromb Haemost. 2019;3(2):234–41.
66. Jarvis KB, LeBlanc M, Tulstrup M, Nielsen RL, Albertsen BK, Gupta R, et al. Candidate single nucleotide polymorphisms and thromboembolism in acute lymphoblastic leukemia – a NOPHO ALL2008 study. Thromb Res. 2019;184:92–8.
67. Jarvis KB, Nielsen RL, Gupta R, Hede FD, Huttunen P, Jónsson ÓG, et al. Polygenic risk score-analysis of thromboembolism in patients with acute lymphoblastic leukemia. Thromb Res. 2020;196:15–20.
68. Mateos MK, Tulstrup M, Quinn MCJ, Tuckuviene R, Marshall GM, Gupta R, et al. Genome-wide association meta-analysis of single-nucleotide polymorphisms and symptomatic venous thromboembolism during therapy for acute lymphoblastic leukemia and lymphoma in caucasian children. Cancers (Basel). 2020;12(5):1285.
69. Athale UH, Mizrahi T, Laverdière C, Nayiager T, Delva YL, Foster G, et al. Impact of baseline clinical and laboratory features on the risk of thrombosis in children with acute lymphoblastic leukemia: a prospective evaluation. Pediatr Blood Cancer. 2018;65(5):e26938.
70. Mizrahi T, Leclerc JM, David M, Ducruet T, Robitaille N. ABO group as a thrombotic risk factor in children with acute lymphoblastic leukemia: a ret-

rospective study of 523 patients. J Pediatr Hematol Oncol. 2015;37(5):e328–32.
71. Klok FA, van der Hulle T, den Exter PL, Lankeit M, Huisman MV, Konstantinides S. The post-PE syndrome: a new concept for chronic complications of pulmonary embolism. Blood Rev. 2014;28(6):221–6.
72. Kuhle S, Spavor M, Massicotte P, Halton J, Cherrick I, Dix D, et al. Prevalence of post-thrombotic syndrome following asymptomatic thrombosis in survivors of acute lymphoblastic leukemia. J Thromb Haemost. 2008;6(4):589–94.
73. Goldenberg NA, Donadini MP, Kahn SR, Crowther M, Kenet G, Nowak-Göttl U, et al. Post-thrombotic syndrome in children: a systematic review of frequency of occurrence, validity of outcome measures, and prognostic factors. Haematologica. 2010;95(11):1952–9.
74. Athale UH, Chan AKC. Thrombosis in children with acute lymphoblastic leukemia Part I. Epidemiology of thrombosis in children with acute lymphoblastic leukemia. Thromb Res. 2003;111:125–31.
75. Dietz AC, Chen Y, Yasui Y, Ness KK, Hagood JS, Chow EJ, et al. Risk and impact of pulmonary complications in survivors of childhood cancer: a report from the Childhood Cancer Survivor Study. Cancer. 2016;122(23):3687–96.
76. Cerveri I, Fulgoni P, Giorgiani G, Zoia MC, Beccaria M, Tinelli C, et al. Lung function abnormalities after bone marrow transplantation in children: has the trend recently changed? Chest. 2001;120(6):1900–6.
77. Gower WA, Collaco JM, Mogayzel PJJ. Lung function and late pulmonary complications among survivors of hematopoietic stem cell transplantation during childhood. Paediatr Respir Rev. 2010;11(2):115–22.
78. Nysom K, Holm K, Olsen JH, Hertz H, Hesse B. Pulmonary function after treatment for acute lymphoblastic leukaemia in childhood. Br J Cancer. 1998;78(1):21–7.
79. Fulgoni P, Zoia MC, Corsico A, Beccaria M, Georgiani G, Bossi G, et al. Lung function in survivors of childhood acute lymphoblastic leukemia. Chest. 1999;116(5):1163–7.
80. Suh E, Stratton KL, Leisenring WM, Nathan PC, Ford JS, Freyer DR, et al. Late mortality and chronic health conditions in long-term survivors of early-adolescent and young adult cancers: a retrospective cohort analysis from the Childhood Cancer Survivor Study. Lancet Oncol. 2020;21(3):421–35.
81. Fidler MM, Reulen RC, Bright CJ, Henson KE, Kelly JS, Jenney M, et al. Respiratory mortality of childhood, adolescent and young adult cancer survivors. Thorax. 2018;73(10):959–68.
82. Garneau AP, Riopel J, Isenring P. Acute methotrexate-induced crystal nephropathy. N Engl J Med. 2015;373(27):2691–3.
83. Skärby T, Jönsson P, Hjorth L, Behrentz M, Björk O, Forestier E, et al. High-dose methotrexate: on the relationship of methotrexate elimination time vs renal function and serum methotrexate levels in 1164 courses in 264 Swedish children with acute lymphoblastic leukaemia (ALL). Cancer Chemother Pharmacol. 2003;51(4):311–20.
84. Christensen AM, Pauley JL, Molinelli AR, Panetta JC, Ward DA, Stewart CF, et al. Resumption of high-dose methotrexate after acute kidney injury and glucarpidase use in pediatric oncology patients. Cancer. 2012;118(17):4321–30.
85. Zobeck MC, Bernhardt MB, Kamdar KY, Rabin KR, Lupo PJ, Scheurer ME. Novel risk factors for glucarpidase use in pediatric acute lymphoblastic leukemia: Hispanic ethnicity, age, and the ABCC4 gene. Pediatr Blood Cancer. 2021;68(8):e29036.
86. Pommert L, Liberio N, Ng JS, Egelund TA, Siver MJ, Katzenstein HM, et al. Concurrent imatinib dosing with high-dose methotrexate leads to acute kidney injury and delayed methotrexate clearance in pediatric patients with Philadelphia chromosome-positive B-cell acute lymphoblastic leukemia. J Pediatr Hematol Oncol. 2021;43(2):e296–300.
87. Skinner R. Late renal toxicity of treatment for childhood malignancy: risk factors, long-term outcomes, and surveillance. Pediatr Nephrol. 2018;33:215–25.
88. Miralbell R, Bieri S, Mermillod B, Helg C, Sancho G, Pastoors B, et al. Renal toxicity after allogeneic bone marrow transplantation: the combined effects of total-body irradiation and graft-versus-host disease. J Clin Oncol. 1996;14(2):579–85.
89. Tarbell NJ, Guinan EC, Niemeyer C, Mauch P, Sallan SE, Weinstein HJ. Late onset of renal dysfunction in survivors of bone marrow transplantation. Int J Radiat Oncol Biol Phys. 1988;15(1):99–104.
90. Kumar M, Kedar A, Neiberger RE. Kidney function in long-term pediatric survivors of acute lymphoblastic leukemia following allogeneic bone marrow transplantation. Pediatr Hematol Oncol. 1996;13(4):375–9.
91. Freycon F, Casagranda L, Trombert-Paviot B. The impact of severe late-effects after 12 Gy fractionated total body irradiation and allogeneic stem cell transplantation for childhood leukemia (1988–2010). Pediatr Hematol Oncol. 2019;36(2):86–102.
92. Bonnesen TG, Winther JF, Asdahl PH, De Fine LS, Gudmundsdottir T, Sällfors Holmqvist A, et al. Long-term risk of renal and urinary tract diseases in childhood cancer survivors: a population-based cohort study. Eur J Cancer. 2016;64:52–61.
93. Toksvang LN, Schmidt MS, Arup S, Larsen RH, Frandsen TL, Schmiegelow K, et al. Hepatotoxicity during 6-thioguanine treatment in inflammatory bowel disease and childhood acute lymphoblastic leukaemia: a systematic review. PLoS One. 2019;14:e0212157.
94. Piel B, Vaidya S, Lancaster D, Taj M, Pritchard-Jones K, Stoneham S, et al. Chronic hepatotoxicity following 6-thioguanine therapy for childhood acute lymphoblastic leukaemia. Br J Haematol. 2004;125:410–1.

95. Robison LL, Hudson MM. Survivors of childhood and adolescent cancer: life-long risks and responsibilities. Nat Rev Cancer. 2014;14(1):61–70.
96. Mulder RL, Bresters D, Van den Hof M, Koot BGP, Castellino SM, Loke YKK, et al. Hepatic late adverse effects after antineoplastic treatment for childhood cancer. Cochrane Database Syst Rev. 2019;4:CD008205.
97. Toksvang LN, De Pietri S, Nielsen SN, Nersting J, Albertsen BK, Wehner PS, et al. Hepatic sinusoidal obstruction syndrome during maintenance therapy of childhood acute lymphoblastic leukemia is associated with continuous asparaginase therapy and mercaptopurine metabolites. Pediatr Blood Cancer. 2017;64(9):1–8.
98. Stanulla M, Schaeffeler E, Möricke A, Buchmann S, Zimmermann M, Igel S, et al. Hepatic sinusoidal obstruction syndrome and short-term application of 6-thioguanine in pediatric acute lymphoblastic leukemia. Leukemia. 2021;35(9):2650–7.
99. Roy Moulik N, Taj M, M. Long-term risk of portal hypertension and related complications in children treated with 6-thioguanine for acute lymphoblastic leukemia: a single-center experience. Pediatr Blood Cancer. 2017;64(10):e26495.
100. Lennard L, Richards S, Cartwright CS, Mitchell C, Lilleyman JS, Vora A. The thiopurine methyltransferase genetic polymorphism is associated with thioguanine-related veno-occlusive disease of the liver in children with acute lymphoblastic leukemia. Clin Pharmacol Ther. 2006;80(4):375–83.
101. De Bruyne R, Portmann B, Samyn M, Bansal S, Knisely A, Mieli-Vergani G, et al. Chronic liver disease related to 6-thioguanine in children with acute lymphoblastic leukaemia. J Hepatol. 2006;44(2):407–10.
102. Nicholls L, Montez J, Pelayo-Katsanis L, Katsanis E. Esophageal varices in adolescent and young adult males with acute lymphocytic leukemia. J Adolesc Young Adult Oncol. 2019;8(2):217–20.
103. Castellino S, Muir A, Shah A, Shope S, McMullen K, Ruble K, et al. Hepato-biliary late effects in survivors of childhood and adolescent cancer: a report from the Children's Oncology Group. Pediatr Blood Cancer. 2010;54:663–9.
104. Bonnesen TG, Winther JF, Andersen KK, Asdahl PH, de Fine LS, Gudmundsdottir T, et al. Liver diseases in Adult Life after Childhood Cancer in Scandinavia (ALiCCS): a population-based cohort study of 32,839 one-year survivors. Int J Cancer. 2018;142(4):702–8.
105. De Pietri S, Ingham AC, Frandsen TL, Rathe M, Krych L, Castro-Mejía JL, et al. Gastrointestinal toxicity during induction treatment for childhood acute lymphoblastic leukemia: the impact of the gut microbiota. Int J Cancer. 2020;147(7):1953–62.
106. Oldenburg M, Rüchel N, Janssen S, Borkhardt A, Gössling KL. The microbiome in childhood acute lymphoblastic leukemia. Cancers (Basel). 2021;13(19):4947.
107. Goldsby R, Chen Y, Raber S, Li L, Diefenbach K, Shnorhavorian M, et al. Survivors of childhood cancer have increased risk of gastrointestinal complications later in life. Gastroenterology. 2011;140(5):1464–71.e1.
108. Schmiegelow K, Müller K, Mogensen SS, Mogensen PR, Wolthers BO, Stoltze UK, et al. Non-infectious chemotherapy-associated acute toxicities during childhood acute lymphoblastic leukemia therapy. F1000Research. 2017;6:444.
109. Docimo R, Anastasio MD, Bensi C. Chemotherapy-induced oral mucositis in children and adolescents: a systematic review. Eur Arch Paediatr Dent. 2022;23:501–11.
110. Sonis ST. The pathobiology of mucositis. Nat Rev Cancer. 2004;4(4):277–84.
111. Cheng KKF, Goggins WB, Lee VWS, Thompson DR. Risk factors for oral mucositis in children undergoing chemotherapy: a matched case-control study. Oral Oncol. 2008;44(11):1019–25.
112. Shafey A, Ethier M-C, Traubici J, Naqvi A, Sung L. Incidence, risk factors, and outcomes of enteritis, typhlitis, and colitis in children with acute leukemia. J Pediatr Hematol Oncol. 2013;35(7):514–7.
113. McCarville MB, Adelman CS, Li C, Xiong X, Furman WL, Razzouk BI, et al. Typhlitis in childhood cancer. Cancer. 2005;104(2):380–7.
114. Sundell N, Boström H, Edenholm M, Abrahamsson J. Management of neutropenic enterocolitis in children with cancer. Acta Paediatr. 2012;101(3):308–12.
115. Cross SJ, Patel JR, Wolf J. Diagnosis and management of typhlitis and neutropenic enterocolitis in children with cancer. Pediatr Infect Dis J. 2022;41(8):e326–8.
116. de Fine LS, Winther JF, Gudmundsdottir T, Holmqvist AS, Bonnesen TG, Asdahl PH, et al. Hospital contacts for endocrine disorders in Adult Life after Childhood Cancer in Scandinavia (ALiCCS): a population-based cohort study. Lancet (London, England). 2014;383(9933):1981–9.
117. Richardson A, Park WG. Acute pancreatitis and diabetes mellitus: a review. Korean J Intern Med. 2021;36(1):15–24.
118. Das SLM, Singh PP, Phillips ARJ, Murphy R, Windsor JA, Petrov MS. Newly diagnosed diabetes mellitus after acute pancreatitis: a systematic review and meta-analysis. Gut. 2014;63(5):818–31.
119. Dixon SB, Chen Y, Yasui Y, Pui C-H, Hunger SP, Silverman LB, et al. Impact of risk-stratified therapy on health status in survivors of childhood acute lymphoblastic leukemia: a report from the Childhood Cancer Survivor Study. Cancer Epidemiol Biomarkers Prev. 2022;31(1):150–60.
120. Kirk JA, Raghupathy P, Stevens MM, Cowell CT, Menser MA, Bergin M, et al. Growth failure and growth-hormone deficiency after treatment for acute lymphoblastic leukaemia. Lancet (London, England). 1987;1(8526):190–3.

121. Shalet SM, Brennan BM. Growth and growth hormone status following treatment for childhood leukaemia. Horm Res. 1998;50(1):1–10.
122. Krull KR, Li C, Phillips NS, Cheung YT, Brinkman TM, Wilson CL, et al. Growth hormone deficiency and neurocognitive function in adult survivors of childhood acute lymphoblastic leukemia. Cancer. 2019;125(10):1748–55.
123. Howard SC, Pui C-H. Endocrine complications in pediatric patients with acute lymphoblastic leukemia. Blood Rev. 2002;16(4):225–43.
124. Haddy TB, Mosher RB, Nunez SB, Reaman GH. Growth hormone deficiency after chemotherapy for acute lymphoblastic leukemia in children who have not received cranial radiation. Pediatr Blood Cancer. 2006;46(2):258–61.
125. Link K, Moëll C, Garwicz S, Cavallin-Ståhl E, Björk J, Thilén U, et al. Growth hormone deficiency predicts cardiovascular risk in young adults treated for acute lymphoblastic leukemia in childhood. J Clin Endocrinol Metab. 2004;89(10):5003–12.
126. Schriock EA, Schell MJ, Carter M, Hustu O, Ochs JJ. Abnormal growth patterns and adult short stature in 115 long-term survivors of childhood leukemia. J Clin Oncol Off J Am Soc Clin Oncol. 1991;9(3):400–5.
127. Clayton PE, Shalet SM, Morris-Jones PH, Price DA. Growth in children treated for acute lymphoblastic leukaemia. Lancet (London, England). 1988;1(8583):460–2.
128. Chow EJ, Liu W, Srivastava K, Leisenring WM, Hayashi RJ, Sklar CA, et al. Differential effects of radiotherapy on growth and endocrine function among acute leukemia survivors: a Childhood Cancer Survivor Study report. Pediatr Blood Cancer. 2013;60(1):110–5.
129. Chow EJ, Friedman DL, Yasui Y, Whitton JA, Stovall M, Robison LL, et al. Decreased adult height in survivors of childhood acute lymphoblastic leukemia: a report from the Childhood Cancer Survivor Study. J Pediatr. 2007;150(4):370–5, 375.e1.
130. Bruzzi P, Predieri B, Corrias A, Marsciani A, Street ME, Rossidivita A, et al. Final height and body mass index in adult survivors of childhood acute lymphoblastic leukemia treated without cranial radiotherapy: a retrospective longitudinal multicenter Italian study. BMC Pediatr. 2014;14:236.
131. van Casteren NJ, Pieters R, Dohle GR, van Baalen M, Neggers S, van den Heuvel-Eibrink MM. Cranial irradiation does not result in pituitary-gonadal axis dysfunction in very long-term male survivors of childhood acute lymphoblastic leukemia. Leukemia. 2009;23:2310–3.
132. Lie Fong S, Laven JSE, Hakvoort-Cammel FGAJ, Schipper I, Visser JA, Themmen APN, et al. Assessment of ovarian reserve in adult childhood cancer survivors using anti-Müllerian hormone. Hum Reprod. 2009;24(4):982–90.
133. van Dorp W, Haupt R, Anderson RA, Mulder RL, van den Heuvel-Eibrink MM, van Dulmen-den BE, et al. Reproductive function and outcomes in female survivors of childhood, adolescent, and young adult cancer: a review. J Clin Oncol Off J Am Soc Clin Oncol. 2018;36(21):2169–80.
134. Overbeek A, van den Berg MH, Kremer LCM, van den Heuvel-Eibrink MM, Tissing WJE, Loonen JJ, et al. A nationwide study on reproductive function, ovarian reserve, and risk of premature menopause in female survivors of childhood cancer: design and methodological challenges. BMC Cancer. 2012;12:363.
135. van Dorp W, Blijdorp K, Laven JSE, Pieters R, Visser JA, van der Lely AJ, et al. Decreased ovarian function is associated with obesity in very long-term female survivors of childhood cancer. Eur J Endocrinol. 2013;168(6):905–12.
136. Chow EJ, Stratton KL, Leisenring WM, Oeffinger KC, Sklar CA, Donaldson SS, et al. Pregnancy after chemotherapy in male and female survivors of childhood cancer treated between 1970 and 1999: a report from the Childhood Cancer Survivor Study cohort. Lancet Oncol. 2016;17(5):567–76.
137. Krawczuk-Rybak M, Solarz E, Wysocka J, Matysiak M, Gadomski A, Kazanowska B, et al. Testicular function after treatment for acute lymphoblastic leukemia (all) in prepubertal and pubertal boys. Pediatr Hematol Oncol. 2009;26(7):504–14.
138. van Dorp W, Mulder RL, Kremer LCM, Hudson MM, van den Heuvel-Eibrink MM, van den Berg MH, et al. Recommendations for premature ovarian insufficiency surveillance for female survivors of childhood, adolescent, and young adult cancer: a report from the International Late Effects of Childhood Cancer Guideline Harmonization Group in collaboration With the PanCareSurFup. J Clin Oncol. 2016;34(28):3440–50.
139. Jahnukainen K, Heikkinen R, Henriksson M, Cooper TG, Puukko-Viertomies L-R, Mäkitie O. Semen quality and fertility in adult long-term survivors of childhood acute lymphoblastic leukemia. Fertil Steril. 2011;96(4):837–42.
140. Levine JM, Whitton JA, Ginsberg JP, Green DM, Leisenring WM, Stovall M, et al. Nonsurgical premature menopause and reproductive implications in survivors of childhood cancer: a report from the Childhood Cancer Survivor Study. Cancer. 2018;124(5):1044–52.
141. Hamre MR, Robison LL, Nesbit ME, Sather HN, Meadows AT, Ortega JA, et al. Effects of radiation on ovarian function in long-term survivors of childhood acute lymphoblastic leukemia: a report from the Childrens Cancer Study Group. J Clin Oncol Off J Am Soc Clin Oncol. 1987;5(11):1759–65.
142. Green DM, Zhu L, Wang M, Chemaitilly W, Srivastava D, Kutteh WH, et al. Effect of cranial irradiation on sperm concentration of adult survivors of childhood acute lymphoblastic leukemia: a report from the St. Jude Lifetime Cohort Study†. Hum Reprod. 2017;32(6):1192–201.

143. Byrne J, Fears TR, Mills JL, Zeltzer LK, Sklar C, Meadows AT, et al. Fertility of long-term male survivors of acute lymphoblastic leukemia diagnosed during childhood. Pediatr Blood Cancer. 2004;42(4):364–72.
144. Nielsen SN, Andersen AN, Schmidt KT, Rechnitzer C, Schmiegelow K, Bentzen JG, et al. A 10-year follow up of reproductive function in women treated for childhood cancer. Reprod Biomed Online. 2013;27(2):192–200.
145. Larsen EC, Müller J, Schmiegelow K, Rechnitzer C, Andersen AN. Reduced ovarian function in long-term survivors of radiation- and chemotherapy-treated childhood cancer. J Clin Endocrinol Metab. 2003;88(11):5307–14.
146. van der Perk MEM, van der Kooi ALF, Bos AME, Broer SL, Veening MA, van Leeuwen J, van Santen HM, van Dorp W, van den Heuvel-Eibrink MM. Oncofertility Perspectives for Girls with Cancer. J Pediatr Adolesc Gynecol. 2022;35(5):523–6. https://doi.org/10.1016/j.jpag.2022.03.005. Epub 2022 Mar 28. PMID: 35358705.
147. Mulder RL, Font-Gonzalez A, Green DM, Loeffen EAH, Hudson MM, Loonen J, et al. Fertility preservation for male patients with childhood, adolescent, and young adult cancer: recommendations from the PanCareLIFE Consortium and the International Late Effects of Childhood Cancer Guideline Harmonization Group. Lancet Oncol. 2021;22(2):e57–67.
148. Mulder RL, Font-Gonzalez A, van Dulmen-den BE, Quinn GP, Ginsberg JP, Loeffen EAH, et al. Communication and ethical considerations for fertility preservation for patients with childhood, adolescent, and young adult cancer: recommendations from the PanCareLIFE Consortium and the International Late Effects of Childhood Cancer Guideline Harmonization Group. Lancet Oncol. 2021;22(2):e68–80.
149. Mulder RL, Font-Gonzalez A, Hudson MM, van Santen HM, Loeffen EAH, Burns KC, et al. Fertility preservation for female patients with childhood, adolescent, and young adult cancer: recommendations from the PanCareLIFE Consortium and the International Late Effects of Childhood Cancer Guideline Harmonization Group. Lancet Oncol. 2021;22(2):e45–56.
150. van der Perk MEM, van der Kooi A-LLF, van de Wetering MD, IJgosse IM, van Dulmen-den Broeder E, Broer SL, et al. Oncofertility care for newly diagnosed girls with cancer in a national pediatric oncology setting, the first full year experience from the Princess Máxima Center, the PEARL study. PLoS One. 2021;16(3):e0246344.
151. Blijdorp K, van Dorp W, Laven JSE, Pieters R, de Jong FH, Pluijm SMF, et al. Obesity independently influences gonadal function in very long-term adult male survivors of childhood cancer. Obesity (Silver Spring). 2014;22(8):1896–903.
152. Chow EJ, Friedman DL, Stovall M, Yasui Y, Whitton JA, Robison LL, et al. Risk of thyroid dysfunction and subsequent thyroid cancer among survivors of acute lymphoblastic leukemia: a report from the Childhood Cancer Survivor Study. Pediatr Blood Cancer. 2009;53(3):432–7.
153. Delvecchio M, Cecinati V, Brescia LP, Faienza MF, De Mattia D, Cavallo L, et al. Thyroid function and thyroid autoimmunity in childhood acute lymphoblastic leukemia off-therapy patients treated only with chemotherapy. J Endocrinol Investig. 2010;33(3):135–9.
154. Iughetti L, Bruzzi P, Predieri B, Paolucci P. Obesity in patients with acute lymphoblastic leukemia in childhood. Ital J Pediatr. 2012;38:4.
155. Marriott CJC, Beaumont LF, Farncombe TH, Cranston AN, Athale UH, Yakemchuk VN, et al. Body composition in long-term survivors of acute lymphoblastic leukemia diagnosed in childhood and adolescence: a focus on sarcopenic obesity. Cancer. 2018;124(6):1225–31.
156. van Waas M, Neggers SJCMM, Pieters R, van den Heuvel-Eibrink MM. Components of the metabolic syndrome in 500 adult long-term survivors of childhood cancer. Ann Oncol. 2010;21(5):1121–6.
157. van Waas M, Neggers SJ, van der Lelij A-J, Pieters R, van den Heuvel-Eibrink MM. The metabolic syndrome in adult survivors of childhood cancer, a review. J Pediatr Hematol Oncol. 2010;32(3):171–9.
158. Pluimakers VG, van Waas M, Neggers SJCMM, van den Heuvel-Eibrink MM. Metabolic syndrome as cardiovascular risk factor in childhood cancer survivors. Crit Rev Oncol Hematol. 2019;133:129–41.
159. Pluimakers V, Fiocco M, van Atteveld J, Hobbelink M, Bresters D, Van Dulmen-den BE, et al. Metabolic syndrome parameters, determinants, and biomarkers in adult survivors of childhood cancer: protocol for the Dutch Childhood Cancer Survivor Study on Metabolic Syndrome (Dutch LATER METS). JMIR Res Protoc. 2021;10(1):e21256.
160. Gibson TM, Ehrhardt MJ, Ness KK. Obesity and metabolic syndrome among adult survivors of childhood leukemia. Curr Treat Options in Oncol. 2016;17(4):17.
161. Nottage KA, Ness KK, Li C, Srivastava D, Robison LL, Hudson MM. Metabolic syndrome and cardiovascular risk among long-term survivors of acute lymphoblastic leukaemia - From the St. Jude Lifetime Cohort. Br J Haematol. 2014;165(3):364–74.
162. Ness KK, DeLany JP, Kaste SC, Mulrooney DA, Pui C-H, Chemaitilly W, et al. Energy balance and fitness in adult survivors of childhood acute lymphoblastic leukemia. Blood. 2015;125(22):3411–9.
163. Skoczen S, Surmiak M, Strojny W. Survivors of acute lymphoblastic leukemia and body mass changes. Expert Opin Drug Saf. 2010;9(1):65–77.
164. Cohen JE, Wakefield CE, Cohn RJ. Nutritional interventions for survivors of childhood cancer. Cochrane Database Syst Rev. 2016;2016(8):CD009678.

165. Boot AM, van den Heuvel-Eibrink MM, Hählen K, Krenning EP, de Muinck Keizer-Schrama SM. Bone mineral density in children with acute lymphoblastic leukaemia. Eur J Cancer. 1999;35(12):1693–7.
166. van der Sluis IM, van den Heuvel-Eibrink MM, Hählen K, Krenning EP, de Muinck K-SSMPF. Altered bone mineral density and body composition, and increased fracture risk in childhood acute lymphoblastic leukemia. J Pediatr. 2002;141(2):204–10.
167. Hartman A, te Winkel ML, van Beek RD, de Muinck K-SSMPF, Kemper HCG, Hop WCJ, et al. A randomized trial investigating an exercise program to prevent reduction of bone mineral density and impairment of motor performance during treatment for childhood acute lymphoblastic leukemia. Pediatr Blood Cancer. 2009;53(1):64–71.
168. Verwaaijen EJ, Ma J, de Groot-Kruseman HA, Pieters R, van der Sluis IM, van Atteveld JE, et al. A validated risk prediction model for bone fragility in children with acute lymphoblastic leukemia. J Bone Miner Res. 2021;36(12):2290–9.
169. Jain S, Jain S, Kapoor G, Virmani A, Bajpai R. No impact of disease and its treatment on bone mineral density in survivors of childhood acute lymphoblastic leukemia. Pediatr Blood Cancer. 2017;64(4).
170. den Hoed MAH, Klap BC, te Winkel ML, Pieters R, van Waas M, Neggers SJCMM, et al. Bone mineral density after childhood cancer in 346 long-term adult survivors of childhood cancer. Osteoporos Int. 2015;26(2):521–9.
171. van der Sluis IM, de Muinck K-SSMPF, Pols HAP, Lequin MH, Krenning EP, Uitterlinden AG. Collagen Ialpha1 polymorphism is associated with bone characteristics in Caucasian children and young adults. Calcif Tissue Int. 2002;71(5):393–9.
172. te Winkel ML, de Muinck K-SSMPF, de Jonge R, van Beek RD, van der Sluis IM, Hop WCJ, et al. Germline variation in the MTHFR and MTRR genes determines the nadir of bone density in pediatric acute lymphoblastic leukemia: a prospective study. Bone. 2011;48(3):571–7.
173. te Winkel ML, van Beek RD, de Muinck K-SSMPF, Uitterlinden AG, Hop WCJ, Pieters R, et al. Pharmacogenetic risk factors for altered bone mineral density and body composition in pediatric acute lymphoblastic leukemia. Haematologica. 2010;95(5):752–9.
174. van Beek RD, de Muinck K-SSMPF, Hakvoort-Cammel FG, van der Sluis IM, Krenning EP, Pieters R, et al. No difference between prednisolone and dexamethasone treatment in bone mineral density and growth in long term survivors of childhood acute lymphoblastic leukemia. Pediatr Blood Cancer. 2006;46(1):88–93.
175. Karaman S, Ercan O, Yildiz I, Bolayirli M, Celkan T, Apak H, et al. Late effects of childhood ALL treatment on body mass index and serum leptin levels. J Pediatr Endocrinol Metab. 2010;23(7):669–74.
176. Kaste SC, Jones-Wallace D, Rose SR, Boyett JM, Lustig RH, Rivera GK, et al. Bone mineral decrements in survivors of childhood acute lymphoblastic leukemia: frequency of occurrence and risk factors for their development. Leukemia. 2001;15(5):728–34.
177. te Winkel ML, Pieters R, Hop WCJ, Roos JC, Bökkerink JPM, Leeuw JA, et al. Bone mineral density at diagnosis determines fracture rate in children with acute lymphoblastic leukemia treated according to the DCOG-ALL9 protocol. Bone. 2014;59:223–8.
178. Gurney JG, Kaste SC, Liu W, Srivastava DK, Chemaitilly W, Ness KK, et al. Bone mineral density among long-term survivors of childhood acute lymphoblastic leukemia: results from the St. Jude Lifetime Cohort Study. Pediatr Blood Cancer. 2014;61(7):1270–6.
179. Cummings EA, Ma J, Fernandez CV, Halton J, Alos N, Miettunen PM, et al. Incident vertebral fractures in children with leukemia during the four years following diagnosis. J Clin Endocrinol Metab. 2015;100(9):3408–17.
180. van Atteveld JE, Pluijm SMF, Ness KK, Hudson MM, Chemaitilly W, Kaste SC, et al. Prediction of low and very low bone mineral density among adult survivors of childhood cancer. J Clin Oncol. 2019;37(25):2217–25.
181. van Atteveld JE, Mulder RL, van den Heuvel-Eibrink MM, Hudson MM, Kremer LCM, Skinner R, et al. Bone mineral density surveillance for childhood, adolescent, and young adult cancer survivors: evidence-based recommendations from the International Late Effects of Childhood Cancer Guideline Harmonization Group. Lancet Diabetes Endocrinol. 2021;9(9):622–37.
182. van Atteveld JE, Verhagen IE, van den Heuvel-Eibrink MM, van Santen HM, van der Sluis IM, Di Iorgi N, et al. Vitamin D supplementation for children with cancer: a systematic review and consensus recommendations. Cancer Med. 2021;10(13):4177–94.
183. Saini A, Saifuddin A. MRI of osteonecrosis. Clin Radiol. 2004;59(12):1079–93.
184. Niinimäki T, Niinimäki J, Halonen J, Hänninen P, Harila-Saari A, Niinimäki R. The classification of osteonecrosis in patients with cancer: validation of a new radiological classification system. Clin Radiol. 2015;70(12):1439–44.
185. te Winkel ML, Pieters R, Hop WCJ, de Groot-Kruseman HA, Lequin MH, van der Sluis IM, et al. Prospective study on incidence, risk factors, and long-term outcome of osteonecrosis in pediatric acute lymphoblastic leukemia. J Clin Oncol. 2011;29(31):4143–50.
186. Kuhlen M, Kunstreich M, Krull K, Meisel R, Borkhardt A. Osteonecrosis in children and adolescents with acute lymphoblastic leukemia: a therapeutic challenge. Blood Adv. 2017;1(14):981–94.
187. te Winkel ML, Appel IM, Pieters R, van den Heuvel-Eibrink MM. Impaired dexamethasone-

related increase of anticoagulants is associated with the development of osteonecrosis in childhood acute lymphoblastic leukemia. Haematologica. 2008;93(10):1570–4.
188. Mattano LAJ, Devidas M, Nachman JB, Sather HN, Hunger SP, Steinherz PG, et al. Effect of alternate-week versus continuous dexamethasone scheduling on the risk of osteonecrosis in paediatric patients with acute lymphoblastic leukaemia: results from the CCG-1961 randomised cohort trial. Lancet Oncol. 2012;13(9):906–15.
189. van Atteveld JE, de Groot-Kruseman HA, Fiocco M, Lequin MH, Neggers SJCMM, Pluijm SMF, et al. Effect of post-consolidation regimen on symptomatic osteonecrosis in three DCOG acute lymphoblastic leukemia protocols. Haematologica. 2021;106:1198–201.
190. den Hoed MAH, Pluijm SMF, te Winkel ML, de Groot-Kruseman HA, Fiocco M, Hoogerbrugge P, et al. Aggravated bone density decline following symptomatic osteonecrosis in children with acute lymphoblastic leukemia. Haematologica. 2015;100(12):1564–70.
191. Janke LJ, Kim J, Payton MA, Jenkins DA, Cai X, Finch ER, et al. Effects of zoledronic acid on osteonecrosis and acute lymphoblastic leukemia treatment efficacy in preclinical models. Pediatr Blood Cancer. 2021;68(10):e29183.
192. Sonis AL, Tarbell N, Valachovic RW, Gelber R, Schwenn M, Sallan S. Dentofacial development in long-term survivors of acute lymphoblastic leukemia. A comparison of three treatment modalities. Cancer. 1990;66(12):2645–52.
193. Kaste SC, Hopkins KP, Jones D, Crom D, Greenwald CA, Santana VM. Dental abnormalities in children treated for acute lymphoblastic leukemia. Leukemia. 1997;11(6):792–6.
194. Immonen E, Nikkilä A, Peltomäki T, Aine L, Lohi O. Late adverse effects of childhood acute lymphoblastic leukemia treatment on developing dentition. Pediatr Blood Cancer. 2021;68(9):e29200.
195. Wilberg P, Kanellopoulos A, Ruud E, Hjermstad MJ, Fosså SD, Herlofson BB. Dental abnormalities after chemotherapy in long-term survivors of childhood acute lymphoblastic leukemia 7-40 years after diagnosis. Support Care Cancer. 2016;24(4):1497–506.
196. Wogelius P, Dahllöf G, Gorst-Rasmussen A, Sørensen HT, Rosthøj S, Poulsen S. A population-based observational study of dental caries among survivors of childhood cancer. Pediatr Blood Cancer. 2008;50(6):1221–6.
197. Kaste SC, Goodman P, Leisenring W, Stovall M, Hayashi RJ, Yeazel M, et al. Impact of radiation and chemotherapy on risk of dental abnormalities: a report from the Childhood Cancer Survivor Study. Cancer. 2009;115(24):5817–27.
198. Baytan B, Evim MS, Güler S, Güneş AM, Okan M. Acute central nervous system complications in pediatric acute lymphoblastic leukemia. Pediatr Neurol. 2015;53(4):312–8.
199. Mateos MK, Marshall GM, Barbaro PM, Quinn MCJ, George C, Mayoh C, et al. Methotrexate-related central neurotoxicity: clinical characteristics, risk factors and genome-wide association study in children treated for acute lymphoblastic leukemia. Haematologica. 2022;107(3):635–43.
200. Banerjee J, Niinimäki R, Lähteenmäki P, Hed Myrberg I, Arola M, Riikonen P, et al. The spectrum of acute central nervous system symptoms during the treatment of childhood acute lymphoblastic leukaemia. Pediatr Blood Cancer. 2020;67(2): e27999.
201. Banerjee JS, Heyman M, Palomäki M, Lähteenmäki P, Arola M, Riikonen PV, et al. Posterior reversible encephalopathy syndrome: risk factors and impact on the outcome in children with acute lymphoblastic leukemia treated with Nordic Protocols. J Pediatr Hematol Oncol. 2018;40(1):e13–8.
202. Khan RB, Sadighi ZS, Zabrowski J, Gajjar A, Jeha S. Imaging patterns and outcome of posterior reversible encephalopathy syndrome during childhood cancer treatment. Pediatr Blood Cancer. 2016;63(3):523–6.
203. Bhojwani D, Bansal R, Wayne AS. Managing therapy-associated neurotoxicity in children with ALL. Hematol Am Soc Hematol Educ Progr. 2021;2021(1):376–83.
204. Bhojwani D, Sabin ND, Pei D, Yang JJ, Khan RB, Panetta JC, et al. Methotrexate-induced neurotoxicity and leukoencephalopathy in childhood acute lymphoblastic leukemia. J Clin Oncol. 2014;32(9):949–59.
205. Badke C, Fleming A, Iqbal A, Khilji O, Parhas S, Weinstein J, et al. Rechallenging with intrathecal methotrexate after developing subacute neurotoxicity in children with hematologic malignancies. Pediatr Blood Cancer. 2016;63(4):723–6.
206. Pryweller JR, Glass JO, Sabin ND, Laningham FH, Li Y, Jacola LM, et al. Characterization of leukoencephalopathy and association with later neurocognitive performance in pediatric acute lymphoblastic leukemia. Investig Radiol. 2021;56(2):117–26.
207. Bond J, Hough R, Moppett J, Vora A, Mitchell C, Goulden N. "Stroke-like syndrome" caused by intrathecal methotrexate in patients treated during the UKALL 2003 trial. Leukemia. 2013;27:954–6.
208. Sabin ND, Cheung YT, Reddick WE, Bhojwani D, Liu W, Glass JO, et al. The impact of persistent leukoencephalopathy on brain white matter microstructure in long-term survivors of acute lymphoblastic leukemia treated with chemotherapy only. AJNR Am J Neuroradiol. 2018;39(10):1919–25.
209. Stuart FA, Segal TY, Keady S. Adverse psychological effects of corticosteroids in children and adolescents. Arch Dis Child. 2005;90(5):500–6.
210. Śliwa-Tytko P, Kaczmarska A, Lejman M, Zawitkowska J. Neurotoxicity associated with treatment of acute lymphoblastic leukemia chemotherapy and immunotherapy. Int J Mol Sci. 2022;23(10):5515.

211. Krull KR, Brinkman TM, Li C, Armstrong GT, Ness KK, Srivastava DK, et al. Neurocognitive outcomes decades after treatment for childhood acute lymphoblastic leukemia: a report from the St Jude lifetime cohort study. J Clin Oncol. 2013;31(35):4407–15.
212. Buizer AI, de Sonneville LMJ, Veerman AJP. Effects of chemotherapy on neurocognitive function in children with acute lymphoblastic leukemia: a critical review of the literature. Pediatr Blood Cancer. 2009;52(4):447–54.
213. Liu W, Cheung YT, Conklin HM, Jacola LM, Srivastava D, Nolan VG, et al. Evolution of neurocognitive function in long-term survivors of childhood acute lymphoblastic leukemia treated with chemotherapy only. J Cancer Surviv. 2018;12(3): 398–406.
214. Kanellopoulos A, Andersson S, Zeller B, Tamnes CK, Fjell AM, Walhovd KB, et al. Neurocognitive outcome in very long-term survivors of childhood acute lymphoblastic leukemia after treatment with chemotherapy only. Pediatr Blood Cancer. 2016;63(1):133–8.
215. Peterson CC, Johnson CE, Ramirez LY, Huestis S, Pai ALH, Demaree HA, et al. A meta-analysis of the neuropsychological sequelae of chemotherapy-only treatment for pediatric acute lymphoblastic leukemia. Pediatr Blood Cancer. 2008;51(1):99–104.
216. Krull KR, Cheung YT, Liu W, Fellah S, Reddick WE, Brinkman TM, et al. Chemotherapy pharmacodynamics and neuroimaging and neurocognitive outcomes in long-term survivors of childhood acute lymphoblastic leukemia. J Clin Oncol. 2016;34(22):2644–53.
217. Iyer NS, Balsamo LM, Bracken MB, Kadan-Lottick NS. Chemotherapy-only treatment effects on long-term neurocognitive functioning in childhood ALL survivors: a review and meta-analysis. Blood. 2015;126(3):346–53.
218. Zhou C, Zhuang Y, Lin X, Michelson AD, Zhang A. Changes in neurocognitive function and central nervous system structure in childhood acute lymphoblastic leukaemia survivors after treatment: a meta-analysis. Br J Haematol. 2020;188(6):945–61.
219. Mavrea K, Efthymiou V, Katsibardi K, Tsarouhas K, Kanaka-Gantenbein C, Spandidos DA, et al. Cognitive function of children and adolescent survivors of acute lymphoblastic leukemia: a meta-analysis. Oncol Lett. 2021;21(4):262.
220. Jacola LM, Krull KR, Pui C-H, Pei D, Cheng C, Reddick WE, et al. Longitudinal assessment of neurocognitive outcomes in survivors of childhood acute lymphoblastic leukemia treated on a contemporary chemotherapy protocol. J Clin Oncol. 2016;34(11):1239–47.
221. Jacola LM, Edelstein K, Liu W, Pui C-H, Hayashi R, Kadan-Lottick NS, et al. Cognitive, behaviour, and academic functioning in adolescent and young adult survivors of childhood acute lymphoblastic leukaemia: a report from the Childhood Cancer Survivor Study. Lancet Psychiatry. 2016;3(10):965–72.
222. Jacola LM, Partanen M, Lemiere J, Hudson MM, Thomas S. Assessment and monitoring of neurocognitive function in pediatric cancer. J Clin Oncol. 2021;39(16):1696–704.
223. Daetwyler E, Bargetzi M, Otth M, Scheinemann K. Late effects of high-dose methotrexate treatment in childhood cancer survivors-a systematic review. BMC Cancer. 2022;22(1):267.
224. Phillips NS, Duke ES, Schofield H-LT, Ullrich NJ. Neurotoxic effects of childhood cancer therapy and its potential neurocognitive impact. J Clin Oncol. 2021;39(16):1752–65.
225. Rodwin RL, Kairalla JA, Hibbitts E, Devidas M, Whitley MK, Mohrmann CE, et al. Persistence of chemotherapy-induced peripheral neuropathy despite vincristine reduction in childhood B-acute lymphoblastic leukemia. J Natl Cancer Inst. 2022;114:1167.
226. Burgess J, Ferdousi M, Gosal D, Boon C, Matsumoto K, Marshall A, et al. Chemotherapy-induced peripheral neuropathy: epidemiology, pathomechanisms and treatment. Oncol Ther. 2021;9(2):385–450.
227. Kerckhove N, Collin A, Condé S, Chaleteix C, Pezet D, Balayssac D. Long-term effects, pathophysiological mechanisms, and risk factors of chemotherapy-induced peripheral neuropathies: a comprehensive literature review. Front Pharmacol. 2017;8:86.
228. van de Velde ME, Kaspers GL, Abbink FCH, Wilhelm AJ, Ket JCF, van den Berg MH. Vincristine-induced peripheral neuropathy in children with cancer: a systematic review. Crit Rev Oncol Hematol. 2017;114:114–30.
229. Goodenough CG, Diouf B, Yang W, Sapkota Y, Finch ER, Lu L, et al. Association between CEP72 genotype and persistent neuropathy in survivors of childhood acute lymphoblastic leukemia. Leukemia. 2022;36(4):1160–3.
230. Verstappen CCP, Koeppen S, Heimans JJ, Huijgens PC, Scheulen ME, Strumberg D, et al. Dose-related vincristine-induced peripheral neuropathy with unexpected off-therapy worsening. Neurology. 2005;64(6):1076–7.
231. Tay CG, Lee VWM, Ong LC, Goh KJ, Ariffin H, Fong CY. Vincristine-induced peripheral neuropathy in survivors of childhood acute lymphoblastic leukaemia. Pediatr Blood Cancer. 2017;64(8).
232. Varedi M, Lu L, Howell CR, Partin RE, Hudson MM, Pui C-H, et al. Peripheral neuropathy, sensory processing, and balance in survivors of acute lymphoblastic leukemia. J Clin Oncol. 2018;36(22):2315–22.
233. Moriyama B, Henning SA, Leung J, Falade-Nwulia O, Jarosinski P, Penzak SR, et al. Adverse interactions between antifungal azoles and vincristine: review and analysis of cases. Mycoses. 2012;55(4):290–7.
234. Jain P, Gulati S, Seth R, Bakhshi S, Toteja GS, Pandey RM. Vincristine-induced neuropathy in childhood ALL (acute lymphoblastic leukemia) survivors: prevalence and electrophysiological characteristics. J Child Neurol. 2014;29(7):932–7.

235. Ramchandren S, Leonard M, Mody RJ, Donohue JE, Moyer J, Hutchinson R, et al. Peripheral neuropathy in survivors of childhood acute lymphoblastic leukemia. J Peripher Nerv Syst. 2009;14(3):184–9.
236. Lieber S, Blankenburg M, Apel K, Hirschfeld G, Hernáiz Driever P, Reindl T. Small-fiber neuropathy and pain sensitization in survivors of pediatric acute lymphoblastic leukemia. Eur J Paediatr Neurol. 2018;22(3):457–69.
237. Hayek S, Dhaduk R, Sapkota Y, Evans WE, Diouf B, Bjornard K, et al. Concordance between Self-reported Symptoms and Clinically Ascertained Peripheral Neuropathy among Childhood Cancer Survivors: the St. Jude Lifetime Cohort Study. Cancer Epidemiol Biomarkers Prev. 2021;30(12):2256–67.
238. Ness KK, Kirkland JL, Monica Gramatges M, Wang Z, Kundu M, McCastlain K, et al. Premature physiologic aging as a paradigm for understanding increased risk of adverse health across the lifespan of survivors of childhood cancer. J Clin Oncol. 2018;36(21):2206–15.
239. Sulicka J, Surdacki A, Mikołajczyk T, Strach M, Gryglewska B, Ćwiklińska M, et al. Elevated markers of inflammation and endothelial activation and increased counts of intermediate monocytes in adult survivors of childhood acute lymphoblastic leukemia. Immunobiology. 2013;218(5):810–6.
240. Ariffin H, Azanan MS, Abd Ghafar SS, Oh L, Lau KH, Thirunavakarasu T, et al. Young adult survivors of childhood acute lymphoblastic leukemia show evidence of chronic inflammation and cellular aging. Cancer. 2017;123(21):4207–14.
241. Chua LL, Rajasuriar R, Azanan MS, Abdullah NK, Tang MS, Lee SC, et al. Reduced microbial diversity in adult survivors of childhood acute lymphoblastic leukemia and microbial associations with increased immune activation. Microbiome. 2017;5(1):35.
242. Felicetti F, Cento AS, Fornengo P, Cassader M, Mastrocola R, D'Ascenzo F, et al. Advanced glycation end products and chronic inflammation in adult survivors of childhood leukemia treated with hematopoietic stem cell transplantation. Pediatr Blood Cancer. 2020;67(3):1–7.
243. Franceschi C, Campisi J. Chronic inflammation (inflammaging) and its potential contribution to age-associated diseases. J Gerontol Ser A Biol Sci Med Sci. 2014;69(Suppl 1):S4–9.
244. Aird WC. Phenotypic heterogeneity of the endothelium: I. Structure, function, and mechanisms. Circ Res. 2007;100(2):158–73.
245. Amarasekera AT, Chang D, Schwarz P, Tan TC. Does vascular endothelial dysfunction play a role in physical frailty and sarcopenia? A systematic review. Age Ageing. 2021;50:725.
246. López-Otín C, Blasco MA, Partridge L, Serrano M, Kroemer G. The hallmarks of aging. Cell. 2013;153:1194.
247. Cupit-Link MC, Kirkland JL, Ness KK, Armstrong GT, Tchkonia T, LeBrasseur NK, et al. Biology of premature ageing in survivors of cancer. ESMO Open. 2017;2(5):e000250.
248. Ness KK, Armstrong GT, Kundu M, Wilson CL, Tchkonia T, Kirkland JL. Frailty in childhood cancer survivors. Cancer. 2015;121(10):1540–7.
249. Qian M, Cao X, Devidas M, Yang W, Cheng C, Dai Y, et al. TP53 germline variations influence the predisposition and prognosis of B-cell acute lymphoblastic leukemia in children. J Clin Oncol. 2018;36(6):591–9.
250. Junk SV, Klein N, Schreek S, Zimmermann M, Möricke A, Bleckmann K, et al. TP53, ETV6 and RUNX1 germline variants in a case series of patients developing secondary neoplasms after treatment for childhood acute lymphoblastic leukemia. Haematologica. 2019;104:e402–5.
251. Kratz CP, Achatz MI, Brugières L, Frebourg T, Garber JE, Greer M-LC, et al. Cancer screening recommendations for individuals with Li-Fraumeni syndrome. Clin Cancer Res. 2017;23(11):e38–45.
252. Levinsen M, Rotevatn EØ, Rosthøj S, Nersting J, Abrahamsson J, Appell ML, et al. Pharmacogenetically based dosing of thiopurines in childhood acute lymphoblastic leukemia: influence on cure rates and risk of second cancer. Pediatr Blood Cancer. 2014;61(5):797–802.
253. Yoshida M, Nakabayashi K, Yang W, Sato-Otsubo A, Tsujimoto S-I, Ogata-Kawata H, et al. NUDT15 variants confer high incidence of second malignancies in children with acute lymphoblastic leukemia. Blood Adv. 2021;5(23):5420–8.
254. Stanulla M, Schaeffeler E, Möricke A, Coulthard SA, Cario G, Schrauder A, et al. Thiopurine methyltransferase genetics is not a major risk factor for secondary malignant neoplasms after treatment of childhood acute lymphoblastic leukemia on Berlin-Frankfurt-Münster protocols. Blood. 2009;114(7):1314–8.

19 Supportive Care During Therapy for Childhood Acute Lymphoblastic Leukemia

Etan Orgel, Sheena Mukkada, Christopher Denton, and Deepa Bhojwani

19.1 Introduction

Improvements in the survival rates for children with acute lymphoblastic leukemia (ALL) would have not been possible without parallel improvements in supportive care over the past several decades. In the early days, the major causes of death in children with ALL were infection in 70% and hemorrhage in 52% [1]. The incidence of *Pneumocystis carinii* pneumonia was 21% without prophylaxis [2]. Access to blood components and antibiotics greatly enabled intensification of chemotherapy. Additionally, a deeper understanding of the pathophysiology of the disease led to prompt recognition and strategies to manage acute manifestations such as hyperleukocytosis and tumor lysis syndrome which in turn led to decrease in the rate of early deaths [3]. Supportive care guidelines undergo continued refinement and optimization. As we move toward targeted agents and immunotherapy, the success of these therapies is also in part dependent on the ability to safely support patients through the anticipated untoward effects.

The goal of supportive care is to minimize the morbidity and mortality associated with the disease and its therapy; effective supportive care strategies allow providers to optimize treatment delivery for cure while maximizing quality of life during and after therapy. Psychosocial supportive care, a crucial component in the care of patients with ALL, is outside the scope of this chapter. Despite an increased focus on supportive care, severe grade 3 or 4 toxicity is reported in ~40–80% of those treated on recent ALL consortia trials [4–6]. Non-disease-related treatment related mortality (TRM) continues to be problematic on current regimens, affecting 1–3% of children treated for ALL irrespective of the specific regimen or consortia [7–11]. While relapse of disease remains the number one cause of death in children with ALL, improvement in disease response has reduced the number of relapse-related deaths. As a result, the relatively constant rate for TRM over the years now constitutes an increasing proportion of mortality; approximately one in five deaths on therapy are now due to TRM rather than the disease itself [12]. Infection remains the primary reason for TRM. The highest risk occurs within the initial Induction phase, with up to 50% of non-disease-

E. Orgel · C. Denton · D. Bhojwani (✉)
Division of Hematology and Oncology, Children's Hospital Los Angeles, Keck School of Medicine, University of Southern California, Los Angeles, CA, USA
e-mail: eorgel@chla.usc.edu; chdenton@chla.usc.edu; dbhojwani@chla.usc.edu

S. Mukkada
Department of Global Pediatric Medicine, St Jude Children's Research Hospital, Memphis, TN, USA

Department of Infectious Diseases, St Jude Children's Research Hospital, Memphis, TN, USA
e-mail: Sheena.Mukkada@stjude.org

G. Escherich, V. Conter (eds.), *Acute Lymphoblastic Leukemia in Children and Adolescents*, Pediatric Oncology, https://doi.org/10.1007/978-3-031-71180-0_19

related deaths occurring within those first 28 days [9, 10]. The induction phase of ALL chemotherapy is therefore not only critical for obtaining a remission for eventual cure [13] but also the period of greatest risk for a life-threatening event.

The overall goal of this chapter is to provide insight into common supportive care issues at presentation, as well as those globally impacting therapy, and to aid the clinician in providing anticipatory supportive care and prompt recognition and intervention for serious adverse effects. Specific treatment-related toxicities, as a consequence of individual chemotherapeutic agents and their management are detailed in chapter "Acute Toxicity and Late Effects Related to ALL Treatment".

19.2 Oncologic Emergencies at Diagnosis

Onset of symptomatic ALL is often accompanied by several, frequently concurrent oncologic emergencies. As such, at time of suspected ALL (i.e., prior to confirmation of diagnosis), it is critical to refer patients for immediate assessment, triage, and stabilization. The goal during this period is *preventive*; due to the typically large and fragile tumor burden, potential extra-marrow nodal aggregates, and overarching severe immunocompromise, even relatively well-appearing children can rapidly decompensate and incur organ injury. Obtaining input from an oncology specialist is essential to gauge the risk for presenting comorbidities and emergencies and develop a care plan to allow for definitive therapy to be initiated safely.

19.2.1 Hyperleukocytosis

Approximately 15% of patients with ALL present with hyperleukocytosis (leukocyte count >100×10^9/L) at initial diagnosis. The incidence is higher in patients with Philadelphia chromosome-positive ALL, *KMT2A* rearrangements and T-ALL [14, 15] Clinical consequences result from hyperviscosity and include pulmonary leukostasis requiring mechanical ventilation, neurologic complications (e.g., intracranial hemorrhage, seizure and confusion), thrombosis, bleeding, and acute kidney injury. These manifestations are most evident in patients with leukocyte counts >400×10^9/L [16]. Leukapheresis can transiently decrease the leukocyte count by 20–50% but can be associated with untoward effects such as electrolyte disturbances, coagulopathy, and catheter dysfunction/thrombosis. The role of leukapheresis in pediatric ALL is not well defined and is generally not recommended. Recent studies show that enhanced supportive care and careful initiation of cytoreductive, low-dose chemotherapy (steroids with or without a dose of vincristine) may mitigate the need for more invasive leukapheresis [15, 17, 18]. Maintaining euvolemia with adequate hydration prior to the initiation of chemotherapy and close monitoring of respiratory and neurologic status (especially in the peri-anesthesia period) are other measures to decrease morbidity and mortality [19]. In patients with hyperleukocytosis, it is imperative to transfuse platelets and optimize coagulation parameters to mitigate the risk of bleeding, but to limit packed red cell transfusions except in case where absolutely required (e.g., hemodynamic unstable, critically poor oxygenation) as increased blood viscosity can increase risk for intracranial hemorrhage [15, 20].

19.2.2 Mediastinal Mass

Routine screening by chest radiograph is standard practice for all patients with a suspected or confirmed diagnosis of ALL. Approximately 10% of patients with ALL are noted to present with an anterior mediastinal mass; the incidence is higher at 50% in T-ALL [21, 22]. Of all patients with mediastinal mass, 42% have tracheal deviation/compression impacting clinical management [21]. Due to limited chest volume in children, an anterior mediastinal mass often causes compression of both the superior vena cava (SVC) and airway, resulting in superior mediastinal syndrome and risk for cardiorespiratory compromise. Many patients are asymptomatic, and common signs and symptoms are non-specific, including cough, dyspnea, orthopnea, noisy breathing and upper body edema. Patients with mediastinal mass must be assessed expeditiously and managed by a multidisciplinary team including an intensivist. These patients should remain in position of maximum comfort with head elevated, or in lateral or prone position. Supine position exacerbates airway and cardiac compression and should be avoided. In cases where it is important to assess the extent of airway impingement (e.g., for intensive care triage or prior to procedures), a rapid computerized tomography (CT) scan, ideally in semi-upright position is helpful to determine the tracheal cross-sectional area (TCA), and a bedside peak expiratory flow rate (PEFR) is a simple measure of airflow obstruction [23]. A critical airway is defined as any of the following: TCA <50% of predicted, PEFR <50% of predicted, severe narrowing or complete occlusion of one or both mainstem bronchi and/or clinical finding of acute respiratory distress [24]. Additionally, all patients should be assessed by upright echocardiogram for cardiac compromise from a pericardial effusion/tamponade or impingement of the ventricles or outflow tract. Hydration is recommended to maintain adequate venous return and cardiac output. Medications that alter intrathoracic pressure (e.g., anxiolytics, analgesics) may result in large masses shifting to more occlusive positions and should be avoided or used with caution only in a controlled setting. Diagnostic workup in these patients can be challenging as sedation and anesthesia are risky in patients with a critical airway. The least invasive method to obtain diagnostic specimen must be pursued. If peripheral blood or pleural fluid are nondiagnostic, bone marrow aspirate or lymph node biopsy can be attempted under local anesthesia [24]. In life-threatening situations, 24–48 h of empiric steroids or radiotherapy may be required to shrink the mass prior to safe biopsy, lumbar puncture, and initiation of definitive therapy.

19.2.3 Tumor Lysis Syndrome (TLS)

Though hyperleukocytosis and other indicators of high tumor burden such as hepatosplenomegaly and elevated LDH are risk factors for tumor lysis, all children with ALL can be considered to have bulky disease as the volume of the bone marrow is approximately 20 mL/kg of the body weight [25]. Spontaneous, osmotic, or chemotherapy-induced blast breakdown and massive release of intracellular metabolites are responsible for the clinical and laboratory consequences of TLS [26]. The Cairo–Bishop definition of laboratory TLS requires elevation of two or more values of serum uric acid, potassium, phosphate or calcium at presentation or an increase of these values by 25% in the period of 3 days prior to 7 days post initiation of chemotherapy [27]. Clinical TLS is defined as renal insufficiency, cardiac arrhythmia or seizure in addition to one or more laboratory parameters.

Close monitoring and prophylactic measures are essential to minimize adverse outcomes of TLS. These include aggressive hydration to maintain urine output of 80–100 mL/m^2/h, judicious use of diuretics (only in the absence of hypovolemia and obstructive uropathy), and rapid intervention to normalize electrolyte imbalance (e.g., hyperkalemia, hyperphosphatemia, and hyperuricemia). Historical practices for alkalinizing of urine to increase the solubility of uric acid are no longer recommended; alkalinization enhances uric acid precursor and calcium phosphate precipitation in the kidneys.

Allopurinol inhibits the formation of uric acid by blocking xanthine oxidase, however the accumulated precursors of uric acid (hypoxanthine and xanthine) can also precipitate in the renal tubules compromising renal function further. Rasburicase (recombinant urate oxidase) is highly effective in converting uric acid to allantoin, a highly soluble compound readily excreted in the urine. The use of rasburicase has significantly decreased the need for dialysis in patients with TLS and hyperuricemia [28]. Rasburicase can cause severe methemoglobinemia and hemolysis in patients with glucose-6-phosphatase dehydrogenase (G6PD) deficiency [29]. Preferably testing for G6PD deficiency is recommended prior to administration of rasburicase, particularly in populations with high incidence.

19.3 Hematologic Supportive Care

Hematologic complications are prevalent in ALL due to the myeloablative effects of chemotherapy as well as characteristics of the underlying disease. Transfusion of platelets and red blood cells can be required at diagnosis and is almost certainly necessary during treatment, therefore transfusion guidelines have been adapted for supportive care. Thrombosis is a less common but still important aspect of ALL care that has received more attention in recent years.

19.3.1 Transfusion Guidelines for Anemia and Thrombocytopenia

Frequent blood transfusion is often required due to therapy-induced pancytopenia [30]. Thrombocytopenic bleeding was a major cause of morbidity and mortality during intensive chemotherapy until prophylactic platelet transfusion was introduced in the 1970s, when a landmark study improved stored platelet function [31, 32]. Most centers have adopted a threshold of $<10 \times 10^3$ cells/μL for prophylactic platelet transfusion [33] while a threshold of $<20 \times 10^3$ cells/μL is used for patients with bleeding, fever, infection, or a rapid fall in platelet count [34]. Despite a paucity of available evidence, the threshold of $<20 \times 10^3$ cells/μL is also used for platelet transfusion prior to central venous catheter placement and lumbar puncture [35], while a higher threshold of $<50–100 \times 10^3$ cells/μL is recommended in the setting of circulating blasts due to the risk of traumatic lumbar puncture worsening event free survival [35, 36].

Red blood cell transfusion is recommended at a hemoglobin threshold of 7–8 g/dL [37]. The strongest evidence for a hemoglobin threshold of 7 g/dL in children comes from a study of transfusion in pediatric intensive care units [38]. A more recent study of adults with acute leukemia revealed no difference in bleeding events using a hemoglobin threshold of 7 g/dL versus 8 g/dL, although the patients transfused at 8 g/dL received more transfused units [39]. Patients of certain religious faiths such as Jehovah's Witness present a therapeutic challenge due to their non-acceptance of blood products, but this is not an absolute contraindication to life-saving intensive chemotherapy as transfusion can potentially be avoided with alternate strategies and a multimodal approach [40].

Modification of blood components can mitigate the acute risks of transfusion. Leukoreduction is universally employed where available due to its effectiveness in preventing infection and transfusion reaction, and limiting platelet refractoriness [41]. Using either CMV-seronegative products or leukoreduced blood components consistently reduces the risk of transmitting CMV such that both methods are considered CMV-safe at most centers [42, 43]. The risk of febrile non-hemolytic transfusion reaction is significantly reduced after universal pre-storage leukoreduction of red blood cells and platelets [44]. There is limited evidence that leukoreduction also alleviates the risk of transfusion-related acute lung injury and transfusion-associated graft-versus-host disease (TA-GVHD) [41]. Irradiation of blood products is more effective in preventing TA-GVHD and is therefore recommended for immunocompromised individuals where available, but red cells must be transfused within 24 h after this procedure due to its effect on shelf life [45]. Single-donor apheresis platelets are preferred to whole blood-derived pooled platelets to limit donor exposure and associated risk of infection [46]. Platelet refractoriness and the development of HLA antibodies is also of concern, and response to transfusion is higher with single-donor platelets [47].

Additional safety measures notwithstanding, judicious use of transfusion is recommended to avoid its associated risks. Transfusional iron overload is an important long-term complication of cancer survivors [48], and patients receiving greater than ten red cell transfusions are at higher risk of cardiac iron deposition [49]. Consequences of iron overload and therapeutic impact of chelation are historically understood in patients with thalassemia [50], particularly with respect to stem cell transplant [51, 52]. Phlebotomy is also effective in removing excess total body iron once patients have completed myelosuppressive therapy and are no longer receiving red blood cell transfusions [53].

19.3.2 Thrombosis

Risk factors for venous thromboembolism (VTE) include cancer type, with higher incidence in leukemia, lymphoma, and sarcoma; age $\geq$ 10 years; intrathoracic disease; and central venous catheter (CVC) dysfunction [54]. Presence of CVC is the primary risk factor for VTE in children with cancer [55], while asparaginase and steroids are therapeutic agents that are well known to induce a hypercoagulable state [56].

Current guidelines recommend systemic thromboprophylaxis in pediatric cancer patients with a history of thrombosis who continue to receive intensive therapy and do not have a contraindication to anticoagulation [57]. In the absence of prior thrombosis, systemic thromboprophylaxis should be considered in the setting of significant risk factors [57]. Short of systemic thromboprophylaxis, mechanical prophylaxis is suggested for older patients in hospital settings associated with prolonged immobility [57] Obesity was demonstrated to more than triple the risk of VTE in patients receiving ALL therapy [58], and a trial of apixaban as thromboprophylaxis in pediatric leukemia/lymphoma was efficacious only in this subgroup [59].

Treatment of SVT or symptomatic VTE historically involves anticoagulation for 3–6 months, which has recently been challenged by the results of a large pediatric study demonstrating a 6-week duration to be noninferior, but children with cancer were notably excluded [60]. Low molecular weight heparin has been the anticoagulant of choice for decades and is recommended over unfractionated heparin in patients with cancer [61], while fondaparinux is a more attractive option due to its once- rather than twice-daily dosing [62]. All of these agents require intravenous access or subcutaneous injections, in addition to multiple venipunctures to monitor drug concentrations [63].

Direct oral anticoagulants (DOACs) were recently approved for use in children after randomized controlled trials of dabigatran and rivaroxaban demonstrated non-inferiority to standard of care [64, 65]. While these pediatric trials included only some patients with active or previous history of cancer, adult studies have shown DOACS to be safe and efficacious in treatment and prevention of VTE in patients with cancer [66].

Thrombocytopenia can be a limiting factor in patients receiving intensive chemotherapy who require anticoagulation. Importantly, the risk of thrombosis in patients with cancer is not reduced in the setting of thrombocytopenia. A retrospective study showed that full-dose anticoagulation is safe with platelet count >50 × 10^3 cells/μL [67]. In patients with severe thrombocytopenia with platelet count <50 × 10^3 cells/uL who require anticoagulation, either transfusion support to maintain platelets above this threshold or dose-modified anticoagulation has been proposed [68]. Current guidelines are based on these adult data due to a paucity of data in children [69]. The optimal approach to anticoagulation is determined by an individual patient's risk of recurrent or progressive VTE. Generally, this risk is highest during the acute period of VTE, or within 30 days of diagnosis [70], so full-dose anticoagulation is indicated during this period in patients with a platelet count >50 × 10^3 cells/μL. In patients with acute VTE and additional high-risk features, such as segmental pulmonary embolism or proximal DVT instituting platelet transfusion support and continuing full-dose anticoagulation should be considered [69]. In patients with lower-risk acute VTE, dose-modified anticoagulation for platelet count 25–50 × 10^3 cells/μL and holding anticoagulation for platelets <25 × 10^3 cells/μL is a reasonable strategy. This low-risk strategy may also be considered in patients with VTE after the 30-day acute period.

19.4 Infections

Infection is a common complication of childhood cancer therapy which contributes to morbidity both through direct effects and interruptions to cancer-directed therapy. Estimates of the burden of infection in acute lymphoblastic leukemia (ALL) vary between treatment regimens and centers, but in general infections are reported less frequently and are of less severity when compared with patients with acute myeloid leukemia or recipients of hematopoietic stem cell transplants. Reports of infection-related mortality range from 0.9 to 2.4 with differences based on the patient population, treatment era, drug regimen, and treatment center [11, 71]. Nevertheless, infection by category is the largest cause of treatment related mortality in childhood ALL patients [5, 9, 10, 71–73]. A retrospective study of patients treated on the Total XV protocol at St. Jude Children's Research Hospital documented infection related mortality in 1% of patients during the course of treatment with 30% of documented infections being upper respiratory tract infections and 12% being bloodstream infections [74]. The availability and types of testing modalities as well as testing practices affect the observed estimates, particularly for viral and fungal infection, however patients with ALL are at risk of bacterial, fungal, and viral infections. These complications result both from the underlying disease state and the chemotherapy delivered to treat it. In addition to the lymphosuppression associated with the disease and treatment, certain chemotherapeutic agents cause myelosuppression which further elevates the risk of infection. Additionally, these patients often have CVCs which pose a risk of infection due to being retained foreign bodies and because of being repeatedly accessed.

The risk of infection is related both to the depth and the duration of observed cytopenias whereas the relative risk of each type of infection is related to the affected cell line. Neutrophil count is an important parameter as it is indicative of the ability to control a bacterial or fungal infection. Nevertheless, a low lymphocyte count has been implicated in greater viral disease severity due to multiple viruses, including respiratory viruses [75, 76]. Additionally, patients with lymphopenia have prolonged viral shedding, which, while often of unclear clinical significance, cause delays and dose reductions which may adversely affect patient outcomes [76].

Clinicians have struggled to identify subgroups of patients at high risk for infectious complications, as risk stratification schema have performed poorly when validated outside of derivation cohorts [77–93]. In general, intensive chemotherapy and relapsed ALL have been described as risk factors for significant adverse outcome and invasive bacterial infection, respectively [94, 95]. While the incidence of fungal infections is lower in patients with ALL relative to patients with AML or HSCT, the morbidity and mortality in infected patients can be high [10, 96]. Subsets of patients with ALL, such as those with relapsed disease and those receiving induction and reinduction therapy, have been identified as having an elevated risk for invasive fungal infection [97].

Corticosteroids, a cornerstone for ALL therapy, are a risk factor for development of serious infection, including invasive fungal infection, however translating this risk factor to clinical practice is complicated because the corticosteroid dose used to define high dose differs between studies [97]. Furthermore, the differences in underlying comorbidities of patients included in studies make it difficult to assess the independent risk of steroids [98]. Nonetheless, in phases of ALL therapy with corticosteroid duration ≥10 days, clinical suspicion for infection should be high in patients presenting with consistent symptoms, even in the absence of fever [99]. The infectious risk associated with newer immunotherapies is not well elucidated.

19.4.1 Infection Prevention

Many infections that arise during cancer-directed therapy cannot be prevented. Bacteremias most often result from a patient's colonizing organisms and arise during periods of neutropenia, particularly when concomitant chemotherapy causes damage to mucosal surfaces [100]. Use of central line maintenance bundles and teaching families to care appropriately for central lines may, however, decrease the incidence of catheter-related infections. To prevent communicable diseases, clinicians should direct patients to practice frequent and thorough hand hygiene, wear masks, and avoid crowds if possible. Patients should receive all age-appropriate vaccines that are not live virus vaccines. Immune response, however, may be decreased compared to immunocompetent individuals and may not be fully protective against infection [101, 102]. Therefore, clinicians should encourage optimal vaccination of families and caregivers to create a cocooning effect and diminish exposure to vaccine-preventable diseases.

Prophylaxis for *Pneumocystis jirovecii* pneumonia (PCP) is routinely utilized based on trials demonstrating that this fatal disease occurs in up to 21% of unprophylaxed patients during childhood cancer treatment, and is dramatically reduced by administration of trimethoprim–sulfamethoxazole (TMP/SMX) during the at risk period [2]. A number of dosing strategies have been performed, including daily, three times weekly, and twice weekly, but evidence on effectiveness does not support one dosing strategy over another [103, 104]. Atovaquone, dapsone, and pentamidine are alternative choices for prophylaxis in patients with a true intolerance to TMP/SMX, however TMP/SMX is the preferred agent due to the demonstrated lack of breakthrough infections with this regimen [105]. Intravenous and aerosolized pentamidine have the advantage of less frequent dosing (every 4 weeks), however the aerosolized route exposes healthcare workers to respiratory side effects [106]. Unlike TMP/SMX and atovaquone, pyrimethamine has no activity against toxoplasmosis, which may be a limitation in seropositive patients requiring anti-Toxoplasma prophylaxis.

Use of prophylactic antimicrobials to prevent development of other infections is more controversial since the risks/adverse effects of drug administration may outweigh the potential benefits of administering medications to all patients. Certain subpopulations of patients with ALL, including those with relapsed disease, as well as those receiving highly myelosuppressive therapy, such as those in induction or reinduction/delayed intensification phases of therapy, may benefit from administration of antibacterial or antifungal prophylaxis during periods of highest risk [107]. There is evidence to suggest that antibacterial prophylaxis is associated with decreased episodes of febrile neutropenia and bloodstream infection compared to an unprophylaxed population [96, 108]. Due to concerns for development of antibiotic resistance with prolonged use, as well as concerns for medication side effects, limiting antibiotic prophylaxis to high risk patients and the at risk period is recommended [107]. An international guideline accordingly issues a weak recommendation to consider using systemic antibacterial prophylaxis in patients with relapsed ALL who are receiving intensive chemotherapy with expected myelosuppression for a minimum of 7 days and institutional practice varies [107]. The same guideline recommends against routine use of antibacterial prophylaxis in patients receiving induction chemotherapy for newly diagnosed ALL [107]. In making this weak recommendation, panelists cited the heterogeneity of patient risk status, which means that the long term effects of resistance and medication side effects may outweigh any theoretical benefit of use [107]. Thus, the decision to implement antibacterial prophylaxis should be guided by local context for the institution, including treatment intensity of the patient population, in consultation with infectious disease specialists. While other agents have been used, fluoroquinolones are most commonly recommended in adults and pediatrics as a prophylactic agent due to their broad spectrum of activity, including activity against Pseudomonas aeruginosa and other gram-negative bacteria [96, 108–111]. Levofloxacin offers additional gram-positive coverage relative to ciprofloxacin so therefore is preferred when available [107].

Like antibacterial prophylaxis, the question of how to use antifungal prophylaxis in children with ALL is an unresolved question. To determine the potential benefit of initiating prophylaxis, the clinician must evaluate the general risk profile for the patient population, considering disease status and treatment regimen administered. International guidelines advise that clinicians consider antifungal prophylaxis in patients with relapsed leukemia or new diagnosis of ALL, who may be at higher risk of invasive fungal infection due to prolonged myelosuppression [112]. Clinicians are advised not to use antifungal prophylaxis routinely in patients without risk factors associated with invasive fungal disease, including use of corticosteroids or therapies causing prolonged profound neutropenia [112]. If systemic antifungals are initiated, prophylaxis strategies should account for regional risk factors and variation in fungal flora.

19.4.2 Infection Management

As patients are at risk for infection and infections may be severe, clinicians should have a low index of suspicion for initiating a diagnostic workup for infection. Due to the risk of bacterial translocation and the presence of foreign bodies, one should always treat a fever as a potential infectious event. Fever management guidelines traditionally differentiate management between a neutropenic and a nonneutropenic host, as the risks of bacterial translocation and bacteremia are greater in a neutropenic host. One should obtain blood culture in any patient presenting with a fever [113]. Clinicians should use history and exam to direct further workup, considering endemic diseases and circulating viruses [113]. In a patient with severe neutropenia, clinicians should initiate antibiotic therapy immediately, as delays in therapy are associated with progression to severe infection For this reason, many institutions use the target of administering the first dose of an antimicrobial within 60 min as a quality measure. In the event that diagnostic workup is delayed, clinicians should start antibiotics without waiting to perform diagnostic studies. Institutional guidelines should recommend antibiotics according to the spectrum of resistance observed in the center, the clinical condition of the patient, the patient's personal microbiologic history, and any clinical foci of infection. In neutropenic patients, the spectrum of activity should be broad enough to cover gram-positive and gram-negative organisms, including antipseudomonal coverage [113]. There are many research opportunities within the field of infection management, including duration of therapy in a patient with unknown source of infection, as well as the definition of patients who may not require inpatient therapy. These strategies are based on risk calculation and require reliable follow up as well as local validation. Selected patients with a neutrophil count above 500 may be managed as outpatients and may not require antibiotic therapy [114, 115].

Treatment options for respiratory viral illnesses are limited in number and efficacy. With the exception of influenza, for which oseltamivir is indicated in all new cases, antiviral therapy is rarely administered. If a patent tests positive for SARS-CoV-2, clinicians should consider the both the extent of a patient's respiratory symptoms as well as the risk of progression to severe illness based on disease, treatment, and laboratory parameters. Patients in induction or reinduction or with a low absolute lymphocyte count may benefit from treatment [116]. If clinicians elect to start antiviral treatment, remdesivir is most often selected due to multiple drug interactions between the oral agent nirmatrelvir–ritonavir and other agents used in childhood cancer patients. Remdesivir is an intravenous agent, so this may limit its use in less ill patients.

Primary management of SARS-CoV-2 and other non-influenza viruses in most patients focuses on managing symptoms, including administration of oxygen as needed. In theory, intravenous immunoglobulin replacement may offer some benefit, particularly in patients with a low baseline immunoglobulin G level; however, evidence of benefit in patients with ALL is lacking [117]. The uncertain benefit must be balanced against significant cost and potential hazards of administration. While a patient may remain symptomatic, viremic or continue to shed the virus, the decision to administer either immunoglobulins or antiviral therapy reflects a balance of host and disease factors which is highly individualized [75, 116]. In general, the variety and efficacy of antivirals is limited compared to antibacterial agents, and their toxicities often prohibit clinicians from using them in children with ALL, unless the patients develop severe illness. Varicella zoster virus and herpes simplex virus can cause skin, mucosal, and central nervous system manifestations and can also disseminate in an immunocompromised host. Infections confirmed or suspected to be due to both viruses should be treated promptly with an acyclovir derivative to reduce morbidity and the risk of dissemination. The role of other systemic viruses is less well understood than in patients following hematopoietic stem cell transplant. Viruses such as cytomegalovirus, Epstein–Barr virus, and adenovirus can be intermittently detected in blood; however, there are no threshold viral loads that correlate with disease. Treatment is not indicated for isolated low-grade viremia but may be indicated in the presence of other clinical signs and symptoms of disease.

19.5 Nutrition and Activity During ALL therapy

Patients receiving ALL therapy are at risk for toxicities resulting from being either malnourished or obese. In ALL, either weight extreme has been associated with greater relapse risk, poorer survival, and/or increased risk of toxicity [118–123]. Goals for optimizing nutrition and activity in the ALL population have therefore focused on all of these endpoints: augmenting chemotherapy efficacy to reduce relapse, and improving resilience to treatment associated toxicities to reduce morbidity and improve quality of life. Multiple strategies are available to treat malnourishment once identified, including appetite stimulation and exogenous oral or enteral supplementation [124]. However, obesity during ALL therapy is increasingly common and often intransigent to intervention. In the United States, almost half the adult population, and one in five children, suffer from obesity [125, 126]. a health challenge that is further exacerbated in patients with ALL due to obesogenic therapy (e.g., glucocorticoids, physical inactivity, etc.) [127, 128]. In a clinical trial of ALL conducted by the Children's Oncology Group, the prevalence of children with overweight or obesity doubled during treatment, with nearly half of the population meeting criteria for overweight or obesity by trial end [129]. To address these adverse impacts on quality of life and treatment outcomes, recent evidence-based clinical guidelines strongly recommend the integration of exercise (American Society of Clinical Oncology [ASCO], 2022 [130]) and nutritional assessment and interventions (European Society for Clinical Nutrition and Metabolism [ESPEN], 2021 [124]) into cancer therapy. In addition to these guidelines for general recommendations, we highlight additional considerations applicable to ALL therapy with an emphasis on the oncologist's role.

19.5.1 General Principles for Nutrition and Exercise Interventions

While nutrition and exercise interventions are subject to institutional differences and capabilities, there are several overarching considerations for integration into ALL treatment (Table 1). Foremost, early screening, and repeated assessments, are critical to prevent and treat malnutrition. At diagnosis, patients with obesity and/or those malnourished should be identified, as well as those at-risk for poor nutrition [124]. Nutritional assessment of patients at diagnosis has been demonstrated to improve health outcomes [131]. The combination of obesogenic

Table 1 General considerations for nutrition and activity interventions

1. Early and serial assessments of nutritional status
2. Identify patient-provider shared treatment goals to guide interventions (i.e., general wellness, reduce specific or global toxicity, potentially augment chemotherapy efficacy)
3. Integration of education and interventions from treatment outset
4. Family-focused or "whole home" interventions for children and adolescents
5. Individualized approaches for each patient and family; reassessment required
6. Referral and/or integration of multidisciplinary expertise into care plans (physical therapy, dietitians, physical medicine and rehabilitation, etc.)

therapy, and conversely, comorbidities resulting in periods of decreased intake, creates a mutable nutritional status [127]; this warrants careful surveillance and serial assessments during the multiple years of ALL treatment. To complement early identification, an early education and intervention plan is crucial. Although historically, patient and provider hesitance over such interventions was a concern, multiple trials over the past several years have demonstrated the feasibility of incorporating early into ALL therapy dietary interventions [132], multimodal dietary and exercise interventions [133], and focused exercise interventions [134, 135]. Self-efficacy is an important consideration for intervention success, and provider-patient discussions to develop mutual goals for diet and exercise interventions are often helpful. For instance, understanding whether the goal is for general wellness, maintaining fitness, prevention of toxicities, or to potentially reduce risk of relapse may lead to different recommendations for the timing and nature of proposed interventions. Once goals are set, the intervention must include the entire family unit, and be customized to account for personal, cultural, and socioeconomic differences in dietary and exercise preferences. As with nutritional status, reassessment is key as capabilities and preferences for diet and exercise often change throughout therapy. Lastly, prompt referral for multidisciplinary care from physical therapists, occupational therapists, dietitians, and related specialists is beneficial to best support treatment goals, as these plans must often accommodate complex chemotherapy schedules and comorbidities.

19.5.2 Nutritional Considerations for ALL Therapy

In general, recommendations for nutritional assessment and interventions during cancer therapy apply to patients receiving ALL regimens [124]. ALL therapy has several unique aspects for providers to consider in ensuring adequate nutritional support. As described above, ALL regimens induce obesity in many patients. However, patients receiving ALL regimens are also at high risk for developing “sarcopenic obesity” [136], the result of concurrent loss of muscle mass and gain in body fat. Providers must therefore be wary of using weight alone as a marker of nutritional status and healthy body composition. Distinct from obesity and sarcopenia, sarcopenic obesity has been independently associated with multiple adverse health outcomes across a range of malignancies, including dose-limiting toxicities, metabolic syndrome, cardiovascular toxicity, and pharmacokinetic differences in chemotherapy exposure [137–140]. Biochemical indices often used to screen for malnutrition, such as hypoalbuminemia, are unreliable during ALL therapy. Repeated doses of the chemotherapy asparaginase is associated with hypoalbuminemia [141], and inflammation and comorbidity both negatively influence serum albumin concentrations [142], complicating its use to assess nutritional status during ALL therapy. Where available, periodic assessment of nutritional intake by dietitians is therefore an essential component to assess and treat malnutrition and obesity during ALL therapy. Optimally, dietitians may be embedded within the ALL multidisciplinary treatment team. Providers should monitor for weight fluctuations (loss or gain) and general assessments of nutritional intake to aid in prompt referral for management as indicated. Restrictive diets should not be routinely recommended by the provider. Specifically, the “neutropenic diet” has been demonstrated to be of no benefit and a cause of potential nutritional harm [143–145], and is not recommended [130].

Proactive dietary guidance is also beneficial to manage specific ALL toxicities. Prolonged and/or high-dose glucocorticoid exposure is common throughout ALL regimens; during Induction, >20% of patients will develop hyperglycemia [146], with adolescents particularly at risk [146–149], and many require insulin sensitizers and/or exogenous insulin. Modulation of dietary intake is a key component for prevention and treatment of steroid-induced hyperglycemia. Similarly, vincristine neuropathy results in significant constipation and slowed transit, often manifesting early in ALL therapy due to dose intensity (with a second peak late due to cumulative vincristine exposure). Dietician input to help families plan high fiber diets, with adequate fluid intake, are an effective first line intervention to reduce the requirement for extensive laxative regimens. Taste changes from ALL chemotherapy are common, with parents facing challenges in balancing healthy menus, particularly for younger children. Dietitians can help families plan individualized menus with appropriate food substitutions, advise on practical interventions to maximize taste (e.g., longer chewing to prolong contact with taste buds), and optimize nutritional intake and parental quality of life. Similar to other cancer regimens, close communication between the dietitian and the oncology provider is essential to identify underlying toxicities impacting nutritional intake, most often manifesting as appetite loss, chemotherapy-induced nausea/vomiting, constipation, and adjustment disorders or depression.

19.5.3 Exercise Considerations During ALL Therapy

Patients receiving ALL therapy are particularly prone to loss of lean muscle mass, most profoundly occurring at treatment outset during the induction phase [134, 136]. Unfortunately, exercise interventions during ALL chemotherapy are particularly challenging. Two prospective trials in ALL piloting intensive exercise interventions during early therapy failed to demonstrate benefit for reduction of muscle loss [133, 134]. Both trials reported nonadherence to the exercise component as the likely key determinant of the intervention's failure to do so. In the IDEAL trial (Improving Diet and Exercise in ALL, NCT02708108), self-reported adherence to exercise recommendations during induction was markedly poorer than adherence to diet (31% vs. 82%) [133]. Moreover, patients in the trial were monitored via wearable fitness trackers, and were found to walk, on average, fewer than 2000 steps per day (<5th percentile of normative steps/day for children and adolescents in the United States [150]). This discrepancy highlights the challenges for incorporating exercise into chemotherapy, even in otherwise highly motivated patients and families. Although not specific to ALL, common themes for barriers to exercise during therapy include fatigue, physical limitations, anxiety over injury, and logistical limitations (e.g., hospitalized, treatment requirements, etc.) [151, 152].

As recently endorsed by ASCO [153], exercise during cancer treatment has numerous benefits for wellness, fitness, obesity management, and quality of life. In pediatric ALL therapy, a trend toward similar benefits from exercise have been observed, though data remains of overall low quality. Coombs et al. summarized the results of 19 studies (508 children), and found exercise interventions to benefit children primarily for range of motion, strength, coordination, physical activity, and fatigue [135]. Nonetheless, adverse events from exercise are low, and exercise is recommended as an integral component to cancer therapy, including for ALL. Early referral to a physical therapist may be beneficial to overcome perceived barriers and to develop an individualized, supervised exercise program. In general, exercise recommendations should include both aerobic and resistance training and occur on multiple days per week. There is insufficient evidence to date to recommend a specific duration or daily/weekly quantity of each component of exercise for children and adolescents during the different phases of ALL therapy. In addition to early referral and reinforcing benefits from exercise, providers should encourage reducing physical inactivity (i.e., "sedentary behavior"). During ALL therapy, inactivity is common and is associated with fat gain and persistent obesity. Inactivity is also associated with increased post-prandial glucose [154], exacerbating ALL phases at risk for steroid-induced hyperglycemia. However, even brief interruptions in inactivity can increase overall caloric expenditure and restore metabolic flexibility [155, 156]. Daily step goals, movement reminders, and reduction of physical inactivity are key complementary recommendations to incorporate alongside exercise during therapy.

19.6 Future Directions in Supportive Care

Supportive care is an integral component of providing increasingly intensive therapies for childhood ALL. Inclusion of appropriate supportive care recommendations has led to important strides in chemotherapy delivery for patients at high risk of complications, such as for infants, patients with trisomy 21, and for older adolescents and young adults. Optimal supportive care reduces treatment-related early deaths, minimizes dose-limiting or treatment-interrupting toxicities, and improves both survival and quality of life during after treatment. Groundbreaking trials have provided a strong basis for supportive care recommendations to prevent multiple common treatment-associated toxicities, including severe infection, venous thromboembolism, neurocognitive deficits, and others. Yet, despite these advances, and despite more than five decades of use for some "conventional" chemotherapy agents, our understanding of the pharmacology and mechanism for typical side effects remains in its infancy. Too often supportive care recommendations are based on maximizing interventions versus targeting pathophysiology. Often, these recommendations have unproven benefit, or even potential harms. Recommendations for prolonged hospitalizations may result in infectious risk, financial toxicity, and/or psychosocial stressors [157, 158]. Similarly, multiple supportive care medication, including antimicrobial prophylaxis and treatment, are associated with potential drug–drug interactions that complicate chemotherapy delivery [159]. Improved understanding of the pathophysiology of treatment-associated toxicities is essential to avoid perpetuating the "kitchen sink" philosophy of supportive care delivery.

To move forward, supportive care researchers must therefore simultaneously take a step back. To complement future intervention trials, supportive care research efforts must also focus on the underlying pathophysiology. New technologies such as the "omics" (genomics, metabolomics, lipidomics, microbiomics, etc.), advanced sequencing techniques, and novel computational network capabilities, offer a previously unattainable range of resolution to understand side effects: from broad population insights to detailed understandings of tissue interactions. Turning these technologies to investigate ALL side effects will allow us to better identify promising supportive care interventions as well as the individuals in whom they will most be required. Emerging data has begun to delineate ethnic, racial, and other population differences in risk for treatment-associated toxicities in ALL [160]; research into these differences will provide both insights into the underlying mechanism as well new opportunities for intervention. With the ever-increasing number of interventions possible, and the burgeoning number of pills and medications we require of patients during high intensity ALL phases, it is now more critical than ever to better identify targeted strategies for side effect risk-stratification and prevention at both the population and patient level.

While we have only recently begun to make leaps toward understanding and using conventional chemotherapies, we must also recognize that we stand at the base of an ever-accelerating development arc for novel molecular and immunological targeted therapies for ALL. It is critical that we learn from past lessons to ensure that these advances are supported by research equally focused on minimizing their side effect profile. One need only look at the advent of chimeric antigen receptor (CAR) T-cell therapy. The fortuitous discovery of tocilizumab rescued the technology and transformed cytokine release syndrome from a technology-halting complication to a manageable side effect [161]. Integrating supportive care research and recommendations into emerging therapies will minimize the risk of losing promising agents in development and concurrently ensure their optimal use once deployed. The welcome wave of new immunotherapies, molecular agents, and antibody-conjugates to treat ALL will bring unique supportive care challenges and opportunities. Vigilance and engagement with supportive care researchers will be required, lest it be decades more before we learn how best to use them.

References

1. Hersh EM, Bodey GP, Nies BA, Freireich EJ. Causes of death in acute leukemia: a ten-year study of 414 patients from 1954-1963. JAMA. 1965;193:105–9.
2. Hughes WT, Kuhn S, Chaudhary S, Feldman S, Verzosa M, Aur RJ, et al. Successful chemoprophylaxis for pneumocystis carinii pneumonitis. N Engl J Med. 1977;297(26):1419–26.
3. Heikamp E, Dreyer ZE. 50 Years ago in The Journal of Pediatrics: prevention and management of acute hyperuricemia in childhood leukemia. J Pediatr. 2017;191:178.
4. Burke MJ, Devidas M, Chen Z, Salzer WL, Raetz EA, Rabin KR, et al. Outcomes in adolescent and young adult patients (16 to 30 years) compared to younger patients treated for high-risk B-lymphoblastic leukemia: report from Children's Oncology Group Study AALL0232. Leukemia. 2022;36(3):648–55.
5. Stary J, Zimmermann M, Campbell M, Castillo L, Dibar E, Donska S, et al. Intensive chemotherapy for childhood acute lymphoblastic leukemia: results of the randomized intercontinental trial ALL IC-BFM 2002. J Clin Oncol. 2014;32(3):174–84.
6. Vora A, Goulden N, Mitchell C, Hancock J, Hough R, Rowntree C, et al. Augmented post-remission therapy for a minimal residual disease-defined high-risk subgroup of children and young people with clinical standard-risk and intermediate-risk acute lymphoblastic leukaemia (UKALL 2003): a randomised controlled trial. Lancet Oncol. 2014;15(8):809–18.
7. Lund B, Åsberg A, Heyman M, Kanerva J, Harila-Saari A, Hasle H, et al. Risk factors for treatment related mortality in childhood acute lymphoblastic leukaemia. Pediatr Blood Cancer. 2011;56(4):551–9.
8. Hargrave DR, Hann II, Richards SM, Hill FG, Lilleyman JS, Kinsey S, et al. Progressive reduction in treatment-related deaths in Medical Research Council childhood lymphoblastic leukaemia trials from 1980 to 1997 (UKALL VIII, X and XI). Br J Haematol. 2001;112(2):293–9.
9. Larsen EC, Devidas M, Chen S, Salzer WL, Raetz EA, Loh ML, et al. Dexamethasone and high-dose methotrexate improve outcome for children and young adults with high-risk B-acute lymphoblastic leukemia: a report from Children's Oncology Group Study AALL0232. J Clin Oncol. 2016;34:2380.
10. Rubnitz JE, Lensing S, Zhou Y, Sandlund JT, Razzouk BI, Ribeiro RC, et al. Death during induction therapy and first remission of acute leukemia in childhood: the St. Jude experience. Cancer. 2004;101(7):1677–84.
11. Slats AM, Egeler RM, van der Does-van den Berg A, Korbijn C, Hahlen K, Kamps WA, et al. Causes of death--other than progressive leukemia--in childhood acute lymphoblastic (ALL) and myeloid leukemia (AML): the Dutch Childhood Oncology Group experience. Leukemia. 2005;19(4):537–44.
12. Hunger SP, Lu X, Devidas M, Camitta BM, Gaynon PS, Winick NJ, et al. Improved survival for children and adolescents with acute lymphoblastic leukemia between 1990 and 2005: a report from the Children's Oncology Group. J Clin Oncol. 2012;30(14):1663–9.
13. Borowitz MJ, Devidas M, Hunger SP, Bowman WP, Carroll AJ, Carroll WL, et al. Clinical significance of minimal residual disease in childhood acute lymphoblastic leukemia and its relationship to other prognostic factors: a Children's Oncology Group study. Blood. 2008;111(12):5477–85.
14. Abla O, Angelini P, Di Giuseppe G, Kanani MF, Lau W, Hitzler J, et al. Early complications of hyperleukocytosis and leukapheresis in childhood acute leukemias. J Pediatr Hematol Oncol. 2016;38(2):111–7.
15. Nguyen R, Jeha S, Zhou Y, Cao X, Cheng C, Bhojwani D, et al. The role of leukapheresis in the current management of hyperleukocytosis in newly diagnosed childhood acute lymphoblastic leukemia. Pediatr Blood Cancer. 2016;63:1546.
16. Lowe EJ, Pui CH, Hancock ML, Geiger TL, Khan RB, Sandlund JT. Early complications in children with acute lymphoblastic leukemia presenting with hyperleukocytosis. Pediatr Blood Cancer. 2005;45(1):10–5.
17. Sondhi V, Sharma A, Taneja M, Arora B, Banavali SD. L-asparginase administration reduces white blood cell count and prevents tumor lysis syndrome in children with hyperleukocytic acute lymphoblastic leukemia. Acta Haematol. 2015;133(1):6–9.
18. Ozdemir MA, Karakukcu M, Patiroglu T, Torun YA, Kose M. Management of hyperleukocytosis and prevention of tumor lysis syndrome with low-dose prednisone continuous infusion in children with acute lymphoblastic leukemia. Acta Haematol. 2009;121(1):56–62.
19. Fong C, Fung W, McDonald J, Dalla-Pozza L, De Lima J. Anesthesia for children with hyperleukocytosis a retrospective review. Paediatr Anaesth. 2009;19(12):1191–8.
20. Lichtman MA, Rowe JM. Hyperleukocytic leukemias: rheological, clinical, and therapeutic considerations. Blood. 1982;60(2):279–83.
21. Smith WT, Shiao KT, Varotto E, Zhou Y, Iijima M, Anghelescu DL, et al. Evaluation of chest radiographs of children with newly diagnosed acute lymphoblastic leukemia. J Pediatr. 2020;223:120–7.e3.
22. Wayne NJ, Li Y, Chung P, Coffan K, Rheingold SR. Outcomes of children and young adults with T-cell acute lymphoblastic leukemia/lymphoma who present in critical status. Pediatr Blood Cancer. 2022;69(4):e29457.
23. Shamberger RC, Holzman RS, Griscom NT, Tarbell NJ, Weinstein HJ, Wohl ME. Prospective evaluation by computed tomography and pulmonary function tests of children with mediastinal masses. Surgery. 1995;118(3):468–71.
24. Perger L, Lee EY, Shamberger RC. Management of children and adolescents with a critical airway due

to compression by an anterior mediastinal mass. J Pediatr Surg. 2008;43(11):1990–7.
25. Sambuceti G, Brignone M, Marini C, Massollo M, Fiz F, Morbelli S, et al. Estimating the whole bone-marrow asset in humans by a computational approach to integrated PET/CT imaging. Eur J Nucl Med Mol Imaging. 2012;39(8):1326–38.
26. Howard SC, Jones DP, Pui CH. The tumor lysis syndrome. N Engl J Med. 2011;364(19):1844–54.
27. Coiffier B, Altman A, Pui CH, Younes A, Cairo MS. Guidelines for the management of pediatric and adult tumor lysis syndrome: an evidence-based review. J Clin Oncol. 2008;26(16):2767–78.
28. Jeha S, Kantarjian H, Irwin D, Shen V, Shenoy S, Blaney S, et al. Efficacy and safety of rasburicase, a recombinant urate oxidase (Elitek), in the management of malignancy-associated hyperuricemia in pediatric and adult patients: final results of a multicenter compassionate use trial. Leukemia. 2005;19(1):34–8.
29. Pirrone I, Farruggia P, Cacciatore F, Giambona A, Guarina A, Marcello AP, et al. Rasburicase-induced methemoglobinemia: a case report and literature review. J Pediatr Hematol Oncol. 2021;43(6):e886–e90.
30. Lieberman L, Liu Y, Portwine C, Barty RL, Heddle NM. An epidemiologic cohort study reviewing the practice of blood product transfusions among a population of pediatric oncology patients. Transfusion. 2014;54(10 Pt 2):2736–44.
31. Murphy S, Gardner FH. Platelet storage at 22 degrees C; metabolic, morphologic, and functional studies. J Clin Invest. 1971;50(2):370–7.
32. Cannas G, Thomas X. Supportive care in patients with acute leukaemia: historical perspectives. Blood Transfus. 2015;13(2):205–20.
33. Pine AB, Lee EJ, Sekeres M, Steensma DP, Zelterman D, Prebet T, et al. Wide variations in blood product transfusion practices among providers who care for patients with acute leukemia in the United States. Transfusion. 2017;57(2):289–95.
34. Schiffer CA, Anderson KC, Bennett CL, Bernstein S, Elting LS, Goldsmith M, et al. Platelet transfusion for patients with cancer: clinical practice guidelines of the American Society of Clinical Oncology. J Clin Oncol. 2001;19(5):1519–38.
35. Schiffer CA, Bohlke K, Delaney M, Hume H, Magdalinski AJ, McCullough JJ, et al. Platelet transfusion for patients with cancer: American Society of Clinical Oncology clinical practice guideline update. J Clin Oncol. 2018;36(3):283–99.
36. Shaikh F, Voicu L, Tole S, To T, Doria AS, Sung L, et al. The risk of traumatic lumbar punctures in children with acute lymphoblastic leukaemia. Eur J Cancer. 2014;50(8):1482–9.
37. Steiner ME, Zantek ND, Stanworth SJ, Parker RI, Valentine SL, Lehmann LE, et al. Recommendations on RBC transfusion support in children with hematologic and oncologic diagnoses from the Pediatric Critical Care Transfusion and Anemia Expertise Initiative. Pediatr Crit Care Med. 2018;19(9S Suppl 1):S149–S56.
38. Lacroix J, Hebert PC, Hutchison JS, Hume HA, Tucci M, Ducruet T, et al. Transfusion strategies for patients in pediatric intensive care units. N Engl J Med. 2007;356(16):1609–19.
39. DeZern AE, Williams K, Zahurak M, Hand W, Stephens RS, King KE, et al. Red blood cell transfusion triggers in acute leukemia: a randomized pilot study. Transfusion. 2016;56(7):1750–7.
40. El Chaer F, Ballen KK. Treatment of acute leukaemia in adult Jehovah's Witnesses. Br J Haematol. 2020;190(5):696–707.
41. Bianchi M, Vaglio S, Pupella S, Marano G, Facco G, Liumbruno GM, et al. Leucoreduction of blood components: an effective way to increase blood safety? Blood Transfus. 2016;14(2):214–27.
42. Vamvakas EC. Is white blood cell reduction equivalent to antibody screening in preventing transmission of cytomegalovirus by transfusion? A review of the literature and meta-analysis. Transfus Med Rev. 2005;19(3):181–99.
43. Ratko TA, Cummings JP, Oberman HA, Crookston KP, DeChristopher PJ, Eastlund DT, et al. Evidence-based recommendations for the use of WBC-reduced cellular blood components. Transfusion. 2001;41(10):1310–9.
44. Paglino JC, Pomper GJ, Fisch GS, Champion MH, Snyder EL. Reduction of febrile but not allergic reactions to RBCs and platelets after conversion to universal prestorage leukoreduction. Transfusion. 2004;44(1):16–24.
45. Foukaneli T, Kerr P, Bolton-Maggs PHB, Cardigan R, Coles A, Gennery A, et al. Guidelines on the use of irradiated blood components. Br J Haematol. 2020;191(5):704–24.
46. Vamvakas EC. Relative safety of pooled whole blood-derived versus single-donor (apheresis) platelets in the United States: a systematic review of disparate risks. Transfusion. 2009;49(12):2743–58.
47. Triulzi DJ, Assmann SF, Strauss RG, Ness PM, Hess JR, Kaufman RM, et al. The impact of platelet transfusion characteristics on posttransfusion platelet increments and clinical bleeding in patients with hypoproliferative thrombocytopenia. Blood. 2012;119(23):5553–62.
48. Ruccione KS, Wood JC, Sposto R, Malvar J, Chen C, Freyer DR. Characterization of transfusion-derived iron deposition in childhood cancer survivors. Cancer Epidemiol Biomarkers Prev. 2014;23(9):1913–9.
49. Unal S, Cetin M, Hazirolan T, Yildirim G, Meral A, Birbilen A, et al. Number of erythrocyte transfusions is more predictive than serum ferritin in estimation of cardiac iron loading in pediatric patients with acute lymphoblastic leukemia. Leuk Res. 2014;38(8):882–5.
50. Taher AT, Saliba AN. Iron overload in thalassemia: different organs at different rates. Hematology Am Soc Hematol Educ Program. 2017;2017(1):265–71.

51. Lucarelli G, Galimberti M, Polchi P, Angelucci E, Baronciani D, Giardini C, et al. Bone marrow transplantation in patients with thalassemia. N Engl J Med. 1990;322(7):417–21.
52. Lucarelli G, Galimberti M, Polchi P, Angelucci E, Baronciani D, Giardini C, et al. Marrow transplantation in patients with thalassemia responsive to iron chelation therapy. N Engl J Med. 1993;329(12):840–4.
53. Franchini M, Gandini G, Veneri D, de Matteis G, Federici F, Solero P, et al. Efficacy and safety of phlebotomy to reduce transfusional iron overload in adult, long-term survivors of acute leukemia. Transfusion. 2004;44(6):833–7.
54. Athale U, Siciliano S, Thabane L, Pai N, Cox S, Lathia A, et al. Epidemiology and clinical risk factors predisposing to thromboembolism in children with cancer. Pediatr Blood Cancer. 2008;51(6):792–7.
55. Journeycake JM, Buchanan GR. Catheter-related deep venous thrombosis and other catheter complications in children with cancer. J Clin Oncol. 2006;24(28):4575–80.
56. Athale UH, Chan AK. Thrombosis in children with acute lymphoblastic leukemia part III. Pathogenesis of thrombosis in children with acute lymphoblastic leukemia: effects of host environment. Thromb Res. 2003;111(6):321–7.
57. Tullius BP, Athale U, van Ommen CH, Chan AKC, Palumbo JS, Balagtas JMS, et al. The identification of at-risk patients and prevention of venous thromboembolism in pediatric cancer: guidance from the SSC of the ISTH. J Thromb Haemost. 2018;16(1):175–80.
58. Prasca S, Carmona R, Ji L, Ko RH, Bhojwani D, Rawlins YA, et al. Obesity and risk for venous thromboembolism from contemporary therapy for pediatric acute lymphoblastic leukemia. Thromb Res. 2018;165:44–50.
59. Rodriguez V, O'Brien SH, Lew G, Orgel E, Derr K, Ranalli MA et al. Apixaban is effective and safe in reducing venous thromboembolism (VTE) in obese patients with newly diagnosed pediatric acute lymphoblastic leukemia/lymphoblastic lymphoma: a sub-study analysis of the PREVAPIX-ALL/ Children's Oncology Group ACL1333 trial. Blood 2023;142(Suppl 1):810. https://doi.org/10.1182/blood-2023-180037.
60. Goldenberg NA, Kittelson JM, Abshire TC, Bonaca M, Casella JF, Dale RA, et al. Effect of anticoagulant therapy for 6 weeks vs 3 months on recurrence and bleeding events in patients younger than 21 years of age with provoked venous thromboembolism: the Kids-DOTT Randomized Clinical Trial. JAMA. 2022;327(2):129–37.
61. Lyman GH, Carrier M, Ay C, Di Nisio M, Hicks LK, Khorana AA, et al. American Society of Hematology 2021 guidelines for management of venous thromboembolism: prevention and treatment in patients with cancer. Blood Adv. 2021;5(4):927–74.
62. Shen X, Wile R, Young G. FondaKIDS III: a long-term retrospective cohort study of fondaparinux for treatment of venous thromboembolism in children. Pediatr Blood Cancer. 2020;67(8):e28295.
63. Jaffray J, Young G. Direct oral anticoagulants for use in paediatrics. Lancet Child Adolesc Health. 2022;6(3):207–14.
64. Male C, Lensing AWA, Palumbo JS, Kumar R, Nurmeev I, Hege K, et al. Rivaroxaban compared with standard anticoagulants for the treatment of acute venous thromboembolism in children: a randomised, controlled, phase 3 trial. Lancet Haematol. 2020;7(1):e18–27.
65. Halton J, Brandao LR, Luciani M, Bomgaars L, Chalmers E, Mitchell LG, et al. Dabigatran etexilate for the treatment of acute venous thromboembolism in children (DIVERSITY): a randomised, controlled, open-label, phase 2b/3, non-inferiority trial. Lancet Haematol. 2021;8(1):e22–33.
66. Agnelli G, Becattini C, Meyer G, Munoz A, Huisman MV, Connors JM, et al. Apixaban for the treatment of venous thromboembolism associated with cancer. N Engl J Med. 2020;382(17):1599–607.
67. Khanal N, Bociek RG, Chen B, Vose JM, Armitage JO, Bierman PJ, et al. Venous thromboembolism in patients with hematologic malignancy and thrombocytopenia. Am J Hematol. 2016;91(11):E468–E72.
68. Kopolovic I, Lee AY, Wu C. Management and outcomes of cancer-associated venous thromboembolism in patients with concomitant thrombocytopenia: a retrospective cohort study. Ann Hematol. 2015;94(2):329–36.
69. Samuelson Bannow BT, Lee A, Khorana AA, Zwicker JI, Noble S, Ay C, et al. Management of cancer-associated thrombosis in patients with thrombocytopenia: guidance from the SSC of the ISTH. J Thromb Haemost. 2018;16(6):1246–9.
70. Lee AY, Levine MN, Baker RI, Bowden C, Kakkar AK, Prins M, et al. Low-molecular-weight heparin versus a coumarin for the prevention of recurrent venous thromboembolism in patients with cancer. N Engl J Med. 2003;349(2):146–53.
71. O'Connor D, Bate J, Wade R, Clack R, Dhir S, Hough R, et al. Infection-related mortality in children with acute lymphoblastic leukemia: an analysis of infectious deaths on UKALL2003. Blood. 2014;124(7):1056–61.
72. Moghrabi A, Levy DE, Asselin B, Barr R, Clavell L, Hurwitz C, et al. Results of the Dana-Farber Cancer Institute ALL Consortium protocol 95-01 for children with acute lymphoblastic leukemia. Blood. 2007;109(3):896–904.
73. Lund B, Asberg A, Heyman M, Kanerva J, Harila-Saari A, Hasle H, et al. Risk factors for treatment related mortality in childhood acute lymphoblastic leukaemia. Pediatr Blood Cancer. 2011;56(4):551–9.
74. Inaba H, Pei D, Wolf J, Howard SC, Hayden RT, Go M, et al. Infection-related complications during treatment for childhood acute lymphoblastic leukemia. Ann Oncol. 2017;28(2):386–92.
75. El Saleeby CM, Somes GW, DeVincenzo JP, Gaur AH. Risk factors for severe respiratory syncytial

virus disease in children with cancer: the importance of lymphopenia and young age. Pediatrics. 2008;121(2):235–43.
76. Mukkada S, Bhakta N, Chantada GL, Chen Y, Vedaraju Y, Faughnan L, et al. Global characteristics and outcomes of SARS-CoV-2 infection in children and adolescents with cancer (GRCCC): a cohort study. Lancet Oncol. 2021;22(10):1416–26.
77. Rondinelli PI, Ribeiro Kde C, de Camargo B. A proposed score for predicting severe infection complications in children with chemotherapy-induced febrile neutropenia. J Pediatr Hematol Oncol. 2006;28(10):665–70.
78. Ammann RA, Hirt A, Luthy AR, Aebi C. Predicting bacteremia in children with fever and chemotherapy-induced neutropenia. Pediatr Infect Dis J. 2004;23(1):61–7.
79. Agyeman P, Aebi C, Hirt A, Niggli FK, Nadal D, Simon A, et al. Predicting bacteremia in children with cancer and fever in chemotherapy-induced neutropenia results of the prospective Multicenter SPOG 2003 FN study. Pediatr Infect Dis J. 2011;30(7):E114–E9.
80. Alexander SW, Wade KC, Hibberd PL, Parsons SK. Evaluation of risk prediction criteria for episodes of febrile neutropenia in children with cancer. J Pediatr Hematol Oncol. 2002;24(1):38–42.
81. Hakim H, Flynn PM, Srivastava DK, Knapp KM, Li C, Okuma J, et al. Risk prediction in pediatric cancer patients with fever and neutropenia. Pediatr Infect Dis J. 2010;29(1):53–9.
82. Santolaya ME, Alvarez AM, Becker A, Cofre J, Enriquez N, O'Ryan M, et al. Prospective, multicenter evaluation of risk factors associated with invasive bacterial infection in children with cancer, neutropenia, and fever. J Clin Oncol. 2001;19(14):3415–21.
83. Klaassen RJ, Goodman TR, Pham B, Doyle JJ. "Low-risk" prediction rule for pediatric oncology patients presenting with fever and neutropenia. J Clin Oncol. 2000;18(5):1012–9.
84. Macher E, Dubos F, Garnier N, Delebarre M, De Berranger E, Thebaud E, et al. Predicting the risk of severe bacterial infection in children with chemotherapy-induced febrile neutropenia. Pediatr Blood Cancer. 2010;55(4):662–7.
85. Dommett R, Geary J, Freeman S, Hartley J, Sharland M, Davidson A, et al. Successful introduction and audit of a step-down oral antibiotic strategy for low risk paediatric febrile neutropaenia in a UK, multicentre, shared care setting. Eur J Cancer. 2009;45(16):2843–9.
86. Green LL, Goussard P, van Zyl A, Kidd M, Kruger M. Predictive indicators to identify high-risk paediatric febrile neutropenia in paediatric oncology patients in a middle-income country. J Trop Pediatr. 2018;64(5):395–402.
87. Miedema KG, de Bont ES, Oude Nijhuis CS, van Vliet D, Kamps WA, Tissing WJ. Validation of a new risk assessment model for predicting adverse events in children with fever and chemotherapy-induced neutropenia. J Clin Oncol. 2011;29(7):e182–4; author reply e185.
88. Rackoff WR, Gonin R, Robinson C, Kreissman SG, Breitfeld PB. Predicting the risk of bacteremia in childen with fever and neutropenia. J Clin Oncol. 1996;14(3):919–24.
89. Baorto EP, Aquino VM, Mullen CA, Buchanan GR, DeBaun MR. Clinical parameters associated with low bacteremia risk in 1100 pediatric oncology patients with fever and neutropenia. Cancer. 2001;92(4):909–13.
90. Madsen K, Rosenman M, Hui S, Breitfeld PP. Value of electronic data for model validation and refinement: bacteremia risk in children with fever and neutropenia. J Pediatr Hematol Oncology. 2002;24(4):256–62.
91. Phillips RS, Lehrnbecher T, Alexander S, Sung L. Updated systematic review and meta-analysis of the performance of risk prediction rules in children and young people with febrile neutropenia. PLoS One. 2012;7(5):e38300.
92. Haeusler GM, Thursky KA, Slavin MA, Mechinaud F, Babl FE, Bryant P, et al. External validation of six pediatric fever and neutropenia clinical decision rules. Pediatr Infect Dis J. 2018;37(4):329–35.
93. Phillips B, Morgan JE, Haeusler GM, Riley RD, PICNICC Collaborative. Individual participant data validation of the PICNICC prediction model for febrile neutropenia. Arch Dis Child. 2020;105(5):439–45.
94. Ammann RA, Bodmer N, Hirt A, Niggli FK, Nadal D, Simon A, et al. Predicting adverse events in children with fever and chemotherapy-induced neutropenia: the prospective multicenter SPOG 2003 FN study. J Clin Oncol. 2010;28(12):2008–14.
95. Santolaya ME, Alvarez AM, Aviles CL, Becker A, Cofre J, Enriquez N, et al. Prospective evaluation of a model of prediction of invasive bacterial infection risk among children with cancer, fever, and neutropenia. Clin Infect Dis. 2002;35(6):678–83.
96. Alexander S, Fisher BT, Gaur AH, Dvorak CC, Villa Luna D, Dang H, et al. Effect of levofloxacin prophylaxis on bacteremia in children with acute leukemia or undergoing hematopoietic stem cell transplantation: a randomized clinical trial. JAMA. 2018;320(10):995–1004.
97. Fisher BT, Robinson PD, Lehrnbecher T, Steinbach WJ, Zaoutis TE, Phillips B, et al. Risk factors for invasive fungal disease in pediatric cancer and hematopoietic stem cell transplantation: a systematic review. J Pediatric Infect Dis Soc. 2018;7(3):191–8.
98. Dix D, Cellot S, Price V, Gillmeister B, Ethier MC, Johnston DL, et al. Association between corticosteroids and infection, sepsis, and infectious death in pediatric acute myeloid leukemia (AML): results from the Canadian infections in AML research group. Clin Infect Dis. 2012;55(12):1608–14.
99. Kimberlin DW, Barnett ED, Lynfield R, Sawyer MH. Red Book: 2021–2024 report of the Committee

on Infectious Diseases. Itasca: American Academy of Pediatrics; 2021.

100. Freifeld AG, Bow EJ, Sepkowitz KA, Boeckh MJ, Ito JI, Mullen CA, et al. Clinical practice guideline for the use of antimicrobial agents in neutropenic patients with cancer: 2010 update by the Infectious Diseases Society of America. Clin Infect Dis. 2011;52(4):E56–93.
101. Caver TE, Slobod KS, Flynn PM, Behm FG, Hudson MM, Turner EV, et al. Profound abnormality of the B/T lymphocyte ratio during chemotherapy for pediatric acute lymphoblastic leukemia. Leukemia. 1998;12(4):619–22.
102. Yen TY, Jou ST, Yang YL, Chang HH, Lu MY, Lin DT, et al. Immune response to 2009 pandemic H1N1 influenza virus a monovalent vaccine in children with cancer. Pediatr Blood Cancer. 2011;57(7):1154–8.
103. Hughes WT, Rivera GK, Schell MJ, Thornton D, Lott L. Successful intermittent chemoprophylaxis for pneumocystis carinii pneumonitis. N Engl J Med. 1987;316(26):1627–32.
104. Lindemulder S, Albano E. Successful intermittent prophylaxis with trimethoprim/sulfamethoxazole 2 days per week for Pneumocystis carinii (jiroveci) pneumonia in pediatric oncology patients. Pediatrics. 2007;120(1):e47–51.
105. Ioannidis JP, Cappelleri JC, Skolnik PR, Lau J, Sacks HS. A meta-analysis of the relative efficacy and toxicity of Pneumocystis carinii prophylactic regimens. Arch Intern Med. 1996;156(2):177–88.
106. Balmes JR, Estacio PL, Quinlan P, Kelly T, Corkery K, Blanc P. Respiratory effects of occupational exposure to aerosolized pentamidine. J Occup Environ Med. 1995;37(2):145–50.
107. Lehrnbecher T, Fisher BT, Phillips B, Alexander S, Ammann RA, Beauchemin M, et al. Guideline for antibacterial prophylaxis administration in pediatric cancer and hematopoietic stem cell transplantation. Clin Infect Dis. 2020;71(1):226–36.
108. Wolf J, Tang L, Flynn PM, Pui CH, Gaur AH, Sun Y, et al. Levofloxacin prophylaxis during induction therapy for pediatric acute lymphoblastic leukemia. Clin Infect Dis. 2017;65(11):1790–8.
109. Al Omar S, Anabtawi N, Al Qasem W, Rihani R. Bacterial infections in children with acute myeloid leukemia receiving ciprofloxacin prophylaxis. J Pediatr Hematol Oncol. 2017;39(3):e131–e5.
110. Laoprasopwattana K, Khwanna T, Suwankeeree P, Sujjanunt T, Tunyapanit W, Chelae S. Ciprofloxacin reduces occurrence of fever in children with acute leukemia who develop neutropenia during chemotherapy. Pediatr Infect Dis J. 2013;32(3):e94–8.
111. Mikulska M, Averbuch D, Tissot F, Cordonnier C, Akova M, Calandra T, et al. Fluoroquinolone prophylaxis in haematological cancer patients with neutropenia: ECIL critical appraisal of previous guidelines. J Infect. 2018;76(1):20–37.
112. Lehrnbecher T, Fisher BT, Phillips B, Beauchemin M, Carlesse F, Castagnola E, et al. Clinical practice guideline for systemic antifungal prophylaxis in pediatric patients with cancer and hematopoietic stem-cell transplantation recipients. J Clin Oncol. 2020;38(27):3205–16.
113. Lehrnbecher T, Robinson P, Fisher B, Alexander S, Ammann RA, Beauchemin M, et al. Guideline for the management of fever and neutropenia in children with cancer and hematopoietic stem-cell transplantation recipients: 2017 update. J Clin Oncol. 2017;35(18):2082–94.
114. Esbenshade AJ, Zhao Z, Aftandilian C, Saab R, Wattier RL, Beauchemin M, et al. Multisite external validation of a risk prediction model for the diagnosis of blood stream infections in febrile pediatric oncology patients without severe neutropenia. Cancer. 2017;123(19):3781–90.
115. Esbenshade AJ, Zhao Z, Baird A, Holmes EA, Dulek DE, Banerjee R, et al. Prospective implementation of a risk prediction model for bloodstream infection safely reduces antibiotic usage in febrile pediatric cancer patients without severe neutropenia. J Clin Oncol. 2020;38(27):3150–60.
116. Chiotos K, Hayes M, Kimberlin DW, Jones SB, James SH, Pinninti SG, et al. Multicenter interim guidance on use of antivirals for children with coronavirus disease 2019/severe acute respiratory syndrome coronavirus 2. J Pediatric Infect Dis Soc. 2021;10(1):34–48.
117. Perez EE, Orange JS, Bonilla F, Chinen J, Chinn IK, Dorsey M, et al. Update on the use of immunoglobulin in human disease: a review of evidence. J Allergy Clin Immunol. 2017;139(3S):S1–S46.
118. Orgel E, Sposto R, Malvar J, Seibel NL, Ladas E, Gaynon PS, et al. Impact on survival and toxicity by duration of weight extremes during treatment for pediatric acute lymphoblastic leukemia: a report from the Children's Oncology Group. J Clin Oncol. 2014;32(13):1331–7.
119. Egnell C, Ranta S, Banerjee J, Merker A, Niinimäki R, Lund B, et al. Impact of body mass index on relapse in children with acute lymphoblastic leukemia treated according to Nordic treatment protocols. Eur J Haematol. 2020;105(6):797–807.
120. Orgel E, Genkinger JM, Aggarwal D, Sung L, Nieder M, Ladas EJ. Association of body mass index and survival in pediatric leukemia: a meta-analysis. Am J Clin Nutr. 2016;103(3):808–17.
121. Meenan CK, Kelly JA, Wang L, Ritchey AK, Maurer SH. Obesity in pediatric patients with acute lymphoblastic leukemia increases the risk of adverse events during pre-maintenance chemotherapy. Pediatr Blood Cancer. 2019;66(2):e27515.
122. den Hoed MA, Pluijm SM, de Groot-Kruseman HA, Te Winkel ML, Fiocco M, van den Akker EL, et al. The negative impact of underweight and weight loss on survival of children with acute lymphoblastic leukemia. Haematologica. 2015;100:62.
123. Martin-Trejo JA, Nunez-Enriquez JC, Fajardo-Gutierrez A, Medina-Sanson A, Flores-Lujano J, Jimenez-Hernandez E, et al. Early mortality in children with acute lymphoblastic leukemia in a

developing country: the role of malnutrition at diagnosis. A multicenter cohort MIGICCL study. Leuk Lymphoma. 2017;58(4):898–908.
124. Muscaritoli M, Arends J, Bachmann P, Baracos V, Barthelemy N, Bertz H, et al. ESPEN practical guideline: clinical nutrition in cancer. Clin Nutr. 2021;40(5):2898–913.
125. Ogden CL, Carroll MD, Kit BK, Flegal KM. Prevalence of childhood and adult obesity in the United States, 2011-2012. JAMA. 2014;311(8):806–14.
126. Stierman B, Ogden CL, Yanovski JA, Martin CB, Sarafrazi N, Hales CM. Changes in adiposity among children and adolescents in the United States, 1999–2006 to 2011–2018. Am J Clin Nutr. 2021;114(4):1495–504.
127. Withycombe JS, Post-White JE, Meza JL, Hawks RG, Smith LM, Sacks N, et al. Weight patterns in children with higher risk ALL: a report from the Children's Oncology Group (COG) for CCG 1961. Pediatr Blood Cancer. 2009;53(7):1249–54.
128. Nottage KA, Ness KK, Li C, Srivastava D, Robison LL, Hudson MM. Metabolic syndrome and cardiovascular risk among long-term survivors of acute lymphoblastic leukaemia - from the St. Jude Lifetime Cohort. Br J Haematol. 2014;165(3):364–74.
129. Withycombe JS, Smith LM, Meza JL, Merkle C, Faulkner MS, Ritter L, et al. Weight change during childhood acute lymphoblastic leukemia induction therapy predicts obesity: a report from the Children's Oncology Group. Pediatr Blood Cancer. 2015;62(3):434–9.
130. Ligibel JA, Bohlke K, May AM, Clinton SK, Demark-Wahnefried W, Gilchrist SC, et al. Exercise, diet, and weight management during cancer treatment: ASCO guideline. J Clin Oncol. 2022;40(22):2491–507.
131. Esfahani A, Ghoreishi Z, Abedi Miran M, Sanaat Z, Ostadrahimi A, Eivazi Ziaei J, et al. Nutritional assessment of patients with acute leukemia during induction chemotherapy: association with hospital outcomes. Leuk Lymphoma. 2014;55(8):1743–50.
132. Walters M, Mowbray C, Jubelirer T, Jacobs S, Kelly KM, Smith K, et al. A bilingual dietary intervention early in treatment is feasible and prevents weight gain in childhood acute lymphoblastic leukemia. Pediatr Blood Cancer. 2021;68(5):e28910.
133. Orgel E, Framson C, Buxton R, Kim J, Li G, Tucci J, et al. Caloric and nutrient restriction to augment chemotherapy efficacy for acute lymphoblastic leukemia: the IDEAL trial. Blood Adv. 2021;5(7):1853–61.
134. Hartman A, te Winkel ML, van Beek RD, de Muinck Keizer-Schrama SM, Kemper HC, Hop WC, et al. A randomized trial investigating an exercise program to prevent reduction of bone mineral density and impairment of motor performance during treatment for childhood acute lymphoblastic leukemia. Pediatr Blood Cancer. 2009;53(1):64–71.
135. Coombs A, Schilperoort H, Sargent B. The effect of exercise and motor interventions on physical activity and motor outcomes during and after medical intervention for children and adolescents with acute lymphoblastic leukemia: a systematic review. Crit Rev Oncol Hematol. 2020;152:103004.
136. Orgel E, Mueske NM, Sposto R, Gilsanz V, Freyer DR, Mittelman SD. Limitations of body mass index to assess body composition due to sarcopenic obesity during leukemia therapy. Leuk Lymphoma. 2018;59(1):138–45.
137. Roh E, Choi KM. Health consequences of sarcopenic obesity: a narrative review. Front Endocrinol (Lausanne). 2020;11:332.
138. Prado CM, Lieffers JR, McCargar LJ, Reiman T, Sawyer MB, Martin L, et al. Prevalence and clinical implications of sarcopenic obesity in patients with solid tumours of the respiratory and gastrointestinal tracts: a population-based study. Lancet Oncol. 2008;9(7):629–35.
139. Bozzetti F. Forcing the vicious circle: sarcopenia increases toxicity, decreases response to chemotherapy and worsens with chemotherapy. Ann Oncol. 2017;28(9):2107–18.
140. Anandavadivelan P, Brismar TB, Nilsson M, Johar AM, Martin L. Sarcopenic obesity: a probable risk factor for dose limiting toxicity during neo-adjuvant chemotherapy in oesophageal cancer patients. Clin Nutr. 2016;35(3):724–30.
141. Heo YA, Syed YY, Keam SJ. Pegaspargase: a review in acute lymphoblastic leukaemia. Drugs. 2019;79(7):767–77.
142. Soeters PB, Wolfe RR, Shenkin A. Hypoalbuminemia: pathogenesis and clinical significance. J Parenter Enter Nutr. 2019;43(2):181–93.
143. Moody KM, Baker RA, Santizo RO, Olmez I, Spies JM, Buthmann A, et al. A randomized trial of the effectiveness of the neutropenic diet versus food safety guidelines on infection rate in pediatric oncology patients. Pediatr Blood Cancer. 2018;65(1):e26711.
144. Gardner A, Mattiuzzi G, Faderl S, Borthakur G, Garcia-Manero G, Pierce S, et al. Randomized comparison of cooked and noncooked diets in patients undergoing remission induction therapy for acute myeloid leukemia. J Clin Oncol. 2008;26(35):5684–8.
145. Ma Y, Lu X, Liu H. Neutropenic diet cannot reduce the risk of infection and mortality in oncology patients with neutropenia. Front Oncol. 2022;12:836371.
146. Sonabend RY, McKay SV, Okcu MF, Yan J, Haymond MW, Margolin JF. Hyperglycemia during induction therapy is associated with increased infectious complications in childhood acute lymphocytic leukemia. Pediatr Blood Cancer. 2008;51(3):387–92.
147. Agnoli C, Berrino F, Abagnato CA, Muti P, Panico S, Crosignani P, et al. Metabolic syndrome and postmenopausal breast cancer in the ORDET cohort: a nested case-control study. Nutr Metab Cardiovasc Dis. 2010;20(1):41–8.

148. Lowas SR, Marks D, Malempati S. Prevalence of transient hyperglycemia during induction chemotherapy for pediatric acute lymphoblastic leukemia. Pediatr Blood Cancer. 2009;52(7):814–8.
149. Roberson JR, Spraker HL, Shelso J, Zhou Y, Inaba H, Metzger ML, et al. Clinical consequences of hyperglycemia during remission induction therapy for pediatric acute lymphoblastic leukemia. Leukemia. 2009;23(2):245–50.
150. Barreira TV, Schuna JM Jr, Mire EF, Broyles ST, Katzmarzyk PT, Johnson WD, et al. Normative steps/day and peak cadence values for United States children and adolescents: National Health and Nutrition Examination survey 2005-2006. J Pediatr. 2015;166(1):139–43.e3.
151. Götte M, Kesting S, Winter C, Rosenbaum D, Boos J. Experience of barriers and motivations for physical activities and exercise during treatment of pediatric patients with cancer. Pediatr Blood Cancer. 2014;61(9):1632–7.
152. Ross WL, Le A, Zheng DJ, Mitchell H-R, Rotatori J, Li F, et al. Physical activity barriers, preferences, and beliefs in childhood cancer patients. Support Care Cancer. 2018;26(7):2177–84.
153. King AC, Whitt-Glover MC, Marquez DX, Buman MP, Napolitano MA, Jakicic J, et al. Physical activity promotion: highlights from the 2018 physical activity guidelines Advisory Committee systematic review. Med Sci Sports Exerc. 2019;51(6):1340–53.
154. Mikus CR, Oberlin DJ, Libla JL, Taylor AM, Booth FW, Thyfault JP. Lowering physical activity impairs glycemic control in healthy volunteers. Med Sci Sports Exerc. 2012;44(2):225–31.
155. Rynders CA, Blanc S, DeJong N, Bessesen DH, Bergouignan A. Sedentary behaviour is a key determinant of metabolic inflexibility. J Physiol. 2018;596(8):1319–30.
156. Swartz AM, Squires L, Strath SJ. Energy expenditure of interruptions to sedentary behavior. Int J Behav Nutr Phys Act. 2011;8:69.
157. Getz KD, Szymczak JE, Li Y, Madding R, Huang YV, Aftandilian C, et al. Medical outcomes, quality of life, and family perceptions for outpatient vs inpatient neutropenia management after chemotherapy for pediatric acute myeloid leukemia. JAMA Netw Open. 2021;4(10):e2128385.
158. Sung L, Aplenc R, Alonzo TA, Gerbing RB, Lehrnbecher T, Gamis AS. Effectiveness of supportive care measures to reduce infections in pediatric AML: a report from the Children's Oncology Group. Blood. 2013;121(18):3573–7.
159. Blower P, de Wit R, Goodin S, Aapro M. Drug-drug interactions in oncology: why are they important and can they be minimized? Crit Rev Oncol Hematol. 2005;55(2):117–42.
160. Lee SH, Yang JJ. Pharmacogenomics in acute lymphoblastic leukemia. Best Pract Res Clin Hematol. 2017;30(3):229–36.
161. Grupp SA, Kalos M, Barrett D, Aplenc R, Porter DL, Rheingold SR, et al. Chimeric antigen receptor-modified T cells for acute lymphoid leukemia. N Engl J Med. 2013;368(16):1509–18.

20 Late Adverse Events Following Stem Cell Transplantation in Childhood Acute Lymphoblastic Leukaemia: State of the Art

Alessandro Cattoni, Silvia Molinari, Maria Laura Nicolosi, and Adriana Balduzzi

20.1 Introduction

Haematopoietic stem cell transplantation (HSCT) has been historically regarded as the standard-of-care for very high-risk, relapsed or refractory acute lymphoblastic leukaemia (ALL) in paediatrics [1, 2].

Even though HSCT-related early- and late-onset complications still expose patients to a remarkable risk of morbidity and mortality, the refinement of supportive therapies and the development of pre- and post-HSCT targeted/tailored strategies resulted in outstanding improvements in post-transplantation survival rates over the last decades [3, 4]. Accordingly, the dramatic increase in the population of transplanted ALL survivors has progressively shed light on the burden of adverse events experienced as years elapse following HSCT, in the setting of a medical scenario focussed on the early detection and management of late effects among ALL survivors.

The expression late adverse events (LAEs) encompasses a wide spectrum of long-term clinical conditions arising years or even decades after HSCT, as a result of the synergetic detrimental action of irradiation, alkylating agents, steroids and graft-versus-host disease (GvHD). LAEs result, per se, in a remarkable increase in the late mortality and morbidity rates recorded after HSCT and affect the overall quality of life (QoL) of long-term transplanted survivors compared to non-transplanted gender- and age-matched peers [5–8].

Both alkylators and total body irradiation (TBI) in the setting of myeloablative conditioning regimens play a detrimental role on long-term health among survivors. Nevertheless, despite its efficacy in reducing the risk of relapse and increasing overall survival, as demonstrated in the randomized For Reducing Radiation at Majority Age (FORUM) Trial [9], patients exposed to TBI experience a remarkably greater burden of late-onset adverse events compared to chemo-only regimens [10].

The reported 10-year cumulative incidence of a chronic health condition among HSCT survivors is as high as 60% overall, while it drops to 35% when considering severe/life-threatening LAEs or death [11].

The growing body of children and adolescents is particularly susceptible to the iatrogenic effects of alkylating agents and TBI and LAEs can potentially affect any system or organ.

Table 20.1 summarizes the LAEs most frequently reported among ALL transplanted survivors.

A. Cattoni (✉) · A. Balduzzi
Department of Pediatrics, Fondazione IRCCS San Gerardo dei Tintori, Monza, Italy

School of Medicine and Surgery, Milano-Bicocca University, Monza, Italy
e-mail: alessandro.cattoni@unimib.it; adriana.balduzzi@unimib.it

S. Molinari · M. L. Nicolosi
Department of Pediatrics, Fondazione IRCCS San Gerardo dei Tintori, Monza, Italy

G. Escherich, V. Conter (eds.), *Acute Lymphoblastic Leukemia in Children and Adolescents*, Pediatric Oncology, https://doi.org/10.1007/978-3-031-71180-0_20

Table 20.1 Late adverse events experienced following HSCT among ALL survivors

Organ or system	Most frequent detailed adverse events	Occurrence rates among transplanted ALL survivors	Critical risk factors	Follow-up	Treatment
Eye	Cataracts	4–70%	Corticosteroids, TBI	Periodic ophthalmological examination	Surgery if functional impairment
	Keratoconjunctivitis sicca	35–75%	Chronic GvHD, TBI		Lubrication, treatment of eventual corneal complications
	Ischaemic microvascular retinopathy	0–10%	TBI, alkylating agents, metabolic syndrome		Treatment of predisposing conditions (diabetes, hypertension, dyslipidaemia)
Cardiovascular system	Metabolic syndrome (dyslipidaemia, hypertension, overweight, hyperglycaemia)	20–50%	TBI, alkylating agents, immunosuppressors, GvHD, nephrotoxic supportive therapy	Periodical blood pressure assessment and blood tests (fasting glucose, Hb1Ac, cholesterol, triglycerides)	Healthy lifestyle; pharmacological treatment of hypertension, hyperglycaemia and dyslipidaemia if needed
	Congestive heart failure	5–10%	Anthracyclines, high-dose cyclophosphamide, TBI	Echocardiography	Pharmacological treatment if needed
	Atherosclerosis	10–20%	TBI, alkylating agents, immunosuppressors, GvHD, nephrotoxic supportive therapy, metabolic syndrome	Periodical blood pressure assessment and blood tests (fasting glucose, Hb1Ac, cholesterol, triglycerides)	Healthy lifestyle; pharmacological treatment of hypertension, hyperglycaemia and dyslipidaemia)
Lung	Bronchiolitis obliterans and bronchiolitis obliterans organizing pneumonia	10–60%	Chronic GvHD, busulfan, methotrexate, lung viral infections	History collection, periodic pulmonary function tests	Corticosteroids, immunosuppressors, azithromycin
Kidney	Nephrotic syndrome	2–20%	TBI, immunosuppressors, GvHD, nephrotoxic supportive therapy	Periodic urinary examination, eventual renal function tests	Discontinuation of nephrotoxic treatments, treatment of hypertension, salt-sparing diet, corticosteroids and immunosuppressants (nephrotic syndrome), plasma exchange and additional medications for thrombotic microangiopathy
	Thrombotic microangiopathy				
	Radiation-induced renal sclerosis				

Skin and mucosae	Poikiloderma, lichen planus, lichen sclerosus, morphea-like lesions; nail dystrophy		Chronic GvHD, TBI	Periodic clinical evaluation	Treatment of GvHD
	Oral lichenoid lesions		Chronic GvHD, TBI, corticosteroids	Periodic clinical evaluation	Treatment of GvHD
Endocrine system	Impaired growth	20–40%	TBI, corticosteroids, untreated hormonal disorders, malnutrition, TKI	Periodic auxological evaluation	Recombinant human GH only in case of demonstrated radio-induced GHD; treatment of
	Thyroid function disorders and nodules	10–30%	TBI, alkylating agents, TKI	Periodic TSH and FT4 assessment, neck palpation and/or thyroid ultrasound	L-thyroxin or anti-thyroid medications if needed
	Gonadal dysfunction	Oligospermia–azoospermia: 75–95%; Testosterone deficiency: 15–55%; Ovarian insufficiency: 44–100%	TBI, alkylating agents, chronic GvHD	Medical history (symptoms consistent with hypogonadism, amenorrhea), periodic LH, FSH and testosterone/oestradiol assessment	Hormonal replacement therapy as needed
	Impaired glucose metabolism	Diabetes mellitus: 5% Insulin resistance: up to 50%	TBI, corticosteroids, immunosuppressants, metabolic syndrome	Blood glucose and HbA1c periodically assessed	Diet; eventual pharmacological treatment of diabetes
Bone	Impaired bone mineral density	20–60%	TBI, corticosteroids, TKI	Periodical DEXA scan; medical history (bone frailty)	Adequate calcium and vitamin D intake; if recurrent fractures, bisphosphonates should be considered
	Osteonecrosis	4–40%	Corticosteroids, dyslipidaemia, TBI	MRI in case of pain	Surgery in case of progression or functional impairment

(continued)

Table 20.1 (continued)

Organ or system	Most frequent detailed adverse events	Occurrence rates among transplanted ALL survivors	Critical risk factors	Follow-up	Treatment
Secondary tumours	Solid malignancies (skin, mouth, thyroid, uterine tumours, glioblastoma)	10–15%	TBI, immunosuppressants, alkylating agents	Screening programmes (dermatological evaluation, neck ultrasound, PAP smear, etc.)	Antineoplastic specific protocols
	Acute myeloid leukaemia	Rarely reported among ALL survivors	TBI, immunosuppressants, alkylating agent	Clinical and biochemical assessment in case of consistent signs or symptoms	
	PTLD	1–10%	Immunosuppression, viral infections (EBV)		Immunosuppression discontinuation, anti-CD20 antibodies, cytotoxic treatment
Psychosocial issues	Post-traumatic stress disorder, social anxiety, poor peer acceptance		Traumatic experience upon diagnosis of ALL, late effects affecting QoL	Psychosocial screening	

TBI total body irradiation, *GvHD* graft-versus-host disease. *TKI* tyrosine kinase inhibitors, *EBV* Ebstein–Barr virus, *PTLD* post-transplantation lymphoproliferative disease, *QoL* quality of life, *GHD* growth hormone deficiency

20.2 Organ- or System-Specific Late Adverse Events

20.2.1 Ocular Complications

HSCT-related iatrogenic factors can affect any part of the eye, with a particular involvement of the lens, the retina and the cornea. Total body irradiation, prolonged administration of steroids and graft-versus-host-disease (GvHD) are commonly regarded as the most detrimental determinants of the potential visual impairment reported among childhood ALL survivors [12, 13].

In detail, TBI alongside long-term exposure to corticosteroids may affect the physiological transparency of crystalline lenses, thus resulting in progressive opacification. The cumulative incidence of *cataracts* among stem cell recipients ranges from 4 to 70% [14, 15], with most of this variability depending on the steroid dose administered prior to HSCT, enrolment criteria of different study cohorts, follow-up programmes and eventual eye shielding protocols upon radiation delivery. Fractionated TBI, the administration of radiation-free conditioning regimens and corticosteroids sparing approaches, when clinically feasible, would represent the pivotal choices in order to minimize cataract occurrence and severity [16].

Surgical correction is the standard-of-care and yearly complete ophthalmological evaluation following HSCT is recommended to identify the best timing to undertake cataracts correction [12]. Bilateral involvement and the severe visual impairment should be regarded as the pivotal factors that prompt dedicated treatment, though no shared acuity thresholds have been established and surgery indication should be tailored based on patient's age and specific needs [17].

Dry eye syndrome, also known as *keratoconjunctivitis sicca*, has been reported in 35–75% of HSCT recipients [14, 18]. The clinical scenario is the result of inadequate tear secretion that leads to a moisturizing disorder of the ocular surface and encompasses photophobia, redness and itching or burning sensations [19]. Histological studies of the lacrimal gland ducts of patients with dry eye syndrome show infiltration of lymphocytes and CD34+ stromal fibroblasts, leading to fibrosis and impaired moisturizing function. Indeed, ocular GvHD represents the primary causative factor of *keratoconjunctivitis sicca* and it is defined as the new onset of dry, gritty, or painful eyes, recurrent conjunctivitis, up to cicatricial conjunctivitis or confluent areas of punctate keratopathy following HSCT [20].

Severe untreated keratoconjunctivitis sicca may result in several complications, such as corneal ulcers and perforation, necrosis, and neovascularization. Early symptoms may not be reported timely and specific questions should be asked to detect scenarios that are still subclinical. Annual ophthalmological evaluation along with intense and frequent lubrication by artificial tears and viscous ointments represent key factors to prevent an unfavourable evolution that would affect patient's QoL [21].

Finally, an overall rarer ocular LAE is represented by *ischaemic microvascular retinopathy* [22, 23]. TBI, cyclosporine, and busulfan may play a direct causative action on retinal health. In addition, diabetes, dyslipidaemia, and arterial hypertension, known as HSCT-related metabolic complications, may increase the occurrence of this condition. The histologic findings encompass cotton-wool patches, vitreous haemorrhage, and optic disc oedema. A periodic assessment is recommended, as patients may be completely asymptomatic during the early stages of disease [24].

20.2.2 Cardiovascular Complications

Transplanted patients present a two- to threefold increase in the risk of cardiovascular-related life-threatening complications *quo* ad vitam [25]. On the one hand, the overall cardiovascular risk experienced by transplanted ALL survivors is the result of factors directly related to HSCT and to antineoplastic protocols, i.e. cardiotoxic effects of anthracyclines and radiation-induced coronary disease. On the other hand, transplantation involves a two- to sevenfold increase in the occurrence of *metabolic syndrome* (MS) in different study population, based on the Country-specific prevalence of this condition among otherwise healthy age- and gender-matched individuals [26–29].

Most of the pathogenic pathways involved in the onset of HSCT-related MS still need to be unveiled, but the detrimental role of TBI, prolonged exposure to corticosteroids and calcineurin inhibitors on insulin secretion and resistance, endothelial function, and cholesterol/triglycerides metabolism have been extensively assessed [30–32]. In addition, *hypertension* has been reported in up to 50% of ALL transplanted survivors and, alongside endothelial dysfunction, kidney damage related to chemotherapy, supportive therapy, mainly anti-viral and anti-fungal prophylaxis/therapy, radiation, and immunosuppressants play a negative synergetic role on blood pressure homeostasis.

The reported incidence of *congestive heart failure* following HSCT achieves 10% in selected cohorts of transplanted survivors [33]. Pre-HSCT exposure to cumulative dose of anthracyclines exceeding 250 mg/m^2 and conditioning regimens including TBI or high-dose cyclophosphamide are the most detrimental risk factors for late-occurring direct heart damage [34]. Early treatment of HSCT-related symptomatic or asymptomatic left ventricular dysfunction follows the general guidelines for the management of otherwise healthy population and is pivotal to prevent survivors from experiencing disease progression [35]. Accordingly, screening by periodic echocardiography for asymptomatic disease may provide opportunities for implementation of interventions to reduce the risk of clinically overt disease.

In addition, *cardiac arrhythmias* are rare but life-threatening transplant-related adverse events. As most arrhythmias occur early after HSCT, long-term guidelines do not commonly recommend systematic routine screening in patients without symptoms or a concerning family history. Nevertheless, clinicians involved in the long-term care of HSCT survivors should lower the threshold for prescribing electrocardiogram or Holter monitoring in case of signs or symptoms potentially recalling heart rhythm disorders [36].

Finally, HSCT survivors experience onset and progression of *atherosclerosis* at a faster pace compared to the general population. Indeed, the reported 15- and 20-year cumulative incidence of either clinically overt coronary artery disease or cerebrovascular events exceeds 10% and 20%, respectively [37]. As screening for subclinical arterial disease is limited due to the lack of standardized and reproducible methods, healthy lifestyle recommendations along with eventual pharmacological treatment of MS-related risk factors (i.e. overweight, dyslipidaemia, hypertension, and hyperglycaemia) are the only shared approach to prevent arterial disease progression [38, 39].

20.2.3 Pulmonary Complications

Following HSCT, patients may experience either infectious or non-infectious pulmonary diseases. Among the latter, late onset respiratory complications, reported in 3–23% of survivors [40, 41], include bronchiolitis obliterans, bronchiolitis obliterans organizing pneumonia, and lung fibrosis.

In wide case studies, the onset of *bronchiolitis obliterans* (BO) has been demonstrated to be strictly related to the occurrence of chronic GvHD, supporting the hypothesis that it may represent a pulmonary involvement by graft-versus-host disease. Additional risk factors include busulfan-based conditioning regimen, the administration of methotrexate as GvHD prophylaxis and antecedent lung viral infections [42].

From a pathogenic perspective, BO is characterized by a primary non-specific inflammatory involvement of smaller airways, initially prompting air trapping and obstructive lung disease and subsequently leading, at more advanced stages of disease, to peribronchiolar fibrosis [43, 44].

The clinical onset of this condition occurs at a median time of 1 year following HSCT and its presentation can be insidious, ranging from dry cough, wheezing, and dyspnoea to completely asymptomatic patients only presenting with pulmonary function tests consistent with an obstructive scenario. Chest radiographs typically show hyperinflation, while mosaic perfusion is a common feature on high-resolution computed tomography, with decreased number and size of vessels causing parenchymal lucencies alongside normal lung tissue [45]. Nevertheless, radiological findings of BO may be minimal and thus they probably underestimate its real-life occurrence following HSCT. Given the overall poor *compliance* to pulmonary function tests performance in younger children, BO is probably severely underreported among transplanted ALL survivors.

Bronchiolitis obliterans organizing pneumonia (BOOP) is a clinicopathological syndrome involving bronchioles, alveolar ducts, and alveoli, often presenting as a non-infectious interstitial pneumonia following HSCT. [46] Though commonly occurring 1–12 months following transplantation, also late-onset BOOP have been rarely reported. Although the pathogenesis of BOOP following HSCT is poorly understood, involvement of an allo-immunologic reaction has been considered [47].

The clinical scenario encompasses dyspnoea, cough, and fever. Upon chest X-ray, ground glass attenuation and nodular opacities can be found. In contrast to BO, the pulmonary function tests show a restrictive pattern [48].

Overall, both obstructive and restrictive lung disorders experienced by transplanted ALL childhood survivors are the result of excessive collagen deposition and fibrosis, involving either the peri-bronchiolar or the interstitial space, respectively.

In order to promptly detect late-onset lung disorders, clinical review and history collection at 6 months and annually thereafter are warranted. Patients exposed to TBI and busulfan-based conditioning regimens and with chronic GvHD would benefit from pulmonary function testing monitoring over time, besides high-density CT scan in case BO syndrome is suspected [49].

20.2.4 Renal Complications

Chronic renal injury has been reported in 20–60% of patients treated with HSCT [50–52]. Given the large glomerular reserve of paediatric patients, renal function markers used in everyday clinical practice, such as glomerular filtration rate (GFR), tend to remain within normal ranges until 50% of nephrons are lost. Accordingly, the renal damage after HSCT may be widely underestimated.

Front-line antineoplastic medications, abdominal radiotherapy, high-dose chemotherapy delivered as a part of conditioning regimens, supportive treatments (antibiotics, as aminoglycosides and vancomycin, anti-virals, as acyclovir, ganciclovir, foscarnet, cidofovir, and antifungals, as amphotericin B, voriconazole), chronic GvHD and prolonged administration of immunosuppressors (calcineurin inhibitors) can be listed as the most nephrotoxic iatrogenic factors experienced by ALL transplanted patients [53–55]. In addition, the increased occurrence of diabetes and hypertension among ALL survivors plays a contributory role on the odd of developing progressive impairment of renal function towards end-stage chronic kidney disease.

About one third of renal function disorders occur within the first 2 years following HSCT. Nevertheless, the cumulative incidence of chronic kidney disease (CKD) shows a progressive increase between 5 and 10 years following transplantation [52]. In this setting, CKD, defined as the finding of persistently impaired GFR <60 mL/min/1.73 m^2, can be the result of a wide spectrum of renal disorders, ranging from vascular to glomerular or tubular-interstitial disorders [56].

Nephrotic syndrome is an overall rare HSCT-related LAE and is commonly regarded as the renal expression of systemic GvHD after allogeneic transplantation [57]. Accordingly, early biochemical signs (hypoalbuminaemia, proteinuria, and hypercholesterolaemia) may occur as soon as systemic immunosuppressors are discontinued [58]. Membranous nephropathy and minimal change disease are the most frequently reported nosographic scenarios.

In addition, HSCT-related CKD can be the late and irreversible outcome of kidney involvement in the setting of systemic *thrombotic microangiopathy*. Indeed, acute platelet aggregation and thrombosis often lead to acute ischaemic kidney injury [56]. Steady-state renal function is only rarely retrieved as time elapses.

Among irradiated survivors, *TBI-induced renal sclerosis* is the expression of vascular degeneration of the glomeruli and tubules, leading to progressive interstitial fibrosis. Accordingly, it has been demonstrated that transplant-related nephropathy can be reduced by renal shielding [59].

As transplanted patients may experience renal damage irrespectively of the conditioning regimen undertaken, periodic monitoring of blood pressure and renal function is warranted for all ALL-HSCT survivors.

20.2.5 Skin and Oral Complications

Late *skin involvement* among ALL transplanted survivors includes a wide spectrum of clinical findings, mostly as a result of chronic cutaneous GvHD. Poikiloderma (skin atrophy and pigmentation), lichen planus (erythematous/violaceous flat-topped papules or plaques) and lichen sclerosus (coalescent greyish or whitish plaques) are the most frequently reported findings. In rare cases, morphea-like lesions represent the expression of skin-limited sclerosis [60, 61].

Nail dystrophy following HSCT encompasses several chronic GvHD-related findings, including longitudinal ridging, nail brittleness, onycholysis, and, ultimately, nail loss.

Finally, *oral mucosa* can be targeted by acute and chronic GvHD. As a result, survivors may experience a wide spectrum of clinical oropharyngeal findings, including xerostomia, dysgeusia, dental disorders, mucosal redness and lichenoid focal lesions [62]. In addition, secondary oral infections such as candidiasis, herpes simplex, and cytomegalovirus can exacerbate such complications. GVHD and TBI play a pivotal detrimental role on oral health following HSCT, as they prompt progressive deterioration of salivary glands secretion.

Lifestyle recommendations to improve oral hygiene include bidaily brushing with fluoride enriched toothpaste and avoidance of sugary diet and smoke.

20.2.6 Endocrine Complications

Endocrinopathies represent a remarkable share of all the medical sequelae of transplantation in paediatrics, with reported incidence rates exceeding 60% of HSCT survivors [63].

Cranial irradiation delivered as a part of frontline treatment protocols, the cumulative dose of alkylators administered, chronic GvHD, prolonged exposure to corticosteroids and TBI represent the most detrimental factors affecting endocrine and auxologic health among ALL survivors [64, 65].

Faltering growth is a common finding among transplanted patients and final height attainment often falls below midparental height expectations in HSCT-ALL survivors [66]. Either endocrine or non-hormonal factors may interplay and negatively affect growth potential. Radiation-induced damage to the growth plates, corticosteroids, malnutrition and psychosocial issues can be listed among the latter. Conversely, endocrine factors include untreated hypogonadism, hypothyroidism and growth hormone deficiency (GHD). GHD commonly represents the only pituitary deficiency experienced following the overall low doses delivered in the setting of prophylactic radiotherapy or TBI [67], while chemotherapy does not play any detrimental action on pituitary secretion, even in case of intrathecal administration. Interestingly, insulin-like growth factor-I (IGF-I) has been demonstrated as a poor predictor of radiation-induced GHD and clinicians should rely on a combination of auxological data and inadequate GH peaks upon GH stimulation tests [68]. As TBI affects growth attainments per se, irrespectively of eventual radiation-induced GHD, several authors have demonstrated that the administration of recombinant human growth hormone among GHD patients fails to restore patients' growth potential, despite its beneficial effects on height velocity [69].

TBI and, to a lesser extent, high-dose alkylating agents have been demonstrated as the most detrimental factors affecting thyroid health among ALL survivors [70, 71]. The spectrum of *thyroid function disorders* includes subclinical and overt non-autoimmune hypothyroidism, Hashimoto thyroiditis and autoimmune hyperthyroidism, with an overall 10-year cumulative incidence exceeding 20–30% [70, 72].

The damaging effects of TBI on thyroid function has been extensively assessed in published literature [73, 74]. On the one hand, radiation involving the neck can trigger autoimmune thyroiditis as a result of the presentation of otherwise unexposed thyroid antigens to the immune system, leading to immune dysregulation and to the onset of Hashimoto thyroiditis or Graves' disease [75–77]. On the other hand, radiation may result in non-autoimmune hypothyroidism as a result of the secretive dysfunction and thyroid volume reduction mediated by radiation-induced apoptosis and necrosis leading to thyrocyte dysfunction and thyroid volume reduction [72].

A growing body of literature has more recently shed light on the detrimental effects of high-dose chemotherapy on thyroid action and busulfan has been identified as the most thyroidotoxic alkylator [72]. In addition, an increased incidence of hypothyroidism has been reported in patients treated with tyrosine kinase inhibitors, although the pathophysiology of this condition remains unclear.

Finally, HSCT is an independent risk factor for the onset of *thyroid cancer*, with a 20-year cumulative incidence exceeding 9% in several national and international studies (see the section dedicated to secondary malignancies for additional information).

According to international guidelines for the early detection of LAE among transplanted survivors, patients exposed to TBI should undergo free T4 and TSH assessment at least yearly. In addition, either neck palpation or thyroid ultrasound should be periodically performed to diagnose nodules and/or thyroid secondary cancer [78–80].

Along with thyroid disease, *impaired gonadal function* represents the most frequently reported endocrine LEA among ALL survivors following HSCT [81, 82]. The clinical expression of the iatrogenic ovarian failure experienced by female survivors encompasses a wide spectrum of conditions ranging from a milder scenario known as diminished oocyte reserve (DOR) to overt endocrine dysfunction and subsequent hypoestrogenism [83, 84]. By DOR we indicate a condition characterized by retained regular menses and normal gonadotropins and oestradiol in the presence of biochemical markers consistent with impaired ovarian reserve, potentially predicting an unfavourable reproductive prognosis including the progression towards infertility. On the other hand, the clinical expression of overt endocrine damage depends on the age and pubertal status upon HSCT [85]. Severe ovarian damage in pre−/peripubertal girls may lead to pubertal delay or pubertal arrest, prompting the need for pharmacological induction to achieve full pubertal attainment and menarche. In post-pubertal patients, primary ovarian insufficiency (POI) is defined as the onset of secondary amenorrhoea, hypoestrogenism and infertility in the setting of an adult-onset hypergonadotropic hypogonadism. Though no pharmacological treatments can restore the oocyte pool and promote retrieved fertility, hormonal replacement therapy is the standard-of-care to provide relief from the symptoms of hypoestrogenism and to prevent adolescents and woman from experiencing clinical consequences of prolonged ovarian insufficiency, such as reduced bone mineral density and increased long-term cardiovascular risks [86].

Both alkylating agents and TBI halt follicle maturation and cause a rapidly progressing depletion of ovarian follicles [87, 88]. The detrimental effect of both radiation and chemotherapy is dose-dependent, while younger age and prepubertal status upon HSCT are protective factors. In female leukaemic patients, POI occurs in almost 100% of adolescents and young adults after TBI- or busulfan-based conditioning, while its incidence is lower following cyclophosphamide or treosulfan [89–91].

Also in males testicular function can be severely affected by radio- and chemotherapy following HSCT. Overall, germ cells are remarkably more radio- and chemo-sensitive than Leydig cells, and the occurrence of HSCT-related azoospermia exceeds 85–90% in cohorts of patients transplanted for haematological malignancies. [92, 93] On the other hand, testosterone deficiency is a rarer occurrence, ranging from 0% following the exposure to chemo-only regimens to 55.6% among patients exposed to TBI [94, 95]. Pubertal delay and pubertal arrest are the clinical expression of testosterone deficiency whenever Leydig cell damage becomes overt before or during the early stages of puberty. In this setting, progressively increasing doses of testosterone are the treatment of choice to induce pubertal progression and mimic physiological sexual maturation.

Adult patients may experience a progressive decrease in testosterone levels after achieving complete spontaneous sexual maturation, as an expression of iatrogenic hypergonadotropic hypogonadism. Symptoms and signs consistent with declining testicular endocrine function can be relieved by hormonal replacement therapy (testosterone).

The detrimental effects of chemotherapy on testosterone secretion tends to be remarkably less overt than following radiation. Indeed, patients conditioned with chemo-only regimens often experience isolated compensatory increase in LH and FSH, with retained circulating testosterone [96]. On the other hand, ALL survivors exposed to radiation (frontline or as a part of conditioning regimen) experience overt hypogonadism and decreased testosterone values in 50–75% of cases [95, 97].

Progression into subclinical and subsequently overt hypogonadism may occur at any age, years or decades following HSCT. Accordingly, lifelong periodical clinical and biochemical assessment should be pursued among all transplanted ALL survivors [78].

Several HSCT-related factors negatively affect *glucose metabolism* among ALL survivors. Firstly, it has been demonstrated that pancreatic volume declines following abdomen irradiation, along with β-cells reserve [98]. In addition, the prolonged exposure to corticosteroids may lead to sarcopenic obesity, defined as an abnormal body composition characterized by increased adipose tissue and decreased lean mass [98]. The synergistic reduction in insulin receptors and impaired insulin secretion may result in an increased occurrence of diabetes mellitus (DM) following HSCT and, in particular, TBI. Ten-year cumulative incidence of DM rates as high as 5% have been reported following transplantation [99].

Healthcare professionals are highly warranted to promote healthy lifestyle modifications in HSCT recipients. In addition, the Children's Oncology Group guidelines recommend yearly monitoring of patients' body mass index and fasting blood glucose and glycated haemoglobin assessment every 2 years [78].

20.2.7 Bone

Bone health is negatively affected in a remarkable share of transplanted ALL survivors. TBI, corticosteroids, chronic GvHD and functional impairment related to prolonged immobilization affect bone mineral density and vascularization, leading to osteoporosis and osteonecrosis [100, 101].

The reported 5-year cumulative incidence of severely *impaired bone mineral density* (BMD) exceeds 20% following HSCT for either malignant or non-malignant disorders, but several authors report variable degrees of osteopenia in up to 60% of survivors [102].

Along with the abovementioned detrimental treatment-related factors, several endocrinopathies may worsen BMD. Indeed, GHD, hypothyroidism, hypogonadism, and hypovitaminosis D may play an additional synergetic negative effect on bone health, especially if inadequately treated [65].

Periodic assessment by dual-energy X-ray absorptiometry (DEXA) scan is crucial to early detect BMD decline over time following HSCT. No shared guidelines have been published in this field, and the best screening timing should be tailored to the patient's risk factors. Adequate calcium dietary intake should be pursued. In addition, serum vitamin D levels should be assessed, in order to identify those patients who may benefit from oral supplementation [103].

Finally, in case of vertebral compression fractures or recurrent long bone fractures in the setting of low BMD, paediatric patients and young adult survivors should be unequivocally candidate to pharmacological treatment with bisphosphonates. On the other hand, given the potential of spontaneous recovery of bone disease in acquired conditions and as high-quality data about the occurrence of fractures in untreated paediatric patients with secondary osteoporosis are lacking, a conservative approach is still advised by the International Society for Clinical Densitometry (ISCD) in paediatric patients with isolated decrease of BMD with no bone fractures. [104, 105]

Furthermore, *osteonecrosis* (ON) is a widespread debilitating iatrogenic complication of ALL, experienced by either transplanted or non-transplanted survivors [65, 106], with adolescents and young adults representing the most at-risk population. Indeed, patients post-pubertal upon HSCT are exposed to a three- to fivefold increase in the occurrence of ON compared to infants and children [107], but incidence differs substantially among studies, as diagnostic approaches can be limited to severely symptomatic patients or extended to patients with mild symptoms or even include screening procedures. In a recent cohort of 256 consecutive children and adolescents diagnosed with ALL, the overall cumulative incidence of ON was 18.5% (standard error, SE, 5.7), with a median of 6 lesions in the affected patients. Seventy-eight percent of the cases were diagnosed during the frontline treatment, when the risk of ON was fivefold higher in high-risk patients and tenfold higher in patients aged $\geq$10 years. Furthermore, the risk of ON was double in patients who experienced relapse; even though HSCT per se was not significantly associated with ON [106].

Although the pathophysiology of this condition still needs to be unveiled, it is hypothesized that persistent or recurrent vaso-occlusive events, facilitated by asparaginase treatment, play a crucial role by leading to blood supply disruption and subsequent tissue hypoxia, inflammation, bone necrosis and collapse [108]. If left untreated, osteonecrosis can be extremely debilitating and may lead to severe pain, loss of function, and degenerative joint changes. Intravascular dissemination and hyperlipemia, often experienced following ALL treatments, may affect bone vascularization and play a contributory role. Nevertheless, corticosteroid-related arteriopathy is unequivocally recognized as the most critical detrimental causative factor and cumulative dose of steroids has been demonstrated as significantly associated with the odds of developing ON [109].

From a clinical perspective, the expression of ON is multifaceted and usually depends on the location of ON. In case of long-bone diaphyseal involvement, patients are asymptomatic. On the other hand, when the major joints are affected, ON leads to chronic pain and functional impairment.

MRI is the gold-standard to detect and monitor ON evolution over time and should be promptly prescribed whenever ALL survivors complain about recurrent bone pain [110].

Pain management and physical therapy represent the first-line treatment for symptomatic ON. In case of disease progression or debilitating pictures, surgery is often considered as a curative option. Surgical procedures range from conservative solutions, such as core decompression, to demolitive solutions, including arthroplasty. Nevertheless, no shared positions have been published and different authors report conflicting data about the potential benefits and pitfalls of each surgical approach [111]. Avoiding lesion progression that could lead to articular collapse should be the aim of early conservative surgery in ON treatment.

20.2.8 Secondary Malignancies

Though relapsed leukemia is the first cause of mortality among transplanted ALL survivors, HSCT is related to a two- to threefold increase in the risk of developing cancer compared to age and gender-matched general population [112], with a 15-year cumulative incidence exceeding 10–15% in several population studies. [113–115]

Among *solid secondary malignant neoplasms* (SMN), skin, oral, thyroid, uterine cancers and glioblastoma represent the most frequently reported histotypes following HSCT. The clinical presentation of HSCT-related solid tumours is superimposable to that reported in the general population. Nevertheless, there is a paucity of data about the biological specificity and the clinical behaviour of SMN following treatment for childhood cancer.

Among known risk factors, radiotherapy and TBI play a pivotal role. In this setting, radiotherapy is a well-known causative factor for breast cancer and remarkably greater occurrence rates have been reported among childhood cancer survivors whenever breast tissue was involved in the irradiation field [116]. Iatrogenic amplification of *c-MYC* locus is a key pathogenic element in a representative share of patients with radiation-induced breast cancer [117].

Similarly, the utmost radiosensitivity of thyroid tissue and the detrimental and oncogenic effects of TBI, radiotherapy of the cervical area and prophylactic cranial irradiation on the developing thyroid gland have been extensively described in the literature [118, 119]. From a histopathologic and biological perspective, radiation-induced secondary thyroid tumours show a more aggressive behaviour. Indeed, radiation may induce oncogenes fusion (such as RET and PTC or ALK and NTRK) resulting in higher degree of dedifferentiation, therapy resistance, and infiltrative patterns [72, 120, 121].

On the other hand, chronic GvHD has been demonstrated as a causative factor for mucocutaneous SMN [122], while the potential contribution of alkylating agents on the onset of secondary bone tumours has been suggested, but this association should be confirmed by additional high-quality studies [123].

Several epidemiologic analyses have shed light on the long-term latencies that often elapse between exposure to ionizing radiation and the onset of SMN. To date, no time *plateau* has been identified and the cumulative incidence rates show progressively increasing trendlines over time. Accordingly, screening protocols for ALL-HSCT survivors recommend a life-long monitoring [78].

Therapy-related *acute myeloid leukaemia/myelodysplasia* (AML/MDS) generally occurs following autologous HSCT among patients exposed to pre-treatment alkylating agents before HSCT. In this setting, heavily treated reconstituting HSCs may carry acquired cytomolecular signatures leading to oncogenesis and subsequent transformation into malignant clones. Occasionally, secondary AML/MDS has been reported among ALL survivors, treated by definition with allogeneic HSCT [123, 124]. In this setting, it has been suggested that the co-occurring of an unfavourable bone marrow microenvironment along with HSC replicative stress may interplay and lead to malignant transformation.

Finally, prolonged immunosuppression leads to a decrease in immune surveillance, potentially resulting in a *spectrum* of disorders classified as *post-transplantation lymphoproliferative disorders* (PTLD). In this setting, often following an infectious trigger (predominantly Epstein–Barr virus), transplanted survivors experience a variable degree of manifestations, ranging from asymptomatic scenarios to life-threatening PTLD with multiorgan dysfunction, fever, malaise, hypotension, and bulky involvement. The cornerstone in approaching these clinical scenarios is represented by anti-CD20 antibodies and discontinuation of immunosuppressors. In acute scenarios, cytotoxic treatment may be required.

20.2.9 Psychosocial Issues and Quality of Life

ALL survivors face social and psychosocial challenges that may negatively interfere with their overall QoL achievements [125, 126]. Along with the traumatic experience of diagnosis and antineoplastic treatments, LAEs represent additional factors playing a detrimental role on both physical and psychological health. Late psychosocial effects include post-traumatic stress disorder, diminished self-esteem, social anxiety and poor peer acceptance issues. The occurrence rates and severity of these clinical scenarios tend to increase with younger age, longer pre-HSCT treatment protocols, and severity of HSCT-LAEs [65].

The long-term monitoring programmes recommended for HSCT survivors should include routine interventions to early detect psychosocial issues and to provide prompt interventions aimed at improving patient's overall QoL [127].

Research in the field of long-term survivorship has recently shed light on the pivotal importance of developing effective interventions focussed on prevention and treatment of psychological/psychosocial LAEs [128].

20.3 Conclusion

Most ALL survivors are expected to experience at least one LAE over a lifetime. Accordingly, healthcare professionals should be trained in early detecting and approaching adverse events along dedicated and mandatory long-term follow-up programmes. In addition, patients should receive satisfactory and complete information following HSCT and should be taught about how taking over responsibilities towards themselves and health issues over time.

Long-term follow-up outpatient clinics are warranted to provide patients with a detailed care plan, tailored on patient-specific risk factors. This promotes self-esteem and autonomy and, in addition, smoothens the process of transitioning towards adult care.

References

1. Hunger SP, Raetz EA. How I treat relapsed acute lymphoblastic leukemia in the pediatric population. Blood. 2020;136(16):1803–12. https://doi.org/10.1182/blood.2019004043.
2. Raetz EA, Rebora P, Conter V, et al. Outcome for children and young adults with T-cell ALL and induction failure in contemporary trials. J Clin Oncol. 2023; https://doi.org/10.1200/JCO.23.00088.
3. Yeshurun M, Weisdorf D, Rowe JM, et al. The impact of the graft-versus-leukemia effect on survival in acute lymphoblastic leukemia. Blood Adv. 2019;3(4):670–80. https://doi.org/10.1182/bloodadvances.2018027003.
4. Francisci S, Guzzinati S, Dal Maso L, Sacerdote C, Buzzoni C, Gigli A. An estimate of the number of people in Italy living after a childhood cancer. Int J Cancer. 2017;140(11):2444–50. https://doi.org/10.1002/ijc.30665.
5. Hierlmeier S, Eyrich M, Wölfl M, Schlegel P-G, Wiegering V. Early and late complications following hematopoietic stem cell transplantation in pediatric patients—a retrospective analysis over 11 years. PLoS One. 2018;13(10):e0204914. https://doi.org/10.1371/journal.pone.0204914.
6. Vrooman LM, Millard HR, Brazauskas R, et al. Survival and late effects after allogeneic hematopoietic cell transplantation for hematologic malignancy at less than three years of age. Biol Blood Marrow Transplant. 2017;23(8):1327–34. https://doi.org/10.1016/j.bbmt.2017.04.017.
7. Uderzo C, Pillon M, Corti P, et al. Impact of cumulative anthracycline dose, preparative regimen and chronic graft-versus-host disease on pulmonary and cardiac function in children 5 years after allogeneic hematopoietic stem cell transplantation: a prospective evaluation on behalf of the EB. Bone Marrow Transplant. 2007;39(11):667–75. https://doi.org/10.1038/sj.bmt.1705652.
8. Landier W, Armenian S, Bhatia S. Late effects of childhood cancer and its treatment. Pediatr Clin N Am. 2015;62(1):275–300. https://doi.org/10.1016/j.pcl.2014.09.017.
9. Peters C, Dalle J-H, Locatelli F, et al. Total body irradiation or chemotherapy conditioning in childhood ALL: a multinational, randomized, noninferiority phase III study. J Clin Oncol. 2021;39(4):295–307. https://doi.org/10.1200/JCO.20.02529.
10. Hoeben BAW, Wong JYC, Fog LS, et al. Total body irradiation in haematopoietic stem cell transplantation for paediatric acute lymphoblastic leukaemia: review of the literature and future directions. Front Pediatr. 2021;9:774348. https://doi.org/10.3389/fped.2021.774348.
11. Sun C-L, Francisco L, Kawashima T, et al. Prevalence and predictors of chronic health conditions after hematopoietic cell transplantation: a report from the Bone Marrow Transplant Survivor Study. Blood. 2010;116(17):3129–39. https://doi.org/10.1182/blood-2009-06-229369.
12. Inamoto Y, Petriček I, Burns L, et al. Non-graft-versus-host disease ocular complications after hematopoietic cell transplantation: expert review from the Late Effects and Quality of Life Working Committee of the Center for International Blood and Marrow Transplant Research and the Transplant. Biol Blood Marrow Transplant. 2019;25(5):e145–54. https://doi.org/10.1016/j.bbmt.2018.11.033.
13. Pellegrini M, Bernabei F, Barbato F, et al. Incidence, risk factors and complications of ocular graft-versus-host disease following hematopoietic stem cell transplantation. Am J Ophthalmol. 2021;227:25–34. https://doi.org/10.1016/j.ajo.2021.02.022.
14. Kinori M, Bielorai B, Souroujon D, Hutt D, Ben-Bassat Mizrachi I, Huna-Baron R. Ocular complications in children after hematopoietic stem cell transplantation without total body irradiation. Graefes Arch Clin Exp Ophthalmol. 2015;253(8):1397–402. https://doi.org/10.1007/s00417-015-2964-8.
15. Horwitz M, Auquier P, Barlogis V, et al. Incidence and risk factors for cataract after haematopoietic

stem cell transplantation for childhood leukaemia: an LEA study. Br J Haematol. 2015;168(4):518–25. https://doi.org/10.1111/bjh.13148.
16. Benyunes MC, Sullivan KM, Joachim Deeg H, et al. Cataracts after bone marrow transplantation: long-term follow-up of adults treated with fractionated total body irradiation. Int J Radiat Oncol. 1995;32(3):661–70. https://doi.org/10.1016/0360-3016(94)00392-X.
17. Teär Fahnehjelm K, Törnquist AL, Olsson M, Bäckström I, Andersson Grönlund M, Winiarski J. Cataract after allogeneic hematopoietic stem cell transplantation in childhood. Acta Paediatr. 2016;105(1):82–9. https://doi.org/10.1111/apa.13173.
18. Giannaccare G, Bonifazi F, Sessa M, et al. Ocular surface analysis in hematological patients before and after allogeneic hematopoietic stem cell transplantation: implication for daily clinical practice. Eye. 2017;31(10):1417–26. https://doi.org/10.1038/eye.2017.78.
19. Pathak M, Diep PP, Lai X, Brinch L, Ruud E, Drolsum L. Ocular findings and ocular graft-versus-host disease after allogeneic stem cell transplantation without total body irradiation. Bone Marrow Transplant. 2018;53(7):863–72. https://doi.org/10.1038/s41409-018-0090-z.
20. Jacobs R, Tran U, Chen H, et al. Prevalence and risk factors associated with development of ocular GVHD defined by NIH consensus criteria. Bone Marrow Transplant. 2012;47(11):1470–3. https://doi.org/10.1038/bmt.2012.56.
21. Tichelli A, Duell T, Weiss M, et al. Late-onset keratoconjunctivitis sicca syndrome after bone marrow transplantation: incidence and risk factors. European Group or Blood and Marrow Transplantation (EBMT) Working Party on Late Effects. Bone Marrow Transplant. 1996;17(6):1105–11. http://www.ncbi.nlm.nih.gov/pubmed/8807122.
22. Bylsma GW, Hall AJ, Szer J, West R. Atypical retinal microvasculopathy after bone marrow transplantation. Clin Experiment Ophthalmol. 2001;29(4):225–9. https://doi.org/10.1046/j.1442-9071.2001.00423.x.
23. Bernauer W, Gratwohl A, Keller A, Daicker B. Microvasculopathy in the ocular fundus after bone marrow transplantation. Ann Intern Med. 1991;115(12):925–30. https://doi.org/10.7326/0003-4819-115-12-925.
24. Lopez PF, Sternberg P, Dabbs CK, Vogler WR, Crocker I, Kalin NS. Bone marrow transplant retinopathy. Am J Ophthalmol. 1991;112(6):635–46. https://doi.org/10.1016/S0002-9394(14)77269-1.
25. Chow EJ, Wong K, Lee SJ, et al. Late cardiovascular complications after hematopoietic cell transplantation. Biol Blood Marrow Transplant. 2014;20(6):794–800. https://doi.org/10.1016/j.bbmt.2014.02.012.
26. Viner Smith E, Tierney AC, Klarica D, Walker P, Avery S. Impact of a lifestyle modification program on the metabolic syndrome and associated risk factors in long-term survivors of stem cell transplantation. Bone Marrow Transplant. 2016;51(5):722–4. https://doi.org/10.1038/bmt.2015.312.
27. Majhail NS, Flowers ME, Ness KK, et al. High prevalence of metabolic syndrome after allogeneic hematopoietic cell transplantation. Bone Marrow Transplant. 2009;43(1):49–54. https://doi.org/10.1038/bmt.2008.263.
28. Ragbourne SC, Crook MA. Metabolic syndrome in long-term survivors of hematopoietic stem-cell transplantation. Clin Lymphoma Myeloma Leuk. 2017;17(6):340–6. https://doi.org/10.1016/j.clml.2017.05.004.
29. Oudin C, Auquier P, Bertrand Y, et al. Metabolic syndrome in adults who received hematopoietic stem cell transplantation for acute childhood leukemia: an LEA study. Bone Marrow Transplant. 2015;50(11):1438–44. https://doi.org/10.1038/bmt.2015.167.
30. Walker BR. Glucocorticoids and cardiovascular disease. Eur J Endocrinol. 2007;157(5):545–59. https://doi.org/10.1530/EJE-07-0455.
31. Paris C, Yates L, Lama P, Zepeda AJ, Gutiérrez D, Palma J. Evaluation of metabolic syndrome after hematopoietic stem cell transplantation in children and adolescents. Pediatr Blood Cancer. 2012;59(2):306–10. https://doi.org/10.1002/pbc.24104.
32. Oudin C, Simeoni M-C, Sirvent N, et al. Prevalence and risk factors of the metabolic syndrome in adult survivors of childhood leukemia. Blood. 2011;117(17):4442–8. https://doi.org/10.1182/blood-2010-09-304899.
33. Armenian SH, Sun C-L, Francisco L, et al. Late congestive heart failure after hematopoietic cell transplantation. J Clin Oncol. 2008;26(34):5537–43. https://doi.org/10.1200/JCO.2008.17.7428.
34. López-Fernández T, Vadillo IS, de la Guía AL, Barbier KH. Cardiovascular issues in hematopoietic stem cell transplantation (HSCT). Curr Treat Options in Oncol. 2021;22(6):51. https://doi.org/10.1007/s11864-021-00850-3.
35. Yancy CW, Jessup M, Bozkurt B, et al. 2017 ACC/AHA/HFSA focused update of the 2013 ACCF/AHA guideline for the management of heart failure: a report of the American College of Cardiology/American Heart Association Task Force on Clinical Practice Guidelines and the Heart Failure Society of America. Circulation. 2017;136(6):e137. https://doi.org/10.1161/CIR.0000000000000509.
36. Majhail NS, Rizzo JD, Lee SJ, et al. Recommended screening and preventive practices for long-term survivors after hematopoietic cell transplantation. Bone Marrow Transplant. 2012;47(3):337–41. https://doi.org/10.1038/bmt.2012.5.
37. Armenian SH, Chow EJ. Cardiovascular disease in survivors of hematopoietic cell transplantation. Cancer. 2014;120(4):469–79. https://doi.org/10.1002/cncr.28444.

38. Oliveira GH, Al-Kindi SG, Guha A, Dey AK, Rhea IB, DeLima MJ. Cardiovascular risk assessment and management of patients undergoing hematopoietic cell transplantation. Bone Marrow Transplant. 2021;56(3):544–51. https://doi.org/10.1038/s41409-020-01080-1.
39. Zamorano JL, Lancellotti P, Rodriguez Muñoz D, et al. 2016 ESC Position Paper on cancer treatments and cardiovascular toxicity developed under the auspices of the ESC Committee for Practice Guidelines. Eur Heart J. 2016;37(36):2768–801. https://doi.org/10.1093/eurheartj/ehw211.
40. Zwaan FE, Hermans J, Barrett AJ, Speck B. Bone marrow transplantation for acute nonlymphoblastic leukaemia: a survey of the European Group for Bone Marrow Transplantation (E.G.B.M.T.). Br J Haematol. 1984;56(4):645–53. https://doi.org/10.1111/j.1365-2141.1984.tb02188.x.
41. Yousem SA. The histological spectrum of pulmonary graft-versus-host disease in bone marrow transplant recipients. Hum Pathol. 1995;26(6):668–75. https://doi.org/10.1016/0046-8177(95)90174-4.
42. Tomas LHS, Loberiza FR, Klein JP, et al. Risk factors for bronchiolitis obliterans in allogeneic hematopoietic stem-cell transplantation for leukemia. Chest. 2005;128(1):153–61. https://doi.org/10.1378/chest.128.1.153.
43. Alkhunaizi M, Patel B, Bueno L, et al. Risk factors for bronchiolitis obliterans syndrome after initial detection of pulmonary impairment after hematopoietic cell transplantation. Transplant Cell Ther. 2023;29(3):204.e1–7. https://doi.org/10.1016/j.jtct.2022.12.001.
44. Afessa B, Litzow M, Tefferi A. Bronchiolitis obliterans and other late onset non-infectious pulmonary complications in hematopoietic stem cell transplantation. Bone Marrow Transplant. 2001;28(5):425–34. https://doi.org/10.1038/sj.bmt.1703142.
45. Gower WA, Collaco JM, Mogayzel PJ. Lung function and late pulmonary complications among survivors of hematopoietic stem cell transplantation during childhood. Paediatr Respir Rev. 2010;11(2):115–22. https://doi.org/10.1016/j.prrv.2010.01.006.
46. American Thoracic Society/European Respiratory Society. American Thoracic Society/European Respiratory Society International Multidisciplinary Consensus classification of the idiopathic interstitial pneumonias. Am J Respir Crit Care Med. 2002;165(2):277–304. https://doi.org/10.1164/ajrccm.165.2.ats01.
47. Majeski EI, Paintlia MK, Lopez AD, Harley RA, London SD, London L. Respiratory reovirus 1/L induction of intraluminal fibrosis, a model of bronchiolitis obliterans organizing pneumonia, is dependent on T lymphocytes. Am J Pathol. 2003;163(4):1467–79. https://doi.org/10.1016/S0002-9440(10)63504-3.
48. Bankier AA, Van Muylem A, Knoop C, Estenne M, Gevenois PA. Bronchiolitis obliterans syndrome in heart-lung transplant recipients: diagnosis with expiratory CT. Radiology. 2001;218(2):533–9. https://doi.org/10.1148/radiology.218.2.r01fe09533.
49. Kenyon M, Murray J, Quinn B, Greenfield D, Trigoso E. Late effects and long-term follow-up; 2018. http://www.ncbi.nlm.nih.gov/pubmed/17438588.
50. Chang A, Hingorani S, Kowalewska J, et al. Spectrum of renal pathology in hematopoietic cell transplantation. Clin J Am Soc Nephrol. 2007;2(5):1014–23. https://doi.org/10.2215/CJN.01700407.
51. Patzer L, Ringelmann F, Kentouche K, et al. Renal function in long-term survivors of stem cell transplantation in childhood. A prospective trial. Bone Marrow Transplant. 2001;27(3):319–27. https://doi.org/10.1038/sj.bmt.1702763.
52. Kersting S, Hené RJ, Koomans HA, Verdonck LF. Chronic kidney disease after myeloablative allogeneic hematopoietic stem cell transplantation. Biol Blood Marrow Transplant. 2007;13(10):1169–75. https://doi.org/10.1016/j.bbmt.2007.06.008.
53. Hingorani S. Chronic kidney disease in long-term survivors of hematopoietic cell transplantation. J Am Soc Nephrol. 2006;17(7):1995–2005. https://doi.org/10.1681/ASN.2006020118.
54. Delgado J, Cooper N, Thomson K, et al. The importance of age, fludarabine, and total body irradiation in the incidence and severity of chronic renal failure after allogeneic hematopoietic cell transplantation. Biol Blood Marrow Transplant. 2006;12(1):75–83. https://doi.org/10.1016/j.bbmt.2005.08.036.
55. Wada F, Arai Y, Jo T, et al. Impact of antimicrobial drug-drug interactions on acute kidney injury after allogeneic hematopoietic cell transplantation. Transplant Cell Ther. 2023;29:634.e1. https://doi.org/10.1016/j.jtct.2023.07.017.
56. Abboud I, Peraldi M-N, Hingorani S. Chronic kidney diseases in long-term survivors after allogeneic hematopoietic stem cell transplantation: monitoring and management guidelines. Semin Hematol. 2012;49(1):73–82. https://doi.org/10.1053/j.seminhematol.2011.10.008.
57. Tichelli A, Rovó A, Passweg J, et al. Late complications after hematopoietic stem cell transplantation. Expert Rev Hematol. 2009;2(5):583–601. https://doi.org/10.1586/ehm.09.48.
58. Kemper MJ, Güngör T, Halter J, Schanz U, Neuhaus TJ. Favorable long-term outcome of nephrotic syndrome after allogeneic hematopoietic stem cell transplantation. Clin Nephrol. 2007;67(01):5–11. https://doi.org/10.5414/CNP67005.
59. Kal HB, van Kempen-Harteveld ML. Renal dysfunction after total body irradiation: dose–effect relationship. Int J Radiat Oncol. 2006;65(4):1228–32. https://doi.org/10.1016/j.ijrobp.2006.02.021.
60. Jagasia MH, Greinix HT, Arora M, et al. National Institutes of Health Consensus development project on criteria for clinical trials in chronic graft-versus-host disease: I. The 2014 Diagnosis and Staging Working Group report. Biol Blood Marrow

Transplant. 2015;21(3):389–401.e1. https://doi.org/10.1016/j.bbmt.2014.12.001.
61. Curtis RE. Impact of chronic GVHD therapy on the development of squamous-cell cancers after hematopoietic stem-cell transplantation: an international case-control study. Blood. 2005;105(10):3802–11. https://doi.org/10.1182/blood-2004-09-3411.
62. Woo S-B, Lee SJ, Schubert MM. Graft-vs.-host disease. Crit Rev Oral Biol Med. 1997;8(2):201–16. https://doi.org/10.1177/10454411970080020701.
63. Hows JM, Passweg JR, Tichelli A, et al. Comparison of long-term outcomes after allogeneic hematopoietic stem cell transplantation from matched sibling and unrelated donors. Bone Marrow Transplant. 2006;38(12):799–805. https://doi.org/10.1038/sj.bmt.1705531.
64. Paetow U, Bader P, Chemaitilly W. A systematic approach to the endocrine care of survivors of pediatric hematopoietic stem cell transplantation. Cancer Metastasis Rev. 2020;39(1):69–78. https://doi.org/10.1007/s10555-020-09864-z.
65. Diesch-Furlanetto T, Gabriel M, Zajac-Spychala O, Cattoni A, Hoeben BAW, Balduzzi A. Late effects after haematopoietic stem cell transplantation in ALL, long-term follow-up and transition: a step into adult life. Front Pediatr. 2021;9:773895. https://doi.org/10.3389/fped.2021.773895.
66. Rodari G, Cattoni A, Albanese A. Final height in growth hormone-deficient childhood cancer survivors after growth hormone therapy. J Endocrinol Investig. 2020;43(2):209–17. https://doi.org/10.1007/s40618-019-01102-w.
67. Darzy KH, Shalet SM. Radiation-induced growth hormone deficiency. Horm Res Paediatr. 2003;59(Suppl 1):1–11. https://doi.org/10.1159/000067834.
68. Cattoni A, Clarke E, Albanese A. The predictive value of insulin-like growth factor 1 in irradiation-dependent growth hormone deficiency in childhood cancer survivors. Horm Res Paediatr. 2018;90(5):314–25. https://doi.org/10.1159/000495760.
69. Isfan F, Kanold J, Merlin E, et al. Growth hormone treatment impact on growth rate and final height of patients who received HSCT with TBI or/and cranial irradiation in childhood: a report from the French Leukaemia Long-Term Follow-Up Study (LEA). Bone Marrow Transplant. 2012;47(5):684–93. https://doi.org/10.1038/bmt.2011.139.
70. Sanders JE, Hoffmeister PA, Woolfrey AE, et al. Thyroid function following hematopoietic cell transplantation in children: 30 years' experience. Blood. 2009;113(2):306–8. https://doi.org/10.1182/blood-2008-08-173005.
71. Cohen A, Rovelli A, Merlo DF, et al. Risk for secondary thyroid carcinoma after hematopoietic stem-cell transplantation: an EBMT Late Effects Working Party Study. J Clin Oncol. 2007;25(17):2449–54. https://doi.org/10.1200/JCO.2006.08.9276.
72. Cattoni A, Molinari S, Riva B, et al. Thyroid function disorders and secondary cancer following haematopoietic stem cell transplantation in pediatrics: state of the art and practical recommendations for a risk-based follow-up. Front Endocrinol (Lausanne). 2022;13:1064146. https://doi.org/10.3389/fendo.2022.1064146.
73. Oudin C, Auquier P, Bertrand Y, et al. Late thyroid complications in survivors of childhood acute leukemia. An L.E.A. study. Haematologica. 2016;101(6):747–56. https://doi.org/10.3324/haematol.2015.140053.
74. Reed NS. Dosimetry and radiation scattered to the thyroid gland from prophylactic cranial irradiation for childhood leukemia. Pediatr Hematol Oncol. 1994;11(1):5–8. https://doi.org/10.3109/08880019409141895.
75. Jereczek-Fossa BA, Zarowski A, Milani F, Orecchia R. Radiotherapy-induced ear toxicity. Cancer Treat Rev. 2003;29(5):417–30. https://doi.org/10.1016/S0305-7372(03)00066-5.
76. Tamura K, Shimaoka K, Friedman M. Thyroid abnormalities associated with treatment of malignant lymphoma. Cancer. 1981;47(11):2704–11. https://doi.org/10.1002/1097-0142(19810601)47:11<2704::AID-CNCR2820471129>3.0.CO;2-G.
77. Inskip PD, Veiga LHS, Brenner AV, et al. Hyperthyroidism after radiation therapy for childhood cancer: a report from the Childhood Cancer Survivor study. Int J Radiat Oncol. 2019;104(2):415–24. https://doi.org/10.1016/j.ijrobp.2019.02.009.
78. Chow EJ, Anderson L, Baker KS, et al. Late effects surveillance recommendations among survivors of childhood hematopoietic cell transplantation: a Children's Oncology Group report. Biol Blood Marrow Transplant. 2016;22(5):782–95. https://doi.org/10.1016/j.bbmt.2016.01.023.
79. Clement SC, Kremer LCM, Verburg FA, et al. Balancing the benefits and harms of thyroid cancer surveillance in survivors of childhood, adolescent and young adult cancer: recommendations from the international Late Effects of Childhood Cancer Guideline Harmonization Group in collaboration with the PanCareSurFup Consortium. Cancer Treat Rev. 2018;63:28–39. https://doi.org/10.1016/j.ctrv.2017.11.005.
80. Children's Oncology Group. Long-term follow-up guidelines for survivors of childhood, adolescent, and young adult cancers, and related health; 2018. www.survivorshipguidelines.org.
81. Barnes N, Chemaitilly W. Endocrinopathies in survivors of childhood neoplasia. Front Pediatr. 2014;2:1–12. https://doi.org/10.3389/fped.2014.00101.
82. Abou-Mourad YR, Lau BC, Barnett MJ, et al. Long-term outcome after allo-SCT: close follow-up on a large cohort treated with myeloablative regimens. Bone Marrow Transplant. 2010;45(2):295–302. https://doi.org/10.1038/bmt.2009.128.
83. Webber L, Davies M, Anderson R, et al. ESHRE guideline: management of women with premature ovar-

ian insufficiency. Hum Reprod. 2016;31(5):926–37. https://doi.org/10.1093/humrep/dew027.
84. Cedars MI. Managing poor ovarian response in the patient with diminished ovarian reserve. Fertil Steril. 2022;117(4):655–6. https://doi.org/10.1016/j.fertnstert.2022.02.026.
85. Pastore LM, Christianson MS, Stelling J, Kearns WG, Segars JH. Reproductive ovarian testing and the alphabet soup of diagnoses: DOR, POI, POF, POR, and FOR. J Assist Reprod Genet. 2018;35(1):17–23. https://doi.org/10.1007/s10815-017-1058-4.
86. Cattoni A, Parissone F, Porcari I, et al. Hormonal replacement therapy in adolescents and young women with chemo- or radio-induced premature ovarian insufficiency: practical recommendations. Blood Rev. 2020;45:100730. https://doi.org/10.1016/j.blre.2020.100730.
87. Jadoul P, Anckaert E, Dewandeleer A, et al. Clinical and biologic evaluation of ovarian function in women treated by bone marrow transplantation for various indications during childhood or adolescence. Fertil Steril. 2011;96(1):126–133.e3. https://doi.org/10.1016/j.fertnstert.2011.03.108.
88. Jadoul P, Anckaert E, Dewandeleer A, et al. Fertility preservation in patients undergoing gonadotoxic therapy or gonadectomy: a committee opinion. Fertil Steril. 2019;112(6):1022–33. https://doi.org/10.1016/j.fertnstert.2019.09.013.
89. Couto-Silva A-C, Trivin C, Espérou H, et al. Bone markers after total body irradiation in childhood. Bone Marrow Transplant. 2010;45(3):437–41. https://doi.org/10.1038/bmt.2009.198.
90. Hirabayashi K, Nakazawa Y, Matsuura H, et al. Risk factors for diabetes mellitus and impaired glucose tolerance following allogeneic hematopoietic stem cell transplantation in pediatric patients with hematological malignancies. Int J Hematol. 2014;99(4):477–86. https://doi.org/10.1007/s12185-014-1536-8.
91. Faraci M, Diesch T, Labopin M, et al. Gonadal function after busulfan compared with Treosulfan in children and adolescents undergoing allogeneic hematopoietic stem cell transplant. Biol blood marrow Transplant. 2019;25(9):1786–91. https://doi.org/10.1016/j.bbmt.2019.05.005.
92. Chatterjee R, Mills W, Katz M, McGarrigle HH, Goldstone AH. Germ cell failure and Leydig cell insufficiency in post-pubertal males after autologous bone marrow transplantation with BEAM for lymphoma. Bone Marrow Transplant. 1994;13(5):519–22. http://www.ncbi.nlm.nih.gov/pubmed/8054905.
93. Anserini P, Chiodi S, Spinelli S, et al. Semen analysis following allogeneic bone marrow transplantation. Additional data for evidence-based counselling. Bone Marrow Transplant. 2002;30(7):447–51. https://doi.org/10.1038/sj.bmt.1703651.
94. Sklar C. Reproductive physiology and treatment-related loss of sex hormone production. Med Pediatr Oncol. 1999;33(1):2–8. https://doi.org/10.1002/(SICI)1096-911X(199907)33:1<2::AID-MPO2>3.0.CO;2-7.
95. Lopez R, Plat G, Bertrand Y, et al. Testosterone deficiency in men surviving childhood acute leukemia after treatment with hematopoietic stem cell transplantation or testicular radiation: an L.E.A. study. Bone Marrow Transplant. 2021;56(6):1422–5. https://doi.org/10.1038/s41409-020-01180-y.
96. Taneja S, Rao A, Nussey S, Leiper A. Leydig cell failure with testicular radiation doses <20Gy: the clinical effects of total body irradiation conditioned haematopoietic stem cell transplantation for childhood leukaemia during long-term follow-up. Clin Endocrinol. 2019;91(5):624–32. https://doi.org/10.1111/cen.14059.
97. Sanders JE, Flournoy N, Thomas ED, et al. Marrow transplant experience in children with acute lymphoblastic leukemia: an analysis of factors associated with survival, relapse, and graft-versus-host disease. Med Pediatr Oncol. 1985;13(4):165–72. https://doi.org/10.1002/mpo.2950130402.
98. Wei C, Thyagiarajan M, Hunt L, et al. Reduced beta-cell reserve and pancreatic volume in survivors of childhood acute lymphoblastic leukaemia treated with bone marrow transplantation and total body irradiation. Clin Endocrinol. 2015;82(1):59–67. https://doi.org/10.1111/cen.12575.
99. Hoffmeister PA, Storer BE, Sanders JE. Diabetes mellitus in long-term survivors of pediatric hematopoietic cell transplantation. J Pediatr Hematol Oncol. 2004;26(2):81–90. https://doi.org/10.1097/00043426-200402000-00003.
100. Buxbaum NP, Robinson C, Sinaii N, et al. Impaired bone mineral density in pediatric patients with chronic graft-versus-host disease. Biol Blood Marrow Transplant. 2018;24(7):1415–23. https://doi.org/10.1016/j.bbmt.2018.02.019.
101. Bhatia S, Ramsay N, Weisdorf D, Griffiths H, Robison L. Bone mineral density in patients undergoing bone marrow transplantation for myeloid malignancies. Bone Marrow Transplant. 1998;22(1):87–90. https://doi.org/10.1038/sj.bmt.1701275.
102. Baker KS, Armenian S, Bhatia S. Long-term consequences of hematopoietic stem cell transplantation: current state of the science. Biol Blood Marrow Transplant. 2010;16(1):S90–6. https://doi.org/10.1016/j.bbmt.2009.09.017.
103. Wasilewski-Masker K, Kaste SC, Hudson MM, Esiashvili N, Mattano LA, Meacham LR. Bone mineral density deficits in survivors of childhood cancer: long-term follow-up guidelines and review of the literature. Pediatrics. 2008;121(3):e705–13. https://doi.org/10.1542/peds.2007-1396.
104. Bishop N, Arundel P, Clark E, et al. Fracture prediction and the definition of osteoporosis in children and adolescents: the ISCD 2013 Pediatric Official Positions. J Clin Densitom. 2014;17(2):275–80. https://doi.org/10.1016/j.jocd.2014.01.004.
105. Marini JC. Do bisphosphonates make children's bones better or brittle? N Engl J Med.

2003;349(5):423–6. https://doi.org/10.1056/NEJMp038103.
106. Brivio E, Cossio A, Borra D, et al. Osteonecrosis in paediatric acute lymphoblastic leukaemia: incidence, risk factors, radiological patterns and evolution in a single-Centre cohort. Br J Haematol. 2022;197(5):602–8. https://doi.org/10.1111/bjh.18147.
107. Kuhlen M, Kunstreich M, Gökbuget N. Osteonecrosis in adults with acute lymphoblastic leukemia: an unmet clinical need. HemaSphere. 2021;5(4):e544. https://doi.org/10.1097/HS9.0000000000000544.
108. Levasseur R. Mechanisms of osteonecrosis. Joint Bone Spine. 2008;75(6):639–42. https://doi.org/10.1016/j.jbspin.2008.10.001.
109. Girard P, Auquier P, Barlogis V, et al. Symptomatic osteonecrosis in childhood leukemia survivors: prevalence, risk factors and impact on quality of life in adulthood. Haematologica. 2013;98(7):1089–97. https://doi.org/10.3324/haematol.2012.081265.
110. Dvorak CC, Gracia CR, Sanders JE, et al. NCI, NHLBI/PBMTC first international conference on late effects after pediatric hematopoietic cell transplantation: endocrine challenges—thyroid dysfunction, growth impairment, bone health, & reproductive risks. Biol Blood Marrow Transplant. 2011;17(12):1725–38. https://doi.org/10.1016/j.bbmt.2011.10.006.
111. Kuhlen M, Kunstreich M, Niinimäki R, et al. Guidance to bone morbidity in children and adolescents undergoing allogeneic hematopoietic stem cell transplantation. Biol Blood Marrow Transplant. 2020;26(2):e27–37. https://doi.org/10.1016/j.bbmt.2019.10.007.
112. Curtis RE, Rowlings PA, Deeg HJ, et al. Solid cancers after bone marrow transplantation. N Engl J Med. 1997;336(13):897–904. https://doi.org/10.1056/NEJM199703273361301.
113. Bhatia S, Ramsay NK, Steinbuch M, et al. Malignant neoplasms following bone marrow transplantation. Blood. 1996;87(9):3633–9. http://www.ncbi.nlm.nih.gov/pubmed/8611687.
114. Socié G, Curtis RE, Deeg HJ, et al. New malignant diseases after allogeneic marrow transplantation for childhood acute leukemia. J Clin Oncol. 2000;18(2):348. https://doi.org/10.1200/JCO.2000.18.2.348.
115. Martin A, Schneiderman J, Helenowski IB, et al. Secondary malignant neoplasms after high-dose chemotherapy and autologous stem cell rescue for high-risk neuroblastoma. Pediatr Blood Cancer. 2014;61(8):1350–6. https://doi.org/10.1002/pbc.25033.
116. Mulder RL, Kremer LCM, Hudson MM, et al. Recommendations for breast cancer surveillance for female survivors of childhood, adolescent, and young adult cancer given chest radiation: a report from the International Late Effects of Childhood Cancer Guideline Harmonization Group. Lancet Oncol. 2013;14(13):e621–9. https://doi.org/10.1016/S1470-2045(13)70303-6.
117. Wade MA, Sunter NJ, Fordham SE, et al. c-MYC is a radiosensitive locus in human breast cells. Oncogene. 2015;34(38):4985–94. https://doi.org/10.1038/onc.2014.427.
118. Albi E, Cataldi S, Lazzarini A, et al. Radiation and thyroid cancer. Int J Mol Sci. 2017;18(5):911. https://doi.org/10.3390/ijms18050911.
119. Cattoni A, Molinari S, Gaiero A, et al. Thyroid disorders following hematopoietic stem cell transplantation in childhood: impact of conditioning regimen on thyroid dysfunction, volume changes, and occurrence of nodules. Transplant Cell Ther. 2022;28(8):506.e1–506.e12. https://doi.org/10.1016/j.jtct.2022.05.040.
120. Hamatani K, Eguchi H, Ito R, et al. RET/PTC rearrangements preferentially occurred in papillary thyroid cancer among atomic bomb survivors exposed to high radiation dose. Cancer Res. 2008;68(17):7176–82. https://doi.org/10.1158/0008-5472.CAN-08-0293.
121. Hamatani K, Mukai M, Takahashi K, Hayashi Y, Nakachi K, Kusunoki Y. Rearranged anaplastic lymphoma kinase (ALK) gene in adult-onset papillary thyroid cancer amongst atomic bomb survivors. Thyroid. 2012;22(11):1153–9. https://doi.org/10.1089/thy.2011.0511.
122. Kolb HJ, Socié G, Duell T, et al. Malignant neoplasms in long-term survivors of bone marrow transplantation. Ann Intern Med. 1999;131(10):738–44. https://doi.org/10.7326/0003-4819-131-10-199911160-00004.
123. Hawkins MM, Wilson LMK, Burton HS, et al. Radiotherapy, alkylating agents, and risk of bone cancer after childhood cancer. JNCI J Natl Cancer Inst. 1996;88(5):270–8. https://doi.org/10.1093/jnci/88.5.270.
124. Au W-Y, Chan EC, Pang A, et al. Nonhematologic malignancies after allogeneic hematopoietic stem cell transplantation: incidence and molecular monitoring. Bone Marrow Transplant. 2004;34(11):981–5. https://doi.org/10.1038/sj.bmt.1704674.
125. Rashid N, Arora M, El JN, et al. Frailty in patients with chronic graft-versus-host disease. Transplant Cell Ther. 2023;29(6):367–74. https://doi.org/10.1016/j.jtct.2023.03.010.
126. Yu J, Khera N, Turnbull J, et al. Impact of chronic graft-versus-host disease on patient employment, income, and informal caregiver burden: findings from the living with chronic GVHD patient survey. Transplant Cell Ther. 2023;29(7):470.e1–9. https://doi.org/10.1016/j.jtct.2023.04.004.
127. Sadak KT, Szalda D, Lindgren BR, et al. Transitional care practices, services, and delivery in childhood cancer survivor programs: a survey study of U.S. survivorship providers. Pediatr Blood Cancer. 2019;66(8):e27793. https://doi.org/10.1002/pbc.27793.
128. Signorelli C, Wakefield CE, McLoone JK, et al. Models of childhood cancer survivorship care in Australia and New Zealand: strengths and challenges. Asia Pac J Clin Oncol. 2017;13(6):407–15. https://doi.org/10.1111/ajco.12700.

Part VIII

Perspectives and Future Directions

21 Access Determines Outcomes for People with Acute Lymphoblastic Leukemia in Low- and Middle-Income Countries

Raul C. Ribeiro and Scott C. Howard

21.1 Causes of Treatment Failure for Children with Acute Lymphoblastic Leukemia Differ Among Low- and Middle-, and High-Income Countries

Pediatric acute lymphoblastic leukemia (ALL) is highly curable when treated with intensive chemotherapy and adequate supportive care. Acute lymphoblastic leukemia is genetically heterogenous, and about 15% of cases are relatively resistant to conventional chemotherapy, requiring alternative approaches for cure, including immunotherapy or hematopoietic stem cell transplantation (SCT). Analyzing the initial clinical features and laboratory biological markers informs ALL risk of relapse and allows adapted therapy that maximizes treatment efficacy and minimizes toxicity. In institutions that can provide modern risk-adapted treatment approaches, the survival of children and adolescents with ALL exceeds 85% [1]. Of the therapeutic failures, half are due to resistant leukemia, and the other half due to treatment-related toxicities. However, survival rates for children with ALL (and all other cancers) are dramatically influenced by where the child is diagnosed and treated. Socioeconomic and cultural variables powerfully influence ALL mortality. For children diagnosed with ALL in many low- and middle-income countries (LMICs) treatment failure is much more frequent than that in high-income countries (HICs). Access to correct diagnosis, ongoing care without abandonment, supportive care to prevent toxic death, and high-quality medications with consistent availability are all needed to improve outcomes in LMICs until they rival those in HICs (Fig. 21.1) [2].

R. C. Ribeiro (✉)
Division of Leukemia/Lymphoma, Department of Oncology, St. Jude Children's Research Hospital, Memphis, TN, USA

Global Pediatric Medicine, St. Jude Children's Research Hospital, Memphis, TN, USA
e-mail: Raul.Ribeiro@StJude.org

S. C. Howard
Hospital Sant Joan de Deu Barcelona, Barcelona, Spain

Yerevan, Armenia

Resonance, Memphis, TN, USA
e-mail: Scott.Howard@ResonanceHealth.org

G. Escherich, V. Conter (eds.), *Acute Lymphoblastic Leukemia in Children and Adolescents*, Pediatric Oncology, https://doi.org/10.1007/978-3-031-71180-0_21

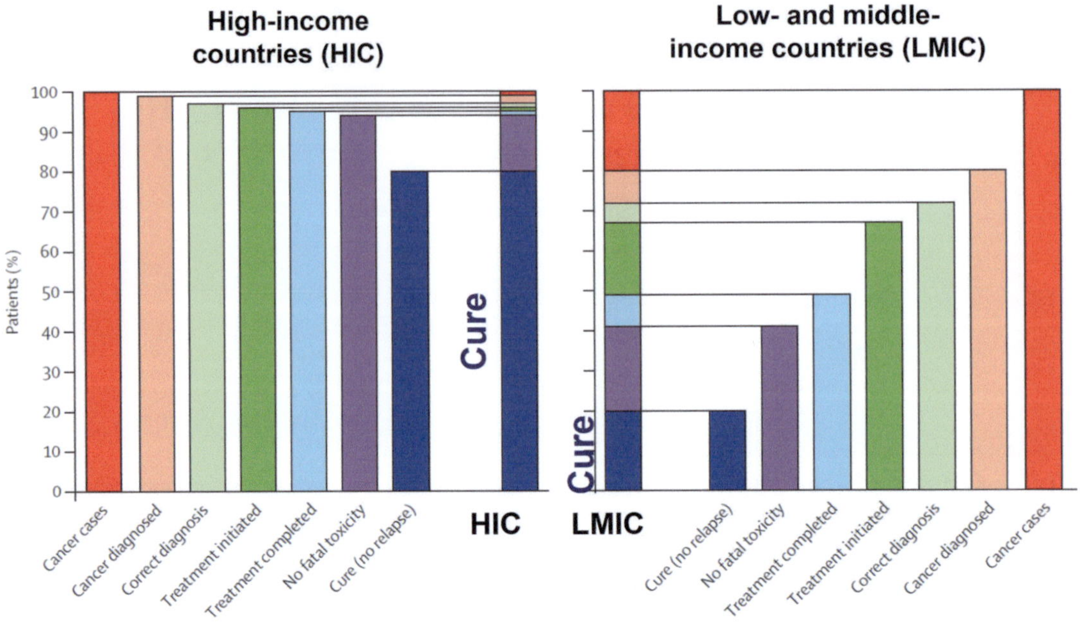

Fig. 21.1 Causes of treatment failure for children with cancer in low- and middle-income countries (LMICs) compared with those in high-income countries (HICs). (Figure used with permission of Scott C. Howard)

21.2 Access to Diagnosis

Lack of diagnosis is defined as death prior to confirmation that the patient has cancer. The diagnosis may be made at autopsy, or the results of a diagnostic evaluation may become available after the patient's death [3]. Examples include a patient succumbing to metabolic complications such as tumor lysis syndrome with acute kidney injury and hyperkalemic cardiac arrest while awaiting the results of pathology evaluation. Worldwide, lack of diagnosis is the most common cause of treatment failure in LMICs [4, 5]. Training of community health workers to recognize early signs and symptoms of childhood cancer, public awareness campaigns, and international twinning partnerships that pair institutions of HICs with those in LMICs have led to improved rates of diagnosis, especially when the efforts and collaborating partners have a long-term commitment and are sustained over time [6]. In addition to enhancing awareness in healthcare providers, it is crucial that once cancer diagnosis is suspected, the child is referred directly to cancer specialty centers to prevent delays in diagnosis and treatment. In some settings, patients must pay for diagnostics, such that clinicians and pathologists must prioritize which specific tests to perform. Patients in lower socioeconomic brackets are less likely to have medical insurance or sufficient funds to pay for healthcare, and costly out-of-pocket private expenditure for healthcare is common [7]. In such settings, basic subsistence needs such as shelter and food may take precedence over expenditure on healthcare, which in turn results in lack of diagnosis and its downstream consequences. Ideally, implementation of a universal healthcare coverage would allow better access to more affordable care, but in some cases, coverage does not extend to all diagnostics needed for people with leukemia. In the absence of universal health coverage, healthcare systems in resource-limited regions must develop strategies to prioritize best practices to fill the needs of cancer management in a cost-effective and timely manner and provide resource-allocation guidance (Fig. 21.2) [2, 6, 8, 9].

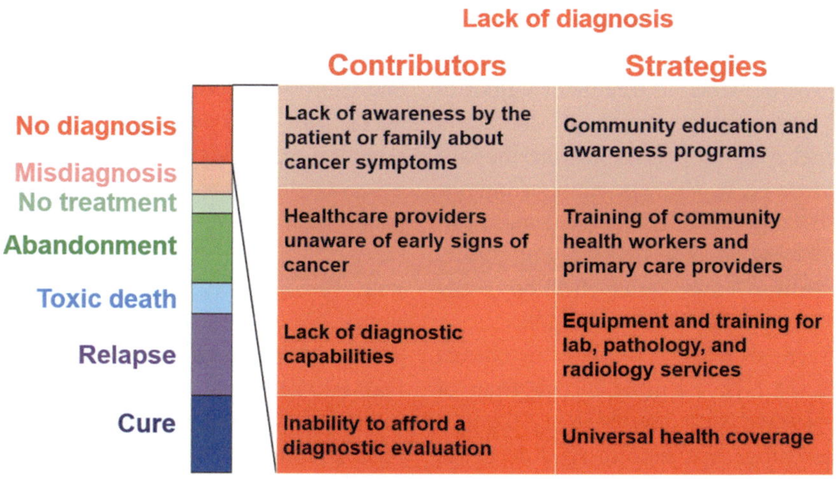

Fig. 21.2 Contributors to lack of diagnosis and strategies to address them. (Figure used with permission of Scott C. Howard)

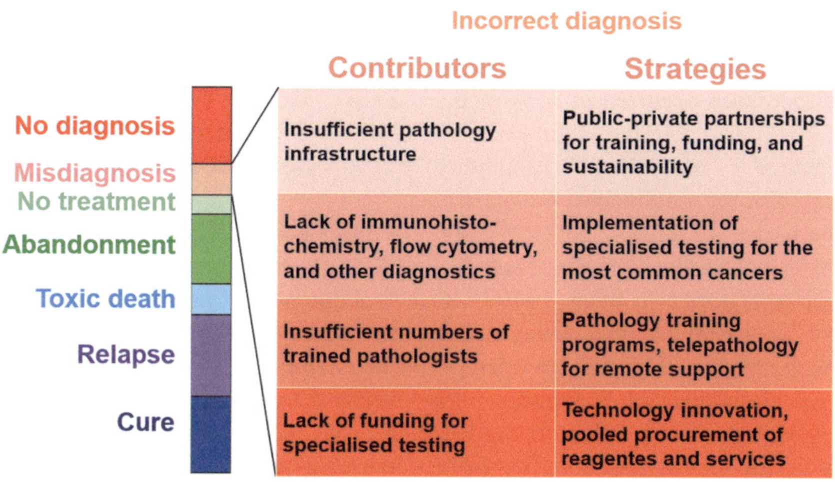

Fig. 21.3 Contributors to misdiagnosis and strategies to address them. (Figure used with permission of Scott C. Howard)

21.3 Access to Correct Diagnosis

Once a patient is suspected to have cancer, the next goal is to achieve a correct diagnosis (Fig. 21.3). Misdiagnosis has serious implications, leading to incorrect treatment plans which inevitably have minimal chance of cure. In countries with effective private healthcare systems, children whose family can afford medical insurance usually receive coverage for specialized testing, whereas funding restrictions often limit the state-funded or subsidized care available to less affluent families. Despite governmental and nongovernmental assistance, the indirect costs of treatment such as loss of income and providing for other family members also affect the ability of the family to pay for expensive diagnostic and staging investigations. An underfunded healthcare system and lack of insurance coverage contribute to misdiagnosis, but also to non-diagnosis, toxic death, abandonment, and relapse. Indeed, in one study that analyzed the major causes of preventable treatment failure in LMICs, the strongest predictor of childhood cancer survival was the per capita total healthcare expenditure [2, 6, 10]. The ideal of universal health coverage for all childhood conditions has been achieved in few LMICs, but efforts have been made to cover more children, especially those with the least resources [10].

Correct diagnosis must be followed by correct risk stratification. For example, a subgroup of ALL can be treated with low-intensity therapy, whereas other subgroups require specific drugs or procedures not available in many LMIC centers [11]. Creating the capacity for the correct diagnosis of pediatric malignancies has been one of the most challenging barriers to overcome. In a report from St. Jude of 705 cases submitted for review by pathologists from LMICs, clinically significant discordance occurred in 25% of the cases [12]. The most common limitations in LMICs include inadequate laboratory infrastructure, lack of equipment, suboptimal quality of the tumor specimens and processing, high cost of reagents, and lack of trained pathologists. Clinical laboratories in many LMIC settings cannot characterize the many ALL subgroups with diverse responses to therapy. Attempting to ship bone marrow samples from one Central American country to St. Jude for leukemia characterization was unsuccessful. Bone marrow samples retained in customs, poor quality of the material on arrival, misplacement of the samples after arrival, and incorrect identification of the samples were some of the difficulties. In contrast, working collaboratively with a local pathologist in Guatemala to perform the diagnosis and classification of ALL for countries in the region of Central America was encouraging. Online interactions between the laboratory in Guatemala and St. Jude provided quality control and further training [13, 14]. In the long term, the Guatemalan laboratory became a training place for individuals from El Salvador and Honduras, resulting in flow cytometric diagnostic capabilities being implemented in these two countries, including measurement of residual disease [13, 14]. The same strategy was used successfully in Recife, Brazil and Cairo, Egypt. Studies in Recife and Cairo revealed that children with progenitor ALL, from 1 to 9 years old, with white blood cell count less than 50×10^9/L, and measurable disease <0.01% after 2 weeks (day 19) of prednisone, vincristine, daunomycin, and L-asparaginase (about 25% of ALL cases), have >90% cure rate with low-intensity therapy [15–17]. An additional 25% of ALL children can be cured with a modest increase of the therapy intensity when Day 19 MRD is <1.0% and negative at the end of induction. Thus, institutions treating pediatric ALL should provide guidelines for the diagnosis of leukemia and be able to have routine blood counts, bone marrow evaluation morphology, and flow cytometry for classification and measurement of residual disease.

21.4 Access to Completion of Treatment Without Abandonment

A third common cause of treatment failure in LMICs is treatment abandonment [18]. Abandonment of treatment is defined as the failure to start or complete medically indicated curative therapy [19, 20]. Missing 4 consecutive weeks of treatment and follow-up while on therapy for cancer is considered abandonment, while in its most extreme form, "refusal" occurs when a patient with cancer does not begin treatment. Risk factors for abandonment include low socioeconomic status, low parental education, and long travel time to the center, and a rarely caused by parental choice [20]. Families are often unable to pay for treatment, cannot forgo income-producing work while taking treatment, live far from the treating center, and may have multiple other factors impacting their ability to continue treatment (Fig. 21.4).

When a parent has to choose between providing for the family or caring for the child with cancer, often the choice is to provide for the family [21]. Efforts to ameliorate financial and logistical barriers have proven effective in reducing the rate of treatment abandonment by fivefold in some

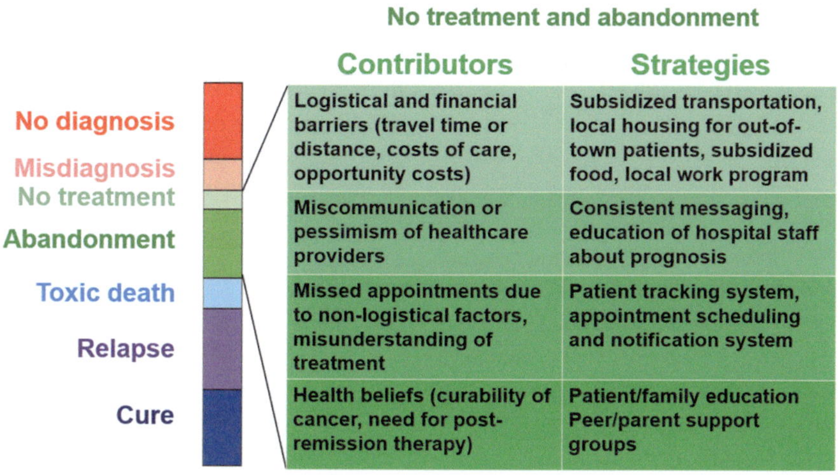

Fig. 21.4 Contributors to abandonment of treatment and strategies to address them. (Figure used with permission of Scott C. Howard)

cases. When cost-free care, subsidized transportation, and free food and local housing were provided to families, abandonment rates were reported to decrease significantly in several LMIC communities [22, 23]. Positive messaging by healthcare providers is also important to make sure that patients and parents understand that their cancer can be cured, and that short-term suffering and costs will be justified by the long-term survival of the child [24].

Less well-defined non-adherence to treatment such as missing appointments or medication doses, may reduce the effectiveness of therapy and increase the risk of abandoning therapy. Patients and parents may misunderstand instructions about repeat visits due to poor health literacy or language barriers and may not trust the medical team. In HICs, the multidisciplinary team includes psychosocial support staff comprised of psychologists and social workers, whose services include not only psychological counseling, but also provision of detailed explanation of treatment protocols and troubleshooting of logistical hurdles, thus acting as a bridge between the patient and medical staff. The addition of psychosocial services may be a feasible starting point to address treatment abandonment in LMICs. At a pediatric oncology unit in Guatemala, a psychosocial services team was created to address abandonment, and after identifying the most at-risk families, the team worked with the families from diagnosis to completion of therapy to address their needs for transportation, financial, nutritional, and psychosocial support. They also implemented a tracking system to detect missed appointments. These combined efforts resulted in a decrease in treatment abandonment from 27% in 2001 to 7% in 2008 [25]. Similar strategies were implemented with increased focus on patient tracking in India and El Salvador, which resulted in significant reduction of treatment abandonment rates in both cohorts [21, 23]. Belief in the incurability of cancer, poor communication, concern about painful or risky procedures, and seeing the death or morbidity of other patients can all contribute to abandonment [19, 25]. Psychosocial services provided by staff of the same culture may help to abate the fear of treatment caused by insufficient understanding of cancer care protocols by the family [26]. Preference for complementary and alternative medicine, and concerns about treatment adverse effects and toxicity also play an important role in not only LMICs but HICs as well [18]. Health systems increasingly recognize that patients need support for non-medical aspects of cancer care, including funding for travel and housing when away from home, but have been slow to include such support in benefits packages [27].

21.5 Access to Supportive Care to Prevent Toxic Death (Treatment-Related Mortality)

Like non-diagnosis, misdiagnosis, and abandonment of treatment, toxic death is another important cause of treatment failure in LMICs, where it occurs far more often than in HICs [3].

Toxic death includes "treatment-related mortality" (TRM) caused by side effects of treatment plus early death which can result from the cancer itself (e.g., tumor lysis syndrome, central airway compression syndrome). Since the cause of early deaths and induction deaths may be difficult to distinguish, the concept of "toxic death" (from any and all causes) is helpful since it serves as a marker of the quality of supportive care. High-intensity treatment is necessary to cure high-risk ALL but requires meticulous supportive care to be delivered safely. Applying the same treatment regimens in LMIC settings may result in toxic death [28]. In HICs, 1–2% of children with ALL die from toxicity of therapy, compared with up to 20% in LMICs if the treatment regimen is not adapted to the local capabilities (Fig. 21.5).

21.5.1 Toxic Death from Infection

Reduction of toxic death requires an established PCU, which becomes a central place for patient care, training, and education for physicians, nurses, students, trainees, and families. Nurses trained in pediatric oncology and dedicated to the PCU are essential. The PCU is also a convergence space for interdisciplinary activities addressing the most common problems associated with poor outcomes in LMICs. Decreasing treatment-related mortality is the primary goal in children with leukemia in LMICs. In some centers, it can be as high as 30%, particularly in the first few weeks after diagnosis. Most deaths are related to infectious or hemorrhagic events and could be avoided with anticipation and planning. It is critical that each institution carefully review all cases of treatment-related deaths to identify areas for improvement, and free tools are available to support continuous quality improvement efforts (Patients.ResonanceHealth.org, project--redcap.org, https://stg-global.stjude.org/en-us/tools/sj-cares-tools/aria-guide.html).

In 2015, a Colorado Children's Hospital study revealed that neutropenic patients who received antibiotics within 1 h from the fever onset had a

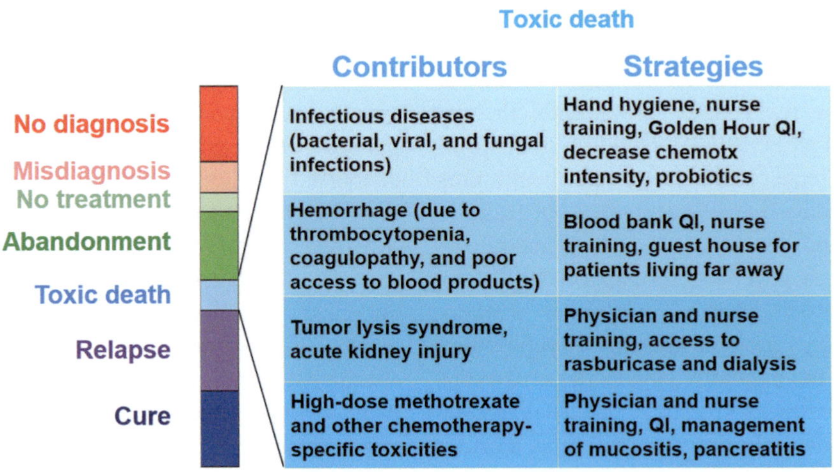

Fig. 21.5 Contributors to toxic death and strategies to prevent it. (Figure used with permission of Scott C. Howard)

mortality rate of 0.7% compared with 3.9% of those who received antibiotics beyond 1 h (the golden hour) [29]. Factors associated with a prolonged time between fever and administration of antibiotics (fever-to-needle) vary from institution to institution and require a careful understanding of the entire process of care for cancer patients with new onset of fever. For example, when arriving at the emergency room, neutropenic patients may not receive urgent attention and venous access, results of laboratory tests may be delayed, preparation and administration of antibiotics can take too long, and transfer of the patient to the hospital ward may take several hours in the best case and much longer when bed shortages occur. Several studies demonstrated the impact of implementing guidelines for managing neutropenic patients to reduce the fever-to-antibiotic time [30].

Because infection in an immunocompromised host can evolve rapidly to shock, the availability of an intensive care unit (ICU) is critical. In many pediatric hospitals in LMICs, the pediatric ICU is overcrowded and understaffed, and children with leukemia are not considered a priority for admission to the ICU. Moreover, the ICU of a public pediatric hospital might not be adequate for immunosuppressed patients. Integrating an ICU into the PCU significantly decreases the mortality of children with leukemia, especially in institutions that perform bone marrow transplantation. It is estimated that 40% of patients with cancer are admitted to the ICU at least once during their anticancer treatment. Another advantage is having an experienced intensive care physician at night to assess patients who develop complications during that period. Other invaluable services needed in the PCU include surgery, nutrition, psychology, social work, and the blood bank. Treatment-related mortality and abandonment decrease when these disciplines are integrated. Finally, central line-associated bloodstream infections can cause severe infection in children treated for cancer and are more likely to occur if there are breaches in aseptic technique during insertion and use, so in some settings it may be safer to use peripheral intravenous access and avoid indwelling cathers [31].

21.5.2 Toxic Death Reduction by Protocol Modification and Management of Chemotherapy Toxicity

Low-risk and "special-risk" ALL can be cured with a three-drug induction followed by a two-drug maintenance with delayed intensification blocks and intrathecal therapy for central nervous system control. Higher-risk ALL requires dose-intensive chemotherapy regimens that should be given in a specialized PCUs with infection prevention measures, antimicrobials, blood products, and intensive care services. Strategies to decrease deaths due to sepsis include the measures mentioned before, but also adapting treatment regimens with decreased chemotherapy intensity [28]. Mucositis from anthracyclines and methotrexate, acute pancreatitis from asparaginase, and other drug-specific toxicities can predispose patients to infections, delay delivery of chemotherapy, and thus increase the risk of both toxic death and relapse [32]. Centers that cannot perform therapeutic drug monitoring may experience higher rates of methotrexate toxicity, leading to sloughing of the mucosa and skin, with subsequent life-threatening sepsis. Alternatively, these centers may elect not to treat patients with high-dose chemotherapy, limiting the ability to cure high-risk disease. Thus, adapting treatment regimens that can be implemented to the local healthcare environment for optimal outcomes is obligatory [28]. Strategies include using lower dosage of chemotherapeutic agents, such as the use of reduced doses of high-dose methotrexate to minimize toxicity and improve long-term outcomes in LIMCs [28].

21.5.3 Toxic Death from Malnutrition

Malnutrition is more common in LMICs, and is associated with higher rates of sepsis and chemotherapy toxicity, with hypoalbuminemia leading to higher concentrations of free (unbound) chemotherapy agents, greater toxicity and prolonged myelosuppression [33, 34]. Malnutrition is also associated with treatment abandonment [35]. Aggressive nutritional support may be given while patients receive a lower dose or less toxic chemotherapy, which can then be followed by more dose-intensive chemotherapy. Nutritional support programs have proven feasible and effective in LMICs [35, 36].

21.5.4 Toxic Death from Bleeding and Renal Complications

Most children with ALL require blood product support during therapy, especially during induction. Hemorrhage due to thrombocytopenia, coagulopathy and limited access to blood products may be fatal. Therefore, the blood bank must not only provide safe blood products, but also have the capacity to rapidly respond to emergencies, especially coagulopathy or thrombocytopenia with life-threatening hemorrhage. Tumor lysis syndrome with acute kidney injury can cause early toxic death, but also can lead to renal dysfunction that interferes with the ability to deliver subsequent therapies like high-dose methotrexate, which can thus increase relapse risk [37, 38]. Death from tumor lysis syndrome is rare, especially when hyperkalemia is prevented, but long-term renal dysfunction can be problematic. Nephrotoxic antibiotics like vancomycin can make things worse but may be required to treat certain infections [39].

21.6 Access to High-Quality Chemotherapy and Adapted Treatment Regimens to Prevent Relapse

Excess, or preventable, relapse is the additional rate of relapse above the expected rate of relapse in a HIC with the best health system and cancer care program [40, 41]. For example, in well-resourced tertiary care centers, the cure rate of ALL may be 90%. Of the 10% who are not cured, 8% of treatment failure is caused by relapse and 2% by toxic death and other causes. If a pediatric cancer program documents a relapse rate higher than 8% for ALL, then any amount greater than 8% is considered avoidable relapse. For example, if patients have a relapse rate of 38%, then the avoidable relapse rate is 30% (38% observed relapse rate minus 8% unavoidable relapse rate). This concept is useful when working to improve cure rates in LMICs, since working to achieve a relapse risk lower than that achieved in HICs would be neither achievable, nor sustainable, nor cost-effective. Therefore, having a disease-specific standard for "unavoidable" (as of 2022) relapse serves as a gold-standard for which to strive in LMICs. A similar standard could be established for non-diagnosis, misdiagnosis, abandonment, and toxic death, but the rates of these problems in HICs are typically 0–2%, so striving for 0% is realistic and disease-specific performance metrics need not be established. As cancer treatment improves and new therapies become standard, the rate of unavoidable relapse inevitably decreases, so the calculation of avoidable relapse requires periodic updates in the rates of expected (unavoidable) relapse for each cancer. Regardless of the rate, the contributing causes and sub-causes have been well documented, and strategies exist to prevent unavoidable relapse (Fig. 21.6). Increased intensity chemotherapy has contributed to improved child-

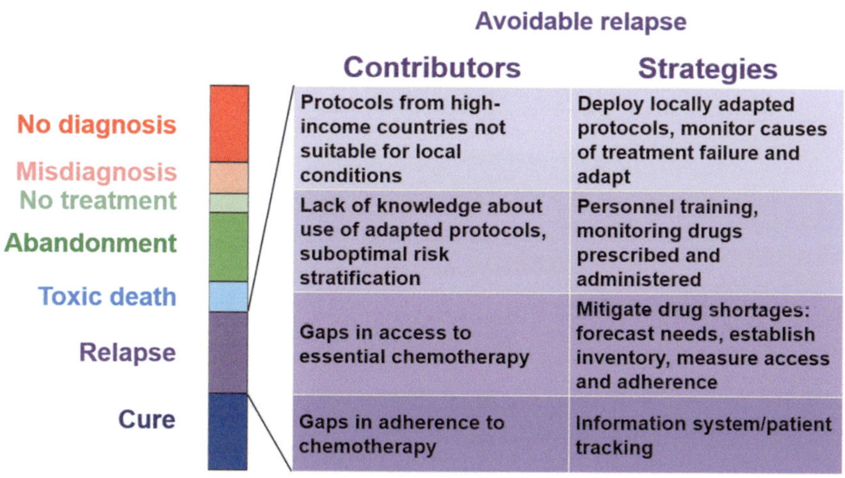

Fig. 21.6 Contributors to avoidable relapse and prevention strategies

hood ALL survival for high-risk patients but may have the opposite effect in LMICs, if toxic death increases more than relapse decreases [40].

21.7 Access to Effective Chemotherapy to Prevent Excess Relapse

Another reason for excess relapse in LMICs is that higher proportion of patients of African and Native American origin, who have higher rates of biologically high-risk ALL subtypes that require more intensive treatment regimens and excellent supportive care, thus representing double jeopardy for these patients, who have more high-risk disease and who are treated in healthcare systems with far fewer resources [2].

21.8 Access to Research: Practical Application of Proven Strategies and Aggressive Drug Discovery and Access Programs That Benefit Children in Both LMICs and HICs

The difference in incidence patterns of pediatric cancer across continents has attracted the attention of the academic community in high-income countries (HICs) because of the research opportunities. However, these initiatives did not intend to address the cancer mortality disparity among LMICs. Although there was the potential to advance knowledge on the basic mechanisms of cancer, they would not improve the survival of children with cancer in those countries that provided the tumor samples and clinical data for correlative analysis. For example, after more than 65 years of the discovery of childhood Burkitt lymphoma in Africa, resulting in information on its sensitivity to cyclophosphamide and the discovery of the Epstein–Barr virus, the outcome of pediatric Burkitt lymphoma in Africa remains dramatically lower than that in HICs [42]. Recent data analysis from 258 cancer registries of 61 countries (CONCORD-3, 2010 and 2014) showed the net survival of children with ALL treated in LMICs has improved some, but continues to be much lower than in HICs, especially among patients 15–19 years of age (Fig. 21.7) [43]. The likely explanation for the improvement in the survival of children with ALL in these countries can be traced back to the consistent efforts of individual pediatric oncologists who raised awareness among the pediatric oncology community of the immense mortality gap between rich and poor regions of the world and the possibility of addressing this disparity [5–9]. These independent observations suggested that humanitarian assistance would be necessary to address the survival inequalities between the rich and poor regions.

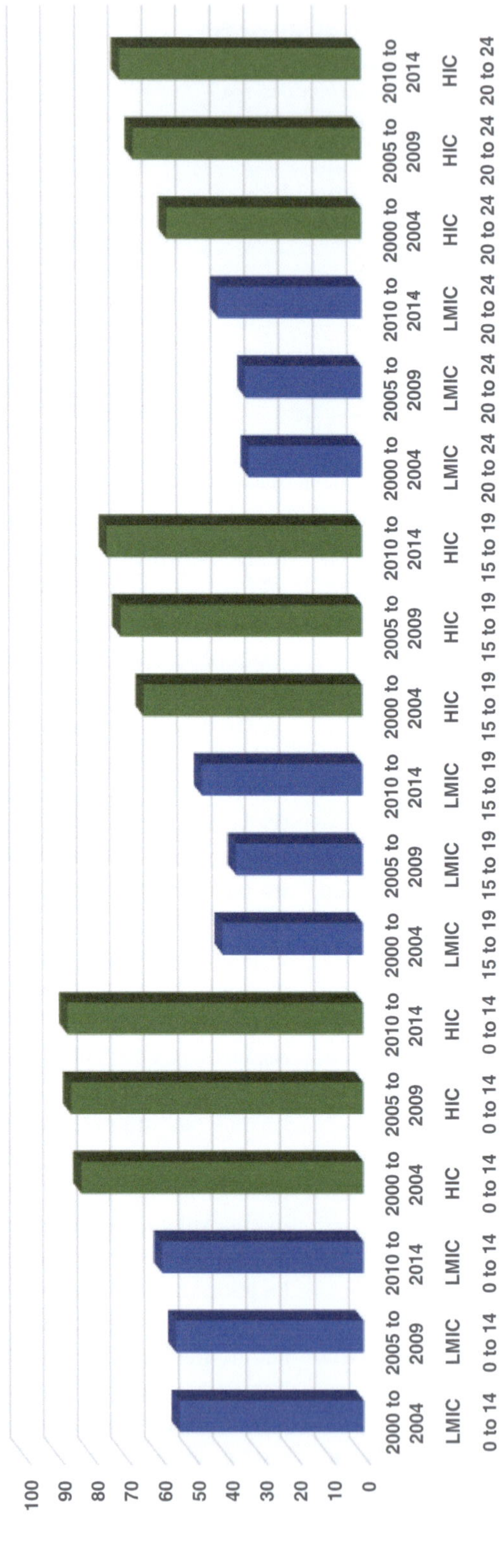

Fig. 21.7 5-Year net survival (%) for all leukemias combined, in patients aged 0–24 years diagnosed during 2000–2014, according to World Bank income group and calendar period of diagnosis (https://www.thelancet.com/pdfs/journals/lanchi/PIIS2352-4642(22)00095-5.pdf). Changes in outcomes for children, adolescents, and young adults with acute leukemia in low- and middle-, and high-income countries

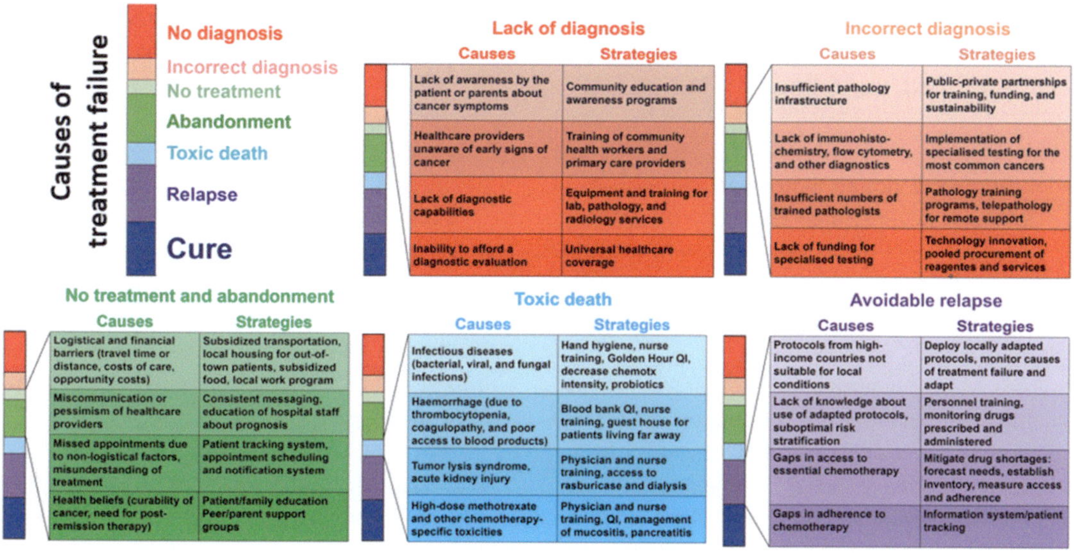

Fig. 21.8 Each cause of treatment failure for children with cancer in low- and middle-income countries can be addressed using proven, published strategies. (Used with permission of Scott C. Howard, MD)

However, contrary to the short-term humanitarian aid to relieve suffering during emergencies, it has been proposed that improving survival for children with cancer in LMICs would require a long-term commitment from the parties involved. Small capacity-building projects demonstrated the feasibility of treating pediatric Burkitt lymphoma [10] and acute lymphoblastic leukemia [11] in Africa and India, respectively. The demonstration that the lives of children with cancer could be saved or prolonged, suffering reduced, families treated with dignity, and local health care providers trained and empowered with relatively small investments provided a compelling rationale for international organizations to include the mortality gap of pediatric cancer in their programmatic agenda resulting in the creation of international and local nongovernmental organizations to share knowledge and resources with LMICs. Locally, it spearheaded initiatives among healthcare providers, including young physicians and nurses, hospital administrators, community groups, and governments, to create conditions to adequately treat children with cancer. To maintain this momentum, research efforts in LMICs should focus increasingly on practical strategies to improve outcomes and reduce known causes of excess treatment failure (Fig. 21.8).

In the early 1980s, multiple bilateral pediatric oncology projects emerged, usually between individuals from countries with historical ties, for example, France and French-speaking African countries [12], South Africa with English-speaking African countries [5], the Netherlands with Indonesia [13], and the National Cancer Institute (United States) with India [11] and English-speaking African countries [10]. The Society of Pediatric Oncology (SIOP) provided support for physicians and nurses from LMICs to attend the annual meeting and a forum for the discussion on topics related to pediatric oncology in limited-resource countries, lead the development of strategies to address specific barriers of institutions in the LMIC. After 20 years, it became clear that pediatric oncology care in LMICs could be improved through partnerships between individuals and institutions in HICs directly with institutions and pediatric oncologists in LMICs.

21.9 The Birth of "AMOR"

In 1986, an initiative between individuals in institutions in Italy and Switzerland with those in a pediatric hospital, "La Mascota" in Nicaragua, provided the conceptual basis for pediatric oncology partnerships between HICs and LMICs, which included the following core principles [14]:

- Multiple individuals from each partner pediatric oncology unit engaged and involved.
- Autonomy and self-determination of the partners in LMICs, including progressive transfer of management responsibilities to local professionals.
- Long-term planning and long-term partnership with periodic reassessments and adjustments of strategies and needs. Many partnerships have lasted 5–25 years.
- Disease-orientated approach that includes training, supply of essential resources, and strengthening of structural facilities to manage each specific cancer plus the associated supportive care issues.
- Adoption of protocols and guidelines adapted for the local situation.
- Financial support from diverse sources to foster independence, flexibility, and sustainability.
- Involvement of community and parent representatives to allow adequate identification of needs and priorities and to harness local resources for psychosocial support, non-medical support (food, housing, transportation) and other needs of families going through childhood cancer care.
- Transparency of project activities with periodic reporting to supporting groups and stakeholders, including government.
- Establishment of research and quality improvement capacity to solve specific local problems that lead to treatment failure. This strategy was summarized by Raul Ribeiro as "helping people become chefs in their own kitchen, not simply providing a recipe book".
  - Adapting cancer treatment protocols to local conditions.
  - Multinational collaborative studies to identify universal strategies to address specific issues in LMICs, like abandonment of treatment and excess relapse.
  - Involvement of multiple partners that specialize in the development of various aspects of pediatric hematology–oncology (e.g., academic institutions, professional societies, nongovernmental organizations, research networks, and guideline development groups).
  - Deployment of information systems to support ongoing analysis, efficacy assessment, and cost-effectiveness assessments.
- Promotion (through publications and ad hoc initiatives) of the wider adoption of the twinning strategy by leading groups.

The term "twinning program" was proposed for the initiative. Historically, a twinning program was defined as a formal and substantive collaboration between two cities in different countries. It was encouraged by the European community following the second world war to improve international relations and reconciliation. More recently, twinning has been defined as a cross-cultural, reciprocal process where two groups work together to achieve joint goals. The World Health Organization (WHO) has used this strategy to reach sustainable development goals. In 1994, St. Jude Children's Research Hospital (St. Jude) partnered with Hospital Benjamin Bloom in El Salvador in response to a request of a Salvadoran mother whose son had died of leukemia at St. Jude. She had created an NGO (Ayúdame a Vivir, https://ayudameavivir.org) in San Salvador to support childhood cancer treatment and raised funds for 2 years before seeking technical and financial assistance from St. Jude. After 3 years of partnership between St. Jude, Ayúdame a Vivir and Hospital Benjamin Bloom, the survival rate of children with acute lymphoblastic leukemia (ALL) had risen from virtually zero to 50%. This experience provided the rationale for creating the St. Jude International Outreach Program (IOP) and established principles for the collaboration (Table 1) [44].

In 1996, investigators from the Pediatric Clinic in Monza (University of Milan-Bicocca) created the Monza International School of Pediatric Hematology Oncology (MISPHO) [15]. The main

Table 21.1 Principles for international oncology collaboration and twinning programs

Elements	Components	Content	Barriers
Commitment by high-income country (HIC) partners	1. Pediatric hemato-oncologists in HICs willing and able to devote time and effort to the program 2. Institutional commitment	A committed leader must define, develop, initiate, implement, and maintain the program. The leader facilitates intra- and inter-institutional communication and engages the hospital to mobilize resources (human, technical, and financial)	The lack of leadership in HICs makes a twinning program unlikely to succeed
Commitment by low- or middle-income (LMIC) partners	1. Pediatric hemato-oncologist leaders in LMICs willing and able to devote time and effort to the program 2. Institutional commitment	A committed leader is necessary to collaborate with the leader in the HICs. The main objectives is to facilitate intra- and inter-institutional communication and engage the hospital and community to mobilize resources (human, technical, and financial)	The lack of leadership in LMICs makes a twinning program unlikely to succeed
Community advocacy and fundraising in LMICs	1. Nonprofit, nongovernmental foundation focused on supporting childhood cancer care	Members of the supporting foundation should include influential members of society, professionals, and parents/relatives of patients	If foundations develop programs for multiple diseases, their message may be diluted, and their ability to raise money and advocate for pediatric cancer diminished
	2. Collaboration with the government to develop a pediatric oncology plan	The foundation works with both government and the medical team to effect change The credibility of foundations is established yearly by independent auditing agencies	
Collaborative principles	1. Respect 2. Trust 3. Humility 4.Collegiality	The partnership must be a culturally sensitive relationship of equals willing to learn from one another. In the best scenario, the association is beneficial and enjoyable on both sides	Focusing on individual accomplishments is less helpful than focusing on the shared mission to cure patients with cancer
Communication	1. Effective	1. Rapid, honest, in the same language	Absent or dishonest communication makes partnership programs impossible
	2. Transparent	2. Addresses programmatic aspects (contracts, financial matters, documentation of activities), patient care (individual cases, supportive care, protocols), continuing education, and hospital infrastructure	
	3. Comprehensive 4. Multimodal	3. E-mail, online meetings, phone conversations, exchange visits of key personnel	
Core activities	1. Based on the needs identified in the LIMC and the capacity of the HIC to address the needs	1. Goals and specific activities must be very well defined and codified in writing. Plans may change over time by mutual agreement	Improvements in cancer diagnosis, infection control, adapted treatment guidelines, education, nursing training, and outcome evaluation
	2. Data collection and analysis must be included	2. Documentation of causes of treatment failure and death is essential to target interventions and measure progress	

(continued)

Table 21.1 (continued)

Elements	Components	Content	Barriers
Capital and operational budget	1. The HIC should seek funding to initiate and maintain the partnership for at least 5 years 2. Increasing local fundraising capacity should be part of the programs 3. Ultimately, an alliance with the government is necessary for sustainability	Funding is needed to support key salaries in the LMIC center (medical director, nurse educator, data manager), to provide some equipment and supplies, and to pay for exchange visits. Expenditures should be tied explicitly to desired outcomes, focusing on developing leaders and implementing simple, effective methods to improve cure rates	Advanced technology or bench research expenditures should be deferred until cancer care is excellent, unless they can be developed using alternative sources of funding that bring additional sustainability and interest to the program
Continuity	A long-term relationship is essential because the goal is to develop an autonomous program	At least a 5-year plan should be developed at the very beginning so that both partners can agree on the partnership's goals and the timing of the included activities	Short-term projects have some value, but a long-term relationship is necessary to realize the full benefits of partnership

Used with permission of Scott C. Howard

goals included educating and training nurses, nutritionists, psychologists, and physicians to provide adequate care for children with cancer in LMICs (Table 1). In 1997, pediatric oncologists in six countries of Central America created an organization named the Central America Association of Pediatric Hematology Oncology (AHOPCA) to promote collaborative initiatives [16], including standard treatment guidelines for the region. Pathologists, surgeons, nurses, and psychosociologists participate in an annual meeting. This multipronged collaborative approach, including two institutions in HICs (St. Jude and the University of Milan) and multiple Latin American institutions, was named AMOR, an acronym for the participants involved (AHOPCA, MISPHO, OutReach of St. Jude). It focuses on initiatives to decrease the mortality from cancer in children in Latin America (Panel 2).

21.10 Critical Pillars to Reduce Treatment Failure

21.10.1 Pediatric Cancer Units

There is strong evidence that pediatric cancer units (PCU) should be established in pediatric hospitals or cancer centers treating children with cancer. Early reports noted that the outcome of children treated for leukemia was significantly better in those treated in pediatric cancer centers, despite use of the same protocol [17]. In 1986, the American Academy of Pediatrics published guidelines for pediatric cancer centers, which have been updated in 1997, 2004, and 2014 [18]. The last report, a policy statement on the standards for PCUs in the United States, specified the need for trained personnel and essential capabilities to provide adequate oncology care to children with cancer and required that the care of the child or adolescent with cancer should be directed by a pediatric hematologist/oncologist who is board certified in this subspecialty. Until the early 2000s, the concept of a separate unit for the care of children with cancer and trained pediatric oncologists to lead the program was not contemplated by most public pediatric hospitals in LMICs.

21.10.2 Trained Pediatric Hematologist-Oncologists

In some LMICs, the pediatric workforce to assist children with cancer is limited or nonexistent. In a recent survey, only nine of 48 African countries offered all three treatment modalities needed for pediatric cancer treatment. Seven of 48 countries did not have pediatric oncology services (surgery, chemotherapy, and radiotherapy), and several countries had no pediatric hematologist-oncologist [19]. In establishing bilateral HIC–LMIC collaborative projects, the first step is identifying individuals willing to be trained in pediatric hematology-oncology, then fully supporting them during training and afterward. The second step is to persuade the public hospital administration to provide facilities and personnel (especially nurses) to implement the program. This may be difficult since creation of a PCU requires consistent financial support and rarely generates net revenue in public hospitals. The concept of having dedicated personnel, including physicians and nurses exclusively dedicated to pediatric oncology, may be met with opposition because of the scarcity of the health workforce in pediatric hospitals and shortages in all subspecialty areas.

21.10.3 Nongovernmental Organizations

Overcoming this significant barrier becomes more feasible when nongovernmental economic resources are available and the pediatric cancer program does not have to compete with other pediatric subspecialties for the meager government budget. Demonstration projects in Managua, San Salvador, Tegucigalpa, Guatemala City, Recife, Campinas, Sao Paulo, and Barretos demonstrated the essential role of nongovernmental foundations that provide financial resources for training of the workforce, supplying anticancer medications and maintaining a dedicated PCU. In addition, these organizations provide financial support to families, care for them during treatment, and develop community projects for public education of early recognition and referral of children with cancer. The project in Guatemala is a notable example of how a nongovernmental entity (https://unop.org.gt/), in collaboration with the government, agreed to an annual budget and 5-year plans for the national Guatemalan PCU. Importantly, medical treatment is free for all children and adolescents in the country [45].

21.11 Conclusion

To improve outcomes, each cause of preventable treatment failure must be systematically identified and addressed using proven, cost-effective strategies that have documented benefits in both LMICs and HICs (Fig. 21.8). Each strategy requires sustained local research and quality improvement efforts in the context of an established pediatric cancer unit that is networked with regional and global collaborators who can support research, provide education, and deploy enabling technologies.

References

1. Biondi A, Conter V, Chandy M, et al. Precursor B-cell acute lymphoblastic leukaemia-a global view. Br J Haematol. 2022;196(3):530–47. https://doi.org/10.1111/bjh.17959.
2. Howard SC, Zaidi A, Cao X, et al. The My Child Matters programme: effect of public-private partnerships on paediatric cancer care in low-income and middle-income countries. Lancet Oncol. 2018;19(5):e252–66. https://doi.org/10.1016/S1470-2045(18)30123-2.
3. Lam CG, Howard SC, Bouffet E, Pritchard-Jones K. Science and health for all children with cancer. Science. 2019;363(6432):1182–6. https://doi.org/10.1126/science.aaw4892.
4. Howard SC, Metzger ML, Wilimas JA, Quintana Y, Pui CH, Robison LL, Ribeiro RC. Childhood cancer epidemiology in low-income countries. Cancer. 2008;112(3):461–74.
5. Parkin DM. The global burden of cancer. Semin Cancer Biol. 1998;8(4):219–35. https://doi.org/10.1006/scbi.1998.0080.
6. Ribeiro RC, Steliarova-Foucher E, Magrath I, et al. Baseline status of paediatric oncology care in ten low-income or mid-income countries receiving My Child Matters support: a descriptive study. Lancet Oncol. 2008;9(8):721–9. https://doi.org/10.1016/S1470-2045(08)70194-3.
7. Gelband H, Jha P, Sankaranarayanan R, Horton S. Cancer. Disease control priorities. Washington, DC: World Bank; 2015.
8. Al-Sukhun S, de Lima Lopes G Jr, Gospodarowicz M, Ginsburg O, Yu PP. Global Health Initiatives of the International Oncology Community. 2017 ASCO educational book. Alexandria: American Society of Clinical Oncology; 2017. p. 395–402.
9. Al LZ. Improving cancer care for children in the developing world: challenges and strategies. Curr Pediatr Rev. 2017;13(1):13–23. https://doi.org/10.2174/1573396312666161230145417.

10. Ribeiro RC. Impact of the Mexican government's system of social protection for health, or Seguro Popular, on pediatric oncology outcomes. Pediatr Blood Cancer. 2013;60(2):171–2. https://doi.org/10.1002/pbc.24355.
11. Lee SHR, Yang W, Gocho Y, et al. Pharmacotypes across the genomic landscape of pediatric acute lymphoblastic leukemia and impact on treatment response. Nat Med. 2023;29(1):170–9. https://doi.org/10.1038/s41591-022-02112-7.
12. Santiago TC, Jenkins JJ, Pedrosa F, Billups C, Quintana Y, Ribeiro RC, Qaddoumi I. Improving the histopathologic diagnosis of pediatric malignancies in a low-resource setting by combining focused training and telepathology strategies. Pediatr Blood Cancer. 2012;59(2):221–5. https://doi.org/10.1002/pbc.24071.
13. Howard SC, Campana D, Coustan-Smith E, et al. Development of a regional flow cytometry center for diagnosis of childhood leukemia in Central America. Leukemia. 2005;19(3):323–5. https://doi.org/10.1038/sj.leu.2403624.
14. Lorenzana R, Coustan-Smith E, Antillon F, Ribeiro RC, Campana D. Simple methods for the rapid exchange of flow cytometric data between remote centers. Leukemia. 2000;14(2):336–7. https://doi.org/10.1038/sj.leu.2401612.
15. Sidhom I, Shaaban K, Youssef SH, et al. Reduced-intensity therapy for pediatric lymphoblastic leukemia: impact of residual disease early in remission induction. Blood. 2021;137(1):20–8. https://doi.org/10.1182/blood.2020007977.
16. Li XY, Li JQ, Luo XQ, et al. Reduced intensity of early intensification does not increase the risk of relapse in children with standard risk acute lymphoblastic leukemia - a multi-centric clinical study of GD-2008-ALL protocol. BMC Cancer. 2021;21(1):59. https://doi.org/10.1186/s12885-020-07752-x.
17. Pedrosa F, Coustan-Smith E, Zhou Y, et al. Reduced-dose intensity therapy for pediatric lymphoblastic leukemia: long-term results of the Recife RELLA05 pilot study. Blood. 2020;135(17):1458–66. https://doi.org/10.1182/blood.2019004215.
18. Friedrich P, Lam CG, Kaur G, Itriago E, Ribeiro RC, Arora RS. Determinants of treatment abandonment in childhood cancer: results from a global survey. PLoS One. 2016;11(10):e0163090. https://doi.org/10.1371/journal.pone.0163090.
19. Mostert S, Arora RS, Arreola M, et al. Abandonment of treatment for childhood cancer: position statement of a SIOP PODC Working Group. Lancet Oncol. 2011;12(8):719–20. https://doi.org/10.1016/S1470-2045(11)70128-0.
20. Weaver MS, Howard SC, Lam CG. Defining and distinguishing treatment abandonment in patients with cancer. J Pediatr Hematol Oncol. 2015;37(4):252–6. https://doi.org/10.1097/MPH.0000000000000319.
21. Salaverria C, Rossell N, Hernandez A, et al. Interventions targeting absences increase adherence and reduce abandonment of childhood cancer treatment in El Salvador. Pediatr Blood Cancer. 2015;62(9):1609–15. https://doi.org/10.1002/pbc.25557.
22. Howard SC, Pedrosa M, Lins M, Pedrosa A, Pui CH, Ribeiro RC, Pedrosa F. Establishment of a pediatric oncology program and outcomes of childhood acute lymphoblastic leukemia in a resource-poor area. JAMA. 2004;291(20):2471–5. https://doi.org/10.1001/jama.291.20.2471.
23. Jatia S, Prasad M, Paradkar A, et al. Holistic support coupled with prospective tracking reduces abandonment in childhood cancers: a report from India. Pediatr Blood Cancer. 2019;66(6):e27716. https://doi.org/10.1002/pbc.27716.
24. Kuerer HM, Eberlein TJ, Pollack RE, et al. Career satisfaction, practice patterns and burnout among surgical oncologists: report on the quality of life of members of the Society of Surgical Oncology. Ann Surg Oncol. 2007;14(11):3043–53.
25. Alvarez E, Seppa M, Rivas S, et al. Improvement in treatment abandonment in pediatric patients with cancer in Guatemala. Pediatr Blood Cancer. 2017;64(10). https://doi.org/10.1002/pbc.26560.
26. Ospina-Romero M, Portilla CA, Bravo LE, Ramirez O, group Vw. Caregivers' self-reported absence of social support networks is related to treatment abandonment in children with cancer. Pediatr Blood Cancer. 2016;63(5):825–31. https://doi.org/10.1002/pbc.25919.
27. Chantada G, Lam CG, Howard SC. Optimizing outcomes for children with non-Hodgkin lymphoma in low- and middle-income countries by early correct diagnosis, reducing toxic death and preventing abandonment. Br J Haematol. 2019;185(6):1125–36.
28. Howard SC, Davidson A, Luna-Fineman S, et al. A framework to develop adapted treatment regimens to manage pediatric cancer in low- and middle-income countries: The Pediatric Oncology in Developing Countries (PODC) Committee of the International Pediatric Oncology Society (SIOP). Pediatr Blood Cancer. 2017;64(Suppl):5. https://doi.org/10.1002/pbc.26879.
29. Salstrom JL, Coughlin RL, Pool K, et al. Pediatric patients who receive antibiotics for fever and neutropenia in less than 60 min have decreased intensive care needs. Pediatr Blood Cancer. 2015;62(5):807–15. https://doi.org/10.1002/pbc.25435.
30. Caniza MA, Odio C, Mukkada S, et al. Infectious complications in children with acute lymphoblastic leukemia treated in low-middle-income countries. Expert Rev Hematol. 2015;8(5):627–45. https://doi.org/10.1586/17474086.2015.1071186.
31. Ardura MI, Bibart MJ, Mayer LC, Guinipero T, Stanek J, Olshefski RS, Auletta JJ. Impact of a best practice prevention bundle on Central Line-associated Bloodstream Infection (CLABSI) rates and outcomes in pediatric hematology, oncology, and hematopoietic cell transplantation patients in

inpatient and ambulatory settings. J Pediatr Hematol Oncol. 2021;43(1):e64–72. https://doi.org/10.1097/MPH.0000000000001950.
32. Raja RA, Schmiegelow K, Henriksen BM, Frandsen TL. Serial ultrasound monitoring for early recognition of asparaginase associated pancreatitis in children with acute lymphoblastic leukemia. Pediatr Hematol Oncol. 2015;32(7):474–81.
33. Israels T, Damen CW, Cole M, et al. Malnourished Malawian patients presenting with large Wilms tumours have a decreased vincristine clearance rate. Eur J Cancer. 2010;46(10):1841–7. https://doi.org/10.1016/j.ejca.2010.03.002.
34. Pedrosa F, Bonilla M, Liu A, Smith K, Davis D, Ribeiro RC, Wilimas JA. Effect of malnutrition at the time of diagnosis on the survival of children treated for cancer in El Salvador and Northern Brazil. J Pediatr Hematol Oncol. 2000;22(6):502–5. http://www.ncbi.nlm.nih.gov/pubmed/11132216.
35. Ladas EJ, Arora B, Howard SC, Rogers PC, Mosby TT, Barr RD. A framework for adapted nutritional therapy for children with cancer in low- and middle-income countries: a report from the SIOP PODC Nutrition Working Group. Pediatr Blood Cancer. 2016;63(8):1339–48. https://doi.org/10.1002/pbc.26016.
36. Murphy AJ, Mosby TT, Rogers PC, Cohen J, Ladas EJ. An international survey of nutritional practices in low- and middle-income countries: a report from the International Society of Pediatric Oncology (SIOP) PODC Nutrition Working Group. Eur J Clin Nutr. 2014;68(12):1341–5. https://doi.org/10.1038/ejcn.2014.122.
37. Ruggiero A, Ferrara P, Attina G, Rizzo D, Riccardi R. Renal toxicity and chemotherapy in children with cancer. Br J Clin Pharmacol. 2017;83(12):2605–14. https://doi.org/10.1111/bcp.13388.
38. Mudi A, Levy CS, Geel JA, Poole JE. Paediatric cancer survivors demonstrate a high rate of sub-clinical renal dysfunction. Pediatr Blood Cancer. 2016;63(11):2026–32. https://doi.org/10.1002/pbc.26132.
39. Wu NL, Hingorani S. Outcomes of kidney injury including dialysis and kidney transplantation in pediatric oncology and hematopoietic cell transplant patients. Pediatr Nephrol. 2021;36(9):2675–86. https://doi.org/10.1007/s00467-020-04842-7.
40. Howard SC, Ortiz R, Baez LF, et al. Protocol-based treatment for children with cancer in low income countries in Latin America: a report on the recent meetings of the Monza International School of Pediatric Hematology/Oncology (MISPHO)--part II. Pediatr Blood Cancer. 2007;48(4):486–90. https://doi.org/10.1002/pbc.20989.
41. Howard SC, Marinoni M, Castillo L, et al. Improving outcomes for children with cancer in low-income countries in Latin America: a report on the recent meetings of the Monza International School of Pediatric Hematology/Oncology (MISPHO)-part I. Pediatr Blood Cancer. 2007;48(3):364–9. https://doi.org/10.1002/pbc.21003.
42. Ribeiro RC, Sandlund JT. Burkitt lymphoma in African children: a priority for the global health agenda? Pediatr Blood Cancer. 2008;50(6):1125–6. https://doi.org/10.1002/pbc.21528.
43. Allemani C, Matsuda T, Di Carlo V, et al. Global surveillance of trends in cancer survival 2000-14 (CONCORD-3): analysis of individual records for 37 513 025 patients diagnosed with one of 18 cancers from 322 population-based registries in 71 countries. Lancet. 2018;391(10125):1023–75. https://doi.org/10.1016/S0140-6736(17)33326-3.
44. Bonilla M, Moreno N, Marina N, et al. Acute lymphoblastic leukemia in a developing country: preliminary results of a nonrandomized clinical trial in El Salvador. J Pediatr Hematol Oncol. 2000;22(6):495–501. https://doi.org/10.1097/00043426-200011000-00004.
45. Wagner CM, Antillon F, Uwinkindi F, et al. Establishing cancer treatment programs in resource-limited settings: lessons learned from Guatemala, Rwanda, and Vietnam. J Glob Oncol. 2018;4:1–14. https://doi.org/10.1200/JGO.17.00082.

Global Disparities in ALL Treatment and Outcome

22

Allen E. J. Yeoh, Shawn H. R. Lee, Sally Blair, and Bernice L. Z. Oh

22.1 Introduction

Despite being the most curable type of childhood cancer, global disparities in treatment outcomes for childhood ALL remain. Globally, these disparities occur at multiple levels: in between continents, World Bank Income Groups, rural-versus-urban residence, and even racial groups within a country [1]. The true scale of these disparities remains unknown because childhood cancer survival data from most low- and middle-income countries (LMICs) simply do not exist. Yet, with 80% of global childhood cancer burden residing in LMICs, majority of the world's children with ALL are not properly diagnosed, let alone cured.

Realising the huge global disparities in ALL outcomes, concerted outreach efforts are made. These efforts are highly cost-effective for many reasons. Firstly, using simple, widely available NCI criteria (age and WBC count at presentation) and day 8 peripheral blood response, we can identify low-risk patients. ALL therapy is metronomic, i.e. need not be myelosuppressive to cure. Secondly, these low-risk patients can be cured with mainly outpatient chemotherapy. Learning to cure childhood ALL with less therapy in LMICs, in return, can help accelerate high-income countries (HICs) find ways to deintensify therapy for their low-risk patients. In this chapter on global disparities, we will review global efforts and lessons learned.

A. E. J. Yeoh (✉)
VIVA-University Children's Cancer Centre, Khoo Teck Puat-National University Children's Medical Institute, National University Hospital, National University Health System, Singapore, Singapore

Department of Paediatrics, Yong Loo Lin School of Medicine, National University of Singapore, Singapore, Singapore

Cancer Science Institute (Singapore), National University of Singapore, Singapore, Singapore
e-mail: allen.yeoh@nus.edu.sg

S. H. R. Lee · B. L. Z. Oh
VIVA-University Children's Cancer Centre, Khoo Teck Puat-National University Children's Medical Institute, National University Hospital, National University Health System, Singapore, Singapore

Department of Paediatrics, Yong Loo Lin School of Medicine, National University of Singapore, Singapore, Singapore
e-mail: Shawnlee@nus.edu.sg; paeolzb@nus.edu.sg

S. Blair
VIVA-University Children's Cancer Centre, Khoo Teck Puat-National University Children's Medical Institute, National University Hospital, National University Health System, Singapore, Singapore

St Jude Global Programme, St Jude Children's Research Hospital, Memphis, TN, USA
e-mail: Sally.blair@stjude.org

G. Escherich, V. Conter (eds.), *Acute Lymphoblastic Leukemia in Children and Adolescents*, Pediatric Oncology, https://doi.org/10.1007/978-3-031-71180-0_22

22.2 Childhood ALL Is Curable

With contemporary therapy, ~90% of children with ALL are cured [2, 3]. Underpinning this high cure rate are decades of collaborative research by cooperative groups and data sharing through consortia such as the Ponte de Legno platform [2]. Together, they helped clearly define the effective components of ALL therapy. Yet this high survival rate for ALL remained largely confined to HICs. Among LMICs, where most of the world's children with ALL reside, survival remains poor.

Even within HICs like the United States, racial disparities in treatment outcome persist. For example, African Americans and Hispanics have lower survival rates compared to Asians and Caucasians [4]. To cure childhood ALL, we need to address the reasons behind these disparities.

22.3 Global Disparities in ALL

The key to tackling global disparities is data. Unfortunately, there are no reliable data of childhood ALL outcome from most LMICs. However, there is budding progress in collecting outcome data. For example, WHO International Incidence of Childhood Cancer, GLOBOCAN, CONCORD [5, 6] and Global Burden of Diseases Study [7] have published reports of childhood cancer incidence and survival data. But only 5–12% of these data are from LMIC registries. The data from majority of LMICs in Asia and Africa simply do not exist.

Based on CONCORD-3 [5], among children and AYA from LMICs and HICs, an ALL-survival gap of 15% remained from 2000 to 2014 (Fig. 22.1a). Although the survival outcomes in South America and Asia improved from 2000–2004 to 2010–2014, they still lagged behind survivals in the North America, Europe and Oceania (Fig. 22.1b).

22.4 Treating ALL Is Cost-Effective

Treating childhood cancer is cost-effective. Atun et al. [1] estimated that for every $1 invested in treating childhood cancer, a lifetime productivity gain of >$3 will be realised. For childhood ALL where treatment is less expensive, more effective and has relatively fewer late effects, we postulate that the lifetime productivity gain is even greater. Most survivors of contemporary ALL therapy can function at their full genetic potential. In Ma-Spore ALL studies [8], where cranial irradiation is restricted only to CNS3 disease, survivors return to normal school and many excel, going to universities and even medical schools.

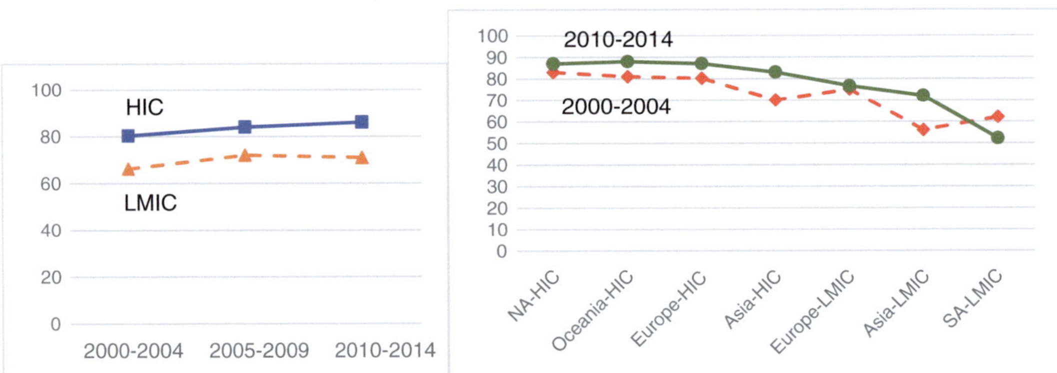

Fig. 22.1 CONCORD-3 data on 5-year net survival outcome for ALL in children and young adults (age 0–24). (**a**) Outcomes between LMICs and HICs show a persistent survival gap of 15%. (**b**) Outcome of ALL across the various continents comparing period 2000–2004 (red dashed) and 2010–2014 (green). Although 5-year net survival of ALL in South American and Asian LMICs are improving from 2000–2004 to 2010–2014, it still lacks behind North America, Europe and Oceania. (Data from Africa not shown. Redrawn from survival data estimates from Ref [5])

To treat ALL effectively, a proper healthcare system is needed. However, most LMICs lack healthcare systems for cancer care. For many MIC, existing healthcare systems can be scaled up quickly to treat ALL; net benefits of treating ALL are immediate and steep [1]. However, because healthcare systems do not exist in LICs, LICs need to scale up by >40% of their current healthcare expenditure before net benefits are realised [1]. However, when realised, these benefits grow exponentially.

Although setting up health systems sounds intimidating, outreach groups like St Jude Global have developed developmental packages that can be adapted to local LMIC use. Reducing complicated jargons and adapting such packages to local needs are keys to success. Complicated jargon-filled packages are intimidating. Implementation should be guided and negotiated. A passionate, talented leader, who can get every hospital level to come and work together, is essential to set up such a health system. Because paediatric oncology is not well recognised, sponsoring organisations like St Jude Global need to help local leaders, who are usually young and inexperienced, to negotiate with hospital and ministerial staff.

22.5 Healthcare System and Levels of Care

Successful treatment of ALL, like all cancers, requires a functional health system [1]. Specifically, there is the need for paediatric oncology centres with the expertise to diagnose, stabilise and safely treat the child with ALL. Because childhood ALL is not common, for most LMICs, it is best to concentrate such centres in urban areas. For example, Vietnam set up seven regional cancer centres to manage childhood ALL, which cater separately for the north, middle and south regions. By dedicating such regional cancer centres, the level 1 and 2 facilities required can be easily set up.

Treatment of ALL is long, spanning at least 2 years. However, despite its length, the intensive treatment phases last only 4–8 months. Most of the remaining maintenance therapy comprise of oral chemotherapy for 18 to 24 months. However, successful treatment of ALL requires uninterrupted access to chemotherapy drugs. Compliance and support are key. The initial diagnosis and intensive phases of therapy are best done centrally in paediatric cancer centres. These cancer centres are best concentrated in major cities or the capital of the LMIC. After completion of intensive therapy, maintenance phase can be continued in regional hospitals with guidance using phone and emails. Taken together, ALL care must be integrated and shared between paediatric cancer centres and regional hospitals.

Initial care needs to be integrated. Patients need to be referred smoothly and cared for in urban paediatric cancer centres (integrated care). After diagnosis and initial intensive phase therapy, patients can be referred back to regional hospitals to continue maintenance therapy (shared care). Setting such a seamless network of integrated and shared care is key for success, especially when patients are interspersed across a large country. This involves dedicated multidisciplinary teams of social workers and doctors. Social workers need to coordinate financial coverage, lodging and transport. In the Ma-Spore Study Group, junior doctors are trained to call up shared-care doctors to track blood counts and doses of chemotherapy during less intensive phases and during maintenance. A standardised method to check for doses of chemotherapy (mercaptopurine every night and methotrexate every week), FBC and toxicity are helpful.

Critically, majority of childhood ALL can be cured within level 1 and 2 care (Table 22.1), making it cost-effective.

Table 22.1 Scaling up level of care needed to treat ALL in LMICs

	Level 1	Level 2 (additional services)
Diagnosis	BM morphology—MGG stain, BCR:: ABL1, ETV6:: RUNX1 CSF cytospin	Flow cytometry—DNA index Cytogenetics Pharmacogenetics: TPMT/NUDT15
Lab	FBC Chemistry—AST/ALT/BU/BC Blood c/s	MTX level Viral CMV, HSV PCR galactomannan levels
Imaging	CXR, ultrasound	CT scan, MRI
Blood	Safe, volunteer donor, screened blood products Red cells. Random platelets	Pheresed platelets
Team	Paed. Oncology leader Paed. Oncology team Dedicated, adequate nursing	Partnering universities—Research Expanding Paed. Oncology and nursing teams
Paed. Cancer Centre	Clean cancer wards with good ventilation and hand wash basins. Isolation rooms ICU with conventional ventilator Day therapy	Sedation for painful procedures ICU with isolation rooms HFOV, broncho-alveolar lavage Dialysis
Chemotherapy	WHO essential med. And chemotherapy list Staff and place to prepare chemotherapy drugs Single-use butterfly needles or IV plugs Single-use infusion sets and fluids	Port-a-cath/Hickman line Clean closed-system infusion sets Self-sealing claves Infusion pumps for chemotherapy delivery
Social	Free cancer care MSW Psychosocial support	
Nongovernmental organisations	Funding support for family Children's cancer foundations Religious organisations	Transport Housing
Shared care	Start with urban centres	Regional hospitals
Twinning with peer and aspirant centres	Paed. Oncology and nursing	Lab support Paediatric subspecialty like ICU, respiratory medicine

CSF cerebrospinal fluid, *FBC* full blood count, *HFOV* high-frequency oscillatory ventilation, *ICU* intensive care unit, *MGG* May Grunwald–Giemsa stain, *MSW* medical social work

22.6 Curing the Curable and Curing the Accessible

HICs took ~30 years before achieving >50% cure for ALL [9]. While we now know the key steps and tools to cure ALL, LMICs need to take time so that the healthcare system can be properly scaled up and not overwhelmed. To do so, we propose starting with curing the curable [10], i.e. identify the children with NCI standard risk ALL (Fig. 22.2), and start with treating children from urban areas and families who can commit to care. This will help reduce initial abandonment and achieve some success. With these initial successes, through publicity and government support, the health system can then be scaled up—both in capacity and capabilities.

In HICs, it costs US$200,000 to cure a child with ALL. Such high costs are due to intensive therapy that needs expensive supportive care. Such expensive supportive care is unaffordable to most LMICs. Because ALL therapy comprises mainly generic drugs which are cheap and widely available, it is now possible to cure 60% of childhood ALL with US$20,000, only 10% of costs in HICs. China successfully piloted funding US$20,000 for every child with ALL.

For NCI SR, intensification of treatment may not improve overall survival. Ma-Spore ALL 2010 standard risk arm showed that an anthracycline-free protocol is less toxic with same survival. COG showed that, in low risk ALL, further intensification with PEG L-asp did not improve outcome [11]. Learning from LMICs

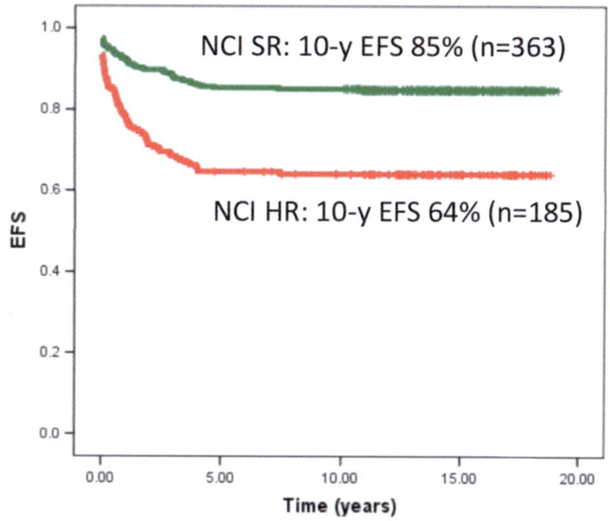

Fig. 22.2 Event-free survival based on NCI risk in Ma-Spore ALL 2003 study. NCI standard risk (age 1–10 years and WBC <50,000/μL at presentation) accounts for 67% of cohort and has survival of 85% compared to NCI HR with significantly poorer outcome of 10-year EFS 64%

Table 22.2 Proposed risk and treatment for LICs (level 1) and MICs (level 2). In LICs where there are few dedicated paediatric oncology healthcare professionals, the focus is on one simple protocol

	LICs (level 1)	MICs (level 1/2)
Risk stratification	NCI SR (age 1-10y) and WBC <50 CNS 1. CXR—No mediastinal mass OFT *BCR::ABL1, ETV6::RUNX1*	NCI SR/HR CNS 1 Flow cytometry T vs. B DNA index OFT *BCR::ABL1, ETV6::RUNX1, MLL::AF4, TCF3::PBX1*
Response	Day 8 PB blast <1 Day 15 BM blast <30% EOI BM blast <5%	Day 8 PB blast <1 Day 15 BM blast <30% EOI BM blast <5% Flow MRD-lite EOI
Protocol	One protocol—Allow familiarity	SR/HR protocol
Induction	Prediction window 1 week Delayed IT to day 8 Two drugs (VCR-Dex) with IT MTX	Prediction window 1 week Delayed IT to day 8 Three drugs (VCR-Dex-Lasp) with IT MTX
CNS directed	Cranial RT 18 Gy or IT MTX for each phase	IT MTX for each phase
Consolidation	MP + MTX oral VCR IV	VCR + escalating MTX (COG)
Delayed intensification ×2	VCR-Dex-Lasp (2–4 weeks) IT MTX	VCR-Dex-LAsp (2–4 weeks) CTX-AraC-MP
Interim maintenance	MP + MTX oral + VCR IV	MP + MTX oral + VCR IV
Maintenance	MP + MTX oral VCR-Dex pulse every 4 weeks IT MTX every 4 weeks for first year	MP + MTX oral VCR-Dex pulse every 8 weeks IT MTX every 8 weeks for first year

COG Children's Oncology Group, *CNS* central nervous system involvement by leukemia, *EOI BM* end of induction bone marrow test (usually 4–5 weeks from start of induction), *OFT* oncogene fusion test by reverse transcription PCR

with regard to low intensity therapy can help the world define the true minimal effective components of ALL therapy. Blinatumomab, an anti-CD19 T-cell engager monoclonal antibody, has been shown to be highly effective when combined with paediatric inspired protocols.

Table 22.3 Single-centre outcome for ALL from India and Indonesia. Abandonment and toxic death account for a significant proportion of failures. Although relapse/resistant disease is a feared complication, it is not the only cause of failures. The Indonesian Jogjakarta improving outcomes are results of wonderful outreach collaboration by Prof. Veerman and the DCOG outreach group [12]

	Chandigarh, India UKALL X [13]	Indo ALL 2013	Indo ALL 2016
N	762	174	188
Abandon (%)	15	11	6
Toxic death	14	13	10
Relapse/resistant (%)	18	30	27
5y EFS	43	37	49
5y OS	46	50	60
Non Leuk event	62%	44%	37%

Blinatumomab is not myelosuppressive but has immune related toxicities like cytokine release syndrome and neurotoxicity that can be managed through training. Even high risk BCR::ABL1 positive ALL can be managed using combination of blinatumomab and tyrosine-kinase inhibitors.

A proposed simple risk stratification and treatment protocol based for LIC (level 1) and MIC (level 2) is summarised in Table 22.2.

22.7 Reducing Non-leukaemia Adverse Outcomes

Although there are limited data from LMICs, non-leukaemia events account for half of the adverse outcomes. Specifically, for centres with ALL survival <50%, abandonment and treatment-related mortality accounts for more events than leukaemia-related events, e.g. Chandigarh and Jogjakarta published experience (Table 22.3). This is because healthcare financing and supportive care are inadequate to support the intensive treatment. HIC treatment protocols are inappropriate for LMICs. A graduated intensity protocol proposed by SIOP PODC or other outreach groups are key.

22.8 Lessons from China [14]

In the last decade, the Chinese government invested significantly to treat childhood ALL. Chinese MOH provided universal health coverage and together with Red Cross Angel Fund made childhood ALL treatment accessible [14]. With treatment universally accessible, astounding results are achieved. Within 7 years, the CCLG published multiple definitive large-scale studies to advance the treatment of ALL—namely on the usefulness of dasatinib in BCR::ABL1 ALL, lack of value of VCR/Dexa pulses during maintenance therapy, and role of delayed initial IT to reduce CNS2. The guidance and support from St Jude Global led by Dr Pui and Chinese VIVA Foundation for Children with Cancer led by Mrs Jennifer Yeo to form an effective cooperative group and collect world class data are lessons we can learn and emulate.

Yet real-world challenges remain. Even with the large investment of resources, rural-urban disparities for a large country like China are difficult to surmount. Travel and affordability of medical care remain important considerations for patients. When China first modernised, unregulated healthcare where doctors had uncontrolled profit from drug prescription, led to families devastated by unaffordable medical bills and poor outcomes. Private insurance led to buffet syndrome and overuse. Peasants paid to donate blood were infected with HIV, HBV and HCV because of shared needles, resulted in blood shortages [14]. To address this, the Chinese government stepped up on healthcare regulations, and ALL treatment was remunerated according to a single disease-related diagnosis package. China's dramatic success demonstrated that cost-effective care on trial protocols is possible even in such a large country like China's. Therefore, with their standardised treatment budget and a national protocol, the CCLG is transforming ALL care not only in China but over the world. With proper regulated healthcare, China has learned well from the world and in turn teaching us new ways to care for childhood ALL [14].

22.9 Paediatric Oncologists and Paediatric Oncology Nurses

As a profession, in LMICs, paediatric oncology is noble but paid poorly. Because they are paid poorly, most paediatric oncologists need to work part time in general paediatrics to supplement their income. This means they are often exhausted and cannot build on improving ALL treatment for the local needs. Concerted efforts are needed to build a cadre of paediatric oncologists. For example, despite declining births, China mandated more paediatric training positions in medical schools and hospitals [14]. St Jude Global funds paediatric oncology leaders by buying their time to lead their programme. St Jude Global also provide training, attachments and teams to support their various alliances throughout the world.

Paediatric oncology nursing also requires trained and dedicated nurses. Nurses need to give chemotherapy safely, good sterile techniques to handle closed loop IV infusions and recognise paediatric oncology emergencies like neutropenic fever and act on it. Dedicated nurses with the heart and passion are crucial in successful oncology programmes. Seeing common faces reduce anxiety among children undergoing chemotherapy. Dedicated paediatric oncology nurses also help to remember which patients are more complicated and need more support. Hospitals should avoid rotating their nurses through various wards. Rather, they should identify, train and support dedicated paediatric oncology nurses. In turn these nurses can do more. For example, in NUH, our nurses take turns to answer a patient hotline. Patients who need admission are directly admitted to the paediatric cancer ward without needing to go to emergency.

22.10 Universal Health Coverage

To avoid families falling into deep, debt traps, WHO advocates a universal health coverage for children with cancer. But such universal coverage needs significant investments by forward looking governments. Many countries now have national insurance. As many LMICs have young, healthy populations, such national insurance schemes are both effective and sustainable. It can be complemented using private insurance.

In Singapore, the government believes health is each individual responsibility. Singapore's national insurance only pay for major illnesses like cancers which are rare but can be financially devastating. In addition, every person and his employer contribute 1% of his pay monthly to the person's own Medisave account. This fund can be used to buy insurance, top up his own extended private insurance and pay for his own care. In Singapore, to avoid abuse, family need to co-pay for treatment. This co-payment is usually 10–30% of standard care. For families who cannot pay, additional funds are available from government or charities.

The problem with private insurance in LMICs is abuse. In Singapore, from 2015 to 2019, the compound annual growth rate of cancer drugs is 25%. That means in 4 years, the cost of treatment of cancer doubled! Singapore government stepped in to regulate the use of expensive, new cancer drugs setting up cost-effective indications and pricing. Adopting a cost-effective approach is key to sustainability.

22.11 UCSF-UMP Vietnam Pediatric Hematology-Oncology Fellowship

In LMICs, there are often no formal paediatric haematology-oncology training programmes. Adult-trained oncologists may be assigned to treat children with cancer. Opportunities for mentorship may be scarce. To advance the specialty of paediatric oncology in these countries, charities and universities should invest and develop specific programmes for specialty training of paediatric oncologists. An example of an ongoing, highly successful programme is in Vietnam, where, in 2018, Dr. Michelle Hermiston from University of California San Francisco (UCSF) started the Vietnamese Pediatric Hematology-Oncology Training programme with funding from Terry Fox Foundation (Vietnam). Dr. Hermiston worked with the leaders of the University of Medicine and Pharmacy (UMP) in Ho Chi Minh City and Ministry of Health to recognise the programme. The backbone of this training is a comprehensive curriculum taught by international volunteer faculty who rotate for 1–2-week blocks. Adapting UCSF fellowship programme to local needs and getting recognition is key.

22.12 Genetic Drivers for Racial Disparities in Incidence of ALL

ALL is biologically heterogeneous. This heterogeneity is driven by at least 21 genetic subtypes of ALL that can be defined by RNA-Seq [15]. The incidence of these genetic subtypes varies with race, and is strongly associated with genetic ancestry [4]. For example, African Americans have high frequency of T-ALL (20% versus 10% in most population) and TCF3-PBX1 and Hispanics have higher frequency of CRLF2 ALL. Asians have higher frequency of DUX4, PAX-5alt and ZNF-384 subtypes (Fig. 22.3). These differences may be driven by germline single-nucleotide polymorphisms (SNPs). For example, there are strong association with ARID5B genotype in Hispanics,

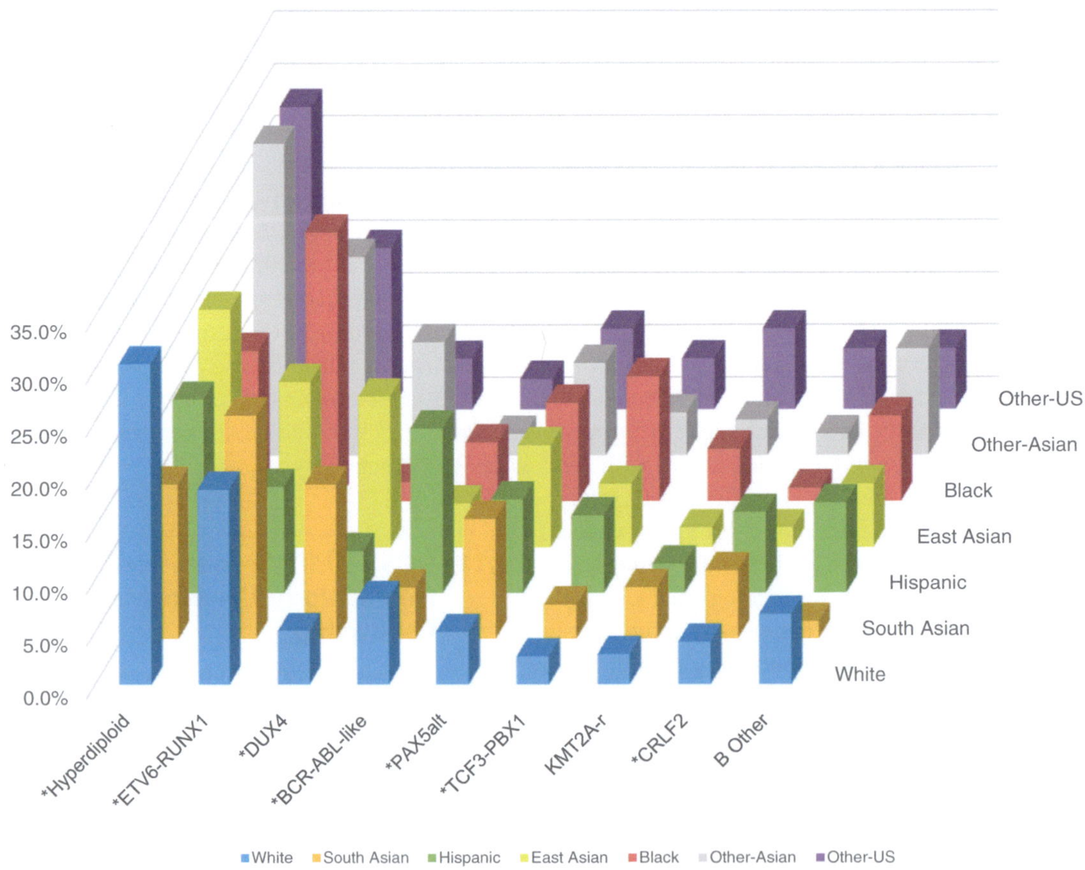

Fig. 22.3 Incidence of major genetic subtypes of B-ALL based on race. Hispanics have a high frequency of BCR-ABL-like ALL, while Asians have a higher frequency of DUX4 and PAX-5alt subtypes

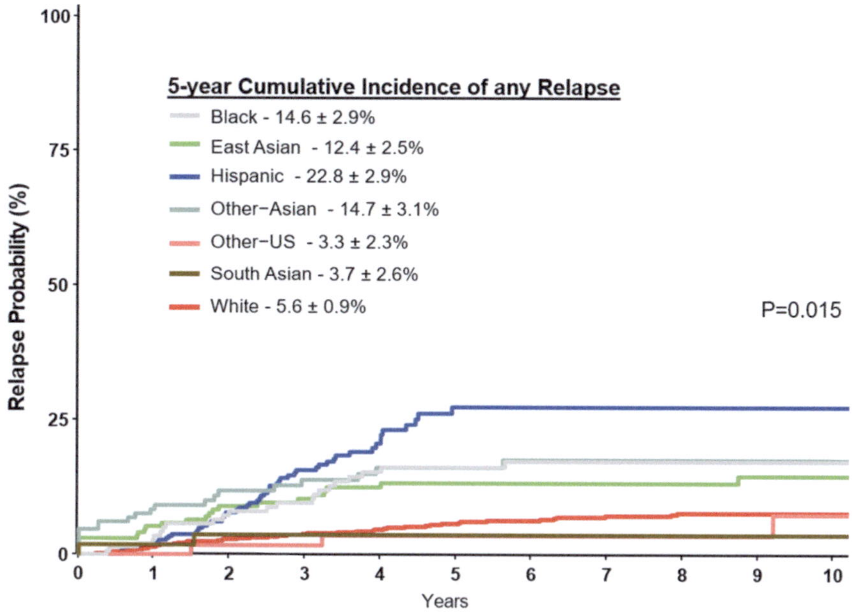

Fig. 22.4 Five-year cumulative incidence of relapse based on race. Hispanics and blacks have the highest risk of relapse [4]

BCL11A-PAPOLG SNP in blacks, and CEBPE SNPs in whites.

By pooling the RNA-Seq data worldwide, we have shown that there are distinct differences incidence of genetic subtypes [4]. But despite controlling for the genetic subtypes, racial difference in outcomes remained (Fig. 22.4), plausibly due to other biological differences, such as in pharmacogenetics between races.

22.13 Pharmacogenomics Across Racial Groups

An example how pharmacogenetics affect cancer care is the use of thiopurines like mercaptopurine and thioguanine. Metabolism of thiopurine drugs like mercaptopurine has important racial variations [16]. Asians are more sensitive to mercaptopurine. In Asians, the recommended starting dose for mercaptopurine is 50 mg/m^2/day compared to in Whites, 75 mg/m^2/day.

TPMT methylates mercaptopurine decreasing its myelosuppressive effect. TPMT variants occur in 10% of whites but only 3% in Asians. However, 20% of East Asians carry variants in the NUDT15 gene which breaks down thio-GTP to thio-GMP. With lower NUDT15 activity because of non-functional variants, Asians are more sensitive to mercaptopurine. More importantly, one in 50 Asians are exquisitely sensitive to mercaptopurine due to either complete loss of NUDT15 or compound heterozygosity of NUDT15 and TPMT. Differences in the incidence of NUDT15 gene accounts for Asian sensitivity to mercaptopurine. While TPMT and NUDT15 exemplify an actionable and race-related pharmacogenomic marker for drug tolerance, variations in thiopurine dosing remain. Moreover, the large majority of drug variation in ALL still remain unexplained. Therefore, further large-scale, whole-genome testing in diverse populations are still needed.

22.14 Conclusion

In conclusion, despite attempts to reduce them, significant global disparities in outcomes of ALL remain. These disparities are due to healthcare expenditure, access to care and genetic variations. Even for cosmopolitan countries like United States, racial differences exist due to difference in genetic drivers of ALL. For LMICs, curing the curable and curing the accessible are the first steps needed before more can be treated. ALL can be treated using metronomic non-intensive protocols which can be given cost-effectively in outpatient settings. Treating childhood ALL is cost-effective in LMICs, but this requires having a stratified road map allows building the appropriate level of care needed. Global disparities in childhood ALL therapy requires outreach programmes that enable mentoring and guiding LMICs to leap-frog to use the key cost-effective elements of ALL treatment.

References

1. Atun R, Bhakta N, Denburg A, et al. Sustainable care for children with cancer: a lancet oncology commission. Lancet Oncol. 2020;21(4):e185–224. https://doi.org/10.1016/S1470-2045(20)30022-X.
2. Pui CH, Yang JJ, Hunger SP, et al. Childhood acute lymphoblastic leukemia: progress through collaboration. J Clin Oncol. 2015;33:2938–48. https://doi.org/10.1200/JCO.2014.59.1636.
3. Hunger SP, Lu X, Devidas M, et al. Improved survival for children and adolescents with acute lymphoblastic leukemia between 1990 and 2005: a report from the children's oncology group. J Clin Oncol. 2012;10(30):1663–9. https://doi.org/10.1200/JCO.2011.37.8018.
4. Lee SHR, Antillon-Klussmann F, Pei D, et al. Association of genetic ancestry with the molecular subtypes and prognosis of childhood acute lymphoblastic leukemia. JAMA Oncol. 2022;8(3):354–63. https://doi.org/10.1001/jamaoncol.2021.6826.
5. Ssenyonga N, Stiller C, Nakata K, et al. CONCORD Working Group. Worldwide trends in population-based survival for children, adolescents, and young adults diagnosed with leukaemia, by subtype, during 2000–14 (CONCORD-3): analysis of individual data from 258 cancer registries in 61 countries. Lancet Child Adolesc Health. 2022;6:409–31. https://doi.org/10.1016/S2352-4642(22)00095-5.
6. Bonaventure A, Harewood R, Stiller CA, et al. Worldwide comparison of survival from childhood leukaemia for 1995–2009, by subtype, age, and sex (CONCORD-2): a population-based study of individual data for 89 828 children from 198 registries in 53 countries. Lancet Haematol. 2017;4:e202–17. https://doi.org/10.1016/S2352-3026(17)30052-2.
7. GBD. Childhood cancer collaborators. The global burden of childhood and adolescent cancer in 2017: an analysis of the global burden of disease study 2017. Lancet Oncol. 2017;2019(20):1211–25. https://doi.org/10.1016/S1470-2045(19)30339-0.
8. Yeoh AE, Ariffin H, Chai EL, et al. Minimal residual disease-guided treatment deintensification for children with acute lymphoblastic leukemia: results from the Malaysia-Singapore acute lymphoblastic leukemia 2003 study. J Clin Oncol. 2012;30:2384–92. https://doi.org/10.1200/JCO.2011.40.5936.
9. Hunger SP, Mullighan CG. Acute lymphoblastic leukemia in children. New Engl J Med. 2015;373:1541–52. https://doi.org/10.1056/NEJMra1400972.
10. Oh BLZ, Lee SHR, Yeoh AEJ. Curing the curable: managing low-risk acute lymphoblastic leukemia in resource limited countries. J Clin Med. 2021;10(20):4728. https://doi.org/10.3390/jcm10204728.
11. Mattano LA, Devidas M, Maloney KW, et al. Favorable Trisomies and ETV6-RUNX1 predict cure in low-risk B-cell acute lymphoblastic leukemia: results from children's oncology. Group trial AALL0331. J Clin Oncol. 2021;39:1540–52. https://doi.org/10.1200/JCO.20.02370.
12. Sutaryo S, Widjajanto PH, Mulatsih S, et al. Childhood acute lymphoblastic leukemia: four years evaluation of protocols 2013 and 2016 in a single center in Indonesia, a lower-middle-income country. Pediatr Blood Cancer. 2022;69(11):e29875. https://doi.org/10.1002/pbc.29875.
13. Kulkarni KP, Marwaha RK, Trhan A, Bansal D. Survival outcome in childhood ALL: experience from a tertiary care centre in North India. Pediatr Blood Cancer. 2009;53:168–73.
14. Chen SL, Zhang H, Gale RP, et al. Toward the cure of acute lymphoblastic leukemia in children in China. JCO Global Oncol. 2021;7:1176–86. https://doi.org/10.1200/GO.21.00049.
15. Li Z, Lee SHR, Chin WHN, et al. Distinct clinical characteristics of DUX4- and PAX5-altered childhood B-lymphoblastic leukemia. Blood Adv. 2021;5(23):5226–38. https://doi.org/10.1182/bloodadvances.2021004895.
16. Moriyama T, Nishii R, Perez-Andreu V, et al. NUDT15 polymorphisms alter thiopurine metabolism and hematopoietic toxicity. Nat Genet. 2016;48(4):367–73. https://doi.org/10.1038/ng.3508.

New Agents

23

Francisco Bautista, C. Michel Zwaan,
and Andrej Lissat

23.1 Introduction

Long-term cure rates for pediatric patients with newly diagnosed acute lymphoblastic leukemia (ALL) are currently above 90% with combination and high-dose chemotherapy [1]. At relapse, up to 85% of patients achieve second complete remission with intensified multi- and high-dose chemotherapy regimens, but still 50% of those will suffer from second relapse. Five-year overall survival (OS) rates for relapsed/refractory (R/R) and high risk (HR) patients with first relapse, including all BCP-ALL and T-ALL leukemia subgroups, approach only 30% [2].

Salvage treatment options for patients with B-cell precursor ALL (BCP-ALL) have increased significantly since blinatumomab and chimeric antigen receptor T cells (CAR-T cells) have obtained marketing authorization, both changing the landscape for treatment options and resulting in a new relapse category after immunotherapy [3]. However, still almost 50% of BCP-ALL patients will suffer from relapse after CAR-T therapy after extended follow-up [4]. The development of inotuzumab ozogamicin may further impact on better outcomes [5].

For patients with T-ALL, the outcome at relapse is particularly dismal for those who do not achieve a second morphological complete remission (CR) and deep minimal residual disease (MRD) response (i.e., $<10^{-4}$) after reinduction. Overall survival of relapsed T-ALL in general is extremely poor; in particular, multiple relapsed patients show resistance to higher line therapeutic approaches which most often do not lead to long-term CR [2].

The use of current molecular and functional profiling technologies has revolutionized our practice in oncology, with dozens of new alterations and matched compounds for selected tumor types successfully developed. The implementation of these technologies into routine practice facilitates the identification of genetic aberrations that may make tumor cells more sensitive to targeted therapies [6–8], some of which are only accessible in the context of clinical trials. The recent experiences of the INFORM and MAPPYACTS molecular platforms reveal that between 70% and 85% of the pediatric cancer patients (4% in these series had ALL) harbor an "actionable event," of which only 4–12% received a matched therapy within a clinical trial [6, 7].

F. Bautista
Princess Máxima Center for Pediatric Oncology, Utrecht, The Netherlands

C. M. Zwaan (✉)
Princess Máxima Center for Pediatric Oncology, Utrecht, The Netherlands

Sophia Children's Hospital/Erasmus MC, Rotterdam, The Netherlands
e-mail: c.m.zwaan@prinsesmaximacentrum.nl

A. Lissat
Charité – Campus Virchow Klinikum, Berlin, Germany

G. Escherich, V. Conter (eds.), *Acute Lymphoblastic Leukemia in Children and Adolescents*, Pediatric Oncology, https://doi.org/10.1007/978-3-031-71180-0_23

The LEAP consortium conducted a dedicated prospective trial for children with leukemias to evaluate the feasibility of rapid identification of targetable mutations by DNA next generation sequencing (NGS) and RNA-based gene fusion testing followed by data review in a multidisciplinary molecular tumor board [9]. Of the 153 patients, 39% had ALL. The program demonstrated to be feasible with rapid turn-arounds of results and reports to the investigators; seven out of the 17 patients who received targeted therapy had relapsed BCP-ALL, mostly with MEK and JAK-STAT inhibitors. In addition, functional approaches, which include drug response profiling (DRP) using high throughput technologies and automated image analysis, represent an additional layer to characterize biology and efficiency of targeted and non-targeted agents [10, 11], although standardization and clinical validation of these assays is key to further understand their potential.

Drug development and approval of new agents for children with cancer has traditionally lagged behind that of the adults, with more than 6 years of delay between first-in-human and first-in-child trials [12], 3 years in case of marketing authorization for its use in children compared to adults and a median of up to 1.5 years between regulatory approval and Health Technology Assessment (HTA) agencies decision on their cost and reimbursement [13], leading to unacceptable delays of making new therapies accessible for children. Changes in regulation in Europe and the United States are encouraging to foster the development of new treatments for pediatric cancer [14] while the multistakeholder platform ACCELERATE has demonstrated to be a powerful tool to harmonize decisions around treatments that need to be prioritized in this population [15]. Still new incentives are needed to promote pediatric specific cancer drug development [16].

Lastly, current standard therapies are associated with significant acute morbidity and mortality and long-term side effects [17]. Replacing elements of current therapies by less toxic and equally effective options remains an important goal [18] and may impact significantly on the quality of life of survivors.

The aim of this chapter is to provide an overview of the current status of drug development for ALL in children, and give a perspective of the future strategies. We focused on the following group of agents due to its current relevance: MEK, JAK, cyclin-dependent kinases (CDK), mTOR, proteasome, KMT2, BCR-ABL inhibitors, and BH3 mimetics. Table 23.1 summarizes studies evaluating agents addressed to these pathways. Figure 23.1 provides an overview on actionable extracellular and intracellular targets. Cellular therapies, including CAR-T, and immunotherapy are covered in detail in chapters "The Role for Immunotherapy in Childhood Acute Lymphoblastic Leukemia" and "CAR T in ALL" of this book and hence not discussed here.

Table 23.1 Studies evaluating new agents in pediatric patients with leukemia

Condition	Molecular criteria	Line	Phase	Investigational agent	Intervention	Status	Sponsor	NCT number
RAS/RAF/MEK/ERK pathway								
T-ALL/B-ALL	RAS activating mutations	R/R	1/2	Selumetinib	Selumetinib oral daily + pulses dexamethasone	Recruiting	University of Birmingham	NCT03705507
T-ALL/B-ALL	RAS activating mutations	R/R	1/2	Trametinib	Trametinib oral daily + dexamethasone + Ara-C and cyclophosphamide	Active, not recruiting	Princess Maxima	NCT05658640
JAK-STAT pathway								
Leukemia	JAK mutations and/or TLSRP surface +	R/R	1	Ruxolitinib	Ruxolitinib single agent	Completed	COG	NCT01164163
ALL/AML	No	R/R	1/2	Ruxolitinib	Ruxolitinib single agent	Terminated	MD Anderson	NCT01251965
Ph like B-ALL	CRLF2 rearrangement JAK pathway alterations	First line	2	Ruxolitinib	Ruxolitinib with chemotherapy	Recruiting	Incyte	NCT02723994
T-ALL/B-ALL	Activation of JAK-STAT signaling	First line	2/3	Ruxolitinib	Ruxolitinib with chemotherapy	Recruiting	St Jude	NCT03117751
Cell cycle: cyclin-dependent kinase inhibitors (CDKs)								
T-ALL/B-ALL	No	R/R	1	Palbociclib	Palbociclib with chemotherapy	Active, not recruiting	COG	NCT03792256
ALL	No	R/R	1	Palbociclib	Palbociclib with chemotherapy	Terminated	St Jude	NCT03515200
ALL	No	R/R	1	Palbociclib	Palbociclib, bortezomib, doxorubicin, and dexamethasone	Recruiting	Stanford University	NCT04996160
ALL	No	R/R	1	Ribociclib	Ribociclib, everolimus, and dexamethasone	Active, not recruiting	Dana-Farber	NCT03740334
Leukemia	Cell cycle and/or PI3K/AKT/mTOR alt	R/R	1/2	Ribociclib	Ribociclib and everolimus (arm B: ESMART)	Completed	Gustave Roussy	NCT02813135
Leukemia	Cell cycle and PI3K/AKT/mTOR alt	R/R	2	Ribociclib	Ribociclib, everolimus, and dexamethasone (arm M: ESMART)	Recruiting	Gustave Roussy	NCT02813135

(continued)

Table 23.1 (continued)

Condition	Molecular criteria	Line	Phase	Investigational agent	Intervention	Status	Sponsor	NCT number
Leukemia	Cell cycle or MLL, FLT3, MYC, HDM2, SMARC, ARID alt	R/R	1/2	Fadraciclib	Fadraciclib and cytarabine (arm L: ESMART)	Recruiting	Gustave Roussy	NCT02813135
PI3K/AKT/mTOR								
ALL	No	R/R	1	Everolimus	Everolimus with chemotherapy	Completed	Dana-Farber	NCT01523977
ALL	No	R/R	1	Everolimus	Everolimus with chemotherapy	Recruiting	Emory Univ	NCT03328104
ALL	No	R/R	1	Temsirolimus	Temsirolimus with chemotherapy	Completed	TACL	NCT01614197
ALL	No	R/R	1	Temsirolimus	Temsirolimus with chemotherapy	Completed	NCI	NCT01403415
ALL	No	R/R	2	Sirolimus	Sirolimus and methotrexate	Completed	CH Philadelphia	NCT01162551
Proteasome inhibitors								
ALL	No	R/R	1/2	Carfilzomib	Carfilzomib with chemotherapy	Recruiting	Amgen	NCT02303821
ALL	No	R/R	1	Ixazomib	Ixazomib with chemotherapy	Withdrawn	Millenium	NCT03888534
ALL	No	R/R	1	Ixazomib	Ixazomib with chemotherapy	Recruiting	TACL	NCT03817320
ALL	No	R/R	1	Bortezomib	Bortezomib single agent	Completed	NCI	NCT00077467
Leukemia	No	R/R	1	Bortezomib	Bortezomib and belinostat	Completed	NCI	NCT00348985
ALL	No	R/R	1	Bortezomib	Bortezomib and vorinostat	Completed	NCI	NCT00994500
ALL	No	R/R	1/2	Bortezomib	Bortezomib with chemotherapy	Completed	TACL	NCT00440726
ALL	No	R/R	2	Bortezomib	Bortezomib and vorinostat	Terminated	Masonic Cancer Center	NCT01312818
ALL	No	R/R	2	Bortezomib	Bortezomib, rituximab, and chemotherapy	Recruiting	CCCG	NCT04224571
ALL	No	R/R	2	Bortezomib	Bortezomib with chemotherapy	Terminated	Children's Mercy Hospital	NCT02535806
ALL	No	R/R	2	Bortezomib	Bortezomib with chemotherapy	Recruiting	Charité	NCT03590171
ALL	No	R/R	2	Bortezomib	Bortezomib with chemotherapy	Completed	NCI	NCT00873093
ALL	No	R/R	2	Bortezomib	Bortezomib with chemotherapy	Recruiting	MD Anderson	NCT03136146
T-ALL	No	R/R	2	Bortezomib	Bortezomib with chemotherapy	Terminated	St Jude	NCT02518750
Leukemia	MLL-rearranged leukemia	R/R	2	Bortezomib	Bortezomib, vorinostat, and chemotherapy	Terminated	St Jude	NCT02419755
ALL	No	First line	2/3	Bortezomib	Bortezomib with chemotherapy	Recruiting	St Jude	NCT03117751
T-ALL	No	First line	3	Bortezomib	Bortezomib with chemotherapy	Active, not recruiting	NCI	NCT02112916

ALL	No	First line	3	Bortezomib	Bortezomib with chemotherapy	Recruiting	AIEOP	NCT03643276
Other agents								
Leukemia	No	R/R	1	AT92832: Aurora kinase inhibitor	AT9283 single agent	Completed	Cancer Research UK	NCT01431664
Mitochondria targeting: BH-3 mimetics								
ALL, AML	No	R/R	1/2	Venetoclax	Venetoclax with chemotherapy	Completed	AbbVie	NCT03236857
ALL	No	R/R	1/2	Venetoclax and navitoclax	Venetoclax and navitoclax with chemotherapy	Completed	AbbVie	NCT03181126
ALL	ABL-class aberration	R/R	1/2	Venetoclax and dasatinib	Venetoclax and dasatinib with chemotherapy	Not yet recruiting	Princess Maxima	NCT05751044
ALL	No	R/R	1/2	Venetoclax, navitoclax, and decitabine	Venetoclax, navitoclax, and decitabine	Not yet recruiting	Princess Maxima	NCT05740449
ALL	IL7-R, JAK and STAT activating mutations	R/R	1/2	Venetoclax and ruxolitinib	Venetoclax, ruxolitinib, and chemotherapy	Not yet recruiting	Princess Maxima	NCT05745714
MLL complex interfering compounds								
ALL, AML	MLLr NUP98r, NPM1c mutation	R/R	1/2	SNDX-5613 (cobicistat)	SNDX-5613 single agent	Recruiting	Syndax Pharmaceuticals	NCT04065399
AML	MLLr, NPM1 mutation	R/R	1/2	Ziftomenib	Ziftomenib single agent	Recruiting	Kura Oncology, Inc.	NCT04067336
BCR-ABL inhibition								
ALL	Ph + ALL	First line	3	Imatinib	Imatinib and chemotherapy	Completed	Rennes University Hospital	NCT00287105
ALL	Ph + ALL	First line	3	Dasatinib	Dasatinib and chemotherapy	Completed	NCI	NCT00720109
ALL	Ph + ALL	First line	3	Imatinib	Imatinib and chemotherapy	Completed	NCI	NCT00022737
ALL	Ph + ALL	First line	3	Imatinib	Imatinib and chemotherapy	Recruiting	COG	NCT03007147
ALL	Ph + ALL (adult)	First line	1/2	Dasatinib	Dasatinib and blinatumomab	Completed	GIMEMA	NCT02744768
ALL	Ph + ALL (adult)	First and higher line	1/2	Ponatinib	Ponatinib and blinatumomab	Completed	MD Anderson	NCT03263572

(continued)

Table 23.1 (continued)

Condition	Molecular criteria	Line	Phase	Investigational agent	Intervention	Status	Sponsor	NCT number
ALL	Ph + ALL	R/R	1/2	Ponatinib	Ponatinib and chemotherapy	Active, not recruiting	Takeda	NCT04501614
ALL, AML, solid tumors	Ph + ALL, mutations of RET, FLT3, KIT, FGFR, PDGFR, TIE2, VEGFR	R/R	1/2	Ponatinib	Ponatinib single agent	Recruiting	Incyte Biosciences	NCT03934372
CML	BCR-ABL+	R/R	1/2	Olverembatinib	Olverembatinib and decitabine	Recruiting	Nanfang Hospital, Southern Medical University	NCT05376852
FGFR1 mutation myeloid and lymphoid neoplasms	FGFR1 mutations	R/R	1/2	Olverembatinib	Olverembatinib single agent	Recruiting	The First Affiliated Hospital of Soochow University	NCT05521204
CML	BCR-ABL+	R/R	1/2	Asciminib	Asciminib single agent	Recruiting	Novartis Pharmaceuticals	NCT04925479

AIEOP Associazone Italiana di Ematologia e Oncologia Pediatrica, *ALL* acute lymhoblastic leukemia, *AML* acute myeloid leukemia, *CCCG* Children's Cancer Group China, *CH* Children's hospital, *COG* Children's Oncology Group, *GIMEMA* Gruppo Italiano Malattie EMatologiche dell'Adulto, *NCI* National Cancer Institute, *Ph + ALL* Philadelphia chromosome-positive ALL, *R/R* relapsed/refractory, *TACL* Therapeutic Advances in Childhood Leukemia Consortium, *TLSRP* thymic stromal lymphopoietin receptor

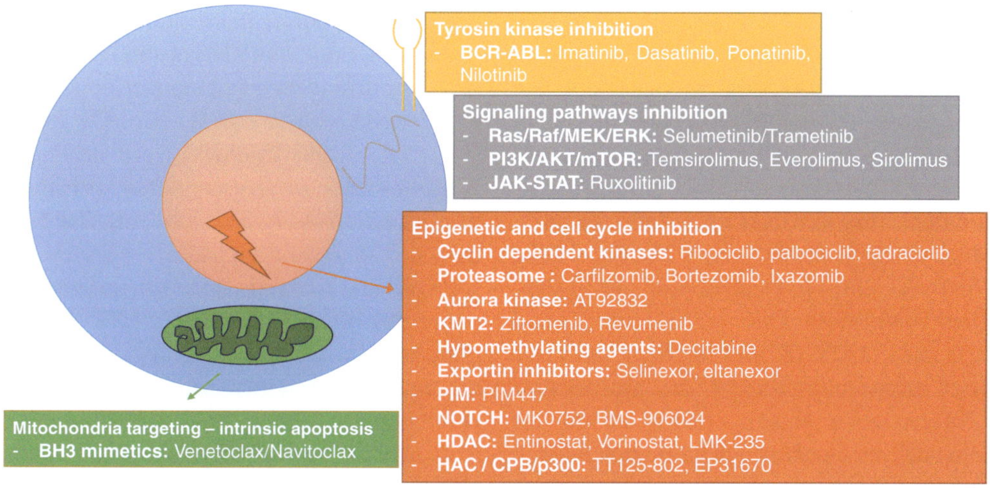

Fig. 23.1 Visual description of actionable extracellular and intracellular targets

23.2 Survival Pathways in Acute Lymphoblastic Leukemia and Potential Targeted Therapies

23.2.1 MEK Inhibition

The RAS/RAF/MEK/ERK or the MAPK/ERK pathway is a critical signal transduction cascade implicated in normal growth, and in the uncontrolled proliferation of many human cancers. In ALL, low-level subclonal mutations of MAPK-pathway genes including *KRAS*, *NRAS*, *PTPN11*, *NF1*, and *FLT3* are found in more than 40% of primary ALL samples, including clonal mutations in around 25% [19, 20]. In the relapsed setting, up to 38% of ALL samples show *RAS* pathway mutations, with complex gains and losses of particular mutations and clonal development of subclones compared to primary disease. *RAS* pathway mutations correlate with inferior prognosis, central nervous system (CNS) positivity, as well as reduced remission rates and—in regard to *KRAS* mutations—reduced overall survival. Clonal and subclonal *RAS* pathway mutations are found in various BCP-ALL subtypes being most frequent in high hyperdiploid (73%) and *MLL-AF4*-positive samples (73%) [20]. In T-ALL, up to 12% of relapsed samples show *RAS* hotspot mutations, mainly affecting *NRAS* and *KRAS*. All of the patients suffering from *RAS*-mutated T-ALL in a cohort of 67 patients died, which indicates treatment resistance [21]. *RAS*-mutations are frequently found in early T-cell precursor (ETP)-ALL and *HOXA*$^+$ subtypes of T-ALL [22]. Importantly, in T-ALL, *RAS* mutations occur in a predominantly mutually exclusive fashion with other IL-7Rα and downstream signaling components such as *JAK*, *AKT* and *PTEN* mutations [23].

Both selumetinib and trametinib have been shown to significantly reduce the viability of RAS-mutant MLL-rearranged ALL cells [24]. In PDX models, the authors demonstrated that bone marrow leukemic burden was reduced in half of the mice, and trametinib effectively reduced ERK phosphorylation in leukemic cells from bone marrows and spleens [25]. In addition, both agents enhance steroid responsiveness by preventing ERK-mediated phosphorylation of BIM in both BCP- and T-ALL, and a synergistic effect has been demonstrated when combining them with dexamethasone [24, 26, 27].

Two studies are ongoing in Europe evaluating selumetinib in combination with dexamethasone (NCT03705507) and trametinib with dexamethasone and low-doses cytarabine and cyclophosphamide (NCT05658640) in molecularly enriched pediatric ALL populations with *RAS* mutations (Table 23.1).

23.2.2 JAK-STAT Inhibition

The Janus kinase (JAK)/signal transducer and activator of transcription (STAT) pathway is central to signaling by cytokine receptors, that regulates cell proliferation, survival, differentiation and immune response and cross-talks to additional surviving pathways (e.g., MAPK, PI3K/AKT/mTOR) [28]. It is composed of ligand–receptor complexes, JAKs (JAK1 to 3 and TYK2), and STATs (STAT1 to 6). JAK/STAT receptors transmit anti-apoptotic, proliferative and differentiation signals, being critical for myeloid and lymphoid lineage development [29]. Up to 25% of pediatric T-ALL patients present with mutations activating the JAK-STAT signaling pathway [22]. *JAK-STAT* activating mutations are frequently associated with concomitant mutations involving additional *JAK-STAT*, *RAS*, or *PI3K-AKT*, which might coexist in the same clone, being of importance for the selection of targeted therapeutic approaches, and the potential for emergence of sub-clones resistant to agents targeting a single pathway [22]. IL-7Rα mutations are present in approximately 9% of pediatric patients with T-ALL [30, 31]. The most common mutations imply insertions and deletions into exon 6 region of the gene, inducing homodimerization of expressed mutated *IL-7Rα* chains that constitutively activate *JAK1* and *STAT5*. Newly diagnosed T-ALL patients have a dismal outcome in presence of *IL-7R* mutations and *JAK* mutations which lead to a reduction in 5-year OS from 80% to 55%. In addition, IL-7R pathway mutated patients showed a higher degree of steroid refractoriness [32]. Activating mutations in the Janus kinases *JAK1* (n = 3), *JAK2* (n = 16), and *JAK3* (n = 1) have been observed in 20 (10.7%) of 187 *BCR-ABL1*-negative, high-risk pediatric B-ALL cases [32]. *JAK2* mutations mainly occur in the poor prognostic subtypes *BCR-ABL1*-like and non-*BCR-ABL1*-like B-other (negative for sentinel cytogenetic lesions) while *JAK2* translocations were restricted to *BCR-ABL1*-like [33].

There is evidence that the kinase mutations described above may lead to enhanced kinase activity and therefore to proliferative advantage in patients harboring these alterations. In T-ALL, ruxolitinib alone inhibited proliferation and survival in a dose-dependent manner *in vitro* in cells transformed with mutant IL-7Rα (D1_hIL7RP1) [34]. The same findings were replicated in Rag1−/− mice *in vivo* engrafted with the same transformed T-ALL cells (D1_hIL7RP1). Mice treated with ruxolitinib had a 2-week increase in survival and slowed leukemic progression in peripheral blood [35]. All six ETP-ALL xenograft models exhibited significantly decreased leukemia burden with ruxolitinib treatment compared with control mice and ruxolitinib efficacy was independent of JAK mutation status. In *CRLF2*-rearranged Philadelphia (Ph)-like BCP-ALL, ruxolitinib was found to enhance the *in vitro* and *in vivo* efficacy of an induction-type regimen consisting of vincristine, dexamethasone, and L-asparaginase in two out of three *CRLF2*-rearranged Ph-like ALL xenografts [36]. On the other hand, there is also preclinical data suggesting that JAK inhibition may be compromised by mutations in alternative survival pathways and microenvironment-induced resistance and that inhibitors induce accumulation of phosphorylated JAK2^{Y1007}, which can result in a profound reactivation of JAK2 signaling upon release of the inhibitors [33].

These findings led to the development of prospective clinical studies to evaluate the role of ruxolitinib in these conditions. In the pediatric phase I ruxolitinib study in patients with relapsed/refractory solid and hematological tumors, 49 patients were enrolled [37]. There were five patients with ALL and 11 with acute myeloid leukemia (AML), but none with the target mutations. The recommended phase 2 dose (RP2D) was 50 mg/m^2/dose, BID (*bis in die*), on a continuous dosing in 28-day cycles. As in adults, most frequent toxicities were hematological (thrombocytopenia and anemia). In a pediatric phase II study, ruxolitinib in combination with BFM-backbone chemotherapy in patients with high-risk BCP-ALL and Ph-like mutations was evaluated [38]. Treatment-emergent adverse events occurred in all patients: anemia (75%), platelet count decrease and/or thrombocytopenia (65%), febrile neutropenia (72.5%), and AST or

ALT increase (57.5%). Thirty-three patients had grade 3/4 events possibly related to ruxolitinib without identified dose-limiting toxicities. The RP2D for ruxolitinib in combination with an iBFM chemotherapy schedule has been defined as 50 mg/m^2 BID applied in a 14 days on/14 days off schedule. Based on these results, two studies are running in newly diagnosed ALL patients combining ruxolitinib and standard chemotherapy for patients with de novo high-risk (HR) Ph-like B-ALL (NCT02723994) and with activation of JAK-STAT signaling (NCT03117751) (Table 23.1).

23.2.3 CDK Inhibition

The cell cycle is regulated by cyclin dependent kinases (CDKs) that are activated by intermittently expressed cyclins. Specific CDK/cyclin partner complexes control each phase of the cycle. For example, the CDK4/6-cyclin D complexes regulate progression through G1, while the CDK2–cyclin E complex regulates progression from G1 to S phase. These complexes phosphorylate the retinoblastoma protein (pRb). Hyperphosphorylation of pRb renders it inactive and allows for the release of E2F transcription factors necessary for initiation of S-phase and cell cycle progression [39]. Cell cycle progression is also negatively regulated by cyclin-dependent kinase inhibitors (CDKIs), and small molecule inhibitors of CDKs (CDKis) have been designed to mimic this negative regulatory activity and to thereby control cell cycle progression and cell proliferation [40]. Several CDKs (CDK2, CDK7, CDK8, and CDK9) also regulate gene transcription by phosphorylating the carboxyl-terminal domain of the large subunit of RNA polymerase II (RNAP II). Genetic or chemical targeting of CDK9 terminates transcriptional elongation by RNAPII and can therefore alter the output of transcription factors such as MYC.

Alterations in the cell cycle genes are frequent abnormalities detected in pediatric cancer, being the most frequent *CDKN2A/B* deletion, and *CCND1* and *CDK4* amplification [7, 41]. In ALL, deletions of the *CDKN2A* and *CDKN2B* genes are found in approximately 70% of childhood T-ALL at first presentation (but also in B-cell precursor) alone or associated with different alterations like *PTEN* loss. On the other hand, CDK9 pathway deregulation results in the increased expression of myeloid leukemia cell differentiation protein (MCL-1), a pro-survival protein from the BCL-2 family and transcriptional inhibitors such as CDK9 inhibitors cause down regulation of the pro-survival and anti-apoptotic proteins from the BCL-2 & IAP families (MCL-1, XIAP, survivin, and others), subsequently leading to cancer cell apoptosis [42].

NOTCH1-mutant and wild-type T-ALL are highly sensitive to pharmacologic inhibition of CDK4/6, which can synergize with glucocorticoids, mTOR and gamma secretase inhibitors [43]. The ESMART trial evaluated the combination of ribociclib (CDK4/6 inhibitor) and everolimus (mTOR inhibitor) in an enriched population of pediatric patients whose tumors harbored cell cycle or PI3K/AKT/mTOR alterations [44]. The RP2D was ribociclib 175 mg/m^2 once a day and everolimus 2.5 mg/m^2 once a day. A patient with T-ALL experienced stable disease with significant blast count reduction. Palbociclib has been investigated in combination with four-drug reinduction chemotherapy in patients with R/R ALL. The RP2D of palbociclib in combination with chemotherapy was 50 mg/m^2 and no dose limiting toxicities (DLTs) were observed [45].

Ribociclib, palbociclib and CDK9 inhibitor fadraciclib are being evaluated in several studies in combination with chemotherapy and corticoids in patients with leukemia (Table 23.1). The role and relevance of this group of agents will be discussed in the upcoming Pediatric Strategy Forum, organized by the ACCELERATE Consortium [15].

23.2.4 mTOR Inhibition

Activation of the PI3K/AKT/mTOR signaling pathway contributes to the proliferative advantage of malignant cells and may confer resistance to chemotherapy in various hematologic and solid malignancies through its fundamental role in regulating cell cycle progression, survival and proliferation [46]. mTOR is a serine/threonine kinase downstream of PI3K/AKT which plays a role in nutrient sensing, insulin signaling, protein translation, and control of growth and metabolism [47]. The PIK3CA-related overgrowth syndrome is the result of a heterozygous mosaic (or rarely, constitutional) activating pathogenic variant in *PIK3CA* [48] and Alpelisib, a PI3K alpha isoform inhibitor, has been approved for this indication.

In T-ALL, dominant genetic aberrations including *NOTCH1* mutations or 9p21 deletion alter the transcriptional programs associated with cellular proliferation and differentiation in which D-type cyclins are highly implicated [49]. Moreover, the intracellular NOTCH1 protein has been found to upregulate the PI3K/mTOR pathway through PTEN degradation [50] and to activate this pathway at multiple levels, regulating cell size, glucose accumulation and glycolysis during T-cell development. Notch inhibitors are currently also being evaluated in children with T-ALL (NCT05464836).

mTOR inhibitors have been found to have additive or synergist effects when they were combined with conventional chemotherapies and to reverse the resistance of certain chemotherapeutics in children with leukemia.

Temsirolimus was evaluated in combination with the UK-ALLR3 backbone in patients with R/R ALL [51]. This combination resulted in excessive toxicity, and DLTs occurred in the three dose levels of temsirolimus, all consistent with safety profile of sirolimus. Despite this, complete responses (CR) were observed in all three levels (seven out of 15 patients). In contrast, the combination temsirolimus with cyclophosphamide and etoposide was found to be feasible and temsirolimus could be escalated up to the higher dose level, and the RP2D was finally identified at 15 mg/m^2 [52]. The overall response rate (ORR) was 47%, with 27% achieving a CR ($n = 4$; 3 of which achieved also complete molecular response). The combination of everolimus and a four-drug backbone therapy in children with late marrow relapse, demonstrated to be feasible and the RP2D of everolimus was identified at 5 mg/m^2 with this combination [53]. Out of the 22 patients included, 19 (86%) achieved a CR, 13 of which presented with deep molecular response ($\leq 10^{-3}$).

Nevertheless, collectively in pediatric cancer, response to single agent mTOR inhibitors or in combination with other agents has been very low, with only a few exceptions (i.e., low-grade glioma). The consensus of the 2023 Accelerate Pediatric Strategy Forum on PI3K, mTOR, AKT, and GSK3B inhibitors, was that no trials should be conducted in children with mTOR inhibitors, unless there is a very strong biological rationale and supportive preclinical data (see Accelerate website).

23.2.5 Proteasome Inhibition

The ubiquitin–proteasome system (UPS) regulates cell growth, cell proliferation, response to oxidative stress and apoptosis; ubiquitination is a posttranslational protein modification that involves the covalent attachment of ubiquitin (UB) [54]. As a result of ubiquitination, proteins can follow different paves, mostly divided in proteolytic and non-proteolytic; within the UPS, the small molecules able to inhibit the proteasome component have been the first to achieve clinical success as therapeutic target. Several generations of proteasome inhibitors have been developed since the initial approval of bortezomib for the treatment of multiple myeloma, particularly those targeting the 20S catalytic core particle, preventing proteasomal degradation of inhibitors of NF-kB.

Bortezomib is a first-in-class proteasome inhibitor and the first of its kind in being evaluated in children. The phase I single agent study in children with leukemia defined the RP2D at 1.3 mg/m^2, twice weekly for 2 weeks and 1 week rest [55]. No objectives responses were seen, indicating the need for combination with other agents. Messinger conducted the phase I/II study of bortezomib added to four-drug-induction chemotherapy (VXLD). The RP2D was 1.3 mg/m^2 and an encouraging 67% of patients achieved CR. The phase II portion included 22 patients

[56]. In this study, three patients died from bacterial complications, showing the additional risks for infections, and the protocol had to be amended to mandate prophylactic bacterial and fungal infections. Responses were only seen in patients with BCP-ALL, where 73% of them achieved a CR. Based on these promising single-arm study results, bortezomib has been evaluated in first line and second line. The COG-AALL1231 trial randomized patients with newly diagnosed T-ALL and T-lymphoblastic lymphoma (T-LL) to receive bortezomib in addition to a modified augmented BFM chemotherapy regimen [57]. The addition of bortezomib did not result in a survival benefit in the T-ALL cohort (4-year progression free survival (PFS) 83.2% vs. 80.1%, with and without), while it increased significantly the PFS in patients with T-LL (86.4% vs. 76.5%), also suggesting that biology between these two subsets may differ. In Europe, two strategies for newly diagnosed and first relapse patients are ongoing. The AIEOP group is evaluating bortezomib added in the consolidation phase for patients with early high risk BCP-ALL (NCT03643276), and the IntReALL consortium investigates the addition of bortezomib during reinduction in a randomized way in patients with high-risk BCP- and T-ALL in first relapse (NCT03590171).

Carfilzomib has also been investigated in children at relapse. The phase IB portion of the study showed that carfilzomib could be safely be combined with the VXLD regimen and the RP2D was identified at 56 mg/m^2 [58]. A total of 50% achieved a CR/CRp (with incomplete platelet recovery) at the end of induction. The study is currently recruiting in the phase II portion (NCT02303821).

Lastly, ixazomib, and oral proteasome inhibitor, is currently being investigated in children with ALL and LL at relapse in combination with four-drug reinduction (NCT03817320) (Table 23.1).

23.2.6 BH-3 Mimetics

Regulation of cell death depends on a complex interaction of intra- and extracellular components including BCL-2 family members. BCL-2, BCL-X_L, BLX-W, and MCL-1 comprise the anti-apoptotic members of the family, the BH-3 only proteins BIM, BIC, PUMA and NOXA are apoptotic enhancers and BAX and BAK the definitive executioners of apoptosis leading to mitochondrial depolarization and cytochrome c release [59]. Cytochrome c binds to APAF9 and induces caspase cleavage and cell death. Up-regulation of anti-apoptotic proteins like BCL-2, who bind BAX and BAK and interfere with mitochondrial depolarization, is found in a variety of hematological disease [59]. In particular chronic lymphocytic leukemia (CLL) is considered as a model for BCL-2 dependent hematologic disease [60, 61]. Promising *in vitro* and *in vivo* data led to stringent drug development of the BCL-2 inhibitor venetoclax which has been granted approval based on high efficacy and safety for CLL and AML through EMA and FDA in 2016 and 2020/2021, respectively.

The regulation of BCL-2 and BIM expression is involved in glucocorticoid (GC) sensitivity. GC-sensitive BCP-ALL cells show BCL-2 downregulation and BIM upregulation through GC-receptor mediated gene regulation [62]. Consequently, BCL-2 inhibition might restore GC sensitivity and apoptosis in these cells. Pediatric BCP-ALL subgroups that are particularly sensitive to BCL-2 inhibition comprise *MLL*-rearranged [63] and *TP53*-mutated BCP-ALL [64]. Interestingly, ALL PDX samples which were treated with chemotherapeutic drugs *in vivo* showed evolving *TP53* mutations as a resistance mechanism as well as up-regulation of BCL-2. These secondary resistant BCP-ALL cells were resensitized to a polychemotherapeutic regimen when combined with venetoclax [64]. However, loss in TP53 expression in AML and pediatric BCP-ALL cell lines did correlate with reduced BCL-2 expression and higher BCL-X_L expression, which might confer resistance to BCL-2 inhibition [65, 66].

The BCL-2 dependency in T-ALL seems to depend on maturation state of malignant leukemic blasts. BCL-2 is highly expressed in early T-cell precursor ALL whereas in more mature phenotypes of T-ALL BCL-X_L as a mediator of resistance to apoptosis is of more importance [67–69]. The dual BCL-X_L and BCL-2 inhibitor navitoclax has been developed to target malignant solid and hematological disease [70]. Due to severe thrombocytopenia in higher doses [71, 72] further development was delayed until recently the combination of venetoclax and navitoclax proofed to be successful in R/R BCP- and T-ALL [73, 74]. Venetoclax has been developed specifically to target BCL-2 thereby optimizing its safety profile sparing thrombocytes [75]. However, analysis of BCL-2 expression and the expression of additional BCL-2 family members at baseline in pediatric trials did not show a clear correlation of BCL-2 expression with objective venetoclax or navitoclax responses [74, 76]. Pullarkat could show that the BCL-2 ad BCL-X_L expression may correlate with functional dependencies analyzed on BH3-profiling and further with clinical responses. However, these observations need to be confirmed in larger patient populations [74].

A phase I/II clinical trial evaluated venetoclax combined with various chemotherapeutic schedules (cyclophosphamide, etoposide (C) and dexamethasone, vincristine, peg-asparaginase (DVP)) in R/R pediatric ALL [76]. The recommended phase II dose (RP2D) in combination with chemotherapy was established as 800 mg adult-equivalent dose venetoclax orally, once daily. Venetoclax serum levels increase significantly if the drug is combined with strong CYP3A4 inhibitors. Consequently, recommended doses were reduced to approximately 1/5 if combined with azoles or comparable strong CYP3A4 inhibitors. Main adverse events included particularly grade 3/4 hematologic toxicities (febrile neutropenia in 52% of patients and anemia in 44% of patients). Hypokalemia (36% of patients) and increased transaminases (32% of patients) have been the most common non-hematologic grade 3/4 toxicities. The combination with DVP showed a promising overall response rate (ORR) of 56% [76].

In a second study, DVP was combined with venetoclax and low-dose navitoclax in R/R adult and pediatric patients [74]. Navitoclax has been combined with venetoclax to prevent resistance due to overexpression and switch of leukemic survival dependency to BCL-X_L [74]. In contrast to dose limiting hematologic toxicity (thrombocytopenia) seen at high doses of single agent navitoclax in trials including patients with R/R lymphoid malignancies and recommending doses >250 mg navitoclax, orally, once daily [71, 77], lowering the navitoclax dose to 25 mg orally, once daily in patients <45 kg and 50 mg orally, once daily in patients ≥45 kg in combination with venetoclax 400 mg adult-equivalent dose, orally, once daily and the DVP regimen, proved to be safe and the combination efficacious. Main grade 3/4 adverse events included neutropenia (32% of patients), febrile neutropenia (19% of patients), and thrombocytopenia (21% of patients) including three of 46 evaluable patients who suffered from a sepsis episode while on trial. The investigators reported a morphologic combined CR in 52.6% and 64% of R/R T-ALL/Lymphoblastic Lymphoma (LBL) and BCP-ALL patients, respectively. 31.8% and 36% of responding R/R T-ALL and BCP-ALL patients achieved MRD negativity [74].

Venetoclax is currently developed in multiple combinations for hematologic diseases. The I-BFM, ITCC and Princess Màxima together with the IntReALL group develop combinations of demethylating agents (decitabine) and targeted drugs (dasatinib, ruxolitinib) with venetoclax and/or navitoclax within the HEM-iSMART master protocol trial (e.g., NCT05658640, NCT05751044). A Chinese group evaluates the safety and efficacy of azacytidine in combination with venetoclax in adults and adolescents >1 years (NCT05376111). The combination of fludarabine, high-dose cytarabine, gemtuzumab ozogamicin, and venetoclax is evaluated in context of a pediatric investigational plan (PIP) (EMEA-002018-PIP02-16-M05) in pediatric AML patients.

23.2.7 KMT2 Inhibition

KMT2 is one of the key transcription factors driving leukemia in 75% of infant leukemia [78]. Depending on the translocation partner, KMT2A confers a poor prognostic marker in childhood

ALL (e.g., KTM2A::AFF4) [78, 79]. The physiological role of MLL is trimethylation at histone 3 lysine 4 (H3K4) residues [80]. Chromosomal rearrangement and breakage of *MLL* leads to loss of the c-terminal methylation site (SET domain). The n-terminal MLL domain of the fusion protein associates with the methylase DOT1L and the DNA binding transcription factor menin, both of them among others forming a protein complex inducing aberrant histone 3 lysine 79 (H3K79) methylation [80]. This leads to upregulation of stem cell programs, in particular induction of *HOXA, MEIS1*, and *MEF2C* gene expression, which renders leukemic blasts resistant to a multitude of compounds including high dose chemotherapy [81].

The observation that MLL-rearrangements confer their oncogenic role within large protein complexes led to development of compounds interfering either with methylation activity of DOT1L [82] or disrupting the complex by interfering with menin–MLL binding [83, 84]. In addition, these complexes include known leukemia drivers like IKAROS1 and LEDGF [85, 86].

Pinometostat (EPZ5676) demonstrated high DOT1L methyltransferase specificity and low *in vitro* IC50, demethylation at H3K79 sites and downregulation of the HOX and MEIS1 gene expression [87]. *In vitro* pinometostat treatment of various MLLr leukemia cell lines and *in vivo* xenograft rat models led to inhibition of apoptosis and complete leukemia regression at a dose of 70 mg/kg/day infused continuously for 20 days [87]. However, the evaluation of safety and preliminary activity of pinometostat in *MLL*r R/R AML and ALL patients demonstrated only modest activity leading to two CR (chronic myelomonocytic leukemia (CMML) and AML) in 54 evaluated patients, despite the pharmacodynamic observation that a variable degree in H3K79 demethylation and *HOXA9* and *MEIS1* downregulation could be observed in most patients while on treatment [82].

Currently, the focus of drug development in *MLLr* leukemia is interfering with complexation of the MLL complex with menin. Krivtsov and colleagues showed that VTP50469, a highly selective menin inhibitor interfering with the MLL–menin binding site and now further developed by Syndax Pharmaceuticals, leads to disruption of the MLL complex, H3K79 demethylation, and downregulation of *MEIS1, MEF2C*, and *PBX3* gene expression [88]. *In vivo* cell line and patient derived xenograft models of AML and ALL demonstrated that VTP50469 is able to induce an almost complete resolution of bone marrow, spleen, and liver leukemia infiltration at day 28 in NSG mice, leading to absence of huCD45+ bone marrow cells and long-term survival of treated animals. This effect was MLL inhibition specific as *in vivo* models with BCR-ABL ALL PDX cells showed rapid progression while on treatment with VTP50469 [88].

Currently, two compounds (ziftomenib, Kura Pharmaceuticals [89, 90] and revumenib (SNDX-5613), a close analog of VTP50469, Syndax Pharmaceuticals [91, 92]) are developed in early phase trials (NCT04065399, NCT04067336).

Preliminary data from adult and pediatric clinical trials on both agents is available. Revumenib as a monotherapeutic agent was evaluated in the Augment-101 trial and included pediatric patients above the age of 30 days [91]. Eleven patients with R/R ALL (16% of the whole cohort) have been included. Pharmacokinetic analysis demonstrated that revumenib levels increase two to threefold if combined with strong CYP3A4 inhibitors, and there are different RP2Ds dependent on concurrent use of azoles. Pharmacodynamic assessment showed that menin binding to DNA was inhibited and gene expression changed as expected. Treatment emergent adverse events were reported as nausea, vomiting and QT prolongation as well as neutropenia with septicemia and thrombocytopenia. Following a median duration of treatment of 18 days, a maximum of grade 2 differentiation syndrome has been observed in 16% of patients which was fully reversable. Thirty percent of patients showed CR/CRh (partial hematological recovery) with 78% of these MRD negative. The ORR (including incomplete count recovery (CRi), CRp and morphologic leukemia free state (MLFS)) was 53%. The analysis did not differentiate between ALL and AML patients. Patients lacking any MLLr or NPM1 mutation lacked an objective response [91].

Ziftomenib is currently evaluated in the KOMET-001 trial in relapsed and refractory AML patients above the age of 18 years [90]. Adverse events were comparable to revumenib and treatment with strong CYP3A4 inhibitors is stated as an exclusion criterion. Differentiation syndrome has been observed in 17% of patients. At the highest dose level of 600 mg, once daily 25% of patients achieved CR/CRh with an ORR of 42% [90].

Combination therapies might further improve efficacy of these compounds and will guide treatments in prospective clinical trials. Preclinical data demonstrated promising synergism between ziftomenib and venetoclax in AML cell lines and PDX models [89]. Furthermore, combination of various FLT3 inhibitors and the menin inhibitor MI-503 demonstrated high synergy on reduction of *MEIS1* and *SOX2* gene expression, apoptosis, induction of morphologic changes, and pFLT3 and pSTAT5 protein expression in *MLLr* and *FLT3* mutated human and murine AML cell lines in vitro. Similar effects were observed with the next generation menin inhibitor VTP-50469. MI-503 in combination with the FLT3 inhibitor quizartinib prolonged life in a *MLLr/FLT3mut* AML cell line PDX model *in vivo* [93]. In addition to *MLLr* AML, menin inhibitors are active in *MEIS1* gene expression dependent *NUP98r* AML (i.e., *NUP98-HOXA9*, *NUP98-JARID1A*, and *NUP98-NSD1*) [94] and in *HOXA9* and *MEIS1* dependent *MN1r* AML [95] *in vitro* and *in vivo*. If menin inhibition is of value in *ETV6-RUNX1* rearranged BCP-ALL, which shows a certain degree of MN1 overexpression [96] or in patients with *NUP98* rearranged BCP-ALL [97], needs to be further investigated.

23.2.8 BCR-ABL Inhibition

Around 5% of pediatric patients present with BCR-ABL fusion, which results from a t(9;22). The protein is found in two isoforms p210, which is expressed mostly in chronic myeloid leukemia (CML) patients and able to transform stem cell in mice to generate CML-like disease and p190 which is mainly observed in BCP-ALL [98].

Biologically related to BCR-ABL leukemias are the Philadelphia (Ph)-like (Children's Oncology Group (COG) definition) and *BCR-ABL*-like (Dutch definition) leukemias, here referred to as Ph-like ALL (reviewed in: [99–102]). These comprise two major subgroups: (1) A diverse group of ABL-class fusion positive ALL and (2) depending on the diagnostic tool applied, a second major group of *CRLF*-rearranged leukemias (COG: 50%; Dutch 15–20% of the Ph-like cohort) which is described in the respective section above. Ph-like ALL affects around 5–10% of children and adolescents at diagnosis. Mechanistically, ABL-class fusion positive leukemias seem to activate similar pathways as in Philadelphia-chromosome positive (Ph+) ALL. Due to the rarity of a single fusion in a particular patient, mechanisms that drive proliferation and transformation by a defined fusion protein are currently not entirely studied. Importantly, dasatinib and imatinib showed efficacy in a subgroup of ABL-class fusion positive Ph-like ALL patients. In an observational study 20 out of 34 BCP-ALL patients with high-risk features after induction presented with ABL class fusion positive ALL, of whom six have been treated with dasatinib, four with imatinib and one patient with imatinib and dasatinib. Both compounds induced rapid and sustained responses in the majority of patients [103].

The classic BCR-ABL fusion protein is a constitutively active tyrosine kinase activating the MAPK pathway [104]. The activation is involved in transformation, proliferation and resistance to chemotherapy. Recently, proteomic analysis in *BCR-ABL* p190 and p210 transformed murine BaF3 cells showed that 147 proteins interact with the BCR-ABL complex. Of these, 56 proteins interact with both isoforms, 30 proteins were only found in the p210 samples and 59 proteins in the p190 samples [105]. Proteins include signaling adaptors (Grb2, Shc1, Dok1, Gab2), E3 ubiquitin ligases (Cbl, Cblb), phosphatases (Inppl1/Ship2 and Ptpn11/Shp2), kinases (Map4k1, Lrrk1), GTPase effector proteins (including the Ras GEFs Sos1/2), and cytoskeleton remodeling proteins [105]. The phosphoproteome revealed marked difference in p210 compared to p190 cells, with 78 proteins to be more highly phosphorylated in p190 compared to the p210 group. Interestingly, the SCR kinase LYN, that interacts more closely with the p190 isoform, was more phosphorylated BCR-ABL p190 compared to BCR-ABL p210 cells. Consequently, in Ph + ALL activation of the SRC pathway might play a more prominent role in comparison to CML, which might rely more on alternative MAPK pathway activation [105].

Pivotal clinical trials examining the safety and efficacy of imatinib and dasatinib in first-line Ph + ALL in combination with chemotherapy in children have been performed by the European EsPhALL group (NCT00287105) and the COG (dasatinib: NCT00720109; imatinib NCT00022737) with the current EsPhALL-COG trial (NCT03007147) ongoing as an international cooperative randomized trial investigating imatinib on the COG and Associazione Italiana di Ematologia Oncologia Pediatrica (AIEOP) BFM chemotherapy backbone. Based on the current amendment this trial is open for pediatric patients with newly diagnosed Ph + ALL and ABLclass fusion positive Ph-like ALL.

The COG trial AALL0622 investigated dasatinib with chemotherapy in first line for children with children, adolescents, and young adults with Ph + ALL [106]. Thirty-nine patients received dasatinib 60 mg/m^2 on a 2-weeks on/2-weeks off schedule and 21 patients were treated on dasatinib continuously. For the 60 evaluable patients, 5-year OS and event free survival (EFS) rates were 86 ± 5% and 60 ± 7%, respectively [106]. The results were comparable with the prior AALL0031 trial investigating imatinib in combination with the same chemotherapy backbone and cranial irradiation [107] and the EsPhALL trial [108]. Since in contrast to imatinib, dasatinib is penetrating the blood–brain barrier, a secondary endpoint of the trial and focus of the investigators was reduction of CNS relapses through dasatinib exposure. However, the (isolated and combined) CNS relapse rate has been 15% in AALL0062 in patients treated on a chemotherapy only regimen (no radiotherapy), compared to a CNS relapse rate of 6% in AALL0031, where all patients underwent cranial irradiation [106, 107]. Based on these data and since clear superiority of dasatinib could not be demonstrated, imatinib in combination with chemotherapy is evaluated in the current COG–EsPhALL consortium (NCT03007147). Both trials and EsPhALL showed that Ph + ALL patients who demonstrate a good MRD response after induction can be treated in the standard risk (SR) group and have good outcome without allogeneic hematopoietic stem cell transplantation (HSCT) which is a significant improvement compared to the pre-tyrosine kinase inhibitor (TKI) era [106–108].

In contrast, Shen et al. reported superior 4-year OS rate and significantly reduced cumulative incidence of relapse (CIR) in a randomized trial comparing efficacy of dasatinib vs. imatinib with chemotherapy in first diagnosed Ph + BCP-ALL Chinese pediatric patients. Compared to the previous three trials discussed above, the dasatinib dose was increased to 80 mg/m^2, once daily, continuously applied in combination with chemotherapy (adapted AIEOP BFM 2009 schedule). Imatinib has been dosed slightly reduced compared to AALL0031 and EsPhALL, 300 mg/m^2, orally, daily. Based on alternative dosing schedules of imatinib and dasatinib, all outcome parameters were in favor of dasatinib compared to imatinib: 4-year EFS 71.0% vs. 49.8%, 4-year OS 88.4% vs. 69.2%, cumulative risk of relapse 19.8 vs. 35.4 for dasatinib vs. imatinib cohorts, respectively [109].

Second line approaches take into account BCR-ABL fusion protein resistance mutations and seek for development of potent TKIs and combinations of the latter with immunotherapeutic and non-targeted compounds, to overcome resistance in second and higher lines of therapy. Pfeifer et al. published a comprehensive analysis of BCR-ABL tyrosine kinase domain mutations in patients while on imatinib therapy over the course of first line therapy compared to salvage treatments [110]. The kinetics and the composition of mutations differed significantly between these two groups. Patients on imatinib salvage treatment showed a significant increase of *BCR-ABL* resistance mutations including T315I,

E255K/V, and Y253H. The proportion of mutated alleles increased over time and exceeded the cut-off of 10E-07 in 23% of patients at start of imatinib treatment, 29% of patients after 2 weeks and 59% patients after 4 weeks of the relapse treatment. This kind of increase has not been observed in first diagnosed BCR-ABL leukemia [110].

Aubert et al. retrospectively analyzed treatment and outcome in a pediatric population of 27 first relapsed Ph + -ALL patients and compared efficacy of imatinib to second and third generation TKI [111]. Twenty-two percent relapsed after allogeneic HSCT performed in first ALL remission. All patients demonstrated a p190 BCR-ABL transcript. Of 17 patients molecularly tested, no resistance mutation was detected in 59% of patients, a T315I in 23%, a Y253H in 12% and an E459K in 6% of patients. All patients received chemotherapy in combination with TKI based on physician's choice. Only the minority of patients received blinatumomab (3 pts) and 1 patient received CAR-T cell therapy. Allogeneic HSCT has been performed in 78% of patients in CR2. Eighty-eight percent changed their TKI at time of relapse compared to front-line treatment, mostly to dasatinib (58%). Ponatinib has been applied in two patients with T315I and in 5 patients of the whole cohort. Outcome analysis demonstrated a 4-year EFS, OS, and CIR rate after first Ph + ALL relapse of 60.9%, 76.1%, and 35.8%, respectively. Three out of three patients treated with imatinib lacking a resistance mutation at relapse survived, one of two treated with nilotinib (one was T315I mutated), four of five treated with ponatinib, and 10/15 treated with dasatinib (one was T315I mutated; $p = 0.58$ for the OS ponatinib vs. dasatinib, and $p = 0.08$ for CIR ponatinib (16.7%) vs. dasatinib (40,8%). The 5-year CIR for treatment with dasatinib was 40.8% and that for ponatinib 16.7% ($p = 0.08$) [111]. Consequently, the authors discuss a tendency for higher efficacy of ponatinib, which might need higher patient numbers to become significant [111].

Abou Dalle retrospectively analyzed the treatment and outcome in adult relapsed Ph + ALL [112]. Compared to the pediatric population, OS has been inferior (20%), as has been the rate of transition to allogeneic HSCT (41%). The transplant-related mortality has been very high (TRM 53%). Of 8 patients demonstrating a T315I mutation, five were treated with ponatinib. Impact of TKI in relapsed adult Ph + ALL demonstrated that a major molecular response could be achieved in 55% ($n = 5/9$) of patients on ponatinib, in 71% ($n = 15/21$) of patients on second generation TKI, in none ($n = 0/4$) of the patients on imatinib, and in only in one patient on no TKI ($n = 1/11$; treated on single agent inotuzumab ozogamicin). The CR2 rate was 100% in patients treated with ponatinib, 92% with second generation TKI (dasatinib, nilotinib, and bosutinib), 80% with imatinib, and 25% with no TKI. In line with the pediatric trial, the authors were not able to demonstrate a significant superiority of ponatinib over second generation TKI [112]. Ongoing early clinical trials of ponatinib in combination with a chemotherapeutic backbone (NCT04501614) or as a monotherapy (NCT03934372) in pediatric hematological conditions including relapsed Ph + ALL will provide data in near future and might enable more insight into the efficacy and safety profile of this agent in the relapsed situation.

Based on very promising results from trials combining dasatinib [113] and ponatinib [114] with immunotherapeutic approaches, future hematologic trials in the pediatric population might focus on these combinations. Foà published promising results of a chemotherapy free treatment regimen of dasatinib in combination with blinatumomab in newly diagnosed Ph + adult ALL patients [113]. The treatment included a short steroid pre-phase of 7 days, dasatinib 140 mg, orally, QD for 31 days in combination with steroid, followed by the combination of dasatinib and blinatumomab for up to five cycles and intrathecal CNS directed therapy. Decision to proceed to HSCT has been made by local investigators. The authors included 63 patients, of whom 98% achieved CR and, after five repetitive cycles of blinatumomab, 72% achieved a molecular response. Disease free survival (DFS) and OS after a median FU of 18 months have been reported as 88% and 95%, respectively. Importantly, patients with IKZF deletion other than IKZFplus showed inferior

DFS and OS of 92% and 64% and 93% and 82% respectively [113]. IKZF deletions were detected in 56.8% of pediatric patients in the COG AALL 0622 clinical trial, conferring an inferior outcome in the SR but not in the HR cohort [106]. Foà reported that 24 patients of the whole cohort, the majority (74%) MRD positive after end of induction, proceeded to HSCT. Only one of these patients received chemotherapy prior to HSCT and 5 patients switched to ponatinib prior to HSCT. Remarkably, transplant related mortality has been very low reported to be 4% [113].

Based on these promising results, Jabbour evaluated ponatinib with blinatumomab in adult newly diagnosed ($n = 40$, 67%) and R/R ($n = 14$, 23%) Ph + ALL patients [114]. Thirty percent of newly diagnosed Ph + ALL patients were pretreated with induction chemotherapy before enrolment and entered the trial in hematologic remission. Ninety-three percent of evaluable patients demonstrated CR after ponatinib/blinatumomab induction and 92% had MRD negativity after one cycle and all patients were MRD negative after the second cycle; 1-year EFS and OS reached 95% and 95%, respectively. In the relapsed and refractory cohort 85% achieved complete response after one cycle and MRD negativity was observed in 93% of patients after two cycles. Only one patient of the newly diagnosed cohort underwent HSCT, 97% of patients in that cohort were in ongoing hematological response without further consolidation chemotherapy. Forty-six percent of the responding patients in the refractory cohort proceeded to allogeneic HSCT. At time of report 38% were in ongoing hematological response. One-year EFS and OS reached 57% and 79%, respectively. Four of the 5 patients with ongoing response >1 year underwent allogeneic HSCT [115].

Based on the very low HSCT rate and promising outcome measures of the TKI and immunotherapy approaches these might be considered for further evaluation in pediatric front- and second line clinical trials. Currently, ponatinib and olverembatinib, representing highly effective multikinase inhibitors, which are active in T315I mutated ALL are evaluated in combination with chemotherapy in an international multicenter clinical trial in pediatric patients with R/R hematologic neoplasms (ponatinib: NCT04501614; [116], olverembatinib: 14 years and older NCT05376852, children NCT05521204). Asciminib, another BCR-ABL targeting compound acting through an alternative binding site to inhibit BCR-ABL function and downstream effects, is currently evaluated in pediatric patients with CML and failure or intolerance to the most recent TKI therapy at enrolment (NCT04925479, [117]). Results of these ongoing trials will be awaited in the upcoming years.

23.3 Perspective

In the era of immunotherapy with highly effective bispecific compounds like blinatumomab [118, 119], chemotherapy coupled antibody conjugates like inotuzumab-ozogamicin [5] and CAR-T cells [120, 121], targeted compounds in treatment of pediatric hematologic disease needs a repositioning and reconsideration. Will there be no further need to specifically target actionable lesions based on a particular alteration in pediatric ALL patients? Will targeted compounds be on retreat based on questionable need and side effects?

As demonstrated in the last section on Ph + and Ph-like (ABLclass) ALL, indeed immunotherapy is on the stage, but targeted treatment has an established role in these leukemias with proven benefit. The current approach in these diseases is focused on eliminating toxic chemotherapeutic elements by TKIs which have been combined with blinatumomab. Indeed, the combinations proved to be highly efficacious in first diagnosed and R/R ALL patients, enabling even substitution of the most intensive current consolidation—allo-HSCT in a subset of adult ALL patients. In addition, proteasome inhibitors are synergistic with daratumumab in multiple myeloma [122]. Venetoclax is improving outcome when combined with DLI in AML [123] and enhances macrophage function in ALL [124], clearly presenting a rationale for further investigation in combination with immunotherapeutic agents. Targeted compounds that inhibit immunotherapeutic function clearly might be less attractive in the future.

However, inhibitory effects of targeted agents rarely effect all types of immune cells [125] and in contrast these compounds might enhance the immune response. The preclinical evaluation focusing on this question will need up to date preclinical models, able to determine the immunogenic effects of targeted compounds in fully immunocompetent organisms.

Based on poor outcome, limited efficacy of immunotherapeutic approaches and/or lack of the latter, *MLLr* Leukemia, extramedullary relapsed ALL and T-ALL will currently stay in the focus of targeted therapy development. Menin inhibitor combinations with immunotherapeutic approaches might be investigated for safety and efficacy in the future, carefully evaluating side effects of simultaneous differentiation syndrome and immune activation in preclinical models.

In T-ALL, CAR-T cell therapy is on the edge [126] and might improve the situation of these patients frequently experiencing a poor prognosis. However, as in BCP-ALL relapses post CAR-T relapses will occur and therapeutic options be requested by patients and parents—a situation targeted therapy could serve as an effective and safe palliation or a bridge allowing second HSCT.

In CNS relapses, more data on CNS PK on most targeted agents is highly needed since crossing of the blood–brain barrier might be of high importance to exert activity in patients refractory to CNS-directed intrathecal treatment or palliative radiation. Moreover, a better understanding of the biology of CNS leukemia including better preclinical models is needed in order to develop new therapeutic options for these patients.

Deep sequencing and molecular stratification, improved outcome of patients treated within first- and second-line trials already led to very small patient populations and ultra-rare, individual medical conditions. International collaboration and collaborative master trials like HEM-iSMART, PEDAL or GloBNHL might allow to improve the situation of these patients with complex medical needs, since they offer clear documentation of toxicity and safety data to avoid ineffective and toxic off-label and compassionate use treatments on an individual basis without proper testing in clinical trials. Intensive collaboration between collaborative groups is needed to rapidly move promising new agents to frontline therapy, as showcased by blinatumomab and inotuzumab which are already integrated in treatment for patients with newly diagnosed ALL.

23.4 Conclusion

The multiplicity of targets and targeted agents defined in the past through rapid development of new techniques enabled significant improvement of prognosis in defined patient subgroups. New developments will mainly follow three pathways. One will focus on optimization of treatment schedules in particular combination of targeted, immunotherapeutic and chemotherapeutic agents of known targeted agents to improve efficacy and reduce toxicity by sparing chemotherapeutic agents. These might be developed in pilot studies providing proof of principle, followed by randomized trials where needed. The second path will further focus on target identification and early drug development. Promising agents in early development which are not discussed in detail here among others are third-generation NOTCH Inhibitors for T-ALL, nuclear exportin inhibitors and PIM inhibitors, HDAC inhibitors, hypomethylating agents in hematologic malignancies and CBP/p300 inhibitors in MLLr ALL. The third may focus on particular areas of need like central nervous system disease or how to tackle the microenvironment role in these conditions.

The development will lead to further stratification into very small well-defined subgroups of leukemia patients which calls for strong collaboration to enable high-quality scientific progress.

References

1. Greaves M. A causal mechanism for childhood acute lymphoblastic leukaemia. Nat Rev Cancer. 2018;18:471–84. https://doi.org/10.1038/s41568-018-0015-6.
2. Eckert C, Parker C, Moorman AV, Irving JA, Kirschner-Schwabe R, Groeneveld-Krentz S, Revesz T,

Hoogerbrugge P, Hancock J, Sutton R, et al. Risk factors and outcomes in children with high-risk B-cell precursor and T-cell relapsed acute lymphoblastic leukaemia: combined analysis of ALLR3 and ALL-REZ BFM 2002 clinical trials. Eur J Cancer. 2021;151:175–89. https://doi.org/10.1016/j.ejca.2021.03.034.
3. von Stackelberg A, Locatelli F, Zugmaier G, Handgretinger R, Trippett TM, Rizzari C, Bader P, O'Brien MM, Brethon B, Bhojwani D, et al. Phase I/phase II study of blinatumomab in pediatric patients with relapsed/refractory acute lymphoblastic Leukemia. J Clin Oncol. 2016;34:4381–9. https://doi.org/10.1200/JCO.2016.67.3301.
4. Laetsch TW, Maude SL, Rives S, Hiramatsu H, Bittencourt H, Bader P, Baruchel A, Boyer M, Moerloose BD, Qayed M, et al. Three-year update of tisagenlecleucel in pediatric and young adult patients with relapsed/refractory acute lymphoblastic leukemia in the ELIANA trial. J Clin Oncol. 2023;41:1664–9. https://doi.org/10.1200/jco.22.00642.
5. Brivio E, Locatelli F, Lopez-Yurda M, Malone A, Diaz-de-Heredia C, Bielorai B, Rossig C, van der Velden VHJ, Ammerlaan ACJ, Thano A, et al. A phase 1 study of inotuzumab ozogamicin in pediatric relapsed/refractory acute lymphoblastic leukemia (ITCC-059 study). Blood. 2021;137:1582–90. https://doi.org/10.1182/blood.2020007848.
6. van Tilburg CM, Pfaff E, Pajtler KW, Langenberg KPS, Fiesel P, Jones BC, Balasubramanian GP, Stark S, Johann PD, Blattner-Johnson M, et al. The Pediatric Precision Oncology INFORM Registry: clinical outcome and benefit for patients with very high-evidence targets. Cancer Discov. 2021;11:2764–79. https://doi.org/10.1158/2159-8290.CD-21-0094.
7. Berlanga P, Pierron G, Lacroix L, Chicard M, Adam de Beaumais T, Marchais A, Harttrampf AC, Iddir Y, Larive A, Soriano Fernandez A, et al. The European MAPPYACTS trial: precision medicine program in pediatric and adolescent patients with recurrent malignancies. Cancer Discov. 2022;12:1266. https://doi.org/10.1158/2159-8290.CD-21-1136.
8. Wong M, Mayoh C, Lau LMS, Khuong-Quang DA, Pinese M, Kumar A, Barahona P, Wilkie EE, Sullivan P, Bowen-James R, et al. Whole genome, transcriptome and methylome profiling enhances actionable target discovery in high-risk pediatric cancer. Nat Med. 2020;26:1742–53. https://doi.org/10.1038/s41591-020-1072-4.
9. Pikman Y, Tasian SK, Sulis ML, Stevenson K, Blonquist TM, Apsel Winger B, Cooper TM, Pauly M, Maloney KW, Burke MJ, et al. Matched targeted therapy for pediatric patients with relapsed, refractory, or high-risk leukemias: a report from the LEAP Consortium. Cancer Discov. 2021;11:1424–39. https://doi.org/10.1158/2159-8290.CD-20-0564.
10. Frismantas V, Dobay MP, Rinaldi A, Tchinda J, Dunn SH, Kunz J, Richter-Pechanska P, Marovca B, Pail O, Jenni S, et al. Ex vivo drug response profiling detects recurrent sensitivity patterns in drug-resistant acute lymphoblastic leukemia. Blood. 2017;129:e26–37. https://doi.org/10.1182/blood-2016-09-738070.
11. Lissat A, Maniotis D, Nosswitz M, Alten J, Jenni S, Tsai Y-C, Cario G, La Starza R, Hrusak O, Kulozik AE, et al. In vitro drug response profiling in BCP- and T-ALL primary samples adds a robust functional layer enabling optimized guidance of individualized therapy in relapsed and refractory pediatric acute leukemia patients. Blood. 2020;136:15–6. https://doi.org/10.1182/blood-2020-142314.
12. Neel DV, Shulman DS, DuBois SG. Timing of first-in-child trials of FDA-approved oncology drugs. Eur J Cancer. 2019;112:49–56. https://doi.org/10.1016/j.ejca.2019.02.011.
13. Schoot RA, Otth MA, Frederix GWJ, Leufkens HGM, Vassal G. Market access to new anticancer medicines for children and adolescents with cancer in Europe. Eur J Cancer. 2022;165:146–53. https://doi.org/10.1016/j.ejca.2022.01.034.
14. Barry E, Walsh JA, Weinrich SL, Beaupre D, Blasi E, Arenson DR, Jacobs IA. Navigating the regulatory landscape to develop pediatric oncology drugs: expert opinion recommendations. Paediatr Drugs. 2021;23:381–94. https://doi.org/10.1007/s40272-021-00455-1.
15. Pearson ADJ, Weiner SL, Adamson PC, Karres D, Reaman G, Rousseau R, Blanc P, Norga K, Skolnik J, Kearns P, et al. ACCELERATE - five years accelerating cancer drug development for children and adolescents. Eur J Cancer. 2022;166:145–64. https://doi.org/10.1016/j.ejca.2022.01.033.
16. de Rojas T, Kearns P, Blanc P, Skolnik J, Fox E, Knox L, Rousseau R, Doz F, Bird N, Pearson AJ, et al. Changing incentives to ACCELERATE drug development for paediatric cancer. Cancer Med. 2023;12:8825–37. https://doi.org/10.1002/cam4.5627.
17. Al-Mahayri ZN, AlAhmad MM, Ali BR. Long-term effects of pediatric acute lymphoblastic leukemia chemotherapy: can recent findings inform old strategies? Front Oncol. 2021;11:710163. https://doi.org/10.3389/fonc.2021.710163.
18. Laetsch TW, DuBois SG, Bender JG, Macy ME, Moreno L. Opportunities and challenges in drug development for pediatric cancers. Cancer Discov. 2021;11:545–59. https://doi.org/10.1158/2159-8290.CD-20-0779.
19. Irving J, Matheson E, Minto L, Blair H, Case M, Halsey C, Swidenbank I, Ponthan F, Kirschner-Schwabe R, Groeneveld-Krentz S, et al. Ras pathway mutations are prevalent in relapsed childhood acute lymphoblastic leukemia and confer sensitivity to MEK inhibition. Blood. 2014;124:3420–30. https://doi.org/10.1182/blood-2014-04-531871.
20. Jerchel IS, Hoogkamer AQ, Aries IM, Steeghs EMP, Boer JM, Besselink NJM, Boeree A, van de Ven C, de Groot-Kruseman HA, de Haas V, et al. RAS pathway mutations as a predictive biomarker for treatment adaptation in pediatric B-cell precursor acute lympho-

blastic leukemia. Leukemia. 2018;32:931–40. https://doi.org/10.1038/leu.2017.303.
21. Richter-Pechanska P, Kunz JB, Hof J, Zimmermann M, Rausch T, Bandapalli OR, Orlova E, Scapinello G, Sagi JC, Stanulla M, et al. Identification of a genetically defined ultra-high-risk group in relapsed pediatric T-lymphoblastic leukemia. Blood Cancer J. 2017;7:e523. https://doi.org/10.1038/bcj.2017.3.
22. Liu Y, Easton J, Shao Y, Maciaszek J, Wang Z, Wilkinson MR, McCastlain K, Edmonson M, Pounds SB, Shi L, et al. The genomic landscape of pediatric and young adult T-lineage acute lymphoblastic leukemia. Nat Genet. 2017;49:1211–8. https://doi.org/10.1038/ng.3909.
23. Cante-Barrett K, Spijkers-Hagelstein JA, Buijs-Gladdines JG, Uitdehaag JC, Smits WK, van der Zwet J, Buijsman RC, Zaman GJ, Pieters R, Meijerink JP. MEK and PI3K-AKT inhibitors synergistically block activated IL7 receptor signaling in T-cell acute lymphoblastic leukemia. Leukemia. 2016;30:1832–43. https://doi.org/10.1038/leu.2016.83.
24. Kerstjens M, Driessen EM, Willekes M, Pinhancos SS, Schneider P, Pieters R, Stam RW. MEK inhibition is a promising therapeutic strategy for MLL-rearranged infant acute lymphoblastic leukemia patients carrying RAS mutations. Oncotarget. 2017;8:14835–46. https://doi.org/10.18632/oncotarget.11730.
25. Kerstjens M, Pinhancos SS, Castro PG, Schneider P, Wander P, Pieters R, Stam RW. Trametinib inhibits RAS-mutant MLL-rearranged acute lymphoblastic leukemia at specific niche sites and reduces ERK phosphorylation in vivo. Haematologica. 2018;103:e147–50. https://doi.org/10.3324/haematol.2017.174060.
26. Jones CL, Gearheart CM, Fosmire S, Delgado-Martin C, Evensen NA, Bride K, Waanders AJ, Pais F, Wang J, Bhatla T, et al. MAPK signaling cascades mediate distinct glucocorticoid resistance mechanisms in pediatric leukemia. Blood. 2015;126:2202–12. https://doi.org/10.1182/blood-2015-04-639138.
27. van der Zwet JCG, Buijs-Gladdines J, Cordo V, Debets DO, Smits WK, Chen Z, Dylus J, Zaman GJR, Altelaar M, Oshima K, et al. MAPK-ERK is a central pathway in T-cell acute lymphoblastic leukemia that drives steroid resistance. Leukemia. 2021. https://doi.org/10.1038/s41375-021-01291-5.
28. O'Shea JJ, Plenge R. JAK and STAT signaling molecules in immunoregulation and immune-mediated disease. Immunity. 2012;36:542–50. https://doi.org/10.1016/j.immuni.2012.03.014.
29. Vainchenker W, Constantinescu SN. JAK/STAT signaling in hematological malignancies. Oncogene. 2013;32:2601–13. https://doi.org/10.1038/onc.2012.347.
30. Zenatti PP, Ribeiro D, Li W, Zuurbier L, Silva MC, Paganin M, Tritapoe J, Hixon JA, Silveira AB, Cardoso BA, et al. Oncogenic IL7R gain-of-function mutations in childhood T-cell acute lymphoblastic leukemia. Nat Genet. 2011;43:932–9. https://doi.org/10.1038/ng.924.
31. Zhang J, Ding L, Holmfeldt L, Wu G, Heatley SL, Payne-Turner D, Easton J, Chen X, Wang J, Rusch M, et al. The genetic basis of early T-cell precursor acute lymphoblastic leukaemia. Nature. 2012;481:157–63. https://doi.org/10.1038/nature10725.
32. Li Y, Buijs-Gladdines JG, Cante-Barrett K, Stubbs AP, Vroegindeweij EM, Smits WK, van Marion R, Dinjens WN, Horstmann M, Kuiper RP, et al. IL-7 receptor mutations and steroid resistance in pediatric T cell acute lymphoblastic leukemia: a genome sequencing study. PLoS Med. 2016;13:e1002200. https://doi.org/10.1371/journal.pmed.1002200.
33. Steeghs EMP, Jerchel IS, de Goffau-Nobel W, Hoogkamer AQ, Boer JM, Boeree A, van de Ven C, Koudijs MJ, Besselink NJM, de Groot-Kruseman HA, et al. JAK2 aberrations in childhood B-cell precursor acute lymphoblastic leukemia. Oncotarget. 2017;8:89923–38. https://doi.org/10.18632/oncotarget.21027.
34. Senkevitch E, Li W, Hixon JA, Andrews C, Cramer SD, Pauly GT, Back T, Czarra K, Durum SK. Inhibiting Janus kinase 1 and BCL-2 to treat T cell acute lymphoblastic leukemia with IL7-Ralpha mutations. Oncotarget. 2018;9:22605–17. https://doi.org/10.18632/oncotarget.25194.
35. Maude SL, Dolai S, Delgado-Martin C, Vincent T, Robbins A, Selvanathan A, Ryan T, Hall J, Wood AC, Tasian SK, et al. Efficacy of JAK/STAT pathway inhibition in murine xenograft models of early T-cell precursor (ETP) acute lymphoblastic leukemia. Blood. 2015;125:1759–67. https://doi.org/10.1182/blood-2014-06-580480.
36. Bhm JW, Sia KCS, Jones C, Evans K, Mariana A, Pang I, Failes T, Zhong L, Mayoh C, Landman R, et al. Combination efficacy of ruxolitinib with standard-of-care drugs in CRLF2-rearranged Ph-like acute lymphoblastic leukemia. Leukemia. 2021;35:3101–12. https://doi.org/10.1038/s41375-021-01248-8.
37. Loh ML, Tasian SK, Rabin KR, Brown P, Magoon D, Reid JM, Chen X, Ahern CH, Weigel BJ, Blaney SM. A phase 1 dosing study of ruxolitinib in children with relapsed or refractory solid tumors, leukemias, or myeloproliferative neoplasms: a Children's Oncology Group Phase 1 Consortium study (ADVL1011). Pediatr Blood Cancer. 2015;62:1717–24. https://doi.org/10.1002/pbc.25575.
38. Tasian SK, Assad A, Hunter DS, Du Y, Loh ML. A phase 2 study of ruxolitinib with chemotherapy in children with Philadelphia chromosome-like acute lymphoblastic leukemia (INCB18424-269/AALL1521): dose-finding results from the part 1 safety phase. Blood. 2018;132:555. https://doi.org/10.1182/blood-2018-99-110221.
39. Asghar U, Witkiewicz AK, Turner NC, Knudsen ES. The history and future of targeting cyclin-dependent kinases in cancer therapy. Nat Rev Drug Discov. 2015;14:130–46. https://doi.org/10.1038/nrd4504.

40. Molenaar JJ, Koster J, Ebus ME, van Sluis P, Westerhout EM, de Preter K, Gisselsson D, Ora I, Speleman F, Caron HN, et al. Copy number defects of G1-cell cycle genes in neuroblastoma are frequent and correlate with high expression of E2F target genes and a poor prognosis. Genes Chromosomes Cancer. 2012;51:10–9. https://doi.org/10.1002/gcc.20926.
41. Harttrampf AC, Lacroix L, Deloger M, Deschamps F, Puget S, Auger N, Vielh P, Varlet P, Balogh Z, Abbou S, et al. Molecular screening for cancer treatment optimization (MOSCATO-01) in pediatric patients: a single-institutional prospective molecular stratification trial. Clin Cancer Res. 2017;23:6101–12. https://doi.org/10.1158/1078-0432.CCR-17-0381.
42. Koumenis C, Giaccia A. Transformed cells require continuous activity of RNA polymerase II to resist oncogene-induced apoptosis. Mol Cell Biol. 1997;17:7306–16. https://doi.org/10.1128/MCB.17.12.7306.
43. Pikman Y, Alexe G, Roti G, Conway AS, Furman A, Lee ES, Place AE, Kim S, Saran C, Modiste R, et al. Synergistic drug combinations with a CDK4/6 inhibitor in T-cell acute lymphoblastic Leukemia. Clin Cancer Res. 2017;23:1012–24. https://doi.org/10.1158/1078-0432.CCR-15-2869.
44. Bautista F, Paoletti X, Rubino J, Brard C, Rezai K, Nebchi S, Andre N, Aerts I, De Carli E, van Eijkelenburg N, et al. Phase I or II study of ribociclib in combination with topotecan-temozolomide or everolimus in children with advanced malignancies: arms A and B of the AcSe-ESMART trial. J Clin Oncol. 2021;39:3546. https://doi.org/10.1200/JCO.21.01152.
45. Raetz EA, Teachey DT, Minard C, Liu X, Norris R, Reid J, Beeles T, Gore L, Fox E, Loh ML, et al. Safety of palbociclib in combination with chemotherapy in pediatric and young adult patients with relapsed/refractory acute lymphoblastic Leukemia and lymphoma: a Children's Oncology Group pilot study. Blood. 2020;136:20–1. https://doi.org/10.1182/blood-2020-141572.
46. Tasian SK, Teachey DT, Rheingold SR. Targeting the PI3K/mTOR pathway in pediatric hematologic malignancies. Front Oncol. 2014;4:108. https://doi.org/10.3389/fonc.2014.00108.
47. Moschetta M, Reale A, Marasco C, Vacca A, Carratù MR. Therapeutic targeting of the mTOR-signalling pathway in cancer: benefits and limitations. Br J Pharmacol. 2014;171:3801–13. https://doi.org/10.1111/bph.12749.
48. Hughes M, Hao M, Luu M. PIK3CA vascular overgrowth syndromes: an update. Curr Opin Pediatr. 2020;32:539–46. https://doi.org/10.1097/mop.0000000000000923.
49. Girardi T, Vicente C, Cools J, De Keersmaecker K. The genetics and molecular biology of T-ALL. Blood. 2017;129:1113–23. https://doi.org/10.1182/blood-2016-10-706465.
50. Palomero T, Sulis ML, Cortina M, Real PJ, Barnes K, Ciofani M, Caparros E, Buteau J, Brown K, Perkins SL, et al. Mutational loss of PTEN induces resistance to NOTCH1 inhibition in T-cell leukemia. Nat Med. 2007;13:1203–10. https://doi.org/10.1038/nm1636.
51. Rheingold SR, Tasian SK, Whitlock JA, Teachey DT, Borowitz MJ, Liu X, Minard CG, Fox E, Weigel BJ, Blaney SM. A phase 1 trial of temsirolimus and intensive re-induction chemotherapy for 2nd or greater relapse of acute lymphoblastic leukaemia: a Children's Oncology Group study (ADVL1114). Br J Haematol. 2017;177:467–74. https://doi.org/10.1111/bjh.14569.
52. Tasian SK, Silverman LB, Whitlock JA, Sposto R, Loftus JP, Schafer ES, Schultz KR, Hutchinson RJ, Gaynon PS, Orgel E, et al. Temsirolimus combined with cyclophosphamide and etoposide for pediatric patients with relapsed/refractory acute lymphoblastic leukemia: a Therapeutic Advances in Childhood Leukemia Consortium trial (TACL 2014-001). Haematologica. 2022;107:2295–303. https://doi.org/10.3324/haematol.2021.279520.
53. Place AE, Pikman Y, Stevenson KE, Harris MH, Pauly M, Sulis ML, Hijiya N, Gore L, Cooper TM, Loh ML, et al. Phase I trial of the mTOR inhibitor everolimus in combination with multi-agent chemotherapy in relapsed childhood acute lymphoblastic leukemia. Pediatr Blood Cancer. 2018;65:e27062. https://doi.org/10.1002/pbc.27062.
54. LaPlante G, Zhang W. Targeting the ubiquitin-proteasome system for cancer therapeutics by small-molecule inhibitors. Cancers (Basel). 2021;13:3079. https://doi.org/10.3390/cancers13123079.
55. Horton TM, Pati D, Plon SE, Thompson PA, Bomgaars LR, Adamson PC, Ingle AM, Wright J, Brockman AH, Paton M, et al. A phase 1 study of the proteasome inhibitor bortezomib in pediatric patients with refractory leukemia: a Children's Oncology Group study. Clin Cancer Res. 2007;13:1516–22. https://doi.org/10.1158/1078-0432.CCR-06-2173.
56. Messinger YH, Gaynon PS, Sposto R, van der Giessen J, Eckroth E, Malvar J, Bostrom BC. Bortezomib with chemotherapy is highly active in advanced B-precursor acute lymphoblastic leukemia: Therapeutic Advances in Childhood Leukemia & Lymphoma (TACL) Study. Blood. 2012;120:285–90. https://doi.org/10.1182/blood-2012-04-418640.
57. Teachey DT, Devidas M, Wood BL, Chen Z, Hayashi RJ, Hermiston ML, Annett RD, Archer JH, Asselin BL, August KJ, et al. Children's Oncology Group trial AALL1231: a phase III clinical trial testing bortezomib in newly diagnosed T-cell acute lymphoblastic leukemia and lymphoma. J Clin Oncol. 2022;40:2106–18. https://doi.org/10.1200/jco.21.02678.
58. Burke MJ, Ziegler DS, Bautista F, Attarbaschi A, Gore L, Locatelli F, O'Brien MM, Pauly M, Kormany WN, Tian S, et al. Phase 1b study of carfilzomib with induction chemotherapy in pediatric relapsed/refractory acute lymphoblastic leukemia. Pediatr Blood Cancer. 2022;69:e29999. https://doi.org/10.1002/pbc.29999.

59. Singh R, Letai A, Sarosiek K. Regulation of apoptosis in health and disease: the balancing act of BCL-2 family proteins. Nat Rev Mol Cell Biol. 2019;20:175–93. https://doi.org/10.1038/s41580-018-0089-8.
60. Anderson MA, Deng J, Seymour JF, Tam C, Kim SY, Fein J, Yu L, Brown JR, Westerman D, Si EG, et al. The BCL2 selective inhibitor venetoclax induces rapid onset apoptosis of CLL cells in patients via a TP53-independent mechanism. Blood. 2016;127:3215–24. https://doi.org/10.1182/blood-2016-01-688796.
61. Huber H, Edenhofer S, Estenfelder S, Stilgenbauer S. Profile of venetoclax and its potential in the context of treatment of relapsed or refractory chronic lymphocytic leukemia. Onco Targets Ther. 2017;10:645–56. https://doi.org/10.2147/OTT.S102646.
62. Jing D, Bhadri VA, Beck D, Thoms JAI, Yakob NA, Wong JWH, Knezevic K, Pimanda JE, Lock RB. Opposing regulation of BIM and BCL2 controls glucocorticoid-induced apoptosis of pediatric acute lymphoblastic leukemia cells. Blood. 2015;125:273–83. https://doi.org/10.1182/blood-2014-05-576470.
63. Fidyt K, Pastorczak A, Cyran J, Crump NT, Goral A, Madzio J, Muchowicz A, Poprzeczko M, Domka K, Komorowski L, et al. Potent, p53-independent induction of NOXA sensitizes MLL-rearranged B-cell acute lymphoblastic leukemia cells to venetoclax. Oncogene. 2022;41:1600–9. https://doi.org/10.1038/s41388-022-02196-y.
64. Wirth A-K, Wange L, Vosberg S, Henrich K-O, Rausch C, Özdemir E, Zeller CM, Richter D, Feuchtinger T, Kaller M, et al. In vivo PDX CRISPR/Cas9 screens reveal mutual therapeutic targets to overcome heterogeneous acquired chemo-resistance. Leukemia. 2022;36:2863–74. https://doi.org/10.1038/s41375-022-01726-7.
65. Findley HW, Gu L, Yeager AM, Zhou M. Expression and regulation of Bcl-2, Bcl-xl, and Bax correlate with p53 status and sensitivity to apoptosis in childhood acute lymphoblastic leukemia. Blood. 1997;89:2986–93.
66. Nechiporuk T, Kurtz SE, Nikolova O, Liu T, Jones CL, D'Alessandro A, Culp-Hill R, d'Almeida A, Joshi SK, Rosenberg M, et al. The TP53 apoptotic network is a primary mediator of resistance to BCL2 inhibition in AML cells. Cancer Discov. 2019;9:910–25. https://doi.org/10.1158/2159-8290.Cd-19-0125.
67. De Smedt R, Morscio J, Goossens S, Van Vlierberghe P. Targeting steroid resistance in T-cell acute lymphoblastic leukemia. Blood Rev. 2019;38:100591. https://doi.org/10.1016/j.blre.2019.100591.
68. Peirs S, Matthijssens F, Goossens S, Van de Walle I, Ruggero K, de Bock CE, Degryse S, Cante-Barrett K, Briot D, Clappier E, et al. ABT-199 mediated inhibition of BCL-2 as a novel therapeutic strategy in T-cell acute lymphoblastic leukemia. Blood. 2014;124:3738–47. https://doi.org/10.1182/blood-2014-05-574566.
69. Van der Meulen J, Van Roy N, Van Vlierberghe P, Speleman F. The epigenetic landscape of T-cell acute lymphoblastic leukemia. Int J Biochem Cell Biol. 2014;53:547–57. https://doi.org/10.1016/j.biocel.2014.04.015.
70. Suryani S, Carol H, Chonghaile TN, Frismantas V, Sarmah C, High L, Bornhauser B, Cowley MJ, Szymanska B, Evans K, et al. Cell and molecular determinants of in vivo efficacy of the BH3 mimetic ABT-263 against pediatric acute lymphoblastic leukemia xenografts. Clin Cancer Res. 2014;20:4520–31. https://doi.org/10.1158/1078-0432.CCR-14-0259.
71. Roberts AW, Seymour JF, Brown JR, Wierda WG, Kipps TJ, Khaw SL, Carney DA, He SZ, Huang DC, Xiong H, et al. Substantial susceptibility of chronic lymphocytic leukemia to BCL2 inhibition: results of a phase I study of navitoclax in patients with relapsed or refractory disease. J Clin Oncol. 2012;30:488–96. https://doi.org/10.1200/JCO.2011.34.7898.
72. Mason KD, Carpinelli MR, Fletcher JI, Collinge JE, Hilton AA, Ellis S, Kelly PN, Ekert PG, Metcalf D, Roberts AW, et al. Programmed anuclear cell death delimits platelet life span. Cell. 2007;128:1173–86. https://doi.org/10.1016/j.cell.2007.01.037.
73. Rubnitz JE, Alexander TB, Laetsch TW, Khaw SL, Pullarkat VA, Opferman JT, Roberts KG, Rosenwinkel L, Tong B, Pesko JC, et al. Venetoclax and navitoclax in pediatric patients with acute lymphoblastic leukemia and lymphoblastic lymphoma. Blood. 2020;136:12–3. https://doi.org/10.1182/blood-2020-134582.
74. Pullarkat VA, Lacayo NJ, Jabbour E, Rubnitz JE, Bajel A, Laetsch TW, Leonard J, Colace SI, Khaw SL, Fleming SA, et al. Venetoclax and navitoclax in combination with chemotherapy in patients with relapsed or refractory acute lymphoblastic leukemia and lymphoblastic lymphoma. Cancer Discov. 2021;11:1440–53. https://doi.org/10.1158/2159-8290.CD-20-1465.
75. Gibson CJ, Davids MS. BCL-2 antagonism to target the intrinsic mitochondrial pathway of apoptosis. Clin Cancer Res. 2015;21:5021–9. https://doi.org/10.1158/1078-0432.CCR-15-0364.
76. Place AE, Karol SE, Forlenza CJ, Gambart M, Cooper TM, Fraser C, Cario G, O'Brien MM, Gerber NU, Barnette P, Reinhardt D, Ramsingh G, Tong B, Unnebrink K, Vishwam D, Loh ML. Pediatric patients with relapsed/refractory acute lymphoblastic leukemia harboring heterogeneous genomic profiles respond to venetoclax in combination with chemotherapy. Blood. 2020;136:ASH abstract.
77. Wilson WH, O'Connor OA, Czuczman MS, LaCasce AS, Gerecitano JF, Leonard JP, Tulpule A, Dunleavy K, Xiong H, Chiu YL, et al. Navitoclax, a targeted high-affinity inhibitor of BCL-2, in lymphoid malignancies: a phase 1 dose-escalation study of safety, pharmacokinetics, pharmacodynamics, and antitumour activity. Lancet Oncol. 2010;11:1149–59. https://doi.org/10.1016/S1470-2045(10)70261-8.
78. Biondi A, Cimino G, Pieters R, Pui C-H. Biological and therapeutic aspects of infant leukemia. Blood. 2000;96:24–33. https://doi.org/10.1182/blood.V96.1.24.

79. van der Linden MH, Valsecchi MG, De Lorenzo P, Möricke A, Janka G, Leblanc TM, Felice M, Biondi A, Campbell M, Hann I, et al. Outcome of congenital acute lymphoblastic leukemia treated on the Interfant-99 protocol. Blood. 2009;114:3764–8. https://doi.org/10.1182/blood-2009-02-204214.
80. Krivtsov AV, Armstrong SA. MLL translocations, histone modifications and leukaemia stem-cell development. Nat Rev Cancer. 2007;7:823–33. https://doi.org/10.1038/nrc2253.
81. Borkin D, He S, Miao H, Kempinska K, Pollock J, Chase J, Purohit T, Malik B, Zhao T, Wang J, et al. Pharmacologic inhibition of the Menin-MLL interaction blocks progression of MLL leukemia in vivo. Cancer Cell. 2015;27:589–602. https://doi.org/10.1016/j.ccell.2015.02.016.
82. Stein EM, Garcia-Manero G, Rizzieri DA, Tibes R, Berdeja JG, Savona MR, Jongen-Lavrenic M, Altman JK, Thomson B, Blakemore SJ, et al. The DOT1L inhibitor pinometostat reduces H3K79 methylation and has modest clinical activity in adult acute leukemia. Blood. 2018;131:2661–9. https://doi.org/10.1182/blood-2017-12-818948.
83. Borkin D, Pollock J, Kempinska K, Purohit T, Li X, Wen B, Zhao T, Miao H, Shukla S, He M, et al. Property focused structure-based optimization of small molecule inhibitors of the protein-protein interaction between menin and mixed lineage leukemia (MLL). J Med Chem. 2016;59:892–913. https://doi.org/10.1021/acs.jmedchem.5b01305.
84. He S, Malik B, Borkin D, Miao H, Shukla S, Kempinska K, Purohit T, Wang J, Chen L, Parkin B, et al. Menin-MLL inhibitors block oncogenic transformation by MLL-fusion proteins in a fusion partner-independent manner. Leukemia. 2016;30:508–13. https://doi.org/10.1038/leu.2015.144.
85. Aubrey BJ, Cutler JA, Bourgeois W, Donovan KA, Gu S, Hatton C, Perlee S, Perner F, Rahnamoun H, Theall ACP, et al. IKAROS and MENIN coordinate therapeutically actionable leukemogenic gene expression in MLL-r acute myeloid leukemia. Nat Cancer. 2022;3:595–613. https://doi.org/10.1038/s43018-022-00366-1.
86. Yokoyama A, Cleary ML. Menin critically links MLL proteins with LEDGF on cancer-associated target genes. Cancer Cell. 2008;14:36–46. https://doi.org/10.1016/j.ccr.2008.05.003.
87. Daigle SR, Olhava EJ, Therkelsen CA, Basavapathruni A, Jin L, Boriack-Sjodin PA, Allain CJ, Klaus CR, Raimondi A, Scott MP, et al. Potent inhibition of DOT1L as treatment of MLL-fusion leukemia. Blood. 2013;122:1017–25. https://doi.org/10.1182/blood-2013-04-497644.
88. Krivtsov AV, Evans K, Gadrey JY, Eschle BK, Hatton C, Uckelmann HJ, Ross KN, Perner F, Olsen SN, Pritchard T, et al. A Menin-MLL inhibitor induces specific chromatin changes and eradicates disease in models of MLL-rearranged leukemia. Cancer Cell. 2019;36:660–673.e611. https://doi.org/10.1016/j.ccell.2019.11.001.
89. Fiskus W, Daver N, Boettcher S, Mill CP, Sasaki K, Birdwell CE, Davis JA, Das K, Takahashi K, Kadia TM, et al. Activity of menin inhibitor ziftomenib (KO-539) as monotherapy or in combinations against AML cells with MLL1 rearrangement or mutant NPM1. Leukemia. 2022;36:2729–33. https://doi.org/10.1038/s41375-022-01707-w.
90. Erba HP, Fathi AT, Issa GC, Altman JK, Montesinos P, Patnaik MM, Foran JM, De Botton S, Baer MR, Schiller GJ, et al. Update on a phase 1/2 first-in-human study of the Menin-KMT2A (MLL) inhibitor ziftomenib (KO-539) in patients with relapsed or refractory acute myeloid leukemia. Blood. 2022;140:153–6. https://doi.org/10.1182/blood-2022-167412.
91. Stein EM, Aldoss I, DiPersio JF, Stone RM, Arellano ML, Rosen G, Meyers ML, Huang Y, Smith S, Bagley RG, et al. Safety and efficacy of menin inhibition in patients (Pts) with MLL-rearranged and NPM1 mutant acute leukemia: a phase (Ph) 1, first-in-human study of SNDX-5613 (AUGMENT 101). Blood. 2021;138:699. https://doi.org/10.1182/blood-2021-146944.
92. Issa GC, Aldoss I, DiPersio J, Cuglievan B, Stone R, Arellano M, Thirman MJ, Patel MR, Dickens DS, Shenoy S, et al. The menin inhibitor revumenib in KMT2A-rearranged or NPM1-mutant leukaemia. Nature. 2023;615:920–4. https://doi.org/10.1038/s41586-023-05812-3.
93. Dzama MM, Steiner M, Rausch J, Sasca D, Schonfeld J, Kunz K, Taubert MC, McGeehan GM, Chen CW, Mupo A, et al. Synergistic targeting of FLT3 mutations in AML via combined menin-MLL and FLT3 inhibition. Blood. 2020;136:2442–56. https://doi.org/10.1182/blood.2020005037.
94. Heikamp EB, Henrich JA, Perner F, Wong EM, Hatton C, Wen Y, Barwe SP, Gopalakrishnapillai A, Xu H, Uckelmann HJ, et al. The menin-MLL1 interaction is a molecular dependency in NUP98-rearranged AML. Blood. 2022;139:894–906. https://doi.org/10.1182/blood.2021012806.
95. Libbrecht C, Xie HM, Kingsley MC, Haladyna JN, Riedel SS, Alikarami F, Lenard A, McGeehan GM, Ernst P, Bernt KM. Menin is necessary for long term maintenance of meningioma-1 driven leukemia. Leukemia. 2021;35:1405–17. https://doi.org/10.1038/s41375-021-01146-z.
96. Yener MD, Numata M, Ekmekci S, Aydın M, Grosveld G, Ozbek U, Gulec C, Anak S, Karaman S, Ozturk G, Akbiyik M, Kandilci A, Az D. Pediatric TEL-AML1-positive acute lymphoblastic leukemia patients show increased MN1 expression. In: EHA Abstract; 2015. p. 100.
97. Liu H. NUP98 rearrangement in B lymphoblastic leukemia with hyperdiploidy. Blood. 2020;136:1011. https://doi.org/10.1182/blood.2020006652.
98. Schultz KR, Prestidge T, Camitta B. Philadelphia chromosome-positive acute lymphoblastic leukemia in children: new and emerging treatment options. Expert Rev Hematol. 2010;3:731–42. https://doi.org/10.1586/ehm.10.60.

99. Tasian SK, Loh ML, Hunger SP. Philadelphia chromosome-like acute lymphoblastic leukemia. Blood. 2017;130:2064–72. https://doi.org/10.1182/blood-2017-06-743252.
100. Pui CH, Roberts KG, Yang JJ, Mullighan CG. Philadelphia chromosome-like acute lymphoblastic leukemia. Clin Lymphoma Myeloma Leuk. 2017;17:464–70. https://doi.org/10.1016/j.clml.2017.03.299.
101. Ofran Y, Izraeli S. BCR-ABL (Ph)-like acute leukemia-pathogenesis, diagnosis and therapeutic options. Blood Rev. 2017;31:11–6. https://doi.org/10.1016/j.blre.2016.09.001.
102. Cario G, Leoni V, Conter V, Baruchel A, Schrappe M, Biondi A. BCR-ABL1-like acute lymphoblastic leukemia in childhood and targeted therapy. Haematologica. 2020;105:2200–4. https://doi.org/10.3324/haematol.2018.207019.
103. Roberts KG, Li Y, Payne-Turner D, Harvey RC, Yang YL, Pei D, McCastlain K, Ding L, Lu C, Song G, et al. Targetable kinase-activating lesions in Ph-like acute lymphoblastic leukemia. N Engl J Med. 2014;371:1005–15. https://doi.org/10.1056/NEJMoa1403088.
104. Deininger MW, Goldman JM, Melo JV. The molecular biology of chronic myeloid leukemia. Blood. 2000;96:3343–56.
105. Reckel S, Hamelin R, Georgeon S, Armand F, Jolliet Q, Chiappe D, Moniatte M, Hantschel O. Differential signaling networks of Bcr-Abl p210 and p190 kinases in leukemia cells defined by functional proteomics. Leukemia. 2017;31:1502–12. https://doi.org/10.1038/leu.2017.36.
106. Slayton WB, Schultz KR, Kairalla JA, Devidas M, Mi X, Pulsipher MA, Chang BH, Mullighan C, Iacobucci I, Silverman LB, et al. Dasatinib plus intensive chemotherapy in children, adolescents, and young adults with Philadelphia chromosome-positive acute lymphoblastic leukemia: results of Children's Oncology Group trial AALL0622. J Clin Oncol. 2018;36:2306–14. https://doi.org/10.1200/JCO.2017.76.7228.
107. Schultz KR, Carroll A, Heerema NA, Bowman WP, Aledo A, Slayton WB, Sather H, Devidas M, Zheng HW, Davies SM, et al. Long-term follow-up of imatinib in pediatric Philadelphia chromosome-positive acute lymphoblastic leukemia: Children's Oncology Group study AALL0031. Leukemia. 2014;28:1467–71. https://doi.org/10.1038/leu.2014.30.
108. Biondi A, Gandemer V, De Lorenzo P, Cario G, Campbell M, Castor A, Pieters R, Baruchel A, Vora A, Leoni V, et al. Imatinib treatment of paediatric Philadelphia chromosome-positive acute lymphoblastic leukaemia (EsPhALL2010): a prospective, intergroup, open-label, single-arm clinical trial. Lancet Haematol. 2018;5:e641–52. https://doi.org/10.1016/s2352-3026(18)30173-x.
109. Shen S, Chen X, Cai J, Yu J, Gao J, Hu S, Zhai X, Liang C, Ju X, Jiang H, et al. Effect of Dasatinib vs imatinib in the treatment of pediatric Philadelphia chromosome-positive acute lymphoblastic leukemia: a randomized clinical trial. JAMA Oncol. 2020;6:358–66. https://doi.org/10.1001/jamaoncol.2019.5868.
110. Pfeifer H, Lange T, Wystub S, Wassmann B, Maier J, Binckebanck A, Giagounidis A, Stelljes M, Schmalzing M, Dührsen U, et al. Prevalence and dynamics of bcr-abl kinase domain mutations during imatinib treatment differ in patients with newly diagnosed and recurrent bcr-abl positive acute lymphoblastic leukemia. Leukemia. 2012;26:1475–81. https://doi.org/10.1038/leu.2012.5.
111. Aubert L, Petit A, Bertrand Y, Ray-Lunven AF, Angoso M, Pluchart C, Millot F, Saultier P, Cheikh N, Pellier I, et al. Therapeutic approach and outcome of children with Philadelphia chromosome-positive acute lymphoblastic leukemia at first relapse in the era of tyrosine kinase inhibitors: an SFCE retrospective study. Pediatr Blood Cancer. 2022;69:e29441. https://doi.org/10.1002/pbc.29441.
112. Abou Dalle I, Kantarjian HM, Short NJ, Konopleva M, Jain N, Garcia-Manero G, Garris R, Qiao W, Cortes JE, O'Brien S, et al. Philadelphia chromosome-positive acute lymphoblastic leukemia at first relapse in the era of tyrosine kinase inhibitors. Am J Hematol. 2019;94:1388–95. https://doi.org/10.1002/ajh.25648.
113. Foa R, Bassan R, Vitale A, Elia L, Piciocchi A, Puzzolo MC, Canichella M, Viero P, Ferrara F, Lunghi M, et al. Dasatinib-blinatumomab for Ph-positive acute lymphoblastic leukemia in adults. N Engl J Med. 2020;383:1613–23. https://doi.org/10.1056/NEJMoa2016272.
114. Jabbour E, Short NJ, Jain N, Huang X, Montalban-Bravo G, Banerjee P, Rezvani K, Jiang X, Kim KH, Kanagal-Shamanna R, et al. Ponatinib and blinatumomab for Philadelphia chromosome-positive acute lymphoblastic leukaemia: a US, single-Centre, single-arm, phase 2 trial. Lancet Haematol. 2023;10:e24–34. https://doi.org/10.1016/s2352-3026(22)00319-2.
115. Leonard JT, Rowley JS, Eide CA, Traer E, Hayes-Lattin B, Loriaux M, Spurgeon SE, Druker BJ, Tyner JW, Chang BH. Targeting BCL-2 and ABL/LYN in Philadelphia chromosome-positive acute lymphoblastic leukemia. Sci Transl Med. 2016;8:354ra114. https://doi.org/10.1126/scitranslmed.aaf5309.
116. Lia Gore ML, Pui C-H, Matloub Y, Hanley MJ, Du J, Hennessy M, Granier M, Biondi A, Silverman L. PB1763 A phase 1/2 study to evaluate ponatinib with chemotherapy in pediatric patients with relapsed/resistant/intolerant Philadelphia chromosome–positive acute lymphoblastic leukemia or with T315I mutation. Hemasphere. 2022;6:S63, 3091.
117. Hijiya N, Kapoor S, Hoch M, Descamps L, Dasgupta K, Ramscar N. ASC4KIDS: a multicenter, open-label, phase Ib/II study to determine the dose and safety of Asciminib in pediatric patients with chronic myeloid leukemia in chronic phase.

Blood. 2022;140:12204–5. https://doi.org/10.1182/blood-2022-162451.

118. Locatelli F, Zugmaier G, Rizzari C, Morris JD, Gruhn B, Klingebiel T, Parasole R, Linderkamp C, Flotho C, Petit A, et al. Effect of blinatumomab vs chemotherapy on event-free survival among children with High-risk first-relapse B-cell acute lymphoblastic leukemia: a randomized clinical trial. JAMA. 2021;325:843–54. https://doi.org/10.1001/jama.2021.0987.
119. Brown PA, Ji L, Xu X, Devidas M, Hogan LE, Borowitz MJ, Raetz EA, Zugmaier G, Sharon E, Bernhardt MB, et al. Effect of Postreinduction therapy consolidation with blinatumomab vs chemotherapy on disease-free survival in children, adolescents, and young adults with first relapse of B-cell acute lymphoblastic leukemia: a randomized clinical trial. JAMA. 2021;325:833–42. https://doi.org/10.1001/jama.2021.0669.
120. Pasquini MC, Hu ZH, Curran K, Laetsch T, Locke F, Rouce R, Pulsipher MA, Phillips CL, Keating A, Frigault MJ, et al. Real-world evidence of tisagenlecleucel for pediatric acute lymphoblastic leukemia and non-Hodgkin lymphoma. Blood Adv. 2020;4:5414–24. https://doi.org/10.1182/bloodadvances.2020003092.
121. Maude SL, Laetsch TW, Buechner J, Rives S, Boyer M, Bittencourt H, Bader P, Verneris MR, Stefanski HE, Myers GD, et al. Tisagenlecleucel in children and young adults with B-cell lymphoblastic leukemia. N Engl J Med. 2018;378:439–48. https://doi.org/10.1056/NEJMoa1709866.
122. Sonneveld P, Chanan-Khan A, Weisel K, Nooka AK, Masszi T, Beksac M, Spicka I, Hungria V, Munder M, Mateos MV, et al. Overall survival with daratumumab, bortezomib, and dexamethasone in previously treated multiple myeloma (CASTOR): a randomized, open-label, phase III trial. J Clin Oncol. 2023;41:1600–9. https://doi.org/10.1200/jco.21.02734.
123. Amit O, On YB, Perez G, Shargian-Alon L, Yeshurun M, Ram R. Venetoclax and donor lymphocyte infusion for early relapsed acute myeloid leukemia after allogeneic hematopoietic cell transplantation. A retrospective multicenter trial. Ann Hematol. 2021;100:817–24. https://doi.org/10.1007/s00277-021-04398-y.
124. Vogiatzi F, Heymann J, Muller K, Winterberg D, Drakul A, Rosner T, Lenk L, Heib M, Gehlert CL, Cario G, et al. Venetoclax enhances the efficacy of therapeutic antibodies in B-cell malignancies by augmenting tumor cell phagocytosis. Blood Adv. 2022;6:4847–58. https://doi.org/10.1182/bloodadvances.2022007364.
125. Vanneman M, Dranoff G. Combining immunotherapy and targeted therapies in cancer treatment. Nat Rev Cancer. 2012;12:237–51. https://doi.org/10.1038/nrc3237.
126. Teachey DT, Hunger SP. Anti-CD7 CAR T cells for T-ALL: impressive early-stage efficacy. Nat Rev Clin Oncol. 2021;18:677–8. https://doi.org/10.1038/s41571-021-00556-3.

Correction to: Acute Lymphoblastic Leukemia in Children and Adolescents

Gabriele Escherich and Valentino Conter

Correction to: Gabriele Escherich and Valentino Conter, *Acute Lymphoblastic Leukemia in Children and Adolescents*, https://doi.org/10.1007/978-3-031-71180-0

The district Hamburg-Eppend was misspelled in the affiliation of Dr. Gabriele Escherich. The district name has been changed to Hamburg-Eppendorf.

The updated version of this book can be found at https://doi.org/10.1007/978-3-031-71180-0

G. Escherich, V. Conter (eds.), *Acute Lymphoblastic Leukemia in Children and Adolescents*, Pediatric Oncology, https://doi.org/10.1007/978-3-031-71180-0_24

MIX
Papier aus verantwortungsvollen Quellen
Paper from responsible sources
FSC® C105338

If you have any concerns about our products,
you can contact us on
ProductSafety@springernature.com

In case Publisher is established outside the EU,
the EU authorized representative is:
Springer Nature Customer Service Center GmbH
Europaplatz 3, 69115 Heidelberg, Germany

Printed by Libri Plureos GmbH
in Hamburg, Germany